MYOCARDIAL INFARCTION

Measurement and Intervention

DEVELOPMENTS IN CARDIOVASCULAR MEDICINE

VOLUME 14

MYOCARDIAL INFARCTION

MEASUREMENT AND INTERVENTION

edited by

GALEN S. WAGNER, M.D.

Duke University Medical Center,
Durham, North Carolina

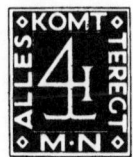

1982

MARTINUS NIJHOFF PUBLISHERS

THE HAGUE/BOSTON/LONDON

Distributors:

for the United States and Canada

Kluwer Boston, Inc.
190 Old Derby Street
Hingham, MA 02043
USA

for all other countries

Kluwer Academic Publishers Group
Distribution Center
P.O. Box 322
3300 AH Dordrecht
The Netherlands

Library of Congress Cataloging in Publication Data   CIP

Main entry under title:
   Myocardial infarction.

   (Developments in cardiovascular medicine; v. 14)
   Includes index.
   1. Heart – Infarction – Measurement. 2. Heart – Infarction – Treatment.
I. Wagner, Galen S. II. Series. [DNLM: 1. Myocardial infarction –
Diagnosis. 2. Myocardial infarction – Rehabilitation. W1 DE997VME v. 14/
WG 300 M99737]
RC685.I6M898   616.1′237   81-18960
                         AACR2

ISBN-13: 978-94-009-7454-8   e-ISBN-13: 978-94-009-7452-4
DOI: 10.1007/ 978-94-009-7452-4

This book is dedicated to
Joseph C. Greenfield, M.D., my mentor and friend,
who has been deeply involved in its preparation.

PREFACE

Patients currently experiencing acute myocardial infarcts are the beneficiaries of information gathered during the 80 years since this clinical phenomenon was described and the 20 years since treatment in coronary care units was introduced. Physicians have gained the ability to minimize inhospital mortality from rhythm disturbances and have gained insight into the importance of optimizing both left ventricular filling pressure and outflow resistance in the management of myocardial failure. Understanding of the pathophysiology of acute myocardial infarcts has matured sufficiently so that now it is possible to consider whether an infarct must evolve to a predetermined size or whether the size could be limited by implementing one or more clinically feasible strategies. Concurrently, it has become evident that patients with acute infarcts are not as 'fragile' as previously supposed, and that they may undergo procedures such as coronary angiography and coronary bypass surgery with acceptable risks.

Clinical trials are currently in progress to assess the possible benefit of various interventions for limiting myocardial infarct size. The outcome of these studies may be used to formulate strategies for clinical care of future patients. If the results are positive, community hospitals may undergo changes even more extensive than those required when they established coronary care units. If the interventions are not proven to provide significant advantages over the course of nature, the current concepts of coronary care may be retained. However, such conclusions will be only as valid as the techniques used to measure infarct size. Therefore, it would have been optimal if trials of interventions, which offer attractive potential for limiting size, were not performed until clinically applicable sizing methods had been developed and tested in experimental animals and in patients. Many potentially useful infarct-sizing methods have already been developed and it is important to ask whether any of these are currently capable of the clinical measurement of infarct size.

Care of patients with acute myocardial infarcts should be in some ways similar to and in some ways different from the care of patients hospitalized for acute coronary insufficiency but without evidence of an infarct. For both groups of patients, pain should be relieved, serious arrhythmias should be prevented, and length of hospital stay should be minimized. Prior to discharge, a stress test may be useful to determine whether critical ischemia persists and requires further management. For patients with an infarct, the clinician might also need to determine whether the involved coronary artery is totally or subtotally occluded, the extent of the myocardium at risk, whether a mural thrombus is present, the degree of infarct expansion, the extent of collateral development, the final size of the infarct, and whether optimal healing is progressing. The rationale for asking these questions and the possible methods for answering them are the themes that course through this book.

This volume was designed for use by the reader who is interested in gaining insight into the pathophysiology of myocardial infarcts, the techniques for estimating infarct size, and the possible strategies for limiting infarct size. Its primary purposes are to provide a detailed account of infarct-sizing methods, presenting both their capabilities and limitations, and to present an extensive bibliography. I selected contributors with proven expertise in specific areas of relevance to myocardial infarct size through their published work. Each was requested to provide a background from experimental studies to give the reader an understanding of the technique or biologic mechanism involved. For some methods such as the electrocardiogram and serum enzymes, points of view have been obtained from two different perspectives. Contributors were also asked to include discussion of the clinical relevance and to provide ample illustrations. The manuscripts were reviewed and sent back to the authors with suggestions for revisions. When the final manuscript was received, I did only the rewriting and cross-referencing that was necessary to develop continuity among chapters. There was no attempt to obtain a consensus about the many points that remain unsettled.

I would like to express my appreciation to those who have been essential to the completion of this project. Jeffrey Smith of Martinus Nijhoff Publishers formulated the concept of the book and has worked closely with me in its development. Nancy Stack coordinated communication with all of the contributors and organized the manuscript drafts and illustrations. Penny Hodgson edited each of the manuscripts and checked each reference. Gail McKinnis prepared the final manuscripts. Judy Berry organized my activities in general and, in particular, my many interactions with the publishers. I would also like to thank Martinus Nijhoff Publishers for providing me with the opportunity for the personal stimulation and education that has accompanied the entire project.

GALEN S. WAGNER, M.D.

CONTENTS

III. INTERVENTIONS FOR LIMITING INFARCT SIZE

IV. AN OVERVIEW

CONTRIBUTORS

Morton F. Arnsdorf, MD, University of Chicago, Department of Medicine (Cardiology), Hospital Box 249, 950 East 59th Street, Chicago, Illinois 60637.

Lewis C. Becker, MD, Department of Cardiology, Johns Hopkins Hospital, Baltimore, Maryland 21205.

Victor S. Behar, MD, Associate Professor of Medicine, PO Box 3012, Duke University Medical Center, Durham, North Carolina 27710.

Harvey J. Berger, Yale University, School of Medicine, 333 Cedar Street, 87 LMP, New Haven, Connecticut 06510.

Charles A. Boucher, Cardiac Unit, Massachusetts General Hospital, Boston, Massachusetts 02114.

Eugene Braunwald, MD, Physician-in-Chief, Peter Bent Brigham Hospital, 721 Huntington Avenue, Boston, Massachusetts 02115.

Frederick R. Cobb, MD, Veterans Administration Hospital, Room C8003, Durham, North Carolina 27705.

James C. Ehrhardt, MD, Department of Radiology, University of Iowa Hospitals and Clinics, Iowa City, Iowa 55242.

John T. Fallon, MD, Massachusetts General Hospital, 32 Fruit Street, Boston, Massachusetts 02114.

Raymundo T. Go, MD, Cleveland Clinic, 9500 Euclid, Cleveland, Ohio 44106.

Herman K. Gold, MD, Massachusetts General Hospital, 32 Fruit Street, Boston, Massachusetts 02114.

Thomas R. Griggs, MD, Cardiology Section, Room 349, Clinical Science Building, University of North Carolina, Chapel Hill, North Carolina 27514.

Donald B. Hackel, MD, Department of Pathology, PO Box 3712, Duke University Medical Center, Durham, North Carolina 27710.

Grover M. Hutchins, MD, Department of Pathology, Johns Hopkins Hospital, Baltimore, Maryland 21205.

Raymond E. Ideker, MD, Department of Pathology, PO Box 3712, Duke University Medical Center, Durham, North Carolina 27710.

Robert B. Jennings, MD, Chairman, Department of Pathology, PO Box 3712, Duke University Medical Center, Durham, North Carolina 27710.

Joseph Kisslo, MD, Associate Professor of Medicine, PO Box 3818, Duke University Medical Center, Durham, North Carolina 27710.

Robert C. Leinbach, Massachusetts General Hospital, 32 Fruit Street, Boston, Massachusetts 02114.

Eric K. Louie, MD, University of Chicago, Department of Medicine (Cardiology), Hospital Box 249, 950 East 59th Street, Chicago, Illinois 60637.

John A. Mantle, MD, Division of Cardiology, University of Alabama in Birmingham, School of Medicine, University Station, Birmingham, Alabama 35294.

Melvin L. Marcus, MD, Department of Internal Medicine, Cardiovascular Division, University of Iowa Hospitals and Clinics, Iowa City, Iowa 35242.

Eric C. McClees, MD, Department of Radiology, PO Box 3808, Duke University Medical Center, Durham, North Carolina 27710.

Huey G. McDaniel, MD, Division of Cardiology, University of Alabama in Birmingham, School of Medicine, University Station, Birmingham, Alabama 35294.

Kenneth G. Morris, MD, Veterans Administration Hospital, Room C8002, Durham, North Carolina 27705.

James E. Muller, MD, Peter Bent Brigham Hospital, 721 Huntington Avenue, Boston, Massachusetts 02115.

Robert H. Murdock, Jr., MAT, Veterans Administration Hospital, Room C8003, Durham, North Carolina 27705.

Robert D. Okada, MD, Cardiac Unit, Massachusetts General Hospital, 32 Fruit Street, Boston, Massachusetts 02114.

Silvio E. Papapietro, MD, Division of Cardiology, University of Alabama in Birmingham, School of Medicine, University Station, Birmingham, Alabama 35294.

Gerald M. Pohost, MD, Cardiac Unit, Massachusetts General Hospital, 32 Fruit Street, Boston, Massachusetts 02114.

Charles E. Rackley, MD, Division of Cardiology, University of Alabama in Birmingham, School of Medicine, University Station, Birmingham, Alabama 35294.

Keith A. Reimer, MD, Department of Pathology, PO Box 3712, Duke University Medical Center, Durham, North Carolina 27710.

Erik L. Ritman, MD, Mayo Foundation, Department of Physiology and Biophysics, Rochester, Minnesota 55901.

Robert Roberts, MD, Barnes Hospital, Washington University School of Medicine, St. Louis, Missouri 63110.

Charles R. Roe, MD, Department of Pediatrics, PO Box 3028, Duke University Medical Center, Durham, North Carolina 27710.

William J. Rogers, MD, Division of Cardiology, University of Alabama in Birmingham, School of Medicine, University Station, Birmingham, Alabama 35294.

Robert E. Rude, MD, Peter Bent Brigham Hospital, 721 Huntington Avenue, Boston, Massachusetts 02115.

Richard O. Russell, Jr., MD, Division of Cardiology, University of Alabama in Birmingham, School of Medicine, University Station, Birmingham, Alabama 35294.

Miguel E. Sanmarco, MD, University of Southern California, School of Medicine, Department of Medicine, Cardiology Section, Rancho Los Amigos Hospital, Downey, California 90242.

Ronald H. Selvester, MD, University of Southern California, School of Medicine, Department of Medicine, Cardiology Section, Rancho Los Amigos Hospital, Downey, California 90242.

Cardiology Section, Rancho Los Amigos Hospital, Downey, California 90242.

Richard S. Stack, MD, Cardiology Division, PO Box 3501, Duke University Medical Center, Durham, North Carolina 27710.

Judith L. Swain, MD, Cardiology Division, PO Box 3828, Duke University Medical Center, Durham, North Carolina 27710.

Frans J.Th. Wackers, MD, Medicine and Radiology, University of Vermont, College of Medicine, Burlington, Vermont 05401.

Galen S. Wagner, MD, Cardiology Division, PO Box 31211, Duke University Medical Center, Durham, North Carolina 27710.

J. William Whitaker, Medical Consultants, 4000 West Woodway Drive, Muncie, Indiana 47304.

Barry L. Zaret, MD, Yale University, School of Medicine, 333 Cedar Street, 87 LMP, New Haven, Connecticut 05610.

I. PATHOPHYSIOLOGY

1. TIME COURSE OF INFARCT AND HEALING

GROVER M. HUTCHINS

After the onset of an event inducing ischemic myocardial necrosis, the heart wall undergoes a stereotyped series of inflammatory and reparative responses. Two distinct types of ischemic myocardial injury can be recognized by pathologic study; each by its presence is indicative of the pathophysiologic event that has occurred. *Coagulation necrosis* results from persistent obstruction to blood flow. *Contraction band necrosis* occurs when coronary reflow follows a period of no perfusion. The overlying endocardium also participates in the response to an infarct and its reaction may be markedly altered depending on the presence or absence of mural thrombus. In individual patients, there may be very different gross topographic changes in infarcted segments of the heart wall, depending on the extent of coronary artery disease, the nature of the coronary occlusion, the size of the myocardial infarct, and the character of the endocardial response. Thus, despite a predictable course of the separate pathological processes in ischemic heart disease, the analysis of the specific case may be very difficult and requires detailed postmortem angiographic, gross, and histologic study of the heart.

COAGULATION NECROSIS

Etiology

Pathologic studies have repeatedly shown that the great majority of myocardial infarcts, about 85%, can be ascribed to occlusions of major epicardial coronary artery branches by thrombus deposited over ulcerations or cracks in atherosclerotic plaques [1–4]. Of the infarcts not accounted for by this mechanism, about two-thirds, or 10% of the total, are explained by coronary thromboembolism [5]. The remainder, where no obstructive lesion can be found, may be secondary to spasm of the coronary arteries [6, 7]. A few studies have failed to confirm the frequent association of coronary lesions with myocardial infarcts [8–10]. Analysis of these reports suggests that the discrepancy lies in a lack of uniformity in the definition of a myocardial infarct. The studies by Mitchell and Schwartz [11] showed that there are two distinct size populations of lesions in

Wagner GS (ed): Myocardial Infarction: Measurement and Intervention, pp 3–20.
© *1982 Martinus Nijhoff Publishers, The Hague/Boston/London.*

which focal destruction of myocardium has occurred. Small lesions, less than 2 cm in any dimension, increased with the patient's age but were unassociated with coronary artery disease. In contrast, large lesions, greater than 3 cm in one dimension, were associated with coronary artery disease. The criterion that infarcts be at least 3 cm in one dimension is very useful. Small lesions are probably frequently of an ischemic nature but they are difficult to correlate with specific blood vessels and are rarely detectable by clinical study. Large lesions are usually secondary to ischemia, but may rarely be caused by something other than ischemia, for example an abscess or neoplasm. The relationship of the myocardial lesions to the coronary arteries and any obstructive lesions present is readily determined with postmortem coronary arteriography [12] (Figure 1).

Morphology

The earliest appearance of diagnostic histologic changes of coagulation necrosis following the onset of coronary obstruction has been difficult to determine. Histochemical methods have been credited with the ability to differentiate necrotic from viable myocardium within short periods of occlusion [13] (see Fallon, p. 373). However, one controlled study of this method has failed to substantiate these claims [14].

At present the hematoxylin—eosin stain may be the most reliable method for early identification of infarcts in humans. Bouchardy and Majno [15] have described the thin wavy fiber change (Figure 2) that they believe to be the earliest discernible histologic change of coagulation necrosis. This phenomenon may be found when death occurs within minutes of the onset of clinical features of an infarct. It is not clear, however, that all infarcts develop thin wavy fibers, so that while their presence may be considered diagnostic, their absence does not rule out infarct. The thinness of the dead fibers probably arises from stretching of the infarcted segment during diastole and the waviness from contraction of the dead segment by the surviving subepicardial muscle during systole. Waviness is a common artifact of preparation of sections so it is important that fiber thinness be identified also.

Within hours, polymorphonuclear leukocytes emigrate to the zone of necrosis. The inflammatory reaction continues and reaches a peak four days after the infarct. Subsequently the cells lyse and leave basophilic debris in the necrotic area. The intensity of the inflammatory reaction varies greatly and the presence of shock tends to suppress the cellular response. The principal cytologic change in the cardiac muscle cells is loss of nuclei, which occurs during the first day. The sarcoplasm becomes more eosinophilic but retains its overall structure until destroyed by macrophagic activity.

Removal of necrotic myocardium is not apparent before seven or eight days after an infarct. Lysis of dead myocytes usually progresses until the necrotic area

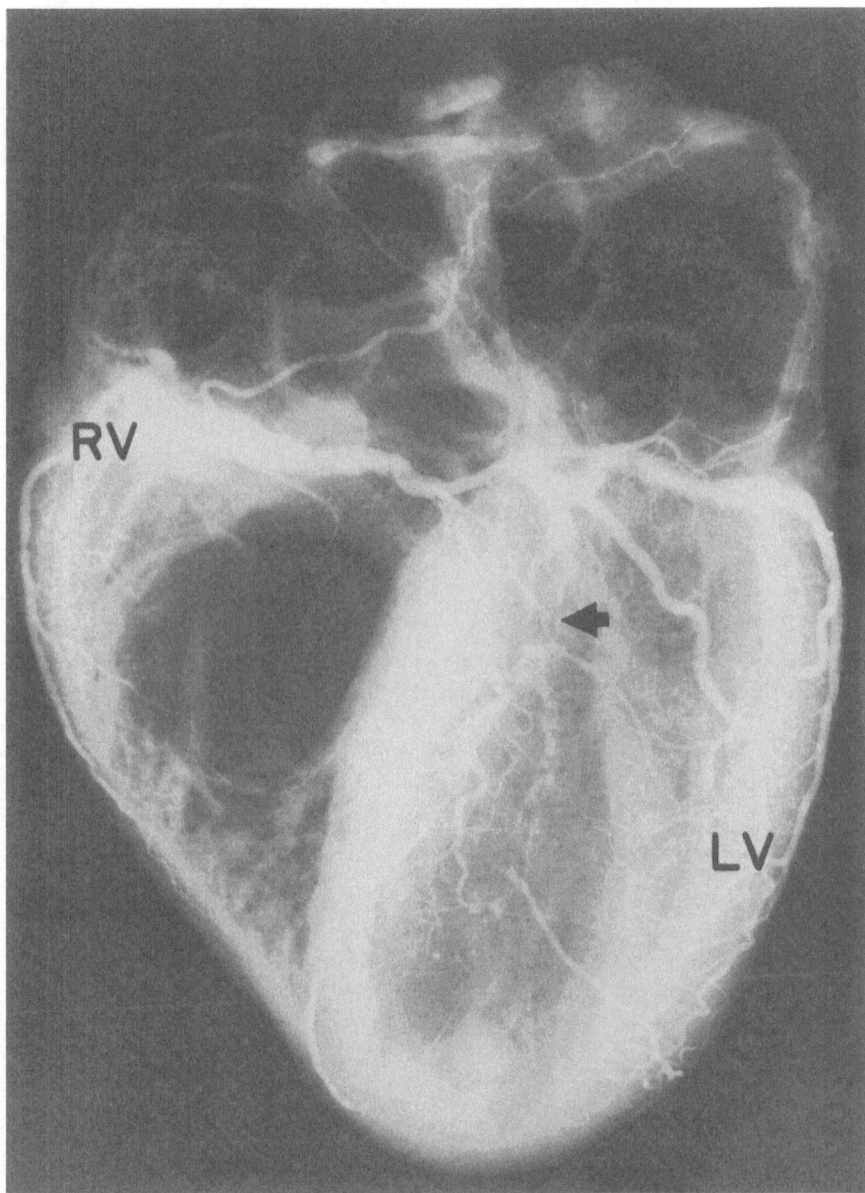

Figure 1. Postmortem coronary arteriogram of a heart with a large anteroseptal myocardial infarct. The left anterior descending coronary artery is occluded (arrow) with what by histology was shown to be a thrombus over an ulcerated atherosclerotic plaque. The infarct in the distribution of the occluded artery has undergone expansion leading to aneurysmal dilatation of the left ventricular cavity; LV, left ventricle; RV, right ventricle.

6

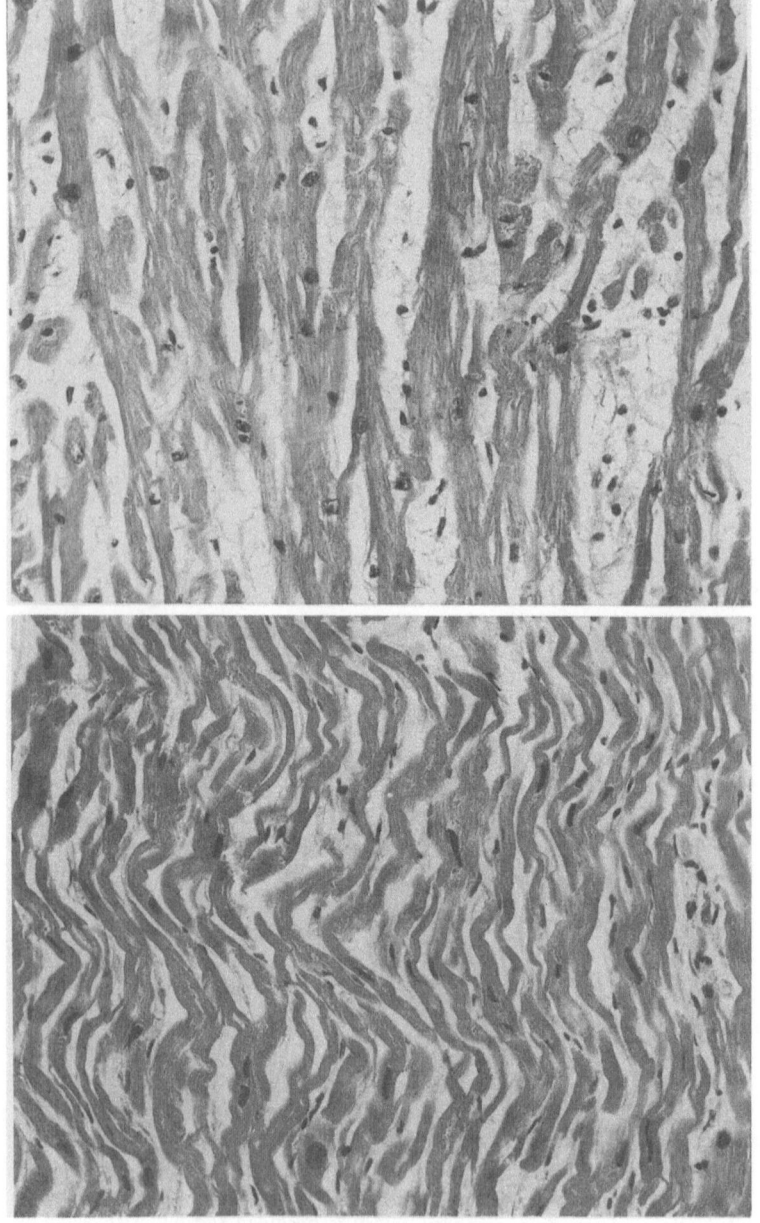

Figure 2. Thin wavy fiber change (left) in the distribution of an acutely occluded left anterior descending coronary artery. The patient died 30 min after onset of symptoms. There is no inflammatory response and the myocyte nuclei are still present. On the right, at the same magnification, the size and arrangement of cardiac muscle away from the area of infarct is shown. Both hematoxylin–eosin, × 250.

is completely removed, which in large infarcts may take several weeks. In very large lesions, connective tissue deposition may overtake the macrophages and entomb a sequestrum of dead muscle in collagenous scar.

As the sarcoplasm of the dead myocytes is removed, the perimysial sheath of connective tissue remains behind. In very small foci of necrosis, these empty sheaths may remain distended, an appearance that has been called myocytolysis. More commonly the connective tissue framework collapses and, with the active fibroblastic and granulation tissue response, begins to create a collagenous scar where the infarct had been. A curious feature of the margin of an infarct of about nine days of age is an attempted regeneration of cardiac muscle cells. Such cells have a basophilic cytoplasm and multiple large nuclei. This process is transient and does not appear to give rise to new myocytes.

Continuing maturation of the replacement fibrosis in an infarct is evident for about a year. The early loose connective tissue with abundant translucent ground substance develops progressively denser collagen fibers. The cellularity of the connective tissue declines and the vascular bed withers away so that by about a year post infarct the replacement fibrosis has attained its permanent appearance with a dense ligament-like collagen arrangement.

CONTRACTION BAND NECROSIS

Contraction band necrosis occurs in those situations in which a period of no flow is followed by reperfusion of the myocardium. It has also been termed 'reflow necrosis.' However, it is now unclear whether the reflow (see Becker, p. 442) actually produces further necrosis or, rather, alters the disposition of previously irreversibly damaged cells. For example, a patient suffering cardiac arrest or an episode of ventricular fibrillation with successful resuscitation may show this form of myocardial necrosis. It was common in patients who died after cardiac surgery under cardiopulmonary bypass [16, 17], but its frequency has declined markedly since the introduction of cold potassium chloride cardioplegia techniques [18]. Spasm of coronary arteries may lead to contraction band necrosis also. This has been noted as a presumably isolated finding [19], associated with coronary artery atherosclerosis [6], and as a coronary artery 'Raynaud's phenomenon' in patients with progressive systemic sclerosis [7, 20]. It is very common to find a narrow zone of contraction band necrosis on the margin of an infarct caused by coronary artery occlusion. An occasional infarct will consist predominantly of contraction band rather than coagulation necrosis. This effect is explainable as the consequence of rapid development of some collateral circulation into the occluded vascular bed from adjacent major vessels. The establishment of an effective collateral supply requires a period of time for growth of the connecting vessels [21].

The importance of the reflow itself in producing necrosis is suggested by a phenomenon observed in some patients receiving coronary artery bypass grafts. Occasionally a vein to artery anastomosis is placed in such a manner that it spans a branchpoint of the artery. Often in this situation, one branch is obstructed or occluded and the other is widely patent [22]. Here the history of the myocardium in the distribution of the two branches has been identical until the moment of reestablishment of blood flow. Following reflow, contraction band necrosis is observed in greater degree in the widely patent branch than in the obstructed branch [16]. This observation suggests that reflow itself produces the necrosis. In the portions of myocardium with inhibition of reflow, the myocytes are seemingly able to repair the injury sustained during the period of no flow. A similar interpretation appears to account for the so-called stone heart syndrome, where massive contraction band necrosis is found in a setting of widely patent coronary arteries [17]. The interpretation of these observations in humans differs from the conclusion drawn from studies in dogs that reperfusion does not increase the extent of necrosis in ischemic tissue [23, 24]. Observations on the left ventricular vent site in patients undergoing cardiac surgery have also suggested that reflow may play an important role in stimulating healing of injured myocardium [25].

It is uncertain how long the period of nonperfusion must be that sets the stage for the appearance of contraction band necrosis during reperfusion. Observations of patients after cardiac surgery would suggest that, without hypothermia, the critical period is 20–30 min [26]. It is also uncertain as to how long a period of nonperfusion is required to produce coagulation necrosis despite the occurrence of reflow.

On gross examination in the early stages, areas of contraction band necrosis are dark red or hemorrhagic. This appearance is caused by the marked distention of the capillary bed in the injured zone. Since the vascular bed has also been injured in the process, extravasation of red cells or even small hemorrhages commonly develop and increase in intensity over the first two days. This appearance has led to use of the terms hemorrhagic necrosis or hemorrhagic infarct for contraction band necrosis. Later the red cells lyse and their hemoglobin diffuses away. As noted above, it is not clear whether the hemorrhage produces further necrosis or, rather, alters the appearance of myocardium that was irreversibly damaged by the period of lack of perfusion. This question becomes extremely important in the presence of clinical interventions as coronary bypass surgery and thrombolytic therapy, performed during the early hours of acute myocardial infarct (see Gold, p. 511).

The histologic appearance of contraction band necrosis is distinctive (Figure 3). The contractile elements form dense irregular transverse masses in the sarcoplasm with intervening cleared areas devoid of cross-striations. The affected cell tends to be swollen. The nuclei undergo lysis and disappear over the first day following injury. This distinctive histologic appearance has also given rise to the term

Figure 3. Contraction band necrosis of myocytes. There are dense irregular condensations of sarcoplasm running transversely in the cells with intervening cleared areas. The patient died two days following cardiac surgery. Hematoxylin—eosin, X 750.

myofibrillar degeneration [26, 27] for the condition. The evolution of the inflammatory response and the reparative process in contraction band necrosis may be identical to that described above for coagulation necrosis. However, no studies have been performed to compare the final appearance of the healed infarct following reperfusion and contraction band necrosis versus no reperfusion and coagulation necrosis. Because of the state of shock existing in many patients with contraction band necrosis, the onset of the acute inflammatory cell response may be delayed or reduced.

The mechanism of development of contraction band necrosis appears to involve two phases: first, an injury to the cell membranes and, second, an influx of calcium into the sarcoplasm, causing contraction band formation and the death of the cell [28]. The first phase, cell membrane injury, can occur from several mechanisms some of which directly, and others presumably indirectly, involve injury to the myocyte membranes. Surgical incision of cardiac muscle cells, for example, typically leads to contraction band necrosis. Potassium solutions of appropriate concentration can produce contraction band injury [29]. The mechanism of catecholamines [27] in producing the lesion as either a direct effect on the cell or mediated through vascular spasm has not been resolved. In the various circumstances discussed previously in this section, the common denominator is a period of anoxia during which the cell continues to be metabolically active. Presumably the anoxic arrest of the myocardium in a setting of no blood flow allows accumulated metabolites to injure the myocyte membrane. In the second phase, the restoration of blood flow allows substances to enter the sarcoplasm through the injured membrane. Calcium appears to be the principal agent producing the distinctive histologic appearance of an exaggerated hypercontraction. This concept is supported by the so-called calcium paradox [30] where, with identical preconditions, reflow with calcium-free solutions fails to produce contraction bands.

ENDOCARDIAL CHANGES FOLLOWING INFARCT

The endocardium undergoes a stereotyped sequence of changes following large myocardial infarcts. The end result of the process is to form a layer of endocardial fibroelastosis over the area of the infarct [31]. This change may be regarded as a nonspecific response to the altered mechanics of the ventricular wall segment that has suffered a loss of a large portion of its functioning myocardium. Fibroelastosis develops in the endocardium and in the intima of blood vessels when there has been an increase in mural tension. Intimal fibroelastosis is the hallmark of hypertensive pulmonary vascular disease caused by left-sided congestive heart failure where pressure increase causes greater mural tension [32]. In the hearts of infants and children, myocarditis leads to ventricular dilatation, which produces increased mural tension. The endocardial response is a diffuse fibroelastic thickening [33]. A similar histologic appearance develops in the normal atrial endocardium [34].

In the early stages after transmural infarct, there is usually a transient inflammatory cell infiltration into the myocardium from the ventricular surface. Within 1—2 weeks, a thickening of the endocardium by proliferating mesenchymal cells becomes apparent and increases until about one month post infarct. Newly formed collagen fibrils are evident and, within 4—6 weeks, elastic fibers are also discernible. Subsequently the elastic tissue increases and becomes arranged in lamellae. The process reaches maturity by about one year post infarct at which time the endocardium has a striking resemblance to the aortic wall, with elastic lamellae alternating with mesenchymal cell layers (Figure 4).

Endocardial fibroelastosis does not develop if mural thrombus forms over the transmural infarct. Instead, granulation tissue develops from the endocardium and progressively organizes the thrombus and converts it to connective tissue. The end result of this process is a large continuous scar that includes replacement fibrosis of the infarcted myocardium, endocardium, and organized thrombus.

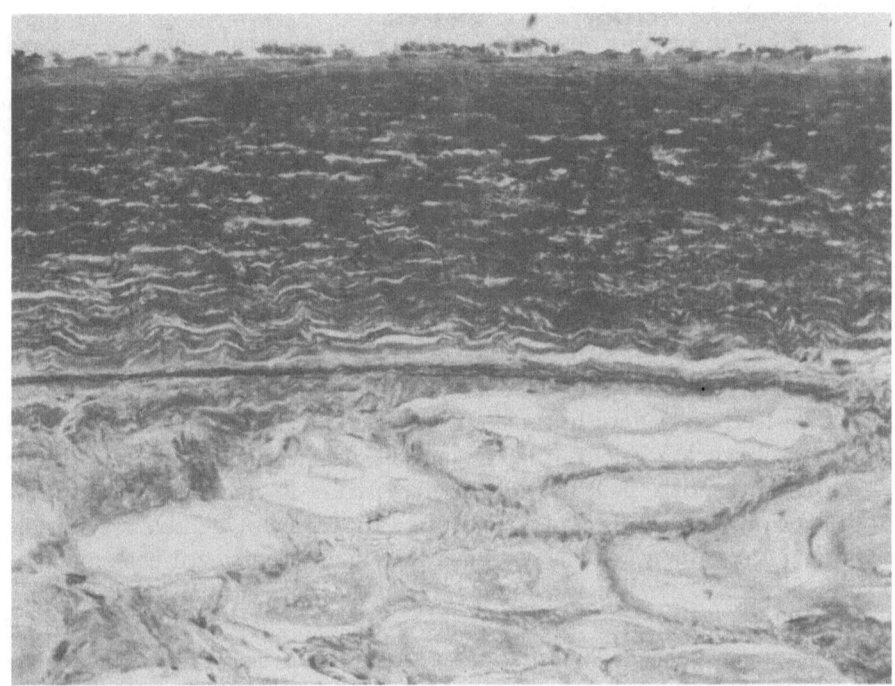

Figure 4. Mature endocardial fibroelastosis overlying a healed transmural myocardial infarct five years old. The myocytes just beneath the markedly thickened endocardium show vacuolar changes. Verhoeff-van Gieson elastic. X 250.

Even the band of myocardium that usually persists beneath the endocardium, kept alive by intracavitary blood, is lost. The mechanical properties of the collagenous scar resulting from organization of mural thrombus are different from the endocardial fibroelastosis that develops when thrombus is not present. Infarcts with a collagenous wall and mural thrombus tend to undergo aneurysm formation while those with fibroelastosis tend to retain the cardiac configuration.

OTHER MORPHOLOGIC CHANGES RELATED TO ISCHEMIA

Ischemic myocardium

Vacuolar change in subendocardial myocytes appears to be the response to inadequate coronary artery perfusion [35]. The affected cells are still alive, as shown by the persistence of normal nuclei, but probably have reduced functional capabilities since the sarcoplasm is pushed to the periphery of the cell by the central vacuolization. These cells seem particularly susceptible to necrosis when a hypotensive episode occurs.

In some patients with very severe diffuse coronary artery atherosclerosis and extensive development of a subendocardial plexus of collateral vessels, atrophy of cardiac muscle cells is found. These fibers retain the general histological characteristics of myocytes but are markedly reduced in diameter. Like the vacuolated myocytes, they seem particularly subject to undergo necrosis from episodes of hypotension.

Small-vessel disease

Specific myocardial injury related to disease of small intramyocardial vessels has been difficult to define. In some rare instances, a relationship can be found between obstructive lesions of intramyocardial arteries and small focal ischemic necroses. Occasional patients with severe vascular amyloid may show such a phenomenon [36]. In contrast, patients with thrombotic thrombocytopenic purpura, a condition in which extremely severe and widespread obstruction of intramyocardial arteries may be found, rarely show evidence of ischemic injury of the myocardium [37]. The situation is unclear for diabetes mellitus; most, if not all, of the ischemic injury found in these patients seems explicable by the accompanying epicardial coronary artery atherosclerosis [38].

COMPLICATIONS OF MYOCARDIAL INFARCT

The immediate effects of infarct on cardiac activity are a function of the amount of myocardium that has been lost. Cardiogenic shock may occur in patients in whom 40%–50% of the myocardium is necrotic [39]. This effect can be found whether the loss of muscle occurs as a single event or as a cumulative loss through several infarcts.

Ruptures of the heart wall typically develop by 4–6 days post infarct. At this time, the inflammatory cell infiltration has peaked and the disintegrated polymorphonuclear leukocytes have released their lytic enzymes into the interstitium. The reparative reactions, on the other hand, have barely begun so that the zone of necrosis is in its structurally weakest state. Free-wall rupture usually produces rapid loss of cardiac output and death of the patient.

Rupture of the interventricular septum may have a more prolonged course in some patients with the clinical effects being dominated by hypotension [40]. Left-sided congestive heart failure is a less prominent or late appearing feature. In these patients, there is usually severe widespread coronary artery disease with relatively poor development of collateral connections.

In contrast, patients who develop ruptures of a papillary muscle complicating myocardial infarct usually have less severe generalized coronary artery atherosclerosis. The affected papillary muscles frequently have contraction band necrosis and the actual rupture may be precipitated by interstitial hemorrhages occurring as a component of the reflow phenomenon [41]. Patients with papillary muscle ruptures commonly develop intractable left-sided congestive heart failure as a consequence of the mitral regurgitation. It seems likely that papillary muscle ruptures would be amenable to surgical correction [42]. The valve replacement would not have to be performed in necrotic tissue since the valve ring is not directly affected by the infarct. This is unlike the situation pertaining with other forms of myocardial rupture where, in the acute stages, the surgeon would have to suture into necrotic tissue.

TOPOGRAPHIC CHANGES IN THE LEFT VENTRICLE AFTER INFARCT

Expansion

An increase in the area of the heart wall that is underlain by an acute infarct may occur by about 4–6 days after the infarct [43]. This expansion of the necrotic tissue does not involve additional new necrosis of myocardium. It is rather a rearrangement of the infarcted area as a result of intramural tearing of the necrotic myocardium. The time frame in which expansion occurs and the character of the infarcted myocardium resemble the circumstances noted above for other types of rupture of the myocardium. The period of 4–6 days post infarct is when the inflammatory reaction is maximal with large number of disintegrated polymorphonuclear leukocytes in the tissue and the reparative reactions have not yet become evident.

Expansion is more frequent with large, transmural, first infarcts and is less apt to be found with severe diffuse coronary artery atherosclerosis, previous infarcts, or a subendocardial infarct. The expansion may occur abruptly and produce a distinct clinical event [44] with an increase in chest pain, hypotension, and left-sided congestive heart failure. There may be electrocardiographic changes and an elevation of cardiac isoenzymes. In some patients, the expansion may occur gradually or at least pass unnoticed by the patient and physician.

In situations in which hypotension follows the expansion, there may be additional foci of contraction band necrosis found in the myocardium, especially in the vascular bed containing the expanded infarct. This *extension* of necrosis may account for some of the clinical features observed in patients with *expansion*. Obviously, infarct extension can occur as a consequence of a hypotensive episode at any time post infarct. The distinctions between expansion and extension are illustrated in Figures 5 and 6. In the individual patient, there may

14

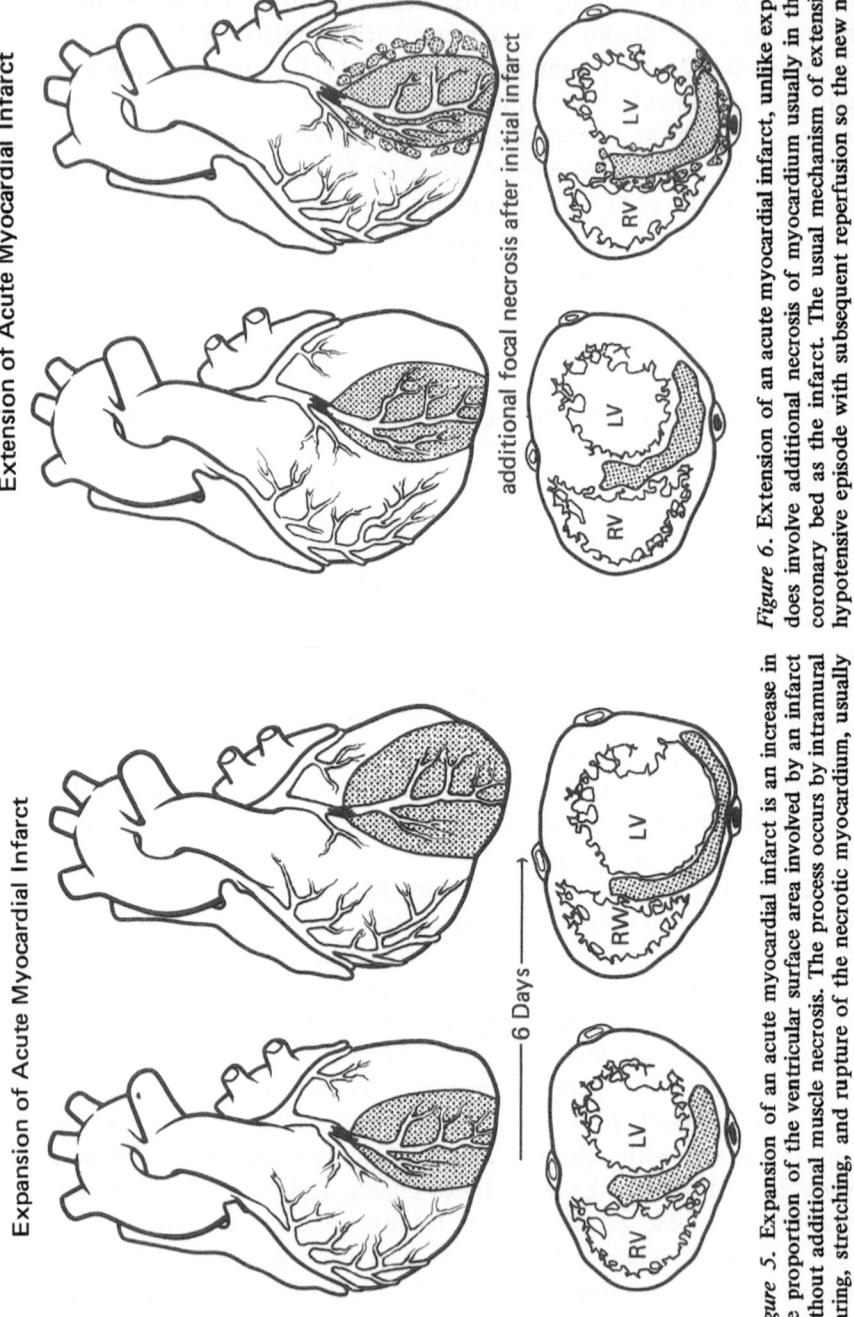

Expansion of Acute Myocardial Infarct

Extension of Acute Myocardial Infarct

6 Days

additional focal necrosis after initial infarct

Figure 5. Expansion of an acute myocardial infarct is an increase in the proportion of the ventricular surface area involved by an infarct without additional muscle necrosis. The process occurs by intramural tearing, stretching, and rupture of the necrotic myocardium, usually by about 4–6 days post infarct. Expansion produces aneurysmal dilatation of the cavity, thinning of the infarcted wall, and rearrangement of the ventricular topography. The effect of the enlargement of the ventricular cavity may be to produce hypotension and/or left-sided congestive heart failure.

Figure 6. Extension of an acute myocardial infarct, unlike expansion, does involve additional necrosis of myocardium usually in the same coronary bed as the infarct. The usual mechanism of extension is a hypotensive episode with subsequent reperfusion so the new necroses are generally of the contraction band type. Expansion may be a cause of extension and in many patients it may be unclear if the pain, serum enzyme elevations, and electrocardiographic changes of a post-acute-infarct event should be attributed to expansion or to extension.

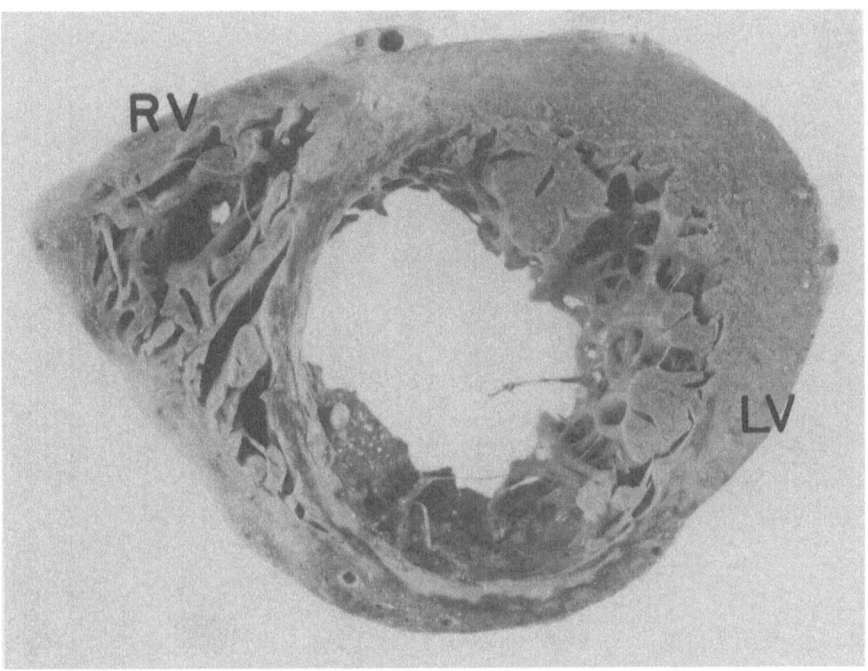

Figure 7. Transverse section of the cardiac ventricles from a patient who suffered a transmural anteroseptal myocardial infarct two weeks before death. The infarct has undergone expansion and shows marked thinning of the infarcted segment and aneurysmal dilatation of the left ventricle in the area of the infarct; LV, left ventricle; RV, right ventricle.

be expansion alone, there may be extension alone, or there could be a combination of the two. Indeed, it seems to be most frequently the case that the two phenomena coexist [43], the expansion probably having given rise to the extension.

The histologic features of the expanded infarct do not differ from those found in other infarcts. On gross examination (Figure 7), it is evident that the infarcted segment is much thinner than would be anticipated from the activities of the reparative response alone. The most important effect of expansion, however, is dilatation of the left ventricular cavity. This is seen as a relative displacement of the internal anatomic landmarks relative to each other.

The expanded ventricle is less effective in converting the tension generated in its wall by muscular contraction into intracavitary pressure [44, 45]. The heart compensates for this functional deficit by developing hypertrophy of the surviving myocardium. The late functional result of expansion is then a propensity to develop hypotension and left-sided congestive heart failure.

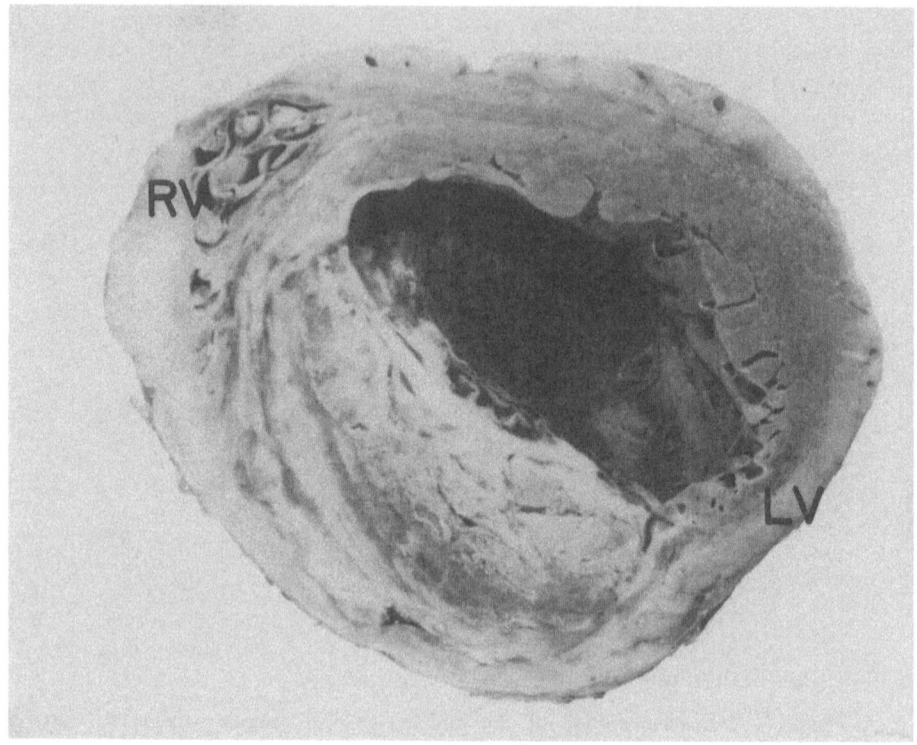

Figure 8. Transverse section of the ventricles from a patient who suffered a transmural anteroseptal myocardial infarct three months before death. Mural thrombus has formed over the area of the infarct and a ventricular aneurysm has developed; LV, left ventricle; RV, right ventricle.

Ventricular aneurysm

There is a problem in the definition of ventricular aneurysm. Many lesions referred to as aneurysms are probably more correctly considered aneurysmal dilatations and are the result of expansion of an infarct. An aneurysm usually produces an irregularity in the external contour of the ventricle, a feature not seen with aneurysmal dilatation [46]. It must be admitted, however, that a number of hearts do not fit readily into one or the other category as defined here.

In a typical aneurysm, the endocardial side of the affected segment is filled with varying amounts of mural thrombus in varying degress of organization (Figure 8). As described above, the effect of deposition of mural thrombus over a healing infarct is to prevent development of endocardial fibroelastosis with its attendant mechanical properties. The effect of organization of mural thrombus is to produce a collagenous scar with very little elasticity of its wall. The result is a progressive irreversible distention of the aneurysmal area. The situation is similar to that observed in aortic aneurysms where replacement of the elastic media by fibrous tissue allows the aneurysm to form.

As with expansion, the functional effect of the aneurysm arises largely as a consequence of left ventricular dilatation and the mechanical disadvantage imposed on the surviving myocardium by the cavity enlargement. Attempts to correct this abnormality by surgery have been less successful than might be expected. Part of the lack of success may arise from a failure to restore appropriate curvature to the remaining ventricular wall after the surgical resection [47].

SUMMARY

Ischemic injury to the myocardium occurs in two morphologic forms. *Coagulation necrosis* results from fixed obstructions to blood flow and is the major component of most myocardial infarcts, namely those that are caused by thrombosis over an ulcerated atherosclerotic plaque. *Contraction band necrosis* is observed when a period of nonperfusion is followed by reflow, for example, after successful resuscitations, with coronary artery spasm, and on the margins of infarcts. The evolution of the processes of *inflammation* and *repair* is the same for both forms of myocardial necrosis and leads eventually to a dense collagenous scar of replacement fibrosis. The endocardium also responds to infarct with a stereotyped nonspecific tissue response that produces fibroelastosis over large infarcts. Rupture is a serious complication of infarcts occurring 4–6 days after the event at a time when inflammation is maximal and repair not begun. A distinct form of intramural rupture may lead to infarct *expansion*, not to be confused with infarct *extension* which consists of additional myocardial necrosis. Expansion produces *aneurysmal dilatation* of the ventricle. Mural thrombus prevents development of endocardial fibroelastosis and predisposes to expansion, aneurysmal dilatation, and the formation of *ventricular aneurysms*. Both aneurysmal dilatations and aneurysms reduce the functional effectiveness of the ventricle by reducing wall curvature and thereby limiting the ability of the myocardium to convert mural tension to intracavitary pressure.

REFERENCES

1. Constantinides P: Plaque fissures in human coronary thrombosis. J Atheroscler Res 6:1–17, 1966.
2. Friedman M, Van den Bovenkamp GJ: The pathogenesis of a coronary thrombus. Am J Pathol 48:19–44, 1966.
3. Chapman I: The cause–effect relationship between recent coronary artery occlusion and acute myocardial infarction. Am Heart J 87:267–271, 1974.

4. Ridolfi RL, Hutchins GM: The relationship between coronary artery lesions and myocardial infarcts: ulceration of atherosclerotic plaques precipitating coronary thrombosis. Am Heart J 93:468–486, 1977.
5. Prizel KR, Hutchins GM, Bulkley BH: Coronary artery embolism and myocardial infarction. A clinicopathologic study of 55 patients. Ann Intern Med 88:155–161, 1978.
6. Maseri A, Mimmo R, Chierchia S, Marchesi C, Pesola A, L'Abbate A: Coronary artery spasm as a cause of acute myocardial ischemia in man. Chest 68:625–633, 1975.
7. Bulkley BH, Klacsmann PG, Hutchins GM: Angina pectoris, myocardial infarction and sudden cardiac death with normal coronary arteries: a clinicopathologic study of 9 patients with progressive systemic sclerosis. Am Heart J 95:563–569, 1978.
8. Ehrlich JC, Shinohara Y: Low incidence of coronary thrombosis in myocardial infarction. A restudy by serial block technique. Arch Pathol 78:432–445, 1974.
9. Roberts WC, Buja LM: The frequency and significance of coronary arterial thrombi and other observations in fatal acute myocardial infarction. A study of 107 necropsy patients. Am J Med 52:425–443, 1972.
10. Silver MD, Baroldi G, Mariani F: The relationship between acute occlusive coronary thrombi and myocardial infarction studied in 100 consecutive patients. Circulation 61:219–227, 1980.
11. Mitchell JRA, Schwartz CJ: Arterial disease. Philadelphia: FA Davis, 1965, pp 109–113.
12. Hutchins GM, Anaya OA: Measurements of cardiac size, chamber volumes and valve orifices at autopsy. Johns Hopkins Med J 133:96–106, 1973.
13. Lie JT, Holley KE, Kampa WR, Titus JL: New histochemical method for morphologic diagnosis of early stages of myocardial ischemia. Mayo Clin Proc 46:319–327, 1971.
14. Knight B: A further evaluation of the reliability of the HBFP stain in demonstrating myocardial damage. Forensic Sci Int 13:179–181, 1979.
15. Bouchardy B, Majno G: Histopathology of early myocardial infarcts. A new approach. Am J Pathol 74:301–330, 1974.
16. Hutchins GM, Bulkley BH: Correlation of myocardial contraction band necrosis and vascular patency: a study of coronary artery bypass graft anastomoses at branch points. Lab Invest 36:642–648, 1977.
17. Hutchins GM, Silverman KJ: Pathology of the stone heart syndrome. Massive myocardial contraction band necrosis and widely patent coronary arteries. Am J Pathol 95:745–752, 1979.
18. Silverman KJ, Moore GW, Brawley RK, Hutchins GM: Analysis of cause of death in coronary artery bypass graft surgery: a clinicopathologic study of 108 patients [abstr]. Lab Invest 42:151, 1980.
19. Hutchins GM, Bulkley BH, Ridolfi RL, Griffith LSC, Lohr FT, Piasio MA: Correlation of coronary arteriograms and left ventriculograms with postmortem studies. Circulation 56:32–37, 1977.
20. Bulkley BH, Ridolfi RL, Salyer WR, Hutchins GM: Myocardial lesions of progressive systemic sclerosis. A cause of cardiac dysfunction. Circulation 53:483–490, 1976.
21. Hutchins GM, Miner MM, Bulkley BH: Tortuosity as an index of the age and diameter increase of coronary collateral vessels in patients after acute myocardial infarction. Am J Cardiol 41:210–215, 1978.

22. Griffith LSC, Bulkley BJ, Hutchins GM, Brawley RK: Occlusive changes at the coronary artery-bypass graft anastomosis: morphologic study of 95 grafts. J Thorac Cardiovasc Surg 73:668–679, 1977.
23. Darsee JR, Kloner RA: The no reflow phenomenon: a time-limiting factor for reperfusion after coronary occlusion? Am J Cardiol 46:800–806, 1980.
24. Fishbein MC, Y-Rit J, Lando U, Kanmatsuse K, Mercier JC, Ganz W: The relationship of vascular injury and myocardial hemorrhage to necrosis after reperfusion. Circulation 62:1274–1279, 1980.
25. Shaw RA, Kong Y, Pritchett ELC, Warren SG, Oldham HN, Wagner GS: Ventricularapical vents and postoperative focal contraction abnormalities in patients undergoing coronary artery bypass surgery. Circulation 55:434–438, 1977.
26. Bulkley BH, Hutchins GM: Myocardial consequences of coronary artery bypass graft surgery: the paradox of necrosis in areas of revascularization. Circulation 56:906–913, 1977.
27. Reichenbach DD, Benditt EP: Myofibrillar degeneration: a response of the myocardial cell to injury. Arch Pathol 85:189–199, 1968.
28. Kloner RA, Ganote CE, Whalen DA Jr, Jennings RB: Effect of a transient period of ischemia on myocardial cells. II. Fine structure during the first few minutes of reflow. Am J Pathol 74:399–422, 1974.
29. Gharagozloo F, Bulkley BH, Hutchins GM, Bixler TJ II, Schaff HV, Flaherty JT, Gardner TJ: Potassium-induced cardioplegia during normothermic cardiac arrest. Morphologic study of the effect of varying concentrations of potassium on myocardial anoxic injury. J Thorac Cardiovasc Surg 77:602–607, 1979.
30. Zimmerman ANE, Daems W, Hulsmann WC, Snijder J, Wisse E, Durrer D: Morphological changes of heart muscle caused by successive perfusion with calcium-free and calcium-containing solutions (calcium paradox). Cardiovasc Res 1:201–209, 1967.
31. Hutchins GM, Bannayan GA: Development of endocardial fibroelastosis following myocardial infarction. Arch Pathol 91:113–118, 1971.
32. Hutchins GM, Ostrow PT: The pathogenesis of the two forms of hypertensive pulmonary vascular disease. Am Heart J 92:797–803, 1976.
33. Hutchins GM, Vie SA: The progression of interstitial myocarditis to idiopathic endocardial fibroelastosis. Am J Pathol 66:483–496, 1972.
34. Hutchins GM, Moore GW, Jones JF, Miller ST: Postnatal endocardial fibroelastosis of the valve of the foramen ovale. Am J Cardiol 47:90–94, 1981.
35. Geer JC, Crago CA, Little WC, Gardner LL, Bishop SP: Subendocardial ischemic myocardial lesions associated with severe coronary atherosclerosis. Am J Pathol 98:663–680, 1980.
36. Smith RRL, Hutchins GM: Ischemic heart disease secondary to amyloidosis of intramyocardial arteries. Am J Cardiol 44:413–417, 1979.
37. Ridolfi RL, Hutchins GM, Bell WR: The heart and cardiac conduction system in thrombotic thrombocytopenic purpura: a clinicopathologic study of 17 autopsied patients. Ann Intern Med 91:357–363, 1979.
38. Vigorita VJ, Moore GW, Hutchins GM: Absence of correlation between coronary arterial atherosclerosis and severity or duration of diabeter mellitus of adult onset. Am J Cardiol 46:535–542, 1980.
39. Page DL, Caulfield JB, Kastor JA, DeSanctis RW, Sanders CA: Myocardial changes associated with cardiogenic shock. N Engl J Med 285:133–137, 1971.

40. Hutchins GM: Rupture of the interventricular septum complicating myocardial infarction: pathological analysis of 10 patients with clinically diagnosed perforations. Am Heart J 97: 165–173, 1979.
41. Wei JY, Hutchins GM: The pathogenesis of papillary muscle rupture complicating myocardial infarction. Hemorrhage accompanying contraction band necrosis. Lab Invest 39:204–209, 1978.
42. Wei JY, Hutchins GM, Bulkley BH: Papillary muscle rupture in fatal acute myocardial infarction. A potentially treatable form of cariogenic shock. Ann Intern Med 90:149–153, 1979.
43. Hutchins GM, Bulkley BH: Infarct expansion versus extension: two different complications of acute myocardial infarction. Am J Cardiol 41:1127–1132, 1978.
44. Silverman KJ, Hutchins GM: Infarct expansion: the 'second event' after myocardial infarction. Am Heart J 100:230–238, 1980.
45. Hutchins GM, Bulkley BH, Moore GW, Piasio MA, Lohr FT: Shape of the human cardiac ventricles. Am J Cardiol 41:646–654, 1978.
46. Dubnow MH, Burchell HB, Titus JL: Postinfarction ventricular aneurysm. A clinicomorphologic and electrocardiographic study of 80 cases. Am Heart J 70:753–760, 1965.
47. Hutchins GM, Brawley RK: The influence of cardiac geometry on the results of ventricular aneurysm repair. Am J Pathol 99:221–230, 1980.

II. METHODS FOR DETERMINING INFARCT SIZE

2. THE ECG: QRS CHANGE

RONALD H. SELVESTER, MIGUEL E. SANMARCO, JOSEPH C. SOLOMON, and
GALEN S. WAGNER

Known and measured cardiac and torso anatomy, electrophysiology, and resistivities have been incorporated into a three-dimensional propagation model of ventricular excitation [1]. This model includes all the first-order effects known to influence the ECG in man. It has been used to generate QRS criteria for the 12-lead ECG in order to locate infarcts in 12 segments of the left ventricle and to predict the amount of infarct in each segment [2, 3]. The ability of these criteria to predict the size of infarct in each of the three main coronary artery distributions is the subject of this chapter.

The formation of a model is an important phase of scientific thinking, serving to demonstrate or explain the workings of an inherently complex natural system in terms that can be more readily understood. In electrocardiography, the simple equivalent dipole as a model of the complex cardiac generator has been used since Einthoven's time [4]. In his early papers, he computed instantaneous cardiac dipoles from the three standard leads using an equilateral triangle to represent the three leads (the Einthoven triangle). It is a simple geometric model of an essentially complex volume conductor, the human torso. Despite many oversimplifications, this model has served for 70 years as a useful reference for a large amount of data and theory.

A more recent model of the cardiac generator was derived from the definitive mapping studies by Scher and Young [5] and by Durrer et al. [6] of the sequence of myocardial depolarization, using isochrone plots of arrival times. This more sophisticated model of a very complex phenomenon has added greatly to our understanding of previously confusing findings in electrocardiography and vectorcardiography. High-speed advanced computer techniques have had wide application in engineering and physical sciences and are currently being utilized to an increasing extent in biology and medicine, making it possible to develop even more sophisticated models, especially nonlinear ones. Such techniques applied to the electric field of the heart could further enhance the contributions of Scher and Durrer and aid our understanding of the relationship between myocardial pathology and observed electrocardiographic and vectorcardiographic changes.

Encouraged by our success with a 20-segment computer simulation of the electric field of the heart [7], we expanded this model [8] to include distance

Wagner GS (ed): Myocardial Infarction: Measurement and Intervention, pp 23–50.
© *1982 Martinus Nijhoff Publishers, The Hague/Boston/London.*

and boundary effects. A set of 20 dipoles distributed in space to represent 20 local segments of myocardium was eccentrically located in a homogeneous sphere. Increasing or decreasing the moment of appropriate sets of these dipoles produced remarkably good simulations of left and right ventricular hypertrophy and typical large myocardial infarcts. The simulation was used to explore the ECG/VCG changes produced by small, medium, and large infarcts in all segments of the myocardium [9].

The potential value of a good mathematical model of the heart and the surrounding volume conductor is clear. An appropriate simulation then would make it possible for a large number of experiments to be run numerically with validation by key experimental observations. Such an approach could minimize nonproductive experimentation and documentation in man by pinpointing the validation studies that are most likely to yield definitive results.

PATHOLOGIC AND ANGIOGRAPHIC CONSIDERATIONS IN DEVELOPING CRITERIA FOR QUANTITATING INFARCT SIZE

The anatomic notations used in discussing localization of infarcts according to coronary distribution are derived as follows: In the cross sections of the heart in Figures 1 and 3, the left ventricle is divided around its long axis into four walls, i.e., anterior (septal), superior, posterior, and inferior (diaphragmatic). The insertion of the right ventricle into the left in these cross sections provides a consistent reference for identifying the anterior (septal) wall. The boundaries of the four walls are defined by two planes at right angles to each other intersecting each other on the long axis of the ventricle. Two additional planes pass through the heart parallel to the AV groove and perpendicular to the long axis of the left ventricle dividing the long axis into three equal parts. In this way, each wall of the left ventricle is further divided from apex to base into three segments (apical, mesial, and basal) of about equal size. The 12 segments thus produced are anteroapical, anteromesial, anterobasal, superoapical, and so forth.

Occlusive coronary artery disease generally occurs in the proximal one-third of the coronary tree. The inferior (posterior) descending coronary artery, which is usually a distal branch of the right coronary artery, is an occasional exception to this rule. The extent of infarct resulting from complete occlusion of any major coronary artery is inversely proportional to the development of collaterals. For single-vessel occlusion, the size of the associated infarct may vary from none (20% of cases) to massive (5% of cases). Even though the occlusion is proximal, the smaller infarcts tend to be in the distal distribution of the involved artery.

Total occlusion of the left superior (anterior) descending coronary artery

Small infarcts tend to localize in the subendocardium at the apex (Figure 2). Moderate-sized infarcts usually exhibit more transmural involvement of the apex

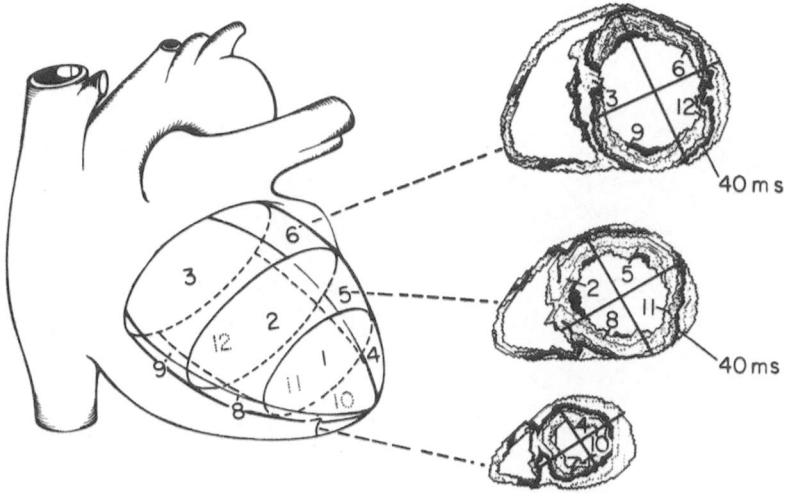

Figure 1. Simulated activation sequence – normal conduction. The segmental divisions of the left ventricle: segments 1–3 are numbered from apex to base in the anterior (septal) wall, segments 4–6 are in the superior wall, 7–9 are in the inferior (diaphragmatic) wall, and 10–12 are posterior. Isochrones of arrival times of the excitation front as generated by the propagation model are shown at 10 ms intervals on the cross sections to the right. Initial 10 ms are shown in solid black. The location of the active front at 40 ms is shown by the heavy line. The cross sections are viewed from the apex, i.e., left anterior oblique view of the patient.

and more of the subendocardial portions of the anteromesial and superomesial segments. Large infarcts extend into all apical segments in a circumferential transmural fashion and involve most or all of the anteromesial and superomesial segements. Massive infarcts involve these same regions and usually extend into the anterobasal and superobasal regions as well. However, complete ablation of these basal segments, even with a massive infarct, is rare.

Total occlusion of the circumflex coronary artery

There are usually three locations of occlusion in the proximal one-third of this artery.

(1) Left main marginal circumflex occlusion usually occurs at or near that vessel's takeoff. The region of perfusion for this artery is the posteromesial segment with some extension into the inferomesial and apical regions. Small infarcts are usually localized at the junction of the inferomesial and posteromesial segments (see Figure 2). Moderate-sized infarcts involve this region and much of the posteromesial region as well. Large or massive infarcts rarely, if ever, occur with occlusion of this artery.

(2) Local occlusions also occur in the distal circumflex at the branch point of the proximal circumflex into the main marginal and distal circumflex branch.

26

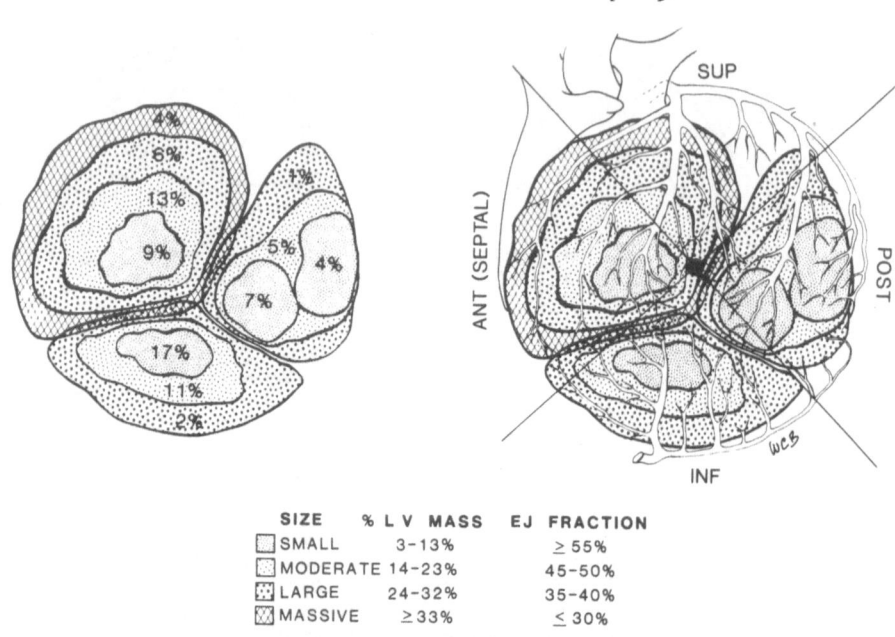

SIZE	% L V MASS	EJ FRACTION
☐ SMALL	3 – 13%	≥ 55%
▨ MODERATE	14 – 23%	45 – 50%
▨ LARGE	24 – 32%	35 – 40%
▨ MASSIVE	≥ 33%	≤ 30%

TOTAL OF 79% OF 580 PATIENTS HAVE A SINGLE VISIBLE INFARCT
NOT INCLUDED ARE 21% OF PATIENTS WITH MULTIPLE INFARCTS

Figure 2. Single visible infarct by size and location. Regional distribution of single infarcts seen on biplane ventriculograms. The numbers shown are the percentage of all ventriculograms showing local dysfunction. In these figures, the left ventricle is seen in a mercator projection as viewed from the apex, the central dark spot of the right-hand figure. The right ventricle has been removed and the anterior wall or septum is to the left. Small infarcts are usually in the distal distribution of each arterial bed, as shown here. Massive infarcts are rare in the posterior wall (circumflex distribution) and in the inferior wall (right coronary distribution). Massive infarcts occur mainly as the result of left anterior (superior) descending occlusion or as the cumulative effect of multiple infarcts.

Total occlusion of this artery produces either no infarct or, at most, small posterobasal infarcts (Figure 2). The small number of patients with left dominant coronary anatomy, in which the inferior (posterior) descending coronary artery is supplied by the distal circumflex, may have a potentially more extensive infarct. This will be discussed under right coronary artery occlusion, from which it is indistinguishable.

(3) Total occlusion of the proximal circumflex produces a combination of the effects of 1 and 2 (Figure 2). Subsequent infarcts may range in size from small (20%) to moderate or large posterior infarcts involving most of the posterior wall with extension usually onto some of the inferior wall. Massive posterior infarct with circumflex occlusion is rare (less than 0.5% of all such occlusions) and usually occurs in the left dominant coronary anatomy variant.

Total occlusion of the right coronary artery

Most occlusions of this artery occur in the proximal one-third, although some patients have occlusion of this artery in the middle one-third or in the distal one-third, where the inferior (posterior) descending artery branches off. The proximal occlusions have a significant incidence of right ventricular involvement, whereas the distal occlusions do not. The effect on the left ventricle of all three locations is similar. One-third of these occlusions occur with little or no infarct. When present, 58% of inferior infarcts are small and are usually in the inferomesial region (see Figure 2). Moderate-sized infarcts (35% of this group) extend into the inferobasal and posterobasal segments. The 6% of the inferior infarcts that are large usually extend into the inferior apex and into the inferior one-third of the anterior (septal) wall and the inferior one-half or two-thirds of the posterior wall, especially at the base. Massive inferior infarcts from right coronary occlusion are rare (0.5% overall). These large to massive lesions are usually associated with a very dominant right coronary system and are indistinguishable, both anatomically and electrocardiographically, from large to massive lesions that are due to total occlusion of a dominant circumflex coronary artery.

Total occlusion of a dominant left circumflex

Only 10% of subjects have a dominant left circumflex in which the inferior descending is a branch of the circumflex. Under these circumstances, the circumflex perfuses about one-half of the left ventricle and the left superior (anterior) descending perfuses the other one-half. Massive infarct would be as likely in about the same percentage of subjects with total occlusion of such a circumflex artery as would be expected with total occlusion of the left superior (anterior) descending. The low incidence of left dominant anatomy, however, accounts for the very low incidence of single-vessel occlusion and massive posterior inferior infarcts (0.5%), as compared with single-vessel occlusion and massive anterior superior infarcts (5%).

In 20% of cases, proximal total occlusion of a left dominant circumflex, like all other major coronary arteries, may not have associated infarct. Small infarcts usually involve the posterior and inferior mesial regions. Moderate-sized infarcts extend into the posterior and inferior base and may extend somewhat toward the apex and into the inferior portion of the anterior (septal) wall of the left ventricle. Large infarcts involve most or all of the inferior and posterior base extending into the anterior (septal) wall and apex. Massive infarcts, while rare, do occur involving most of the posterior and inferior walls. These massive lesions extend well into the anterior (septal) wall as well.

The relationships of size and location and the percentage of distribution in each of the major areas of coronary distribution are shown in Figure 2.

Total occlusion of multiple vessels

While total occlusion of two or three vessels does occur without visible infarct or demonstrable ventricular dysfunction, this is uncommon. In patients with documented coronary disease, 5% have two vessels and 1% have three vessels totally occluded without visible infarct on angiograms. Not unexpectedly, it is much more usual for multiple-vessel occlusion to be associated with significant infarct. These multiple lesions account for 21% of all patients with coronary disease and localized abnormal wall motion on biplane angiograms. They produce a spectrum of changes from two small, discrete localized infarcts (6% of all infarcts) to 15% with multiple but localized larger infarcts. Another 4% of coronary patients will have diffuse hypocontractile ventricles with no clearly localized defects in regional wall motion at ventriculography. The latter have diffuse extensive scarring on pathologic examination.

In summary, single infarcts due to right coronary or circumflex occlusion are usually small (28% of all infarcts), are often moderate in size (16%), and only rarely large or massive (3%). On the other hand, single anterior superior infarcts from left superior descending occlusion are about equally distributed between small (9% of all infarcts), moderate (13%), and large to massive (10%). These probabilities must be taken into account when interpreting ECGs and VCGs.

THE FORWARD MODEL OF PROPAGATION OF VENTRICULAR EXCITATION IN AN INHOMOGENEOUS TORSO (The development of QRS criteria for quantitating infarct size)

Because we desired to explore in detail the effects of infarction, hypertrophy, and conduction abnormalities in various combinations, we were led to the development of a comprehensive forward simulation that would include all the first-order variables that influence the surface ECG. The building blocks of the model are: (1) anatomy of the viable myocardium, (2) model of the electromotive surface, (3) simulation of the wave of excitation, (4) multiple-segment multiple-dipole subdivision of the heart, and (5) effects of the inhomogeneous bounded torso volume conductor.

Anatomy of viable myocardium

The shape, size and location, and direction of any local activation front are a function of the Purkinje programming and the anatomy of viable myocardium. Specific inputs to the simulation are size and location of papillary muscles, size and location of local scars or infarcts, ventricular wall thickness, and local variations in regional wall anatomy. Once the geometry is accurately specified by serial cross sections of an appropriate thickness, inline digitizing tables simplify the introduction of complex geometries into the simulation. We digitized 2 mm cross sections of a normal heart that had been filled to normal diastolic volumes with formalin agar and sliced parallel to the AV groove. The digitized geometry was then interpolated to 1 mm cross sections. Thus, any accurately specified pathologic change, i.e., multifocal or confluent, infarct, septal hypertrophy, left or right ventricular dilatation and/or hypertrophy, becomes an anatomic input parameter of the model.

Model of the electromotive surface

We concluded from previously reported studies [10] that the dipole layer hypothesis, as a model of the electromotive surface in the heart, is inconsistent with the predominantly monophasic waveforms observed on the bipolar intramyocardial electrodes in this study.

A more appropriate model was developed in which the activation front is considered a diffuse collection of microscopic current dipoles distributed in the region undergoing depolarization [11]. These current dipoles are assumed to arise from the depolarization of myocardial cells generating currents over a short distance. It is assumed that macroscopic depolarization can be represented by macroscopic current dipoles. This model of the active surface provides a good fit to the average waveform seen on intramural bipolar electrode pairs having a 1 mm separation. Actual measurements from dog, baboon, or man can now be used to define the electrical properties of a local action region of myocardium in each species.

Simulation of wave of excitation

Our approach to the problem of simulating the pathway of ventricular depolarization was to develop a numerical method analogous to Huygen's method of wavefront construction in a three-dimensional region. Briefly, Huygen's method consists of approximating the propagating wavefront by a large number of spherical wavelets. The area of the wavefront is taken to be the tangent planes connecting the spherical wavelets. The location of the wavelets for each successive time increment is determined by the product of the velocity of propagation and time increment. The distance to successive wavefronts is the radius of the spherical wavelets whose centers lie on the previous wavefronts.

To simulate Huygen's method with a resolution of 1 mm requires a computer with a large core capacity. Our present digital program replicates Huygen's method by using isotropic and homogeneous propagation velocities. The method used to define the regions in which the wavefront propagates results in the core capacity of the computer being the only limit on the resolution of the simulation. We define these regions of viable myocardium by their boundary on a three-dimensional Cartesian coordinate system. These can be plotted as hard copy. By designating appropriate areas of the inner 1 mm of the cardiac geometry as the peripheral Purkinje network, the subendocardial Purkinje system with its more rapid spread is introduced into the simulation. It is run first at a more rapid propagation velocity and then introduced in a second pass as start points to the subendocardial regions of the myocardium. Typical examples of normal conduction with and without an infarct are shown in Figures 1 and 3.

Multiple-segment multiple-dipole subdivision

This is a convenient, although not necessary, method of transferring electrical analogues of local myocardium to the body surface. The sum of all these local contributions over time to each body surface point is, of course, the surface scalar QRS electrocardiogram at that point. The myocardial subdivision is arbitrary and is a compromise between the accuracy with which a local dipole represents the local region and the time required to generate a transfer impedance from that dipole to the surface body. While each cubic millimeter of myocardium could be referenced by an orthogonal set of transfer numbers to each of the 1000 or so points on the body surface, the time needed to obtain such a large set of transfer numbers makes this impractical. Our simulations typically contain a cardiac subdivision of 17, 20, and 22 segments.

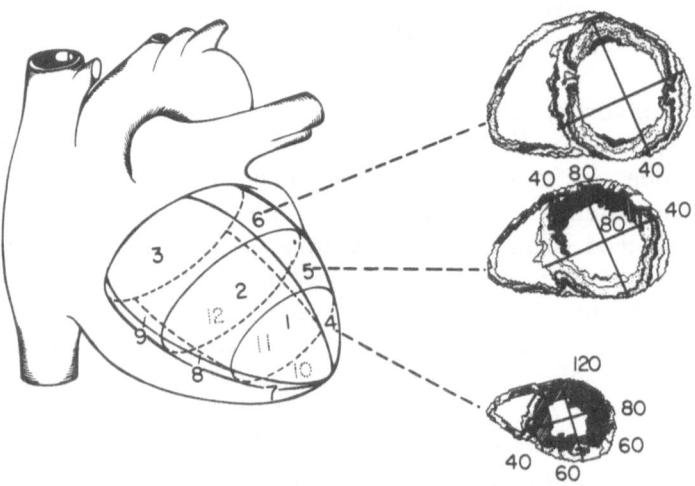

Figure 3. Simulated activation sequence – anterior apical infarct (normal conduction). The anatomical conventions in this simulation are the same for Figure 1. The diagonally shaded area in the heart cross sections to the right represent a moderate to large anterior superior infarct involving most of the apical segments. Arrival times are shown around the periphery. Small fronts persist over the infarct in this case for over 120 ms. Because these subepicardial wavefronts are approaching each other from around the periphery of this infarct, there is a great deal of local cancellation and these excitation fronts are generally poorly seen in surface ECG leads.

Effects of the inhomogeneous bounded torso volume conductor

We use the Galernter–Swihart model [12] to simulate the inhomogeneous torso. This simulation of the volume conductor is cumbersome and time consuming to change. To significantly change torso shape, heart size, or torso conductivities requires that the transfer numbers from the heart to the body surface be computed for each change. The Gelernter–Swihart method is a complex, iterative numerical procedure; convergence for each orthogonal set of dipoles typically requires 3–4 h computer time. A quick, noninvasive method of measuring these transfer impedances from local heart regions to the body surface is needed. A large number of important numerical experiments can be performed, however, with the normal male torso geometry and resistivities. With a set of orthogonal (x, y, z) components to each of the body surface points, it is now possible to generate a total ECG body surface map at 2.5 ms intervals for any combination of ventricular enlargement, conduction abnormalities, and local myocardial infarcts.

Experiments with the forward model

Because the early simulations of normals, large infarcts, and right and left ventricular hypertrophy were quite satisfactory, we began to look at sensitivity and resolution, as well as to explore the effects of various-sized lesions in any portions of the heart [9, 13–15]. The important insight gained was that small scars 8 mm in diameter and 2 mm thick would produce a small notch in the QRS no matter where they were located. Small infarcts involving 3%–9% of the left ventricle in general produce notches, slurs, or borderline Q wave changes. In this sense, most subendocardial infarcts were smaller than the 10%–12% of the left ventricle needed to produce the classic Q waves (or abnormal initial R waves) of transmural infarct, although all produced significant QRS changes when compared with preinfarct controls. When normal human excitation was simulated, large scars produced larger departures of the infarct QRS from the preinfarct QRS. Initial R wave losses, when large enough, produced classic Q waves. Infarct of more than 9%–12% of the LV mass near the midregion or apex was usually required before these classic changes occurred. Furthermore and predictably, even much larger basal infarcts failed to generate abnormal Q waves (or abnormally wide initial R waves) since these regions depolarize after 40 ms and produce mid and terminal QRS change. It became clear early in the simulations that the degree of QRS change was related to the degree of heart change (infarct, in this case). It became equally obvious why criteria that relied exclusively or mainly on Q waves would be only 55%–60% sensitive in detecting infarcts. The failure to include mid and late QRS forces in the usual diagnostic criteria for infarct accounted for much of this poor showing, and is undoubtedly responsible for the consensus promoted for years that little or nothing can be said about infarct size from the ECG.

The desire to study the interactions of peri-infarct geometry and conduction defects led to the development of the more comprehensive simulations. We used the propagation model with a $1\,mm^3$ descretization of the heart geometry to produce the excitation sequence in residual viable myocardium (see Figure 3). Gelernter–Swihart simulation of the inhomogeneous male torso provided the transfer impedances from cardiac sources to body surface electrodes. Damage to local segments of the proximal left bundle, i.e., superior, middle, or inferior fascicular blocks in any combination, was simulated by omitting (or delaying) peripheral Purkinje start points in the region supplied by the fascicles. Infarcts ranging in size 1%–2% of the left ventricle to 50% were simulated in normal and abnormal conduction.

Here one of the major advantages of a validated simulation became quite evident. To explore the effect of many-sized infarcts in normal conduction and with superior and inferior fascicular block, for example, took only a few days to run through the computer simulation. It would be a very lengthy data-gathering mission to collect such combinations in patients going to angiography or to autopsy. It might well take years to accumulate all the combinations that could reasonably be expected in clinical practice, whereas only key examples would be needed to confirm the quantitative interactions involved as defined by the computer simulation.

With the pathologic and angiographic data about location of infarcts of various sizes in each primary arterial distribution and with the comprehensive simulations described earlier, we are now in a position to define infarcts in detail for each artery distribution in the appropriate location for each size of lesion simulated. From these data, a set of criteria involving initial, middle, and terminal QRS forces was developed for each arterial distribution [2, 3].

ECG criteria for anterior superior (and apical) infarct from left superior (anterior) descending coronary occlusion

Infarcts associated with diagonal occlusion may be limited to the superior and apical (lateral) regions. These are so-called hi-lateral, lateral, or superior infarcts with abnormal Q waves in 1, AVL and/or V_5, and V_6. In some patients, the wraparound of the left superior (anterior) descending coronary artery onto the inferior apex is quite prominent. Under these circumstances, the small anteroapical infarct may occasionally be associated with significant inferior extension and produce additional abnormal Q waves in inferior leads. Larger anterior superior infarcts generally involve the apex extensively and produce major R wave losses (and/or abnormal Q waves) in 1, AVL, and $V_1 - V_6$. Table 1

Table 1. Terms (in parentheses) commonly used for the spectrum of infarcts associated with left superior (anterior) descending coronary artery occlusion and their equivalent size modifiers

Abnormal Q, 1, AVL	Small	Anterior superior (hi-lateral)
Abnormal Q, V_5, V_6, 1	Small	Anterior superior (apical or lateral)
Abnormal Q, V_1, V_2, V_3, V_4)	Small	Anterior superior (anteroseptal)
Abnormal Q (or loss of R) 1, V_3-V_6	Small–mod.	Anterior superior (anteroapical or anterolateral)
Abnormal Q-QS V_3-V_6 with loss of mid to late R	Large	Anterior superior (extensive anteroapical)
Abnormal QS V_1-V_6 (1, AVL)	Massive	Anterior superior (massive anterolateral)

summarizes terms (in parentheses) commonly used for the spectrum of infarcts associated with left superior (anterior) descending coronary artery occlusion and their equivalent size modifiers, based on the current proposed terminology. These changes are all manifestations of left superior (anterior) descending coronary artery occlusion. When changes are limited to a few of the leads looking at anterior, superior, and leftward vectors, the infarcts are small. When they involve several leads, the infarcts are moderate to large. When they involve most or all of these leads, and specifically if there is major loss of mid to late R wave forces, the infarcts are large to massive. Therefore, we believe it is clinically more useful and more appropriate to the angiographic findings to use the size modifiers from Table 2 to quantitate the size of the anterior superior infarct. A horizontal-plane vector loop and 12-lead ECG criteria for quantitating anterior superior infarct are shown in Figure 4 and are enumerated in detail in Table 3, along with localization criteria.

Table 2. Size modifiers that are clinically useful and appropriate to angiographic findings in quantifying the size of anterior superior infarct

ECG points	Diagnostic statement	Pathol. % LV	Cathet. % Ej. Fr.	Probability Cor. art. dis.	Probability Normal
1	Consider small (location) infarct	3	65	10–24	10–24
2	Possible small (location) infarct	6	65	25–49	5–9
3	Probable small (location) infarct	9	60	50–94	3
4	Small (location) infarct	12	55	95–97	< 1
5–7	Moderate (location) infarct	15–21	45–50	98	< 1
8–10	Large (location) infarct	24–30	35–40	> 99	< 1
> 11	Massive (location) infarct	≥ 33	≤ 30	> 99	< 1

Increase diagnostic statement for points 1–3 by one level if patient has persistent or recurrent chest pain, decrease by one level if reason for taking ECG was screening of all hospital admissions, and decrease two levels if female under age 60 or male under age 35 years.

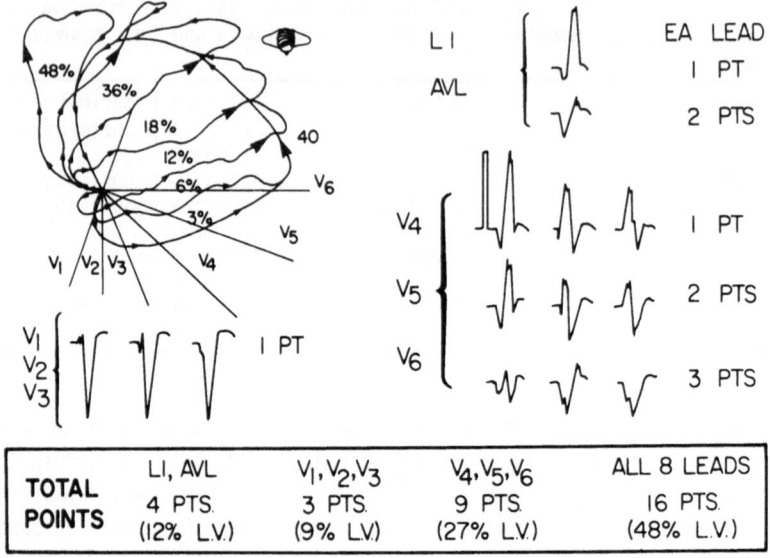

TOTAL POINTS	LI, AVL 4 PTS. (12% L.V.)	V_1, V_2, V_3 3 PTS. (9% LV.)	V_4, V_5, V_6 9 PTS. (27% LV.)	ALL 8 LEADS 16 PTS. (48% L.V.)

Figure 4. ECG criteria for left superior (anterior) descending coronary artery occlusion and infarct size. ECG point scoring criteria below describe graphic changes in the figure. Each point represents 3% of the left ventricular (LV) mass.

Superior (hi-lateral) leads
Lead 1, AVL   Q ≥ 30 ms   1 point (3% LV) each lead
              *R/Q ≤ 1   1 point (3% LV)
   2 points max. each lead; 4 points total (12% LV)

Anterior (septal) leads
Leads $V_1 V_2 V_3$ any Q (QS)   1 point (3% LV) each lead
   1 point max. each lead; 3 points total (9% LV)

Anteroapical (anterolateral) leads
Leads $V_4 V_5 V_6$ Q ≥ 30 ms   1 point (3% LV) each lead
              *R/Q, or R/S
   ≤ 1 in V_4, 2 in V_5, 3 in V_6 1 point (3% LV) each lead
   ≤ 0.5 in V_4, 1 in V_5, 1 in V_6 2 points (6% LV) each lead
   3 points max. each lead; 9 points total (27% LV)

All anterior (and apical or lateral) points
   16 points total (48% LV)

(*Q duration must be ≥ 30 ms to count R/Q points.)

Posterior infarcts from circumflex coronary occlusion

A typical example of the horizontal-plane vector loop and 12-lead ECG criteria for posteromesial infarcts from occlusion of the main marginal branch and/or proximal occlusion of the circumflex coronary artery is shown in Figure 5. Lesions in this location may extend onto the inferior surface and produce small to significant Q waves in AVF. Significant Q waves in lead 2 are usually not present. Large infarcts of the posterior wall may extend well onto the apex. In this case, initial leftward forces are lost, producing prominent and abnormal initial rightward anterior vectors that meet criteria for apical infarct described under anterior superior infarct above. The 30 ms vector will be rightward in the transverse and frontal plane, and abnormal Q waves and/or loss of mid to late R waves will appear in V_6, lead 1, and sometimes AVL and V_5.

Right coronary occlusion and typical inferior infarcts

The right coronary artery supplies the prominent AV nodal artery in 90% of patients. The AV nodal artery takes off from the crux or 'U-turn' in the right coronary at the origin of the inferior (posterior) descending branch. It terminates in a T, one limb of which supplies the AV node while the other supplies the His bundle and the first 1–2 cm of the left bundle [16]. Thus, transient AV nodal block is common with right coronary artery occlusion. A variable dual blood supply is provided by the first septal perforator from the left superior descending coronary artery. The proximal left bundle is more often supplied by the AV nodal or the interior septal branches of the right coronary. Wellens has shown that recent-onset left bundle branch block is associated with recent inferior infarct three times as often as with anterior superior infarct [17]. Right bundle branch block, on the other hand, is five times more common with recent-onset anterior superior infarct, suggesting that the proximal portion of the right bundle is supplied by the first septal perforator of the left superior coronary system more often than by the AV nodal branch or inferior septal arteries. The inferior fascicles of the left bundle, however, are supplied throughout their course by septal branches of the inferior (posterior) descending right coronary artery, or from distal inferior wall branches of the right cononary artery. Thus, disruption of the proximal portion of the inferior fascicles is common (95% of cases) in patients with right coronary occlusion and inferomesial and inferobasal infarct. This group of patients has the following evidence of inferior fascicular block:
(1) The QRS is slightly prolonged to 100–110 ms, which often occurs intermittently in the early stages of acute inferior infarct.
(2) Patients with very small infarcts have an open frontal-plane loop with the ECG/VCG changes associated with inferior fascicular block.
(3) The initial forces are in a smooth arc superior and leftward with no high-frequency notches, which is consistent with early, unopposed propagation through normal superior wall.
(4) The high-frequency notching and irregularities are in the mid and terminal vectors, which is consistent with late activation of the infarcted inferior wall.

Table 3

Myocardial infarct sizing criteria – all vessels[a]

Lead	Morphology	Q dur. (ms)	R amp. (mV)	R dur. (ms)	S amp. (mV)	Ratios	Points[c] Ea. crit	Points[c] Lead max	Ant. LAD 1	2	3	Sup. 4	5	6	Inf. RCA 7	8	9	Post. circ. 10	11	12
I		>30	<0.3			R/Q <1	1	2				2	1							
							1					1	2							
L		>30				R/Q <1	1	2				2	1							
							1					2	1							
II		>30					1	2								2	1			
		>40					2								2	2	2			
F		>30					1	5								2	1			
		>40					2								2	2	2			
		>50					3								3	3	3			
	Abn. Q and noted R or					R/Q <2	1									2	1			
	Abn. q and					R/Q >1	2									3	3			
V₁	↓R; notch or qr or QS or	Any					1	2	1	1	1									
	↑S and QRS 100 ms and				>1.8		1			2			1							
	↑R dur. or amp.		>0.6	>40			1	4											2	1
			>1.0	>50			2											2	2	2
						R/S, R'/S >1	1												1	1
	↓Sc rSr' or				<0.4		1												1	2
V₂	↓R; notch or qr or QS or	Any	<0.1	<20			1	1	1	2										
	↑R dur. or amp.		>1.0	>50			1												1	2
			>1.5	>60			2											2	2	2
						R/S, R'S >1	1												1	2
	↓S with SS' or rSr' or				<0.6		1													
V₃	↓R; notch or qr or QS or	Any	<0.2	<30			1	1	1	2										

Table 3 (continued)

Myocardial infarct sizing criteria – all vessels[a]

Lead	Morphology	Q dur. (ms)	R dur. (ms)	R amp. (mV)	S amp. (mV)	Ratios	Points[c] Ea. crit.	Points[c] Lead max.	Ant. LAD 1 2 3	Sup. LAD 4 5 6	Inf. RCA 7 8 9	Post. circ. 10 11 12
V_4	↓R; slur or notch or rSr' or	> 20		< 0.7		R/Q, R/S < 1	1		2 1			
							1	3	2	1		
						0.5	2		2 2	1 1		
V_5	↓R; slur or notch or rSr' or	> 30		< 0.7		R/Q, R/S < 2	1		1 1	1		1
							1	3	1 1			1
						< 1	2		1	2 1	1	1
V_6	↓R; slur or notch or rSr' or	> 30		< 0.6		R/Q, R/S < 3	1			1	2	1
							1	3	1		1	1
						< 1	2			2	2	1 1

[a] QS V_1, V_2 not applicable in LV overload. ↑ and broad R V_1, V_2, and R/S ratios V_5–V_6 not applicable in RV overload.
[b] Numbers in the right-hand columns represent percent of LV assigned by each criteria to each LV segment.
[c] 1 point = 3% LV.
R < RV_1 or RV_2.

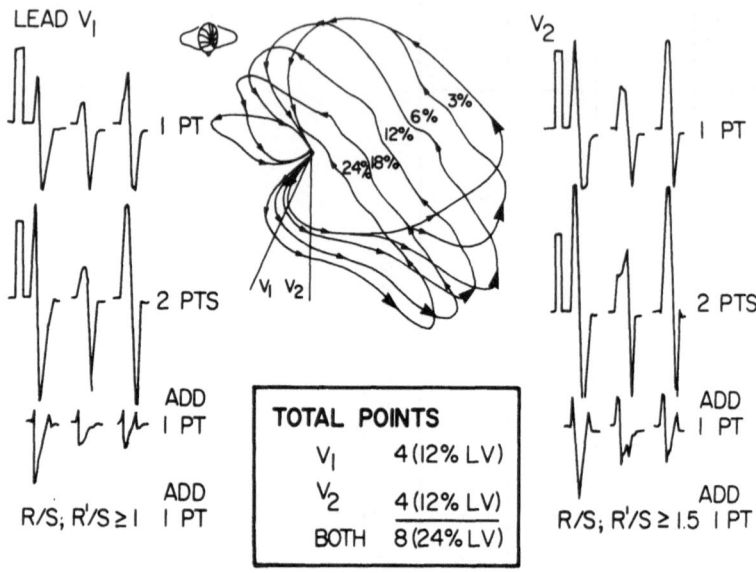

Figure 5. ECG criteria for left posterior circumflex coronary occlusion and infarct size. ECG point scoring criteria below describe graphic changes in the figure. Each point represents 3% of the left ventricular (LV) mass.

Anterior posterior leads

V_1	R dur. > 40 ms but < 50 and/or	
	R amp. > 0.5 mV but < 1.0 mV	1 point (3% LV)
	R dur. > 50 ms and/or amp. > 1 mV	2 points (6% LV)
	RSR' and/or S < 0.4 mV add	1 point (3% LV)
	R/S or R'/S > 1 add	1 point (3% LV)
	Max. in V_1 —	4 points *total* (12% LV)
V_2	R dur. > 50 ms but < 60 and/or	
	R amp. > 1 mV but < 1.5 mV	1 point (3% LV)
	R dur. > 60 ms and/or amp. > 1.5	2 points (6% LV)
	RSR', S-notched and/or < 0.6 mV add	1 point (3% LV)
	R/S or R'/S > 1.5 add	1 point (3% LV)
	Max. in V_2	4 points *total* (12% LV)

All posterior points V_1 and V_2　　　　　　8 points *total* (24% LV)

Note: If right atrial overload is present, right ventricular overload is more likely as a cause of these changes in V_1 and V_2.

(5) Finally, it has been observed for years that the classic Q waves of inferior infarct will sometimes disappear. When the inferior Q waves disappear, the QRS usually returns to a more normal duration of 80–90 ms, and the axis shifts superiorly. These findings support our hypothesis that the inferior fascicular block has now disappeared. The superior axis shift and the decrease in QRS duration are due to the return to normal conduction.

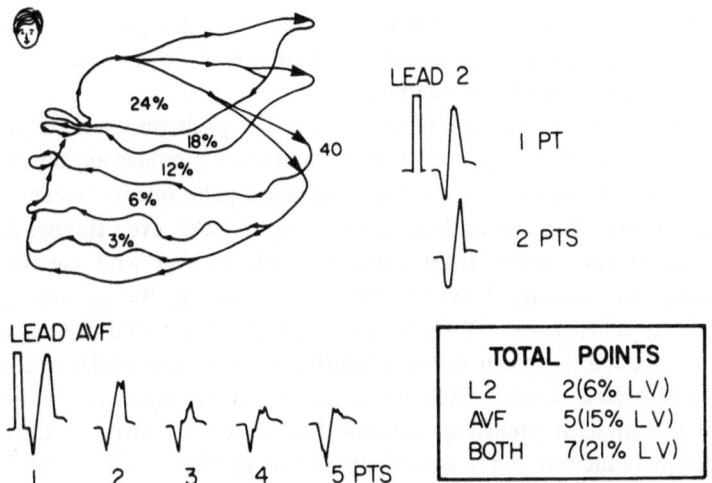

Figure 6. ECG criteria for right coronary artery occlusion and infarct size (with inferior fascicular block). ECG point scoring criteria below describe graphic changes in the figure. Each point represents 3% of the left ventricular (LV) mass.

Inferior leads

Lead 2	$Q \geqslant 30$ ms but < 40	1 point (3% LV)
	$Q \geqslant 40$ ms	2 points (6% LV)
Lead AVF	$Q \geqslant 30$ ms but < 40	1 point (3% LV)
	$Q \geqslant 40$ ms but < 50	2 points (6% LV)
	$Q \geqslant 50$ ms	3 points (9% LV)
	*R/Q $\leqslant 2$ but K 1	1 point (3% LV)
	*R/Q $\leqslant 1$	2 points (6% LV)

All inferior points   7 points *total* (21% LV)

(*Duration must be $\geqslant 30$ ms to count R/Q points.)

Note: An inferior conduction delay, i.e., inferior fascicular block and/or peri-infarction block, is assumed in developing these criteria for the reasons stated in the text. If QRS duration is less than 100 ms, the inferior point score (and the % LV) should be decreased by 50%.

Typical changes of various-sized inferior infarcts due to right coronary occlusion with associated inferior fascicular block are shown in Figure 6.

THEORETICAL BASIS – USEFULNESS OF ECG CRITERA FOR INFARCT SIZE

The most attractive aspect of using 12-lead ECG criteria to size a recent or old myocardial infarct is the routine availability of these data in even the smallest community hospital. The technique is noninvasive, of reasonable cost, and can be readily repeated even in very sick patients. Furthermore, the criteria are easily adapted to automated ECG diagnostic programs or may be used manually. If systematically applied, they will provide the basis for comparing data from a large number of centers.

The best prevention of false negatives and false positives is a baseline preinfarct ECG. A routine ECG taken in young adulthood provides an important aid to diagnosis when years later the patient has 'chest pain, rule out recent myocardial infarct.' Under these conditions, an unchanged ECG, even though it may have met one or two criteria from Table 4, would predict with greater than 95% reliability an unchanged ventriculogram and no significant new infarct. An increase in point score of 2 points (6% LV) or more would predict new infarct with the reliability shown in the validation section. Knowledge of the extent of infarct damage is fundamental to the assessment of cardiac reserve and rehabilitation potential. If preinfarct baseline ECGs are not available, then there is a significant reduction in the specificity and sensitivity of a single ECG to predict new infarct. Since 2% of a large normal series [18] met three criteria (or 9% LV), 3 or more points from the ECG scoring system would be 98% accurate in predicting new infarct, but 1–2 points would be associated with a 5%–20% or greater likelihood of being a false positive.

Theoretically, a changing QRS point score for infarct would indicate a changing degree of infarct. It is possible for large numbers of myocardial cells to be so ischemic that they do not respond to nearby excitation and yet recover to

Table 4. Simplified QRS scoring system

Lead	Duration (ms)		Amplitude ratios		Max. pts.
I	Q ⩾ 30	(1)	R/Q ⩽ 1	(1)	2
II	Q ⩾ 40	(2)			
	Q ⩾ 30	(1)			2
aVL	Q ⩾ 30	(1)	R/Q ⩽ 1	(1)	2
aVF	Q ⩾ 50	(3)	R/Q ⩽ 1	(2)	
	Q ⩾ 40	(2)			
	Q ⩾ 30	(1)	R/Q ⩽ 2	(1)	5
V_1	Any Q	(1)			
	R ⩾ 50	(2)			
	R ⩾ 40	(1)	R/S ⩾ 1	(1)	4
V_2	Any Q or R ⩽ 20	(1)			
	R ⩾ 60	(2)			
	R ⩾ 50	(1)	R/S ⩾ 1.5	(1)	4
V_3	Any Q or R ⩽ 30	(1)			1
V_4	Q ⩾ 20	(1)	R/Q or R/S ⩽ 0.5	(2)	
			R/Q or R/S ⩽ 1	(1)	3
V_5	Q ⩾ 30	(1)	R/Q or R/S ⩽ 1	(2)	
			R/Q or R/S ⩽ 2	(1)	3
V_6	Q ⩾ 30	(1)	R/Q or R/S ⩽ 1	(2)	
			R/Q or R/S ⩽ 3	(1)	3

The number of points awarded for meeting each criterion is in parentheses.

fire synchronously later. In this instance, assuming 3% or more of the left ventricle was involved, the point score would improve, indicating a decrease in infarct size. Likewise, if extension of infarct occurred, an increase in point score would be expected. The potential application of these methods to patients in whom interventions are being tried with the hope of decreasing infarct size is self-evident. The ability to repeat the test whenever desired is a strong argument in favor of using such a simple, noninvasive technique.

When prior infarct has been documented by ECG changes and prior ECGs are available for comparison, a change in ECG point score would be proportional to the extent of new infarct unless a defect in intraventricular conduction has supervened. Theoretically, a decrease in point scores, in V_1 and V_2 for example, from a new anterior superior infarct masking some of the ECG changes of a prior posterior inferior infarct, would have the same significance as an increase in points, suggesting new infarct or extension of an old one. The major pathologic validation studies reported below have been for single infarcts. It is unknown how often significant cancellation effects occur and how reliable these criteria are in the 25%–30% of patients who have multiple infarcts.

Both left superior (anterior) and inferior (posterior) fascicular block without infarcts in the simulations results in an ECG point score of 1 point each from the criteria in Table 4. If the modifier schedule proposed in Table 2 is followed, these tracings would be read as consider small anterior superior or inferior infarct. Since in middle-aged adults the statistical association of these changes with coronary disease and infarct is greater than 10%, this is an appropriate diagnostic modifier and statement. When infarct is added to the simulations, additional criteria for infarct in Table 3 appear and the extent of these changes relate to the size of infarct being simulated.

Complete right bundle branch block produces a minor superior and anterior shift of the initial one-half of the QRS and might be expected to increase the sensitivity of the criteria for inferior and posterior infarcts and, by masking changes, decrease the sensitivity of the criteria for anterior superior infarcts. In practice, the criteria for posterior infarcts are met in most patients with classic complete right bundle branch block unless associated with an obvious anterior superior infarct. The diagnosis or quantification of posterior infarcts is, therefore, not possible in the presence of this conduction defect. However, this combination is statistically unlikely and was not observed in our biplane angiographic series. The diagnosis and quantitation of inferior and anterior superior infarcts based on the simulations would be only minimally affected by the presence of complete right bundle branch block.

VALIDATION STUDIES

Recent animal studies

Most of the current Q wave criteria for the diagnosis of classic infarct have been developed from a large body of experimental data mostly involving canine models. Changes in epicardial unipolar leads were used to establish the ECG criteria for 'transmural infarct' that have been in routine use for years. Flowers et al. have recently recorded ECG body surface maps before and after myocardial infarct in the dog [19]. They found good correlation between size of infarct at autopsy and the volume of change in 'departure maps' (postinfarct map subtracted over time from the control map). They also noted late force changes on many of these departure maps that they thought might represent changes in intraventricular conduction or peri-infarct delay.

Using the McFee–Parungao lead system, Wickline and McNamara [20] noted in a small number of baboons that a change in spatial magnitude after an infarct was highly correlated ($r = 0.89$) with infarct size determined by planimetry at autopsy.

Ejection fraction and ECG criteria for infarct size in man

Ideker and associates [21] found that when akinesis or dyskinesis was seen on ventriculogram, there was a high degree of correlation ($r = 0.88$) with infarct size determined by using planimetric methods in patients evaluated on detailed postmortem examination. They found poor correlation when the ventriculogram showed hypokinesis. However, these infarcts were mainly subendocardial and small, which might have biased the data. In 1978, we reported on serial ECG and VCG changes in patients undergoing serial selective coronary angiography and biplane angiography [22]. An unchanged ECG/VCG was associated with an unchanged ventriculogram with a 98% reliability. A changed ECG/VCG represented a changed ventriculogram, and the magnitude and duration of QRS change on a McFee VCG correlated well ($r = 0.90$) with the change in ventriculographic ejection fraction.

More recently we have looked at 85 patients with single-vessel total occlusion of the left superior (anterior) descending coronary artery. All other arteries had less than 75% narrowing. We examined the reliability of the proposed ECG criteria to predict ejection fraction on biplane ventriculograms. The coefficient of correlation in patients with normal conduction was 0.82. When patients with hypokinesis and ECG changes of superior fascicular block, right bundle branch block, and left ventricular hypertrophy were included, the correlation was not significantly changed ($r = 0.81$). These data are summarized in Figure 7.

Wagner and associates [18] simplified the scoring system as shown in Table 4. This system differed from that of Table 3 in two respects. Only quantitative criteria were used, and R–Q and R–S amplitude ratio criteria were included, while criteria utilizing absolute amplitude measurements were excluded. They then tested the specificity of this simplified scoring system by using the ECGs of 349 normal subjects. The subjects included 243 normal volunteers and 106

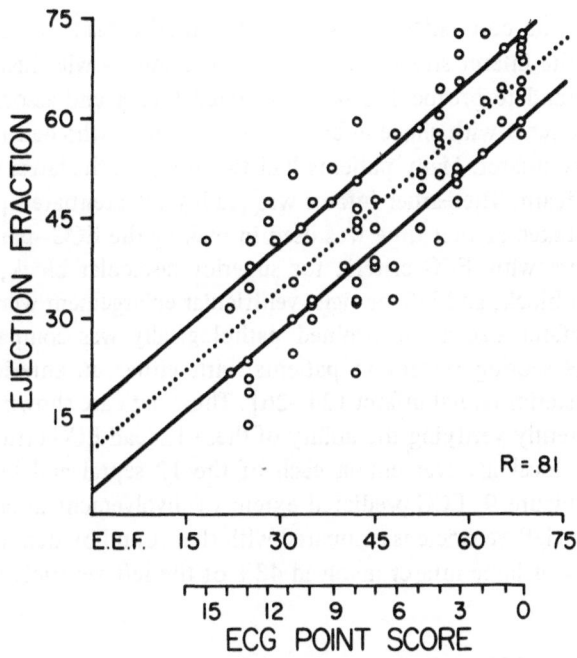

Figure 7. Shown in this scattergram are 85 consecutive patients with total occlusion of the left anterior descending coronary and less than 75% narrowing in the other two coronary arteries. Estimated ejection fraction and ECG point score based on criteria generated from the simulation are shown on the abscissa and observed ejection fraction by left ventricular angiogram is on the ordinate. All patients were included regardless of the presence or absence of ECG criteria for conduction abnormality or ventricular hypertrophy (see text). No cases of typical left bundle branch block were observed in this group of patients.

patients who had undergone diagnostic cardiac catheterization. The criteria in the simplified system all achieved a specificity greater than or equal to 97%. When a score greater than 2 points was required for identification of a myocardial infarct, the scoring system as a whole achieved a 98% specificity.

In a recent study that excluded conduction abnormalities and left ventricular hypertrophy, Palmeri and associates found good correlation ($r = 0.91$) between these modified QRS scoring criteria for infarct size (Table 4) and radionuclide angiographic ejection fraction [23]. Except for the exclusions above, all patients with a documented recent infarct were studied before discharge without regard to the number of prior infarcts or other clinical variables.

Pathological studies and ECG criteria for infarct size in man

The National Multicenter Study of Ischemic Heart Disease has been collecting and examining hearts on a standard protocol for a number of years. Postmortem angiograms of the coronaries and serial 'bread loaf' cross sections of the heart are done and the infarct size is determined by planimetry with histologic confirmation by a standard protocol. This has enabled Ideker and associates to select hearts from patients with single infarcts of various sizes, who had ECGs taken at the time of the infarct. Many patients had two infarcts, the latest one contributing to their death. The earlier infarct was readily differentiated pathologically and the ECG taken at that time was used in making the ECG—pathology correlations. Patients with ECG criteria for superior fascicular block, right or left bundle branch block, and left or right ventricular enlargement were excluded in this study. Infarct size as determined pathologically was compared with the modified QRS scoring system in patients with either an anterior (superior), inferior, or posterior lateral infarct [24—26]. These data are shown in Figure 8.

We are currently verifying the ability of these 12-lead ECG criteria to predict the extent of local involvement in each of the 12 septal and left ventricular segments. In Figure 9, ECG-predicted extent of involvement in each of the 12 segments of the left ventricle is compared with that found by detailed pathologic examination. This large infarct involved 43% of the left ventricle in the typical

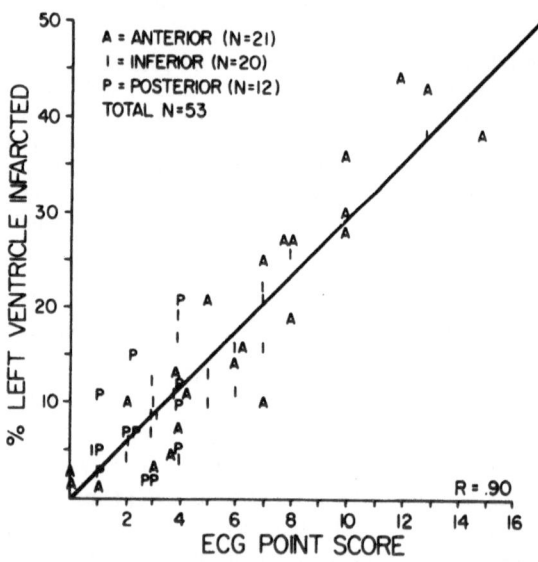

Figure 8. Pathologic infarct size and ECG changes (all location). Patients from the Multicenter Study of Ischemic Heart Disease with single infarcts at autopsy and no ECG evidence of hypertrophy or conduction abnormalities are shown here. Infarcts occurred more than a week before death. No posterior and only two inferior infarcts exceeded 24% of the left ventricle (or 8 ECG points), whereas nine (45%) anterior infarcts showed this degree of change upon quantitative pathologic examination. Modified after Ideker, Wagner, Alonso, Bishop, Bloor, Fallon, Gottlieb, Hackel, Phillips, Reimer, Roark, Rogers, Ruth, Savage, Selvester, and Ward.

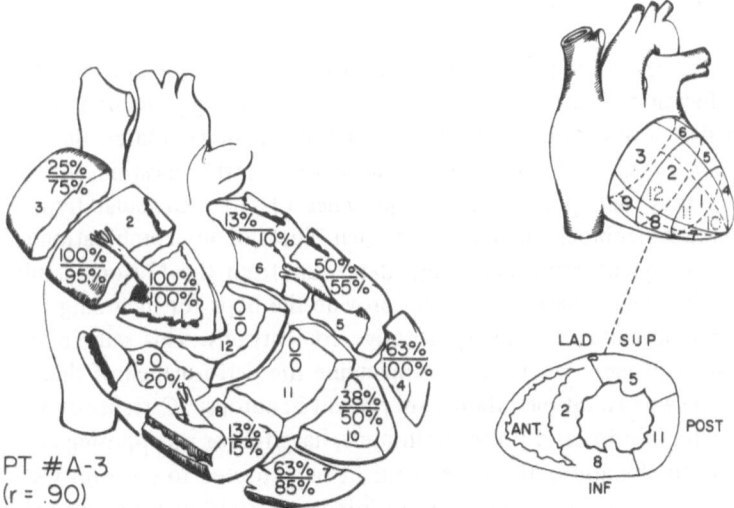

Figure 9. Percentage of segment infarcted (ratio of ECG prediction–pathology found). The distribution of infarct into each of the 12 segments of the left ventricle as predicted by the ECG is shown in the numerator. The amount of infarct found at autopsy is shown in the denominator. The localization by each ECG criterion is in accordance with the right-hand columns of Table 4. The patient is from the anterior infarct group shown in Figure 8. Courtesy of Dr. Ideker and associates.

distribution of the left superior(anterior) descending coronary artery, and is similar to others of this group. An average correlation of 0.91 for the distribution into these 12 segments was found for the four largest infarcts in this series. A similar average correlation of 0.93 for the distribution by location in the 11 smallest infarcts in this series was found. The correlation by location for the inferior and the posterior infarcts appears similar, but detailed analysis has not yet been done.

RECOMMENDATIONS FOR CURRENT CLINICAL UTILIZATION

These criteria would appear to be quite satisfactory for first infarcts. To what degree they deteriorate in various combinations of infarcts needs to be examined before they can be applied with confidence to all patients with suspected coronary artery disease. The finding by Palmeri et al. of good performance of the criteria in a general population of recent infarcts, when nuclear angiograms were used as the standard, suggests that their performance may not deteriorate significantly when applied 'across the board'. This will have to be verified in a pathologic series before final judgment is rendered.

FUTURE DIRECTIONS

A large area exists for refining the 12-lead ECG criteria for quantifying infarct size and location. While the current computer-simulation-generated criteria have performed well in carefully selected populations of single infarcts limited to the distribution of each of the three coronary arteries, the question remains as to how well they will perform in the presence of left ventricular hypertrophy, superior fascicular block, right bundle branch block, or any combination of these. The existing quantitative pathology data base from the National Multicenter Study of Ischemic Heart Disease can provide the basis for including these conduction abnormalities in the quantitative comparisons. This same quantitative pathology data base can be used to examine the performance of these 12-lead ECG criteria when multiple infarcts are present in autopsy. Certain combinations, for example, inferior and posterior infarcts, have few or no opposing effects and with such combinations the criteria might be expected to perform well. When anterior superior and either posterior or inferior infarcts coexisted in preliminary computer simulations, cancellation effects were significant. In this case, the criteria would underestimate the extent of left ventricular damage.

There are two avenues of approach to this dilemma that might utilize the existing forward simulation or existing ECG criteria. Other local leads on the chest might be more sensitive to the differences between opposing walls. From published data [27], it would seem that preferential weighting of high left precordial leads for superior wall damage, back leads for posterior wall damage, and low right precordial leads for inferior wall damage might effect better correlations even when infarcts occur on opposing walls of the left ventricle. Statistical methods, such as multistage multiple-regression techniques, applied to the existing 12-lead ECG criteria from patients with multiple infarcts at autopsy, can be expected to find weighting factors for certain criteria that would be less sensitive to infarcts on the opposite wall and still preserve reasonable sensitivity and accuracy for the primary wall involvement.

Future computer simulation with the forward model

Programs are now being written to simulate Purkinje reentry when the entire activation of Purkinje cells on one side or the other is blocked or not activated as in complete left or right bundle branch block, epicardial ectopics, or myocardial reentry arrhythmias. When the programs are complete, it will be a simple matter to explore all combinations of hypertrophies, bundle branch blocks, and infarctions. Atrial geometry, SA node function, AV node, and His bundles can all be modeled in the same general way that the ventricular myocardium and Purkinje system have been simulated.

It is a large numerical task, but local recovery properties can be included similar to the Miller–Geselowitz model [28] at each mm^3 region. Such parameters as injury, ischemia, and inhomogeneity of spatial distribution of recovery can be explored. Boineau et al. [29] have done early work with such a model for local regions of myocardium and have demonstrated simulated reentrant ventricular tachycardia and fibrillation. Since in reality the whole heart participates in these malignant arrhythmias, it would seem prudent to try to include the whole heart (including atria and AV conduction system) in the simulation. To the degree that the simulation includes the relevant parameters involved in these arrhythmias, the model can become a powerful tool to explore the complex interactions of these variables.

Inverse models and inverse solutions

The forward simulation can be formulated by the matrix equation

$$V = AD$$

where V is the body surface potential distribution over time, A is the transfer matrix from the heart to the surface, and D is the history of current dipole moment from each of the local regions of myocardium.

The solution of the inverse model relates directly to the diagnostic problem in electrocardiography where the objective is to define the condition of the myocardium from surface ECG measurements. If one knows the A matrix accurately for any given patient and records V, then the current dipole moment D in local regions of myocardium is described by the inverse matrix equation

$$D = A^{-1} \cdot V$$

In the 17-dipole model described, this matrix equation requires at least 51 simultaneous surface ECG potentials to solve the 51 simultaneous equations needed to obtain three orthogonal components for each of the 17 local current dipoles representing 17 local myocardial regions. This is a huge computational task. In practice, a smaller number of local regions is sought and overdetermination is used to simplify the numerical problem. Typically, 140 or more simultaneous ECG leads have been used to look for 10–12 local regions [30] .

The dipole time histories contain information about the activation order and integrity of local segments of myocardium. An accurate inverse solution would contain explicit information about fascicular delays, bundle branch blocks, and so on. It would also specify explicitly the local increase in current moment (hypertrophy) and local losses (infarction). Theoretically, any increase or local loss would be specified regardless of activation order. Thus, hypertrophy or infarct can be quantitated as accurately in abnormal conduction, such as Walff–

Parkinson—White syndrome, premature ventricular contractions, fascicular blocks, and bundle branch blocks, as it is in normal conduction. The major problem in producing accurate inverse solutions is that of having an accurate individual set of transfer numbers to specify the A matrix in any given patient.

Research in our laboratory and a number of other centers is going on at the present time to establish a simple method of measuring individual transfer numbers. If this can be done, the inverse matrix equations described can be used to eliminate the effects of various torso shapes and inhomogeneities. Then these measurements plus ECG surface data can be used to look directly and quantitatively at the electrical activity in local segments of the heart. The forward model suggests that changes in local regions of 7—10 mm in diameter can be seen in the surface ECG. It remains to be seen to what degree these changes can be resolved by some form of direct inverse solution.

Acknowledgment. This work has been supported in part by NHLBI grants RO1 HL 17532—04 and RO HL 14688—05; and Specialized Centers of Research in Atherosclerosis USC HL 14138—05S1.

REFERENCES

1. Solomon JC, Selvester RH: Simulation of measured activation sequence in the human Heart. Am Heart J 85:518, 1973.
2. Selvester RH: Criteria for atrial enlargement and infarct size (applicable to computer diagnostic programs). In: Conference proceedings on computerized interpretation of the electrocardiogram. Bull US Dept HEW, 1975, p 81.
3. Selvester RH, Solomon JC, Sapoznikov D: Computer simulation of the electrocardiogram. In: Cady LH (ed) Computer techniques in cardiology. New York: Marcel Dekker, 1979, 9:417.
4. Einthoven W, Fahr G, de Waart A: Ueber die Richtung und die manifeste Grösse der Potentialschwankungen im menschlichen Herzen und über den Einfluss der Herzlage auf die Form des Elektrokardiogramms. Pfluegers Arch Ges Physiol 150:275, 1913.
5. Scher AM, Young AC: The pathway of ventricular depolarization in the dog. Circ Res 4:461, 1956.
6. Durrer D, van Dam RT, Meijler FL, Arzbaecher RC, Müller EJ, Freud GE: Electrical activation and membrane action potentials of a perfused, normal heart [abstr]. Circulation 34:III-92, 1966.
7. Selvester RH, Collier CR, Pearson RB: Analog computer model of the vectorcardiogram. Circulation 31:45, 1965.
8. Selvester RH, Kalaba R, Kagiwada H, Collier CR, Bellman R: Simulated myocardial infarction with a mathematical model of the heart containing distance and boundary effects. In: Vectorcardiography 1965. Amsterdam: North-Holland, p 403, 1966.
9. Selvester RH, Kalaba R, Collier CR, Bellman R, Kagiwada H: A digital computer model of the vectorcardiogram with distance and boundary effects: simulated myocardial infarction. Am Heart J 74:792, 1967.

10. Solomon JC, Selvester RH: Current dipole moment density of the heart. Am Heart J 81:351, 1971.
11. Solomon JC, Selvester RH, Kirk WL, Pearson RB: New theoretical model of the electromotive surface in the heart. In: Engineering in medicine and biology, Proceedings of the 19th annual conference, 1966.
12. Gelernter HL, Swihart JC: A mathematical–physical model of the genesis of the electrocardiogram. IBM Res RC 99, 1963.
13. Collier CR, Selvester RH: Vector lead system evaluation by computer simulation. In: Engineering in medicine and biology, Proceedings of the 19th annual conference, 1966.
14. Selvester RH, Wagner JO, Rubin HB: Quantitation of myocardial infarct size and location by electrocardiogram and vectorcardiogram. In: Snellen HA, et al (eds) Quantitation in cardiology. The Hague: Leiden University Press, 1972, p 31 (in the USA by Williams and Wilkins).
15. Selvester RH, Rubin HB, Hamlin JA, Pote WW: New quantitative vectorcardiographic criteria for the detection of unsuspected myocardial infarction in diabetics. Am Heart J 75:335, 1968.
16. James TN: Anatomy of the coronary arteries. New York: Paul B Hoeber, 1961.
17. Lie KI, Wellens HJJ, Schullenberg RM: Bundle branch block and acute infarction. In: Wellens HJJ, Lie KI, Janse MJ (eds) The conduction system of the heart: structure, function, and clinical implications. Philadelphia: Lea and Febiger, 1976, p 666.
18. Flowers NC, Horan LG, Johnson JC: Anterior infarctional changes occurring during mid and late ventricular activation detectable by surface mapping techniques. Circulation 54:906, 1976.
20. Ideker RE, Behar VS, Wagner GS, Starr JW, Starmer CF, Lee KL, Heckel DB: Evaluation of asynergy as an indicator of myocardial fibrosis. Circulation 57:715, 1978.
21. Selverster RH, Sanmarco ME: Infarct size in hi-gain, hi-fidelity serial VCG's and serial ventriculograms in patients with proven coronary artery disease. In: Proceedings of the 4th world congress on electrocardiography, 1977.
22. Palmeri ST, Harrison DG, Upton MT, Morris KG, Wagner GS, Selvester RH: The electrocardiographic prediction of left ventricular ejection fraction following myocardial infarction [abstr]. Circulation 60:II-187, 1979.
23. Ward RM, Ideker RE, Wagner GS, Alonso DR, Bishop SP, Bloor CM, Fallon JT, Gottlieb GJ, Hackel DB, Phillips HR, Reimer KA, Roark SF, Rogers WJ, Ruth WK, Savage RM, Selvester RH: Myocardial infarcts in the lateral third of the left ventricle: size and ECG recognition [abstr]. Am J Cardiol 45:473, 1980.
24. Ruth WK, Ideker RE, Wagner GS, Alonso DR, Bishop SP, Bloor CM, Fallon JT, Gottlieb GJ, Hackel DB, Phillips HR, Reimer KA, Roark SF, Rogers WJ, Savage RM, Selvester RH, Ward RM: Estimation of myocardial infarct size using the QRS scoring system [abstr]. Circulation 60:II-189, 1979.
25. Ideker RE, Wagner GS, Hackel DB, Bishop SP, Bloor CM, Fallon JT, Phillips HR, Reimer KA, Roark SF, Savage RM, Selvester RH: Evaluation of the QRS complexes in leads V_4-V_6 as indicators of the size of anterior myocardial infarcts defined at necropsy [abstr]. Am J Cardiol 43:351, 1979.

26. Selvester RH, Gillespie TL: Simulated ECG surface map's sensitivity to local segments of myocardium. In: Lepeschkin E, Rush S (eds) Proceedings, advances in cardiology, vol 10: Body surface mapping of cardiac fields. Basel: Karger, 1974.
27. Miller WT III, Geselowitz DB: Simulation studies of the electrocardiogram. I. The normal heart. II. Ischemia and infarction. Circ Res 43:301, 1978.
28. Boineau JP, Farlow W: Use of a computer model to understand mechanisms of ventricular fibrillation [abstr]. Circulation 52:II-162, 1975.
29. Barnard ACL, Hold JH Jr, Lynn MS: Models of the cardiac electrical source: adequacy and clinical usefulness [abstr]. J Electrocardial 2:215, 1969.

3. THE ECG: THE SPATIAL AND NONSPATIAL DETERMINANTS OF THE EXTRACELLULARLY RECORDED POTENTIAL WITH EMPHASIS ON THE TQ-ST SEGMENT

MORTON F. ARNSDORF and ERIC K. LOUIE

The importance of understanding the relationship between bioelectricity and the electrocardiogram has been underscored by the recent attempts to correlate QRS (R) wave and TQ-ST segment amplitudes with myocardial ischemia and injury and the controversy that has resulted from such attempts [1–5]. Myocardial ischemia, injury, and infarct may influence the electrocardiogram by altering the spatial and nonspatial determinants of the extracellularly recorded potential. Spatial determinants include the boundary or boundaries between normal and injured tissue as well as the relationship of the recording electrodes to these boundaries. Nonspatial determinants include the transmembrane voltages of cardiac cells as well as the flow of ions into, through, and around cardiac tissues. Therapeutic interventions also may affect transmembrane voltages or ionic conductivities rather than spatial determinants. It follows, therefore, that electrophysiologic measurements, such as the amplitude of the R wave or the magnitude of the TQ-ST segment, cannot be expected to bear a simple relationship to the boundaries between normal and damaged cells, much less to the zone at risk for infarct which contains tissues that may be salvageable.

Despite theoretical and practical limitations, we would postulate that arrays of epicardial and precordial electrograms are capable of defining an electrophysiologic boundary or series of boundaries. The accuracy with which these electrophysiologic boundaries can be related empirically to the border between normal and reversibly injured tissue in the zone at risk, or perhaps between the zone at risk and the infarcted area, will determine the usefulness of the electrophysiologic index. If an electrophysiologic index were capable of defining the spatial extent of the myocardium at risk for infarct, it might then be possible to use independent techniques to assess the ultimate fate of this tissue after an intervention.

Our postulate can be summarized in terms of four basic assumptions that will be considered in detail in this Chapter.

Assumption 1. An array of voltage measurements obtained from epicardial sites can uniquely determine an electrophysiologic boundary or series of boundaries caused by the difference in transmembrane voltages and conductivities between normal and reversibly damaged tissue and perhaps between reversibly and irreversibly damaged tissues.

Wagner GS (ed): Myocardial Infarction: Measurement and Intervention, pp 51–106.
© *1982 Martinus Nijhoff Publishers, The Hague/Boston/London.*

Assumption 2. It is possible to predict epicardial voltage distributions and hence boundaries from precordial recording, or it is possible in some other way to identify heretofore unidentified information from the surface electrogram that may relate to the zone at risk and the zone of infarct.

Assumption 3. The electrophysiologic boundary or boundaries can be related empirically to the biochemically, biophysically, or anatomically determined extent of tissue that is at risk for eventual death.

Assumption 4. Independent techniques can be used subsequently to determine the ultimate fate of the electrophysiologically and otherwise defined zone at risk of infarct, thereby enabling the efficacy of interventions designed to limit infarct size to be tested. These independent techniques must accurately reflect changes in the extent of infarct in the region at risk and not be influenced spuriously by the interventions being tested.

THE DISTRIBUTED DIPOLE MODEL (SOLID ANGLE THEORY)

General considerations

Newton [6], Gauss [7], Maxwell [8], and others [9, 10] have utilized forms of the distributed dipole model in studies on gravitation, electrical phenomena, magnetics, optics, and radiation. We have recently reviewed several biophysical theories, including the distributed dipole model, that relate cardiac bioelectricity to the extracellularly recorded potential [5]. The distributed dipole model has long been of interest to electrophysiologists and electrocardiographers [11—23] and has been found useful in the interpretation of electrocardiographic data in vitro [20] and in vivo [21—23]. We will consider this model in some detail since it is relatively easy to comprehend and includes many of the considerations important in even more complicated theories.

The membrane can be considered a dipole layer with a relatively uniform dielectric constant and thickness (Figure 1). The charge stored per unit area of membrane surface area is proportional to the transmembrane voltage. The dipole layer, of course, encloses the cell, so at rest or during uniform activation the dipoles on one surface are balanced by equal but oppositely directed dipoles on the opposite surface and, therefore, no extracellular potential is recorded. The low resistance at the gap junctions between cells facilitates intercellular electrotonic communication and, in effect, causes aggregates of cells to act as a single large cell. As a result, a difference in the transmembrane voltage or charge between two areas, as, for example, during the propagation of an action potential when resting and activated tissues are juxtaposed (Figure 2A and B), creates a boundary across which are unopposed positive and negative charges. This

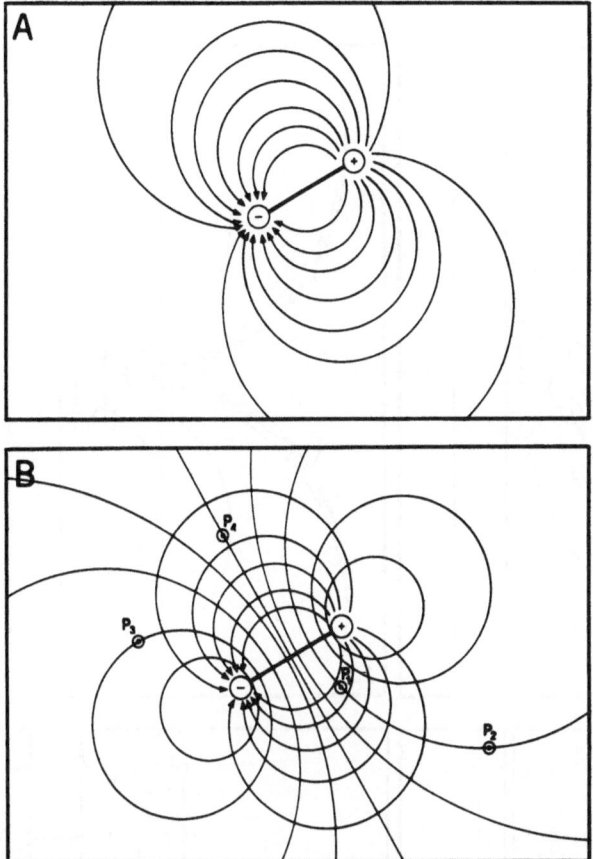

Figure 1. A dipole is an electrical generator consisting of two equal but opposite charges held a short distance apart. Current flows from the positive to the negative pole (*A*) and establishes an electrical field that can be recorded by electrodes (P_{1-4}) placed in the field (*B*). Adapted from Arnsdorf with the permission of the American Physiological Society [25].

separation of charge creates a distributed dipole layer across the boundary composed of an infinite number of dipoles representing infinitely small portions of the boundary which, in turn, establish current flow within cells, between cells through gap junctions, and outside cells in the extracellular space (Figure 2C). This current flow creates the electrical field perceived by the extracellular electrode (Fig. 2D).

Approximation 1. *The distributed dipole layer across the boundary established by the different transmembrane voltages (or charges) is the source of current flow that is responsible for establishing the electrical field in the thorax detected by the electrocardiograph. At a distance from the boundary, the dipoles on opposite sides of the cell tend to cancel each other out.*

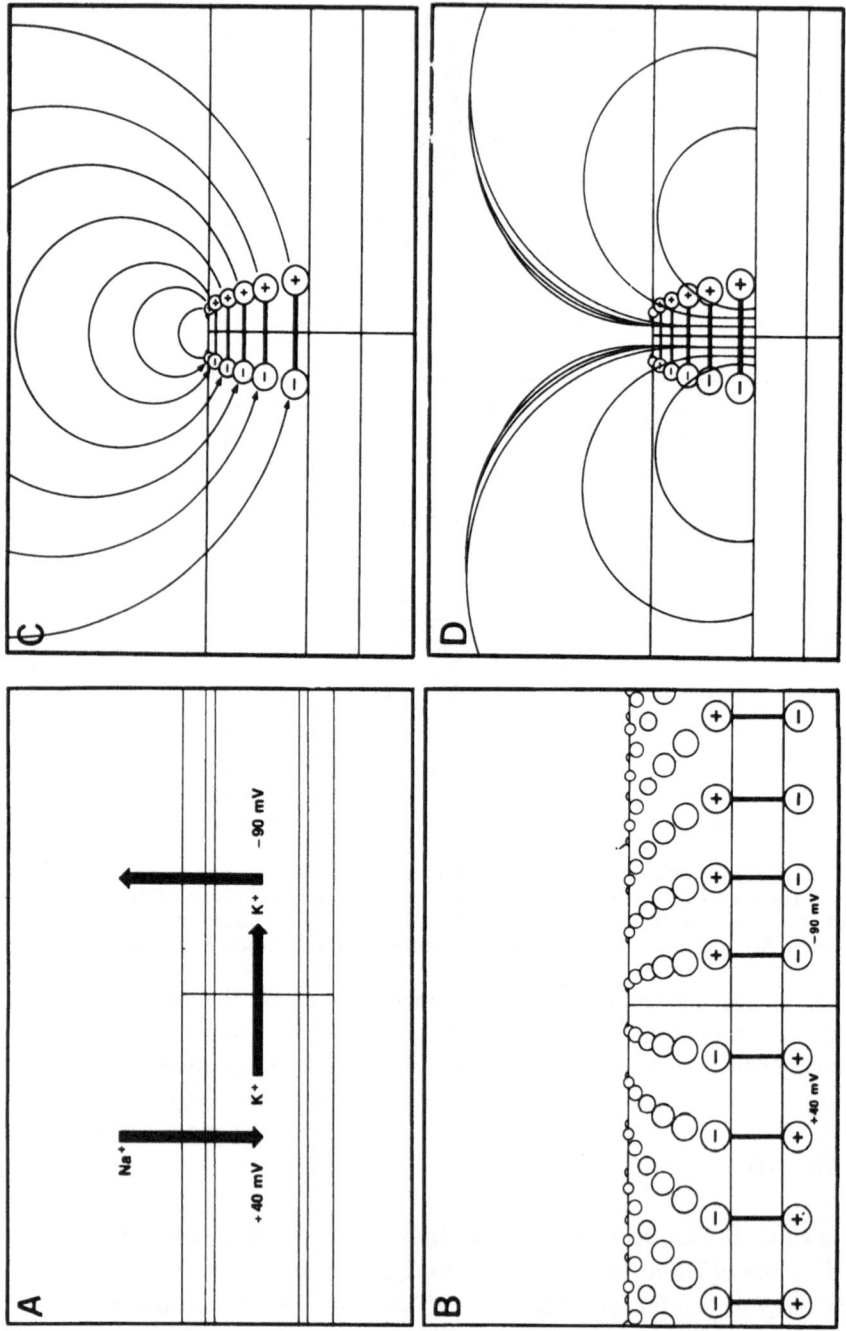

Figure 2. The juxtaposition of resting and activated tissue produces local current flow within, between, and outside cells (*A*). In the resting segment, the negative poles of the membrane dipole layer are inside the cell; in the activated segment, the positive poles of the membrane dipole layer are inside the cell (*B*). A separation of charge exists at the boundary while the dipoles at a distance from the boundary are canceled by opposing dipoles on the opposite surface of the membrane, resulting in current flow from the positive to negative poles of the dipoles across the boundary (*C*). The current establishes an electrical field (*D*). Adapted from Arnsdorf with the permission of the American Physiological

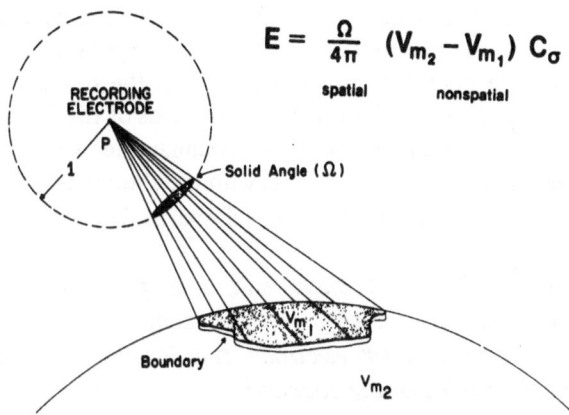

$$E = \frac{\Omega}{4\pi} \ \underset{\text{spatial}}{(V_{m_2} - V_{m_1})} \ \underset{\text{nonspatial}}{C_\sigma}$$

Figure 3. A schematic representation of the spatial and nonspatial determinants of the extracellularly recorded potential (E) according to the distributed dipole theory. The solid angle (Ω) is defined as the area of spherical surface cut off a unit sphere that surrounds the electrode P by radii constructed from every point along the boundary to the electrode. The separation of charge across the boundary is created by the difference in the transmembrane voltages which, in turn, establishes the flow of current that is responsible for the electrical field detected by the electrode. The conductivity term, C_σ, accounts for current flow within, between, and outside cells. See text for discussion of the spatial and nonspatial terms. Adapted from Holland and Arnsdorf, with permission [1].

> *It is primarily the boundary, then, that is perceived or 'seen' by the extracellular electrode.*

In reality, the action potentials throughout an area of tissue such as the ventricle are not identical. Nevertheless, this is a useful first approximation.

Spatial determinants of the extracellular potential

The extracellular recorded potential (ϵ) is determined both by spatial and nonspatial factors. The spatial determinants (Figure 3) include the geometry of the boundary separating areas with different transmembrane voltages (V_{m_1}, V_{m_2}), the position of the extracellular recording electrode relative to this boundary, and the nature and extent of the surrounding volume conductor. In a large homogeneous volume conductor, the spatial term may be quantified by the solid angle (Ω) that includes both electrode position and a measure of the apparent geometry of the boundary. As seen in Figure 3, the solid angle is determined by drawing radii from the site of the electrode P to all points of the boundary, thereby forming an irregular cone. A unit sphere is inscribed about P. The area of the unit sphere cut off or subtended by the cone is termed the solid angle. Remembering that a unit sphere has an area of 4π steradians, the maximum value of the solid angle is $\pm 4\pi$ steradians. The spatial determinants in this situation can be described by $(\Omega/4\pi)$. The solid angle, then, varies directly with the radius of the boundary and inversely with the distance between the electrode and the boundary. One of the major strengths of the distributed dipole model is that it mathematically accounts for boundary geometry and electrode position which, as discussed later, contrasts with the simplified single equivalent dipole model that accounts only poorly for such spatial determinants.

> Approximation 2. *The solid angle and, therefore, the extracellularly recorded potential vary directly with the radius of the boundary as perceived by the extracellular electrode and inversely with the distance between the electrode and the boundary.*

Nonspatial determinants of the extracellular potential

The nonspatial determinants include the polarity and magnitude of the difference in the transmembrane voltage across the boundary, a quantity we have termed the transmembrane potential gradient (TPG). The transmembrane voltage, in turn, is determined by the flow of ions through the cardiac membrane. The determinants of the flow depend on the driving force and the permeability or conductance of the membrane to a given ionic species. The driving force is established by the difference between the transmembrane voltage and the equilibrium potential for the given ionic species (E_i), the latter being approximated by the Nernst equation. Membrane conductance is determined by voltage-dependent, and in some instances, time-dependent activation and inactivation variables as well as by the geometry and integrity of the membrane channel itself. To this must be added the influence of the various energy-requiring ionic pumps that maintain ionic gradients.

The flow of ions inside, between, and outside the cardiac cells also depends on the characteristics of the electrical circuit. For example, the flow of ions between cells depends on both the driving force across and the characteristics of the gap junction. The resistance of the gap junction to the flow of ions is influenced by a variety of factors such as pH, intracellular calcium concentration, and drugs. The properties of the volume conductor, that is, the thorax, have long been recognized to influence the extracellular recorded signal. Recently, elegant theoretical considerations have been presented by several investigators including Rudy and Plonsey [19, 24].

> Approximation 3. *The nonspatial determinants of the extracellular potential depend on neither the geometry of the boundary nor the position of the extracellular recording electrode. These factors include the*

transmembrane potential gradient and the characteristics of ionic flow within, between, and outside cardiac cells.

The relationship between the extracellular potential and its spatial and nonspatial determinants

Given the assumptions of the distributed dipole model, the relationship between the extracellular potential (ϵ) and its spatial and nonspatial determinants can be approximated by the following:

$$\epsilon \qquad = (\Omega/4\pi) \qquad \times [\text{TPG} \cdot C_\sigma] \qquad (1)$$

| extracellular | spatial | nonspatial |
| potential | determinants | determinants |

where the abbreviations are as previously defined and C_σ is a conductivity term that includes consideration of the ionic flow within, between, and around cells.

The transmembrane potential gradient

Since the transmembrane potential gradient (TPG) equals the difference in V_m across the boundary, Eq. 1 becomes:

$$\epsilon = \frac{\Omega}{4\pi} (V_{m_2} - V_{m_1}) C_\sigma \qquad (2)$$

The determinants of V_{m_1} and V_{m_2} are those active and passive membrane properties and conductivities that determine the resting transmembrane voltage (V_r) and the action potential [1, 2]. Since the boundary is defined by the separation in charge, the change in the TPG can be temporal, configurational, or both. A *temporal* change results from an altered sequence of activation or repolarization without a significant change in V_r or in the change of the action potential on one or both sides of the boundary. A *configurational* change results from a change in V_r or the shape of the action potential on one or both sides of the boundary. Figure 4 is an experimental example of these types of change caused by altering the extracellular potassium concentration. The TPG can be eliminated by making V_m identical on both sides of the boundary so that $V_{m_1} - V_{m_2} = 0$.

Approximation 4. *A configurational and/or temporal change in the transmembrane potential gradient will affect the extracellular potential. The transmembrane potential gradient becomes zero in Eq. 2 when* V_{m_1} *changes to equal* V_{m_2}*, when* V_{m_2} *changes to equal* V_{m_1}*, and when both change to equal each other.*

58

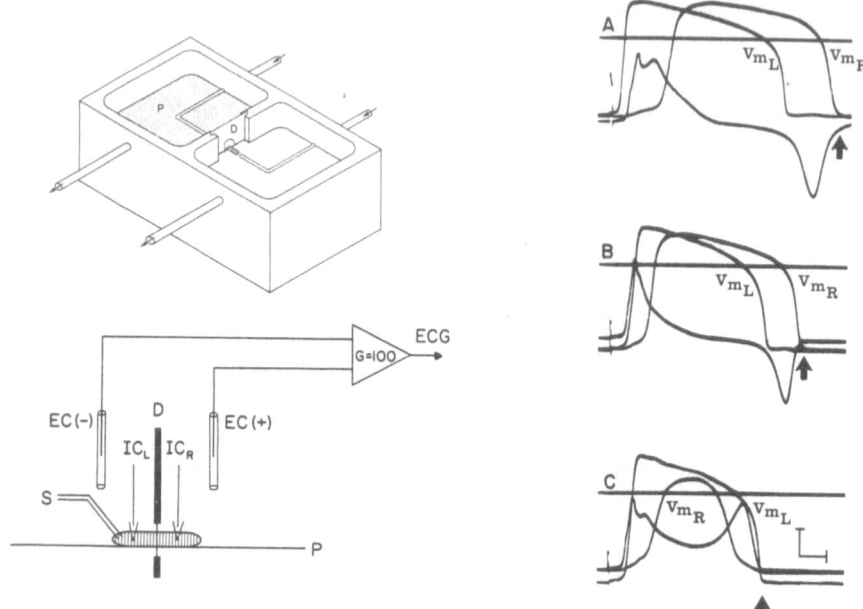

Figure 4. (*Left*) The experimental arrangement. (Top) The tissue bath is partitioned with a latex diaphragm (D) through which is drawn a strip of guinea pig ventricle. Each half of the chamber can be perfused with normal or modified Tyrode's solution. (Bottom) The extracellular electrodes, EC (−) and EC (+), are positioned on opposite sides of the partition. Intracellular microelectrodes (IC_L and IC_R) are inserted in the tissue on the left and right sides of the diaphragm, respectively. S is a Teflon-coated extracellular bipolar stimulating electrode; G is a low-noise preamplifier; and P is the paraffin base in the chambers. (*Right*) Temporal and configurational changes in the TQ-ST segment caused by hyperkalemia. The experimental records show the transmembrane potentials from the left and right portions of the tissue (V_{m_L}, V_{m_R}) and the extracellular electrogram. Both halves of the fiber were bathed in Tyrode's solution containing an extracellular potassium concentration of 12 mM. The arrow indicates the end of the QT interval. *A* and *B* were recorded on consecutive beats and *C* within 10 s of *B*. *A* and *B* demonstrate different conduction delays and action potential durations, but the action potential configurations are essentially identical on both sides of the partition. In *C*, a difference in action potential shape as well as a conduction delay were observed between the two sides. Note the effects that these configurational and temporal changes have on the R, TQ-ST, and T deflections of the electrogram. The vertical calibration bar equals 20 mV and 1 mV for the intracellular and extracellular potentials, respectively; the horizontal bar equals 100 ms. Adapted from Holland and Arnsdorf, with permission [20].

The conductivity term

The extracellular potential is also proportional to a conductivity term, C_σ, that considers the flow of ions inside, between, and outside the cell. As described by Plonsey [17], C_σ can be described by the relationship:

$$C_\sigma = \left[1 + \frac{\sigma_o}{\sigma_i} \cdot (S/A - 1) \right]^{-1} \tag{3}$$

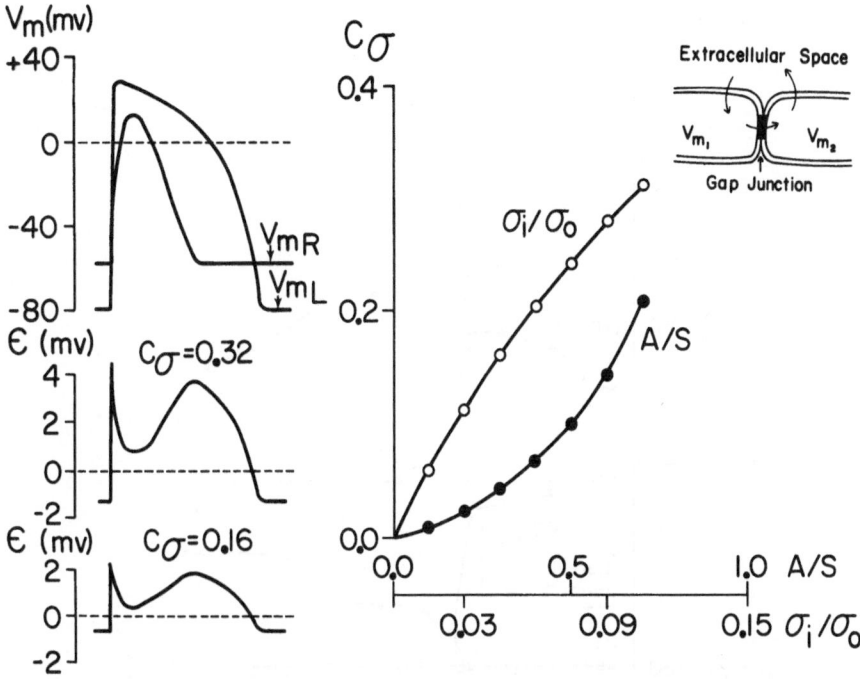

Figure 5. The effect of alterations in the conductivity term on the extracellularly recorded potential. (*Inset*) Diagrammatic representation of current flow into, between, and outside two cells. (*Left*) The upper portion depicts the transmembrane voltage recordings on the right (V_{m_R}) and left (V_{m_L}) of the boundary that is responsible for the current flow leading to the TQ-ST segment changes in the middle panel. If the conductivity term (C_σ) is halved, the extracellularly recorded potential is decreased accordingly (*middle*). Note that the R wave and the TQ-ST segments are decreased equally, and have the same relationship to each other that they had in the middle panel. (*Right*) Theoretical calculations as to the effect that alterations in the determinants of the conductivity term would have on C_σ. See text for abbreviations and discussion. Adapted from Holland and Arnsdorf, with permission [20].

where σ_i and σ_o are the respective intracellular and extracellular conductivities, A is the cross-sectional area of the cardiac fiber, and S is the area of the fiber plus its associated interstitial space. Figure 5 depicts the type of change in ϵ anticipated if C_σ or its components (σ_i, σ_o, A, and S) were altered. Figure 6 is an experimental example of a change in the extracellular potential thought to be due to a change in the conductivity term.

> *Approximation 5. A change in the conductivity term, due to alterations in the determinants of ionic flow within, between, and outside cells as well as aggregates of cells, will affect the extracellular potential.*

Interrelationships

Together, Eqs. 2 and 3 describe most of the variables that need to be considered when attempting to correlate electrocardiographic changes with physio-

60

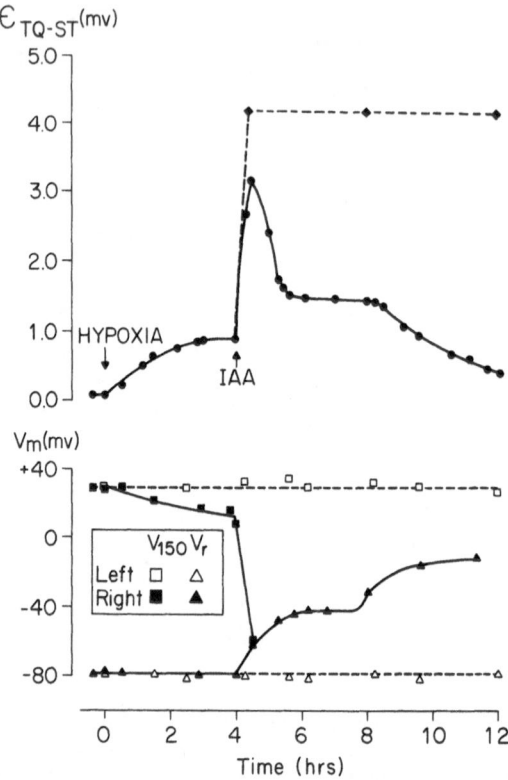

Figure 6. A graphic representation of the effects of hypoxia and the metabolic poison, iodoacetic acid (IAA), on the guinea pig ventricle by using the experimental arrangement depicted in Figure 4. The right portion of the preparation was bathed with hypoxic Tyrode's solution for 4 h after which IAA was added. (*Top*) The TQ-ST segment deflection is plotted against time. The theoretically predicted change in the TQ-ST segment is indicated by the dashed line, and the experimentally observed change in the TQ-ST segment by the solid line. Note the deviation of observation from prediction shortly after the addition of IAA. (*Bottom*) The transmembrane voltages at rest (V_r) and 150 ms after the stimulus (V_{150}) on both the left (open symbols) and right (closed symbols) are plotted against time. The decline in the TQ-ST segment after IAA was initially rapid (about $4\frac{1}{2}$ h) and then much slower (about 8 h). The failure to quantitatively parallel the transmembrane potential gradient in amplitude after the application of IAA suggests that the conductivity term (C_σ) has changed. Adapted from Holland and Arnsdorf, with permission [20].

logic, pathologic, or pharmacologic alterations and lead to the next approximation.

Approximation 6. *The relationship between the extracellular potential and the most important spatial and nonspatial determinants can be approximated by the relationship:*

$$\epsilon = \frac{\Omega}{4\pi} \; (V_{m_2} - V_{m_1}) \cdot \left[1 + \frac{\sigma_o}{\sigma_i} \cdot (S/A - 1) \right]^{-1} \qquad (4)$$

spatial   nonspatial determinants

determinants

Each term in Eq. 4, moreover, has itself several determinants. The amount of information included in the extracellularly recorded signal, then, is immense.

In the past, there has been a tendency to consider each electrocardiographic deflection an isolated event. Little attention has been paid to the interrelationship between these deflections or between the determinants of ϵ. Note, for example, the experimental result in Figure 7 in which the *apparent* total R wave amplitude may be determined in part from the ϵ_{TQ} potential which, in turn, arises from differences in the configuration of the action potential across the boundary [20]. Similarly, we have observed T wave changes to be caused by the same configurational and temporal factors that influenced the ϵ_{ST}.

Approximation 7. *The determinants of ϵ are interrelated and thus must be considered when any index of ϵ is used to assess changes in the myocardium.*

Advantages and limitations of the distributed dipole model

The advantages of the distributed dipole model include the following: (a) it physiologically and mathematically describes the relationship between cardiac bioelectricity and the extracellularly recorded potential; (b) it accounts for spatial factors by considering each boundary to be composed of an infinite number of dipoles that are enabled to move in the direction of the wavefront, thereby enabling an accurate mathematical description of the geometry of the boundary and its relationship to the recording electrode; (c) it is valid at *all* distances from the heart; and (d) it accounts for nonspatial factors that, in turn, have their own determinants.

Although the biophysical theory included in the distributed dipole model is correct and valid, the practical question remains as to whether it is appropriate to analytically and quantitatively describe biologic events. This question, of course, must be addressed to any biophysical theory. The problem is that we know little of the details concerning the action potentials of individual cells, the characteristics of communication between cells, the nature and influences of

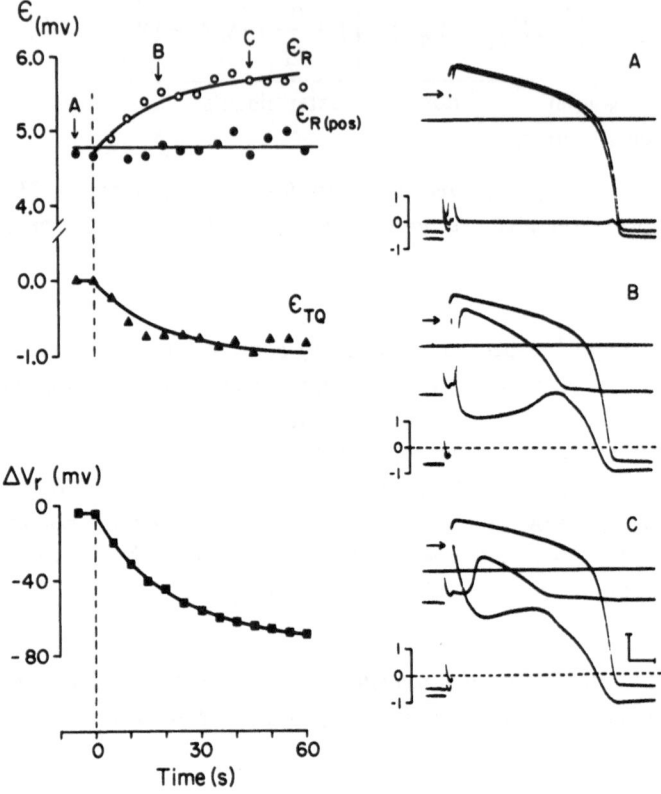

Figure 7. The interrelationships between the TQ-ST segment and the R wave in the guinea pig ventricle by using the experimental arrangement depicted in Figure 4. The effects of a sudden infusion of $1.0\,M$ KCl into the right chamber on the diastolic transmembrane potential gradient (ΔV_r), the TQ segment (ϵ_{TQ}), and the components of the R wave are shown graphically on the left and the experimental tracings on the right. In the control period (A), the action potentials on both sides of the partition are virtually superimposable and non TQ-ST segment deflection is seen. The peak of the R wave is indicated by the arrow. B and C were recorded at 20 and 45 s, respectively, after KCl infusion. Both ΔV_r and the ϵ_{TQ} can be seen to increase. The experimental records show that the positive portion of the R wave, $\epsilon_{R(pos)}$, as measured from the isoelectric (dashed) line to the peak of the R wave (arrow), did not change at 20 and 45 s after KCl infusion. The *total or apparent* R wave amplitude, ϵ_R, as measured from the TQ segment to the peak of the R wave, however, increased. As shown graphically on the left, the increase in ϵ_R was identical to the change in ϵ_{TQ} which, in turn, paralleled ΔV_r. The vertical calibration bar equals 20 mV; the horizontal calibration bar equals 100 ms. The extracellular voltage scale in mV is to the left of the experimental records. Adapted from Holland and Arnsdorf, with permission [20].

extracellular factors, the nature of the boundary between normal and abnormal cells, and similar issues. Spach et al. [26] correctly have challenged a simplifying assumption of the solid angle theory: namely, the assumed constancy of the transmembrane voltage within an area of cardiac tissue such as the ventricle.

Without doubt, Eq. 4 remains unacceptably simplified and can, at best, afford only semiquantitative data. It is not clear, however, how much information is lost by the simplifying assumptions contained in the distributed dipole model. Perhaps the model and the equation can be modified to account for the various populations of action potentials that occur in both normal and diseased myocardium and are responsible for the distribution of potentials described by Spach et al. (compare, for example, Figure 8A and B).

Of enormous importance is the fact that the solid angle theory, as well as more complex theory, enables predictive statements that can be tested. Figure 8 illustrates the predicted solid angle (and hence potential) that should pertain as the wavefront sweeps by a given point: for example, at the boundary between juxtaposed tissues having different transmembrane voltages. Although the fit of experimental observation to theory is not perfect, the sharp rise in ϵ to a maximum at a border of an ischemic area and the subsequent decline on both sides of the boundary have been documented quite convincingly [22, 23, 27]. Subsequently, new hypotheses may be developed to better fit observations and to more accurately predict the general case. An ampliation of these hypotheses results from the predictions arising from appropriately applied biophysical theory and provides new postulates for experimental testing as discussed in detail later in this chapter.

Approximation 8. *Despite the constraints placed upon theory by biologic realities, biophysical theory enables the development of predictive statements that can be experimentally tested. To date, all models have been inadequately tested by experiment.*

All models, including the distributed dipole model, are limited by the thorax being neither homogeneous nor infinite, which, of course, makes mathematical descriptions more difficult. This tends to affect the absolute rather than the relative distribution of the extracellularly recorded potential. Even when inhomogeneities in the volume conductor, boundary effects between different structures such as the heart and intracavitary blood mass, a distribution of action potential characteristics and asymmetric cardiac cell geometry are taken into account, calculation presents a formidable problem.

Approximation 9. *Although the distributed dipole model contains a wealth of information and enables prediction that can be experimentally tested, a great practical limitation is the difficulty of calculation. For this reason, simplified theory such as the single equivalent dipole model has been commonly used. The assumptions involved in such simplification, however, decrease the amount of information obtained.*

64

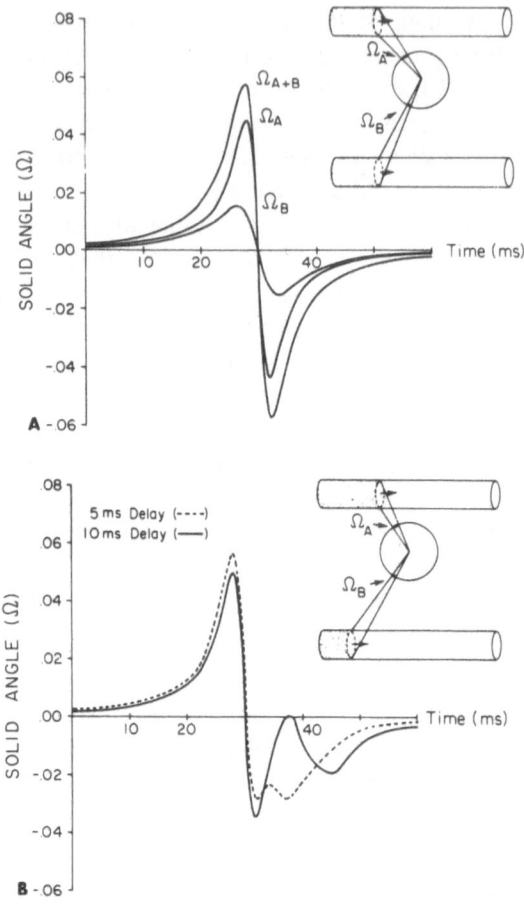

Figure 8. The influence of synchronous (*A*) and asynchronous (*B*) fiber activation on the computed solid angle (Ω). The total solid angle represents the sums of the contributions from fibers A and B (Ω_A and Ω_B, respectively). Note that the morphology of the solid angle, and hence the extracellular potential, can be modified by slightly increasing the delay. More complex modifications of the basic model can recreate virtually any type of waveform. Adapted from Holland and Arnsdorf with permission [1].

THE SINGLE EQUIVALENT DIPOLE MODEL: THE PROBLEMS OF OVERLY SIMPLIFIED THEORY

By summing dipoles or their equivalent vectors, the distributed dipole model can be converted to a single equivalent dipole model. In the classic single equivalent dipole model, cardiac electrical activity is represented by a dipole that is fixed in position but allowed to vary in both magnitude and direction during the cardiac cycle. The limitations of this model are well recognized, but a few comments are in order. For the reasons already discussed, it should be apparent that the electrical activity of the heart cannot be considered a true single dipole. Throughout the inscription of the P, QRS, and T waves, as well as during the diastolic periods, tissues are being activated or repolarized while others are at rest or in intermediate states. Multiple boundaries exist, therefore, that separate areas with differing transmembrane voltages and influence the extracellular potential as summarized in Eq. 4. For the single dipole model to be a relatively good approximation of the observed extracellular potential, the distance between the heart and the recording site must be at least five times the radius of the heart [28].

> Approximation 10. *The advantage of the single dipole model is the ease of calculation, but the mathematical description is quite qualitative. The qualitative description is empirically useful and easily comprehended. The price, however, is the loss of information and precision. For the single equivalent dipole to accurately account for the observed extracellular potential, the recording site must be at least five times the radius of the heart from the wavefronts of interest: a requirement not met by epicardial, intracavitary, esophageal, or precordial recording sites.*

It is difficult to assess the approximate error introduced by the simplifying assumptions of the single equivalent dipole model. Most estimates are based on mirror-pattern cancellations, the theory of which assumes that if the heart behaves as a single equivalent dipole, an extracellularly recorded potential at one point must have a mirror image at some other point. If an electrode is moved along a line that passes through a fixed dipole position, ϵ would remain relatively constant until the dipole is approached. As the dipole is approached, ϵ would rise rapidly; while at the dipole, ϵ would decline to zero and then reverse in sign and morphology as the dipole is passed. Presumably, there is a point at which a mirror image of the original potential exists, and the line connecting these two points should pass through the single equivalent dipole. Schmitt et al. [29] assumed that if surface recordings had the same shape, were of opposite polarity, and were in phase, they could be used to define an isoelectric line. They used a bridge circuit to investigate such mirror-pattern cancellations. When cancellation failed to produce an isoelectric line, the degree of cancellation was expressed by a coefficient. If ϵ as recorded on the precordium was derived primarily from the underlying myocardium, it would be difficult to explain the manner in which the identical ϵ was recorded at another point. Schmitt et al. found that only 9% of any pair of mirror patterns failed to cancel either in normal subjects or in patients with myocardial infarcts. Patients with ventricular hypertrophy had poorer cancellations while those with bundle branch block were poorer yet.

Frank [30] concluded that there was 95% accuracy in normals when the heart was considered a single fixed dipole. Morton et al. [31], however, analyzed not only peak-to-peak cancellations, but also instantaneous cancellations. They concluded that excellent peak-to-peak cancellations do not necessarily imply a true dipolar distribution. Brody and Copeland [32] observed in an elegant study that good cancellation occurred even when there was movement of the cardiac dipole. Furthermore, good cancellation was observed between surface and esophageal electrograms. The proximity of the esophageal electrogram excluded interpretation in terms of a single fixed dipole. Several theories for these results have been proposed and the interested reader should consult Pozzi [33]. In any event, cancellation does not seem to be a good test of the single equivalent dipole hypothesis. Indeed, the single equivalent dipole model must be rejected for quantitative electrocardiographic investigations.

> Approximation 11. *The error in using the single equivalent dipole model is probably between 5% and 25%. Qualitatively, this magnitude of error is acceptable. Quantitatively, it is not acceptable since the error excludes experimentally verifiable quantitative predictions.*

RECENT MULTIPOLAR AND MAPPING APPROACHES

Electrocardiograms from multiple sites on the body surface contain both redundant and unique information, the latter reflecting local myocardial events. Probably up to 25% of ϵ is not accounted for by the single equivalent dipole model. The problem has been in the extraction of this unique information. Computerization enables the analysis of a great deal of data, statistical manipulation, and useful display within a short period of time. The computer therefore, provides the tools for multipolar and other types of mapping approaches.

> Approximation 12. *The developments in computer technology present an enormous opportunity for retrieving previously unidentified data from the extracellularly recorded potential.*

The multiple dipole model

The multiple dipole model enables more quantitative description than the single dipole model, but less than the distributed dipole model. The boundary is represented by a finite number of dipoles, each of which represents a certain anatomic portion of the myocardium. As an example of this approach, Holt and his co-workers divided the heart into 12 segments and assigned a dipole to each [34]. The direction of the dipole was fixed and approximated the average direction of the activation pathway in each section. The magnitude of the dipoles was allowed to vary in time. The magnitude rose from zero as the moving boundary entered the segment and returned to zero as it left the segment. In this way, the model accounted for the influence of thick and thin segments of myocardium. The magnitude of the dipole also corresponded to the area of the activation boundary normally present in the segment. The potential recorded at each electrode site was equal to the sum contributed by each dipole. The model was sufficiently accurate to account for changes seen in hypertrophy and infarction [34] and has been used successfully to correlate electrically and angiographically determined left ventricular mass [35].

General considerations of mapping techniques

In the future, the extraction of unique from redundant electrocardiographic information will probably depend on some method employing the computer analysis of body surface potentials. A good deal of work is under way to define a convenient, yet comprehensive, electrode system. Information from multiple electrodes has been displayed in several formats including the projection of isopotential on a grid system representing thoracic locations, and the translation of the information into tracings that resemble electrocardiographic deflections.

Although several techniques show promise for quantifying myocardial infarction and injury, three are of particular interest: departure mapping, inverse mapping, and QRST area maps.

Departure mapping

Some form of departure mapping may be of clinical importance. This method, as suggested by Flowers and associates [36], consists of the establishment of a data bank of statistically normal electrograms at many thoracic sites, comparison of the electrogram in a patient having cardiac disease with the statistically normal electrogram by electronically subtracting one from the other, and finally displaying the difference as part of a departure map (Figure 9). The departure potential is an expression of the unique information in the signal. In this manner, the component of the extracellular potential that is due to local, regional myocardial events can be analyzed. If all nonspatial determinants of ϵ have remained constant, departures from the normal extracellularly recorded potential can be conceptualized as substractions of the normal from the measured solid angle at each electrode site. Subtraction of solid angles is depicted in Figure 10. The departure potential, then, reflects the deviation from normal of the spatial determinants of ϵ.

68

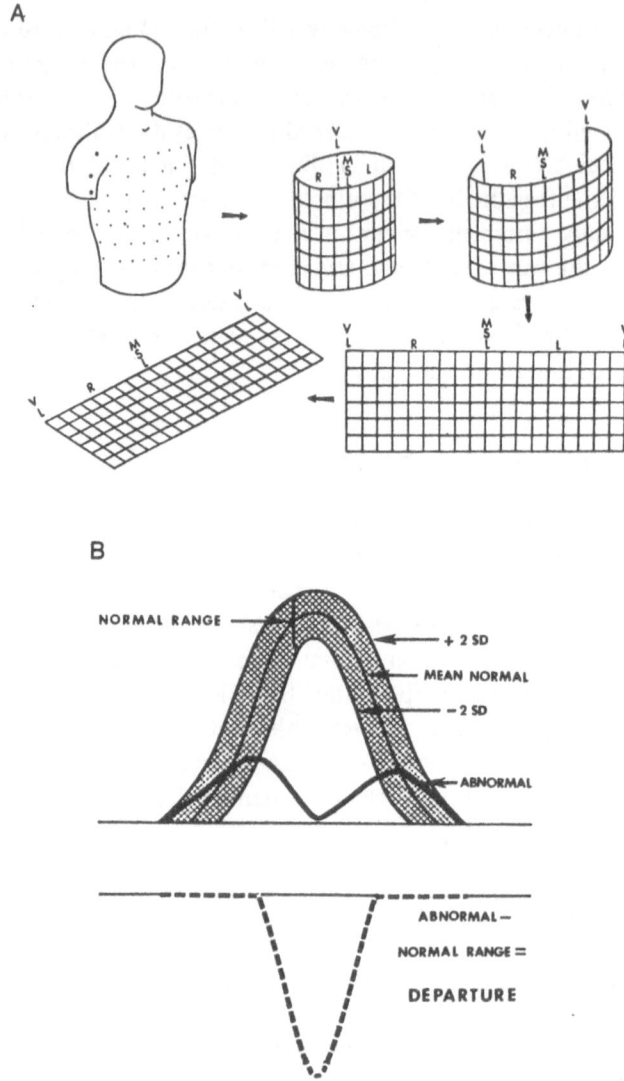

Figure 9. Body surface and departure mapping. (*A*) The recording locations on the torso are indicated by the dots. The body surface representation may be considered to be divided along the spine posteriorly, unrolled and tilted using an isometric projection format to enable three-dimensional viewing. Anatomic landmarks are the vertebral line (VL), the midsternal line (MSL), the right midaxillary line (R), and the left midaxillary line (L). (*B*) The normal range (mean ± 2 SD) for the extracellularly recorded potential in normal subjects is indicated by the cross-hatched area in the upper diagram. An electrogram taken from a hypothetical subject with cardiac disease is labelled 'abnormal.' The departure potential in the lower tracing is derived by subtracting the abnormal from the normal for each instant in time. The unique information in the abnormal electrogram in this case is displayed as a negative departure potential. Adapted and reproduced from Flowers et al. with permission of the *American Journal of Cariology* [36].

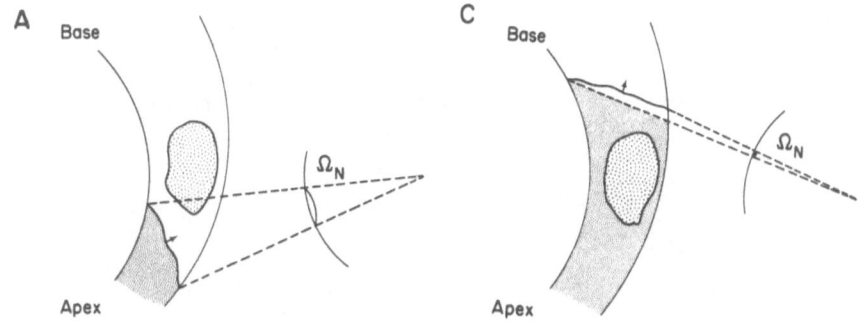

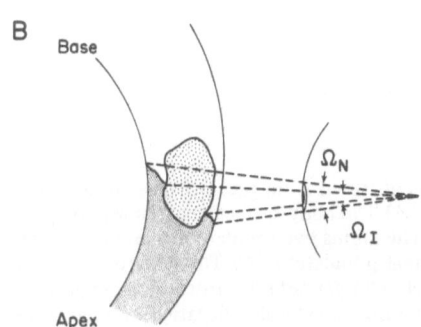

Figure 10. The effect of infarcted tissue in the free wall of the left ventricle on the solid angle subtending the activation wavefront. The infarcted tissue is indicated by the dotted area, the depolarized tissue by the shaded area, and the resting tissue by the white area. The boundaries of interest are between these three areas. (*A*) The wavefront approaching the electrode site subtends the normal solid angle (Ω_N). (*B*) The activation boundary now comes in contact with infarcted tissue, so the solid angle normally subtended is decreased by the quantity Ω_I. (*C*) After the wavefront has swept past the infarcted area, the complete boundary and solid angle are reestablished. Adapted from Holland and Arnsdorf with permission [1].

Approximation 13. *Although departure mapping has not been discussed in terms of distributed dipole theory, conceptually this technique can be envisioned as the subtraction of the solid angle perceived by a recording electrode from a statistically determined normal solid angle. The resulting solid angle reflects the departure from normal which, in turn, is the unique information arising from the local myocardium.*

Clinically relevant data exist throughout the cardiac cycle. For example, it follows that areas of the heart that are infarcted may affect various portions of the QRS complex: that is, areas that normally are activated early should alter

Inferior MI

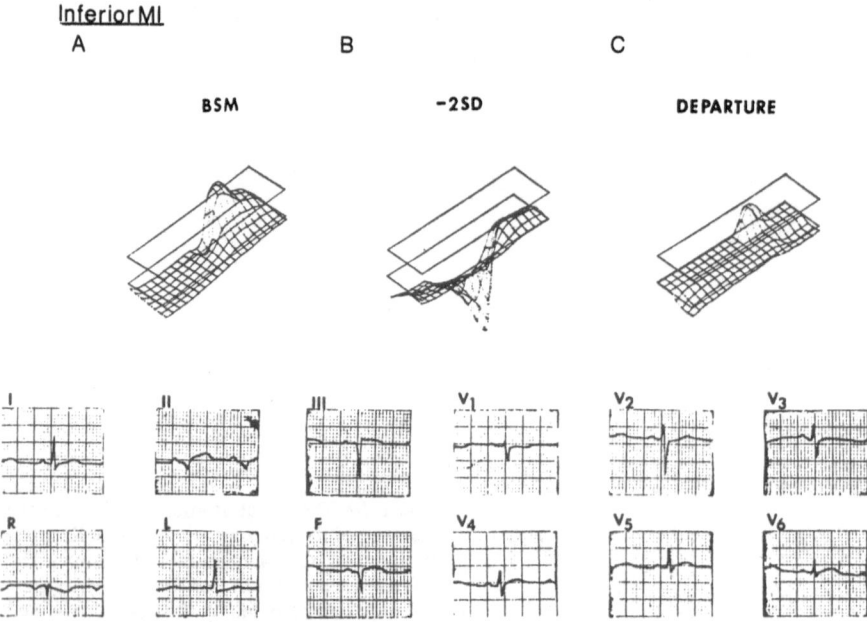

Figure 11. The body surface and departure maps obtained from precordial recordings in a patient with an inferior wall myocardial infarct. (*A*) The body surface map (BSM) obtained 45 ms into the QRS complex of the patient. (*B*) The minus two standard deviation (− 2 SD) map at 45 ms into the QRS complex for a normal population. (*C*) The departure map at 45 ms into the QRS complex for the patient in *A*. The patient's electrocardiogram appears in the lower portion of the illustration. The departure map reveals a negativity that exceeds the normal range along the inferior edge of the map and a region of characteristic positivity that appears high on the left anterior chest. More than 90% of patients with an inferior wall myocardial infarct have departure map abnormalities exceeding ± 2 SD even though the convention electrocardiographic and vectorcardiographic criteria may be disappeared. Adapted and reproduced from Flowers et al. with the permission of the *American Journal of Cardiology* [36].

the initial components of the QRS complex; areas that are activated late should alter the terminal portion of the QRS complex. This hypothesis has been tested and quite convincingly validated in the experimental animal (see review [2]). Flowers et al. have used the difference or departure mapping technique to obtain information from the early, mid-, and late portions of the QRS complex in the experimental animal [37] and in man [36]. The potentials recorded from patients with a documented inferoposterior myocardial infarct were studied with departure mapping. The maps revealed consistent mid- and late activation changes in these patients, including some who no longer had diagnostic Q waves on the electrocardiogram (Figure 11). Subsequently, this group has extended its studies with departure mapping to patients with myocardial infarcts in different locations and with other types of heart disease.

Departure mapping of the repolarization sequence may provide important information.

The departure mapping technique also seems to be useful in chronic heart disease. The quantitative power of the technique in acute myocardial ischemia, injury, and infarct remains to be tested fully. We suspect that there may be problems with the interpretation of the departure map since the extracellularly recorded potential is influenced by alterations both in spatial and in nonspatial factors during ischemia, injury, and infarct. Nonetheless, it may draw our attention to alterations in the extracellularly recorded potential during activation or repolarization sequences that may be of clinical relevance.

Inverse maps

The estimation of the distribution of epicardial potentials from body surface mapping has been termed an 'inverse' map. McFee and Baule [38] have reviewed many of these attempts at inverse calculation. Most investigations have employed a multipolar representation of the heart. Barr, Spach, and their co-workers, however, have employed a model using epicardial potential distributions [26, 39–43]. The problem, of course, is to deal with the problem of the loss of information from the epicardium through the thorax to the body surface. Barr and Spach studied this problem by comparing essentially simultaneous epicardial and body surface recordings throughout the cardiac cycle in chronically instrumented animals. The inverse map was based on the definition of 'inverse transfer functions' that mathematically relate the epicardial to the surface recordings. Generalized inverse transfer functions were developed that enabled the *prediction* of epicardial potential distributions from potentials *measured* at the body surface. The correlation coefficients between epicardial potentials predicted from the body surface potentials and the directly measured epicardial potentials were in the range of 0.6–0.8. The inverse epicardial map convincingly displayed the major features of depolarization and repolarization. Refinement of the calculations promises greater quantitative accuracy and predictive power.

These and other experiments indicate that many electrical events of importance are reflected on the body surface by potentials having a low amplitude ($> 250 \mu V$). These techniques are giving us some knowledge as to the normal state of the cardiac source, information essential to understanding the changes observed in ischemia and infarct. For example, studies in dogs and chimpanzees showed that the amplitude of normal precordial ST segments in chronic animals was greater than the 0.1 mV value used in dog experiments as an index of the extent of myocardial ischemic injury in the studies of Maroko et al. [44].

Recent measurements of total thoracic distributions of repolarization potentials utilizing 100 anterior torso electrodes and 50 posterior torso electrodes have been made in patients experiencing acute myocardial infarcts. As anticipated, this extensive electrode system detected significant additional torso sites of positive repolarization potentials (TQ-ST deflection) when compared with a conventional 35-precordial-electrode array utilized by many investigators [44]. This discrepancy persisted even when analysis was restricted to the subgroup of patients with anterior myocardial infarcts. Clearly more clinical studies are required to evaluate the trade-off between the enhanced sensitivity achieved with extensive electrode arrays and the increasing inconvenience of such systems. Of potential importance was the observation that there was marked temporal overlap between activation and repolarization patterns at torso sites demonstrating positive repolarization potentials. These repolarization forces were detected as early as 54 ms prior to the end of the QRS. Mirvis [45] suggests that this early onset of repolarization potentials may be characteristic of isopotentials measured in patients experiencing a myocardial infarct. This observation raises questions concerning the appropriateness of measuring TQ-ST voltage deflections at an arbitrary time interval after the QRS, if the evolving ischemic process can alter the temporal relation between the activation and repolarization potentials. On the other hand, if subsequent investigation substantiates the hypothesis that early onset of repolarization is a unique characteristic of ischemic injury, this may provide a means of excluding other extraneous influences on the TQ-ST deflection. Though the torso isopotential maps in these patients with acute infarcts exhibited single extrema during repolarization, Mirvis [45] points out that this does not ensure a similar pattern at the epicardium. Hopefully the work of Barr, Spach, et al. [39–42] will eventually enable us to translate surface isopotential measurements into epicardial measurements.

Approximation 14. *The development of inverse transfer functions and other mathematical translations may enable an accurate and quantitative construction of inverse epicardial maps from body surface potentials.*

Barr, Spach, and their co-workers correctly questioned a central assumption of the solid angle theory, namely, the constancy of the transmembrane voltage within an area of cardiac tissue such as the ventricle. Their approach has been to consider the ST segment potentials to be determined by the difference in the spatial distribution of intracellular potentials (the so-called difference 'cardiac sources'). These sources differ in normal adults and seem to change with age. Therefore, it is necessary to measure the total cardiac electrical field on the body surface to account for the effects of the currents from all these electrical sources [26,43]. This, of course, challenges methods that use primarily proximity effects as, for example, the commonly employed precordial map for the assessment of ischemic injury. The approach of Barr, Spach, and their co-workers extends the problems involved with the quantitative analysis beyond those associated with the nonspatial terms in Eq. 4 since it necessitates consideration of the preexisting spatial arrangement of the intracellular action potentials throughout the atrium and ventricle that is 'normal' for a given individual.

Approximation 15. *Measurement of the total electrical field on the body surface may be required to account for the spatial distribution of intracellular potentials, suggesting additional constriants on the acceptance of precordial mapping procedures that use primarily proximity effects.*

Although this method deals with some of the terms in Eq. 4 (such as extracellular conductivity), other terms in the equation are not fully considered. Nevertheless, a combination of approaches may enable a more inclusive assessment of the determinants of the potential recorded at the body surface.

QRST area maps

Determination of the maps of the QRST area is yet another approach in the extraction of unique from redundant information. Wilson et al. [46] postulated that the QRST area, the 'ventricular gradient,' should be independent of the sequence of ventricular activation so long as the repolarization properties are constant. As reviewed by Abildskov [47], there is some controversy as to whether the QRST area is independent of the activation sequence and the constancy of recovery properties with varied activation sequences. Recently, Abildskov et al. [48] have presented evidence, based on the studies of QRST area maps in dogs, suggesting that the QRST area tracks changes in refractory period. They concluded that the QRST area is largely independent of activation and suggested that it depends primarily on intrinsic recovery properties. This technique, then, many be useful in identifying areas that are disparate in their recovery properties. Anatomic definition of the sources of such disparities may eventually enable the use of this type of map in the estimate of ischemia, injury, and infarct.

Approximation 16. *QRST area mapping, or similar techniques, may be capable of tracking alterations in the recovery properties of tissue, thereby providing a marker of underlying electrophysiologic and possibly anatomic change.*

MYOCARDIAL ISCHEMIA, INJURY, AND INFARCT

General considerations

A decrease or interruption in the blood supply to the myocardium produces varying degrees of damage to the tissues of the heart. Traditionally, an area of tissue necrosis has been depicted as being surrounded by area of injury and both these zones by yet another zone of ischemia. Textbooks often suggest that necrosis causes the changes in the QRS morphology, injury the change in the TQ-ST segment, and ischemia the change in T waves. This concept implies that the degree of myocardial damage is greatest in the zone of necrosis, intermediate in the zone of injury where 'leaky' membranes cause diastolic and systolic current flow, and least in the zone of ischemia where alterations in repolarization predominate. Myocardial damage is considered to be irreversible in the zone of necrosis, but potentially reversible in the zones of injury and ischemia.

We have reviewed many of the basic principles relating cardiac bioelectricity to the extracellularly recorded potential. The interrelationships between the spatial and nonspatial determinants of the extracellular potential force us to reject investigations on ischemia and infarct that utilize overly simplistic views of the electrocardiographic signal as a measure of tissue injury, ischemia, and death. Very little experimental validation of the assumptions underlying the use of the electrocardiographic signal as an index of ischemia and reversible injury has been forthcoming.

It would now seem appropriate to review the effects that ischemia, injury, and infarct should have on the spatial and nonspatial determinants of the electrocardiogram according to the principles outlined previously. Perhaps such a consideration would suggest potentially fruitful areas for investigation.

Anatomic considerations and the electrocardiogram

Although it is attractive to relate three areas of supposedly different degrees of cell damage to three different components of the electrocardiogram, little ultrastructural and electrophysiologic evidence supports such a separation. Since all electrocardiographic deflections result from the normal or abnormal flow of currents during systole and diastole, and since the effects of systolic and diastolic current flow on the electrocardiogram are interdependent, it would be most unlikely that such anatomic–electrophysiologic correlations exist.

Pathologists can define tissue death with reasonable accuracy so long as classic findings are present, but the problem of definition becomes troublesome in the several hours immediately following a myocardial infarct. Various states of irreversible tissue injury cannot be differentiated with certainty from one another, although ultrastructural and other types of studies may eventually enable such distinctions.

Correlative radionuclear and anatomic studies suggest the infarcted area to be surrounded by a substantial zone of risk consisting of cells that presumably may recover or die. The relationship between the zone at risk and the electrophysiologic boundary responsible for alterations in the R wave, the TQ-ST segment, and the T wave is uncertain; and, although the geometry of the boundary resulting from juxtaposed normal and abnormal tissue importantly influences the extracellular potential, our knowledge of that geometry is incomplete.

These and other uncertainties in the anatomic and electrophysiologic definitions of myocardial ischemia, injury, and infarct lead to the next approximation.

> Approximation 17. *Problems exist in both the anatomic and electrophysiologic definitions of myocardial ishemia, injury and infarct. It is unreasonable, therefore, to accept unverified assumptions that correlate or otherwise link a specific anatomic change with a specific electrocardiographic measurement.*

SPATIAL DETERMINANTS OF THE EXTRACELLULAR POTENTIAL IN MYOCARDIAL ISCHEMIA, INJURY, AND INFARCT

Relation of the boundary to the recording electrode

It is apparent that the position of the heart in the thorax and the configuration of the chest are constant in a given individual but may vary between individuals. The techniques of departure mapping and inverse mapping may be useful in minimizing the influences of these spatial determinants. Similarly, precise positioning of precordial electrodes is required for sequential surface maps in a given individual and some standards need be developed when comparing one patient with another. Again, recent studies suggest that such standards can be developed and that the number of leads required may be reduced to between 24 and 32 [see discussion in Spach et al. [43].

The extracellularly recorded potential is not a simple function of geometry and distance (see Figure 8). The function is complex, and the simple addition of ST segments or similar procedures clearly have little theoretical justification. Let us consider two types of problems concerned in relating precordial to epicardial events in ischemia. On the epicardium, the boundary between normal and ischemic myocardium can be identified with precision as that area in which polarity of the solid angle and, therefore, the recorded potential, quickly changes. The idealized situation is depicted in Figure 8. The relationship between a change in potential and the boundary is more tenuous for precordial recordings, so TQ-ST segment maps constructed at the body surface are less likely to define the ischemic boundary than are maps constructed at the epicardium. A second problem is the often complex relationship between extracellular potentials recorded on the epicardium and the immediately overlying precordium. For example, a number of studies have demonstrated

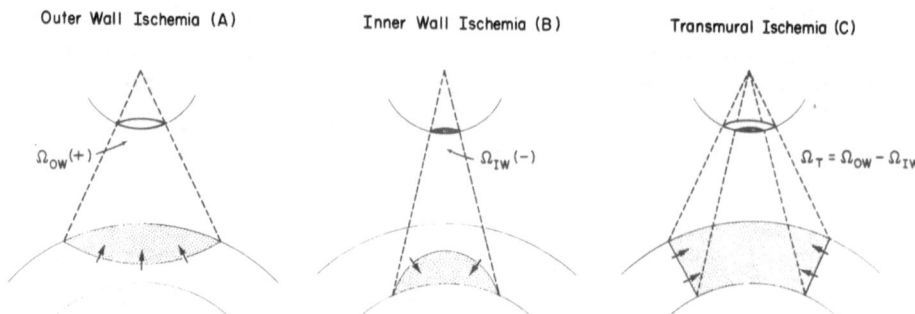

Figure 12. The effect of the shape of the ischemic area on the solid angle. The positive to negative flow of current across the ischemic boundary at midsystole is indicated by the arrows. Ischemia involving the outer wall (subepicardial) results in a positive solid angle, $\Omega_{ow}(+)$ (*A*) while ischemia of the inner wall (subendocardial) results in a negative solid angle, $\Omega_{iw}(-)$ (*B*). Transmural ischemia with the shape depicted in *C* results in a solid angle Ω_I, that is essentially the difference between Ω_{ow} and Ω_{iw}. The absolute magnitude of the TQ-ST deflection, then, will be smaller for the transmural ischemia than for either the subepicardial or subendocardial ischemia, despite the fact that the mass or volume of the ischemic tissue is greatest with transmural ischemia. From Holland and Arnsdorf [1].

experimentally that an increase in ischemic area may increase the solid angle at precordial locations and decrease it at epicardial locations overlying the ischemic region [1, 2]. Techniques such as inverse mapping may be capable of mathematically relating surface and epicardial recording in a quantitatively useful manner.

The shape and location of the damaged tissue

The shape of the ischemic or otherwise damaged area also influences the extracellularly recorded potential [1, 2]. For example, as perceived by a precordial electrode over the center of the ischemic area, subepicardial ischemia subtends a positive solid angle, subendocardial ischemia a negative solid angle, and transmural ischemia a combination of positive and negative solid angles. The implication is that although transmural ischemia may involve a greater mass of tissue than either subendocardial or subtraction of solid angles in transmural ischemia. These concepts are depicted schematically in Figure 12.

Janse et al. [49] recorded transmembrane action potentials with floating microelectrodes from cells within the border zone of myocardial ischemia in the isolated perfused pig heart. They found cells with low resting potentials in close proximity to cells with nearly normal action potentials. Notwithstanding the technical difficulties of making intracellular recordings in this preparation, these workers found a rather sharp and distinct transition from electrophysiologically abnormal to normal cells.

Much investigation has concerned the nature of the boundary between normal tissue and reversibly ischemic (presumed salvageable) tissue. Theoretic possibilities include: (a) a zone of tissue with homogeneous properties intermediate between normal tissue and infarcted tissue, (b) islands of abnormal tissue scattered amidst normal tissue, or (c) fingers of abnormal tissue interdigitating with the normal myocardium. Uncertainty exists as to which parameters predict the ultimate fate of injured myocardial tissue. The accuracy of a given biophysical and biochemical technique, therefore, to define the spatial extent of injury and ischemia is uncertain. The result has been confusing data and conflicting interpretations. For example, although biochemical determinations of lactate, creatine phosphate, and ATP has shown intermediate values from tissue samples from border zone areas [49–51], histologic assessment of glycogen depletion [49] and nicotinamide adenine dinucleotide fluorescent staining techniques [52, 53] suggest that the line of demarcation between normal and abnormal tissue may be very sharp. Unfortunately we do not know which of these indices of metabolic function most closely parallels tissue viability. Furthermore it is uncertain as to whether a quantitative relationship exists between the degree of derangement in any of these parameters and eventual tissue survival. Finally, one often is uncertain as to whether intermediate values in a metabolic index reflect values from tissue with an intermediate degree of injury or the averaging of small amounts of entirely normal tissue with infarcted tissue. An example of the latter is tissue creatine kinase depletion at the lateral border zone [54].

Cox et al. [55] used dehydrogenase staining to delineate the changing geometry of the infarct border between 18h and one week after infarct. They defined a zone of intermediate injury characterized by 'large dot mitochondrial swelling and A-band swelling' but otherwise normal architecture. At 18h, the area encompassed by the necrosis and the intermediate zone was maximal, but with time the region of necrosis enlarged at the expense of the intermediate zone. A recent pathologic study employing reconstructions of serial sections from the border zone of infarcted tissue in *one* section could be shown to have continuity with the central mass of infarcted tissue *outside* the plane of section. This study proposed that, at 24h after infarct, the anatomic borders consisted of complex interdigitations of normal and infarcted tissue. The relevance of these anatomic studies to the precise geometry between potentially viable and nonviable tissue in the *acute* period of ischemia when the electrophysiologic boundary is determined is conjectural.

Clearly we do not have a precise enough knowledge of the geometric relationships at the ischemic boundary to enable the complex calculation of solid angles required for an analytic prediction of the measured R wave amplitude or TQ-ST voltage. For this reason, attempts at establishing an empiric correspondence between the electrophysiologic boundary and the underlying biochemical and biophysical properties of the border zone are needed.

In addition to electrode location, ischemic shape, and ischemic location, one must consider the thickness of the wall involved in the ischemic process. A thicker wall will tend to produce a larger boundary and hence a larger solid angle. It has been shown experimentally that the TQ-ST deflections recorded over ischemic areas of the right ventricle are smaller than those over an ischemic portion of the left ventricle, and that the TQ-ST deflection differs over the aplical and basilar portions of the ischemic left ventricle [22].

The persistence and geometry of the boundary can also be influenced by alterations in conduction velocity (physiologic and pharmacologic influences), in the sequence of activation (anatomic, pathologic alterations), and in the size of the boundary related to the mass of the tissue as (myocardial infarct, fibrosis, and hypertrophy). Some of these spatial problems perhaps can be assessed by the development of normal data banks in the manner employed in departure or difference mapping.

Approximation 18. *Spatial determinants that influence the extracellular potential in myocardial ischemia, injury, and infarct include the relation of the boundary to the electrode site, the shape and location of the damaged tissue, and the persistence of the boundary.*

Irreversible and reversible cellular injury

For the purpose of discussion, let us consider the effects that irreversible and reversible cellular injury may have on the TQ-ST segment. The boundary responsible for the ionic flow that eventuates in the TQ-ST segment can be abolished by (a) electrotonic uncoupling due to cell death, (b) electrotonic uncoupling in reversibly injured cells, and (c) survival of reversibly injured cells that regain normal electrophysiologic properties. The first represents a change in spatial factors; and the second and third, alterations due primarily to nonspatial changes.

Dead cells are no longer coupled to viable cells and they behave as part of the volume conductor. The manner in which infarcted tissue affects the extracellular potential is schematically depicted in Figure 10.

Injured cells, however, presumably will either die or recover. A zone at risk consisting of cells that may survive or perish has been described anatomically and physiologically, and recent studies using correlative radionuclear and anatomic techniques suggest that the zone of risk may include a relatively large mass of myocardial tissue. We feel that the electrophysiologic boundary responsible for the change in the R wave and TQ-ST segment is probably rather *narrow* and of uncertain relationship to the borders of the zone at risk. Injured cells rapidly uncouple from normal cells, presumably due to an increase in intracellular calcium and a decrease in intracellular pH [57]. The requirements for normal coupling are quite tight, and an increase in the intracellular calcium concentration from $10^{-7} M$ to $10^{-5} M$ is sufficient for electrotonic uncoupling. Uncoupling will have the same effect on the electrocardiogram as electrotonic dissociation due to cell death (Approximation 6, Eq. 4), yet it does not imply irreversible cellular damage.

Injured cells that survive and recover normal electrophysiologic properties will be indistinguishable from normal cells, resulting in the abolition of the boundary (Approximation 4).

Approximation 19. *The zone of risk around an area of myocardial infarct bears an uncertain relationship to the presumably narrow electrophysiologic boundary responsible for alterations in the extracellular potential.*

Approximation 20. *In tissues with irreversibly and reversibly injured cells, identical changes in the extracellular potential may result from cellular uncoupling due to tissue death (spatial), uncoupling due to reversible injury (nonspatial), and the recovery of normal electrophysiologic function (nonspatial).*

The implication of Approximations 19 and 20 for clinical studies is that a therapeutic intervention may profoundly affect the TQ-ST segment by altering the properties within a relatively narrow boundary zone which, in turn, bears an uncertain relationship to the zone at risk and that a decrease in the TQ-ST segment may reflect an increase or decrease in the viability of a group of cardiac cells.

NONSPATIAL DETERMINANTS OF THE EXTRACELLULAR POTENTIAL IN MYOCARDIAL ISCHEMIA, INJURY, AND INFARCT

Samson and Scher in 1960 presented experimental evidence that the ST segment elevation had both systolic and diastolic components [58]. We, therefore, prefer to use the term TQ-ST segment change. This point is schematically illustrated in Figure 13. Magnetocariography indicates that, in early ischemia, the deflection is primarily a diastolic event [59]. Experimentally, TQ-ST segment changes occur within seconds of coronary occlusion. The evidence that the agent producing these early changes is the release of potassium from ischemic cells has been summarized by Holland and Brooks [2]. A release of only 1% of the intracellular store would raise the potassium concentration in the local extracellular space sufficiently to produce large diastolic and systolic electrophysiologic changes including depolarization of the membrane from a V_r of $-95\,mV$ to $-71\,mV$

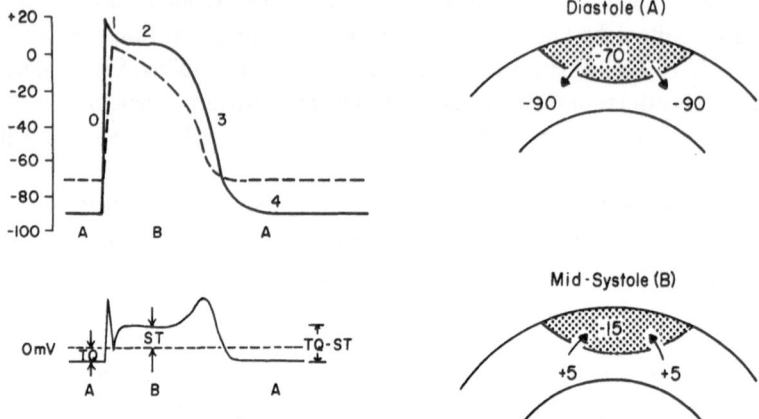

Figure 13. Nonspatial determinants of the TQ-ST segment. (*Left*) The upper portion depicts the superimposed action potentials of normal (solid line) and ischemic (broken line) myocardium. The phases of the action potential are indicated. The lower portion shows the electrocardiogram recorded by an electrode overlying the ischemic tissue. The TQ segment is below the isoelectric potential (interrupted line) and the ST segment above the isoelectric potential. The transmembrane potential gradient is determined by the difference in the transmembrane voltages across the boundary (Eq. 4). (*Right*) The transmembrane potential gradient during diastole and midsystole are depicted in *A* and *B*, respectively. The flow of current (positive to negative) at the boundary is indicated by the arrows. Adapted from Holland and Arnsdorf with permission [1].

and a marked shortening of the action potential. A less negative than normal V_r would also influence the state of sodium inactivation, and active membrane generator properties [such as the maximal rate of rise of phase 0 ($\dot{V}_{max}$), the overshoot, and the conduction velocity] would decrease. As a result, changes in the extracellular potassium concentration would produce configurational and temporal changes in the transmembrane potential gradient (Approximation 3) and alter not only the TQ-ST segment, but the QRS complex and T wave as well. Table 1 includes the factors that influence the balance of K^+ in the myocardial cell.

Downar et al. found an unidentified substance present in the venous effluent of the ischemic pig heart that was capable of depressing normal myocardial cells in a manner similar to an extracellular potassium concentration of $16\,mM$ [60]. Recently, lysophosphatides have been isolated from ischemic heart muscle and the effluent of anoxic hearts that have electrophysiologically depressant effects on normal cardiac cells [61, 62]. Arnsdorf and Sawicki reported that one of these compounds, lysophosphatidylcholine (LPC), may increase or decrease cardiac excitability, depending on the net effect of altered passive, active, and repolarization properties [63]. LPC influences not only the action potential shape and conduction, but also intracellular longitudinal resistance presumably

Table 1. A selected list of factors common in myocardial ischemia and infarct that directly influence the net potassium balance in the myocardial cell[a]

Net increased potassium loss	Net decreased potassium loss
Physiologic factors	*Physiologic factors*
Inotropy	Potassium
Chronotropy	K^+, Mg^{++}-aspartate
Preload	K^+-hyaluronidase
Afterload	Acetylcholine
Hyperthermia	Hypothermia
Catecholamines	Insulin
Calcium	Glucose
ATP inhibition	Taurine
Anoxia and ischemia	Hypoxia
Acidosis	Alkalosis
Adrenal corticoids including cortisol, aldosterone, deoxycorticosterone	
Noxious metabolites such as lysophosphatides[b]	
Pharmacologic factors	*Pharmacologic factors*
Ouabain	Quinidine
Furosemide	Procaine amide
Ethacrynic acid	Lidocaine, phenytoin (mechanism 2)[c]
Calcium, adrenal corticoids, catecholamines, or drugs that produce effects such as those listed under 'physiologic factors' above	Spironolactone
	Triamterene
	Alkalosis
Lidocaine, perhaps phenytoin (mechanism 1)[c]	
Other factors	*Other factors*
Paired pacing	Interventions that influence the 'physiologic factors' listed above
Interventions that influence the 'physiologic factors' listed above	

[a]These factors may *independently and directly* influence the K^+ balance in the myocardial cell. Some interventions may have indirect actions such as hormones and drugs that influence the renal handling of electrolytes, drugs and the like. Some factors, such as catecholamines, may influence a number of physiologic variables. Drugs such as quinidine, procaine amide, and propranolol have a negative inotropic effect while others such as digitalis preparations have a positive inotropic effect. Many of the antiarrhythmic drugs also affect vascular and autonomic tone which, in turn, could affect many of the physiologic variables. See review by Holland and Brooks for an extensive bibliography on this topic [2].
[b]This is probable rather than documented. Disruption of the membrane by such detergent agents would be expected to increase the K^+ leak.
[c]Lidocaine, and perhaps phenytoin, may at times increase the net potassium loss while at other times decrease the net posassium loss. These mechanisms are discussed more extensively in the recent reviews by Arnsdorf and Hsieh [72].

at the gap junction. Both the TPG and the C_σ would influence ϵ as summarized by Eq. 4 in Approximation 6. These actions would influence all components of the electrocardiogram (Approximation 7). Initially, at least, the effects of lysophosphatides are reversible. Without doubt, other compounds also influence the electrophysiologic properties of the membrane such as, for example, acyl

Table 2. Selected factors that vary during myocardial ischemia and infarct and potentially may alter the transmembrane voltage in the normal and/or ischemic tissue

Metabolic factors
Hypoxia, anoxia
Oligemia, ischemia
Altered substrate levels (e.g., glucose, glycogen, lactate)
Altered oxidation-reduction state (e.g., NADH accumulation)
Altered levels of energy storage forms (e.g., creatine phosphat, adenosine triphosphate)
Acidosis
Noxious metabolites (e.g., lysophosphatides; the substance described by Downar et al. [61])

Physiologic factors
Electrolyte changes (e.g., potassium [see Table 1], calcium)
Temperature changes
Autonomic mediators (e.g., acetylcholine and catecholamines via humoral and neural mechanisms)
Altered cellular coupling at the gap junction
Altered extracellular conductance
Changes in global inotropic and chronotropic state
Changes in regional inotropic state

Pharmacologic factors
Antiarrhythmic drugs
Digitalis glycosides
Psychotropic drugs
Sympathomimetic agents
Parasympathomimetic agents
Others

carnitine [64]. The correlation between the accumulation of these compounds and irreversible or reversible tissue damage remains to be defined.

Other factors are commonly present in ischemia and infarct that may influence the transmembrane voltage and/or conductivity term (Table 2). Later in ischemia, the relative balance of the electrophysiologic determinants may change. The changes in time have been reviewed by Lazzara et al. [65] and include alterations in the V_r and action potential configuration as well as the appearance of unusual oscillatory activity. Recently, Spear et al. [66] have observed similar abnormalities of action potentials in the ventricular tissue of patients after aneurysmectomy or mitral valve replacement.

Figure 14 diagrammatically illustrates the manner in which an identical change in the TQ-ST segment can be caused by an alteration in either the size of the ischemic area (spatial determinant) or the transmembrane potential gradient (nonspatial determinant) assuming a constant conductivity term.

Approximation 21. *Numerous factors are present in myocardial ischemia that may affect the transmembrane potential gradient (TPG) by changing configurational or temporal determinants. Since the TPG determines in part the extracellularly recorded potential (Approximation 4; Eq. 4 in Approximation 6), the TQ-ST segment, and any other portion of the electrogram may be affected by alterations in this nonspatial factor (Approximation 7).*

$$\epsilon_{\text{TQ-ST}} = \underbrace{\frac{\Omega}{4\pi}}_{\text{Spatial}} \quad \times \quad \underbrace{(V_{m_N} - V_{m_I})C_\sigma}_{\text{Nonspatial}}$$

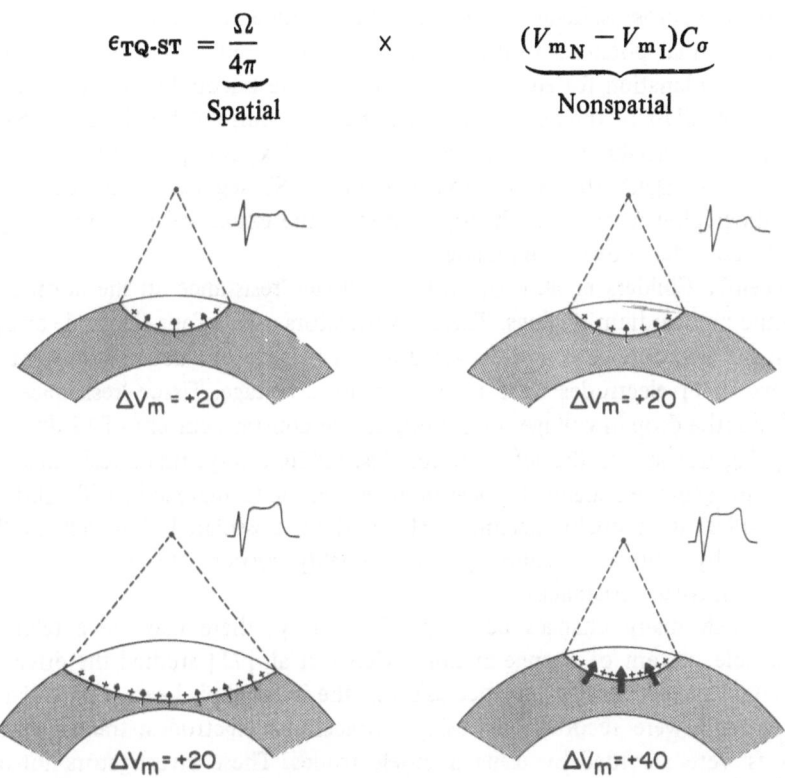

Figure 14. The influence of spatial (*left*) and nonspatial (*right*) factors on the extracellularly recorded TQ-ST deflection ($\epsilon_{\text{TQ-ST}}$). The direction of current flow (positive to negative) across the boundary during midsystole is depicted by the arrows. The intensity of current flow is indicated by the size of the arrows. The difference in the transmembrane potentials (ΔV_m) between normal (V_{m_N}) and ischemic (V_{m_I}) myocardium is indicated by the number. (*Left*) An increase in the ischemic area results in an increase in the solid angle and in the TQ-ST segment. C_σ and ΔV_m remain constant. (*Right*) An increase in ΔV_m results in an increased flow of current, solid angle, and TQ-ST segment deflection. C_σ and the geometry of the boundary remain constant. Reproduced with permission from Holland and Arnsdorf [1].

Myocardial injury and infarct may result in the loss of electrical activity. The loss of manifest electrical activity may result from tissue death and from damaged tissue being electrotonically uncoupled from its neighbors (Approximation 20). The former is irreversible; the latter will be reversible. Engelmann [67, 68] in the 1870s observed that the current of injury declined with time, an observation that led to his statement that 'cells live together, but die singly'. Currently, we believe that cells first uncouple from their neighbors due to changes in the intracellular calcium concentrations and pH [57]. They may then recover, or die. Anderson and his co-workers [69] recently measured systolic and diastolic current flow across ischemic boundaries in the canine heart and found change in the extracellular potential to diverge from the measured current flow. The most probable explanation for such an observation is the uncoupling of cells prior to death. Regardless of the explanation, the change in current flow is related to the change in extracellular potential in some complex, and presently undefined, manner. Once again, the assumption that the TQ-ST segment or any other electrocardiographic measure is directly related to the extent of ischemia or injury must be considered overly simplistic.

Recently Childers et al. [70] measured tissue 'resistance' in the normal and ischemic myocardium of dogs. These investigators used a four-electrode array in which the two outer electrodes were used for passage of a constant current and the two inner electrodes were used to measure voltage. Tissue 'resistance' was defined as the drop in voltage for a subthreshold constant current of 1 s duration. Following ligation of the left anterior descending artery, tissue resistance rose progressively in the ischemic myocardium and reached a plateau in 150–200 min, after which it gradually declined. The authors postulated that cell swelling followed by cellular uncoupling was probably responsible for the biplasic response in tissue resistance.

Although many changes occur simultaneously, there may be a relatively predictable pattern of change in time. Kléber et al. [71] studied the effects of left anterior descending artery occlusion in the isolated pig heart. Epicardial DC electrograms were recorded by using extracellular electrodes; transmembrane voltages were recorded by using microelectrodes. These investigators not only found a consistent spatial distribution, but also observed that the electrical changes seemed to follow a characteristic time course.

> Approximation 22. *Although the nonspatial changes after myocardial ischemia, injury, and infarct are complex, one may tentatively establish the hypothesis that such electrical changes follow a characteristic time course and design experiments to further test this hypothesis.*

Pharmacologic interventions can influence the extracellular potential by influencing nonspatial terms (Table 2). We recently reviewed many of the electrophysiologic effects of pharmacologic agents [72, 73]. A great deal is known about the effects of drugs on the characteristics of the action potential, but relatively little is known about their effects on cellular coupling.

TECHNIQUES FOR VALIDATING ELECTROPHYSIOLOGIC INDICES

General considerations

This section will consider the last two assumptions of the postulate discussed in the introductory section, both of which concern the validation of electrophysiologic indices by other techniques. The majority of studies to date have related electrophysiologic measurements at a given site to histologic, biochemical, and biophysical characteristics of the immediately underlying myocardium [74–84]. Relatively few studies have examined the transitions in electrophysiologic measurements with respect to the distance from an ischemic border [23, 27, 49, 50, 84] to enable a spatial estimate of the extent of ischemia. Many of the studies have been reviewed recently and the controversies presented [2, 5]. We shall focus, therefore, on the techniques that seem particularly well suited to testing our hypothesis and its underlying assumptions.

Techniques for quantitating eventual myocardial necrosis

Histologic and pathologic estimates of the extent and severity of myocardial infarct have served as our reference for judging all other techniques. The evaluation of these histologic and pathologic features is well known and described in classic works such as that of Mallory in 1939 [86] and in chapters of this book (see Fallon, p. 374 and Ideker, p. 347). We will concentrate on the application of these techniques to experimental models of myocardial ischemia and infarct as they have been used to validate electrophysiologic measurements. In a carefully studied model of canine posterior papillary muscle infarct resulting from controlled periods of left circumflex artery occlusion followed by reperfusion, early histologic evidence of subendocardial injury has been demonstrated after periods of ischemia as brief as 20 min [87, 88]. With progressively longer periods of left circumflex artery occlusion, a predictable pathologic pattern was described by these investigators that included: (a) a central zone with well-preserved architecture free of hemorrhage or inflammation but containing myocytes with pale nuclei and glassy cytoplasm, (b) a hemorrhagic midzone, and (c) a peripheral zone of coagulation necrosis and inflammation. Reimer and his co-workers also sampled longitudinal transmural sections through the posterior papillary muscle that was at the center of the zone of infarct and quantitated the amount of infarcted myocardium as a percent of tissue in the sample by separating histologically normal from abnormal tissue on a photograph of a Mallory stained section. While this technique does not size the boundaries of an infarct, it does enable quantitation of the progression of transmural spread of infarct from the endocardium to the epicardium. Recent work by Reimer and his co-workers has suggested that the anatomic infarct size may be overestimated due to disproportionate swelling of the infarcted tissue [87, 89]. Maroko et al. [74] and Ginks et al. [76], using a semiquantitative grading system for histologic necrosis 24 h or six days after occlusion of the left anterior descending artery in dogs, presented evidence suggesting that the presence or absence of ST segment elevation 15 min after occlusion predicted the subsequent presence or absence of

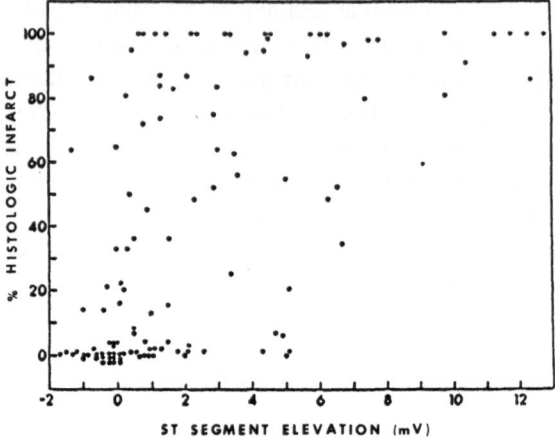

Figure 15. Percent histologic infarct as a function of ST segment elevation. In 13 dogs, epicardial ST segment elevation was measured 15 min after occlusion of the left anterior descending coronary artery and six days later histologic infarct was quantified from plani-metric measurements of hematoxylin—eosin-stained sections from transmural myocardial specimens subjacent to each epicardial electrode. Sites demonstrating conduction disturb-ances were excluded from the analysis. (*Ordinate*) Percent of area of section showing histologic infarct. (*Abscissa*) Epicardial ST elevation (mV) above the TP segment 100 ms from the beginning of the QRS complex. Note the wide scatter in the extent of infarct for any given magnitude of ST segment elevation (correlation coefficient 0.59). Adapted with permission from Irvin and Cobb [84].

histologic necrosis in the immediately underlying myocardium. A quantitative relationship between the ST segment magnitude and the extent of histologic necrosis was not demonstrated, however. Subsequently, Irvin and Cobb [84] studied the relationship between histologic change and electrophysiologic events in dogs with permanent occlusion of the left anterior descending artery (Figure 15). The extent of histologic necrosis, as estimated by planimetry six days after occlusion, correlated poorly with ST segment elevation measured 15 min after occlusion.

In an effort to develop an alternative method of quantifying myocardial necrosis, Kjekshus and Sobel [90] measured creatine kinase (CK) activity in the supernatant from tissue homogenates and found the CK level to be depressed significantly in the supernatant from infarcted as compared with normal tissues. They assayed CK with the spectrophotometric kinetic Rosalki assay and measured the 'back reaction' of creatine phosphate to creatine with the generation of adenosine triphosphate and expressed this as micromoles of substrate converted per minute per milligram of supernatant fraction protein as determined by the biuret technique. They also performed experiments to exclude enzyme inhibitors in the infarcted tissue, differences in recoverability of CK in infarcted as com-pared with noninfarcted tissue, and differences in reference protein determination from infarcted as compared with noninfarcted tissue. Histologic data from Ginks et al. [76] suggest an inverse relationship between myocardial CK activity and the severity of histologic injury. One might anticipate, however, that factors other than tissue viability may influence tissue CK activity, including factors governing enzyme release and clearance from the ischemic tissue. The acceptance of CK measurements as a quantitative index of the severity of myocardial injury at a given site, therefore, must be considered tentative at best. Hirzel et al. [54] have used CK assays of biopsy samples to map out the region of infarct and have emphasized the problems encountered in defining a border zone with a technique requiring tissue biopsies of finite dimensions.

Early studies demonstrated correlation between epicardial ST segment elevation 15 min after coronary occlusion in the dog and the logarithm of the CK activity at 24 h ($r = -0.79$) or seven days ($r = 0.66$) [73, 74]. The inclusion of ischemic with nonischemic tissue in the regression analysis has been criticized on statistical grounds by Holland and Brooks [2]. Subsequently, Heng [83] could not confirm the earlier results, finding a correlation coefficient of only -0.36 for epicardial ST segment voltage 15 min after occlusion versus CK activity in subjacent myocardium 24 h later.

The lack of consistent correlations between histologic or enzymatic estimates of myocardial injury and the magnitude of the TQ-ST segment is not surprising if we remember that in each study the electrophysiologic measurements were correlated with parameters assessed in the immediately underlying myocardium. A more productive approach might be a correlation between the electrophysiologic boundary as predicted from a distribution of epicardial potentials and the topography of pathologic injury. The tissue CK technique is limited in its ability to resolve boundaries due to the requirement for a biopsy specimen of finite dimensions. By contrast, definition of the boundary of infarct by anatomic techniques does not suffer from this limitation. An approach to this problem in the rat has been presented [91].

Techniques for quantitating a region at risk of infarct

Regional myocardial blood flow (RMBF) is considered a major determinant of the ultimate viability of ischemic tissue. Techniques to quantify RMBF, therefore, have been used to define a region at risk of infarct (see Cobb and Murdoch, p. 286). Rudolph and Heymann [92] introduced a method for quantifying the distribution of cardiac output and have recently reviewed this technique [93]. They measured the distribution to organ capillary beds of carbonized radioactive microspheres (50μ) that had been administered systemically. The administration of these microspheres did not cause grossly detectable alterations in hemodynamic performance. Subsequently, several authors suggested that smaller

$(9-15\mu)$ microspheres per tissue sample are required for accurate determinations [96], a condition that limits the spatial resolution of the technique. A systemic dose of over 10^7 microspheres causes hemodynamic deterioration [93]. Marcus et al. [97] have analyzed other sources of variability in the technique. About 8% of the error is introduced by scintillation counting, variation in the number of microspheres per tissue sample, weighing errors, and the inclusion of counts from nonmyocardial tissue from the endocardial and epicardial surfaces. Other factors may differentially influence the microsphere activity measured in the infarcted and normal myocardium. After 12 h of ischemia, Jugdutt et al. [98] found that infarcted tissue failed to retain all its microspheres, presumably due to damage of the microcirculation. The weight of tissue against which RMBF is referenced (the anatomic reference base) may vary with expansion due to tissue edema in early infarcts (2–4 days) and contraction in late infarcts (28 days) [89]. The loss of microspheres and expansion of the anatomic reference base due to edema results in an underestimation of the RMBF expressed per unit weight of tissue in experiments using early infarcts.

Despite these limitations, investigators have been able to correlate RMBF to the eventual extent of infarct as assessed by histologic criteria. Irvan and Cobb [84] attempted to correlate RMBF and histologic criteria in a canine model after occlusion of the left anterior descending artery. RMBF was measured 15 and 120 min after occlusion and histologic examination was performed after six days. The correlation coefficients of RMBF was measured after 15 and 120 min with the histologic criteria were -0.83 and -0.89, respectively (Figure 16). Rivas et al. [99] occluded the left circumflex artery in dogs and correlated the RMBF 45 s and 2 h after occlusion with histologic change after six days. The results for transmural tissue specimens were similar to those of Irvin and Cobb [84]. Endocardial specimens, however, showed more histologic necrosis than did epicardial specimens, with equivalent degrees of ischemia suggesting perhaps that factors other than perfusion contributed to the ultimate fate of ischemic myocardium. Reimer and Jennings [88] used a canine model with left circumflex artery occlusion and correlated histologic necrosis at four days with RMBF corrected for the effects of microsphere loss from the infarct and changes in the 'anatomic reference base.' They found that subepicardial RMBF 20 min after occlusion correlated well with histologic evidence of transmural progression of necrosis four days later ($r = -0.85$).

These data suggest that RMBF determined by the microsphere technique is a major, though not sole, determinant of the extent of subsequent infarction and, therefore, may be a useful early marker of myocardium at risk of infarct (see Cobb and Murdock, p. 286). Attempts at validating the use of the TQ-ST segment deflection as an index of the ischemic myocardium have compared the ST segment elevation above the TQ segment as measured from an epicardial electrogram with the simultaneously determined RMBF (microsphere technique)

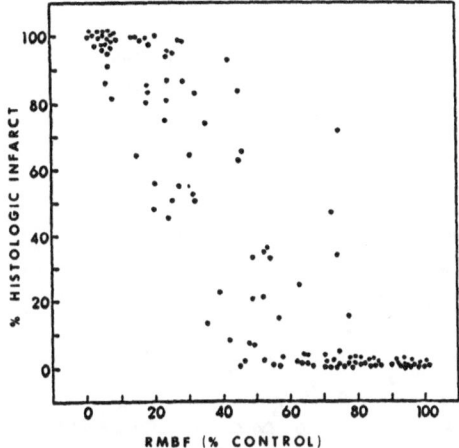

Figure 16. Percent histologic infarct as a function of regional myocardial blood flow (RMBF). In 13 dogs, RMBF was determined with 7- to 10-μ, radioactive microspheres for transmural myocardial specimens within and outside the distribution of the left anterior descending coronary artery 2h after occlusion. As in Figure 15, the percent of histologic infarct was quantified in these specimens six days after occlusion. (*Abscissa*) RMBF expressed as a percent of flow to the nonischemic posterior left ventricular wall. (*Ordinate*) Percent of area of sections showing histologic infarct. Note the inverse relationship between myocardial infarct and RMBF (correlation coefficient − 0.89). Adapted with permission from Irvin and Cobb [84].

in the immediately subjacent myocardium. Heng et al. [83] occluded the left anterior descending artery in dogs, and found a weak although significant inverse correlation between the ST voltage and transmural RMBF assessed 15 min after occlusion ($r = -0.41$) (Figure 17). Irvin and Cobb [84] found little improvement in the correlation coefficient when epicardial RMBF was compared with the ST voltage ($r = -0.57$); Timogiannakis et al. [79] and Smith et al. [82] reported similar results. Although it can be argued that RMBF is not the sole determinant of tissue injury and thus cannot serve as an absolute indicator of jeopardized tissue, we propose that close correlations between the TQ-ST deflection and RMBF in the directly subjacent myocardium *would not be expected* since the magnitude of the TQ-ST segment is influenced by electrophysiologic events remote from the subjacent myocardium. The electrophysiologic boundary should be defined from the epicardial distribution of R and TQ-ST potentials, and this boundary should be correlated with the zone of regional ischemia. This would define the relationship of the electrophysiologic boundary to the zone at risk of infarct.

A variety of metabolic and physiologic parameters have been measured in an attempt to define the region at risk of infarct, and some correlations have been made with electrocardiographic measurements. Intramyocardial oxygen tension

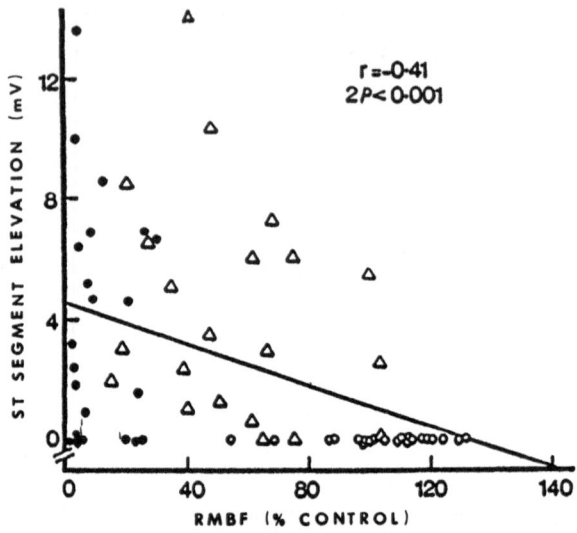

Figure 17. ST segment elevation as a function of regional myocardial blood flow (RMBF). In 11 dogs, epicardial ST segment elevation was measured 15 min after occlusion of the left anterior descending artery. Sites with abnormal QRS prolongation were excluded. RMBF was determined with 15 μ radioactive microspheres for transmural specimens subjacent to the epicardial recording sites 15 min after occlusion. (*Abscissa*) RMBF as percent flow to the nonischemic posterior wall of the left ventricle. (*Ordinate*) Epicardial ST elevation (mV) above the TP segment 60 ms after the end of the S wave. Note the wide scatter of ST voltages for any given degree of ischemia (correlation coefficient −0.41). Open circles: sites peripheral to the zone of ischemia. Open triangles: sites at the border zone of ischemia. Closed circles: sites in the center of the zone of ischemia. Adapted and used with permission from Heng et al. [83].

as determined polarographically [72, 80], intramyocardial oxygen and carbon dioxide tension as determined by mass spectrometry [81], the myocardial content of lactate, creatine phosphate, or adenosine triphosphate (ATP) [50, 51, 78] have been evaluated in ischemic myocardium and compared with ST segment measurements from epicardial electrodes. Since definite studies relating these early parameters of tissue oligemia to eventual anatomic infarct size or histologic indices of necrosis are not available, the quantitative relationship to the jeopardized myocardium is inferential and unproven. Angell et al. [80] found linear correlation coefficients ranging from −0.581 to −0.767 between polarographically determined intramyocardial oxygen tension and the magnitude of ST segment elevation in overlying epicardial electrodes. By contrast, Khuri et al. [81] reported no ST segment elevations in two of seven experiments comparing epicardial electrograms with intramyocardial oxygen and carbon dioxide tensions in subjacent ischemic myocardium. They did find correlations with *intramyocardial* ST segment elevations ($r = 0.732$ for carbon dioxide tension and −0.655 for oxygen tension). While Karlsson et al. [78] demonstrated lactate accumulation, ATP depletion, and creatine phosphate deplection at sites of depletion at sites of ST segment elevation in ischemic myocardium, they could demonstrate no relationship between the magnitude of the ST segment elevation and the degree of biochemical derrangement.

Electrophysiologic definition of the ischemic boundary

We are unconvinced that a strict quantitative relationship has been established between the magnitude of the epicardial TQ-ST deflection and a variety of nonelectrophysiologic validation techniques applied to the immediately subjecent myocardium. For the theoretical reasons discussed in this chapter, we would suggest that such relationships would not be expected and much experimental evidence supports our view. A few investigators have begun to examine the distributions of epicardial potentials. If the electrophysical boundary as defined by the distribution of potentials can be correlated with the borders of the ischemic myocardium (as defined by metabolic markers or the microsphere techniques) or the infarcted myocardium (as defined biochemically or pathologically), we have have a useful approach to infarct sizing.

Ginks et al. [76] noted a correlation between the area of epicardial cyanosis following acute coronary occlusion in the dog and the distribution of epicardial sites with ST segment elevation. Others have used NADH fluorescence stains to delineate ischemic tissue with altered oxidation-reduction potential and have found a characteristic variation in the ST voltage with respect to the distance from the boundary of the flourescent tissue [27] (Figure 18). Richeson et al. [23] distinguished normal from infarcted myocardium with the fluorescent vital stain, Thioflavin S. They reconstructed the anatomic borders of infarcts and demonstrated a pattern of TQ-ST segment deflections in relation to the infarct border that correspond with predictions from solid angle theory (Figure 19). Hearse et al. [50] mapped metabolic gradients (intramyocardial lactate, ATP, creatine phosphate, and glycogen as assayed in multiple rapidly sampled tissue biopsies) at the border of ischemic myocardial tissue. The border was defined by the limits of visible tissue cyanosis at the epicardium and the microsphere technique. The contours for each of the metabolic gradients follow closely a transition in the TQ-ST deflection at the border zone.

Janse et al. [49] studied the isolated perfused pig heart after occlusion of the left anterior descending coronary artery. Multiple epicardial DC electrograms were obtained from regularly spaced sites in and about the area of ischemia. Tissue levels of adenosine triphosphate (ATP), creatine phosphate (CP), and magnitude of the TQ-ST deflection varied inconsistently with the changes in these metabolites, an electrophysiologic boundary could be defined with epicardial electrograms that correspond to the border of the zone of accumulation

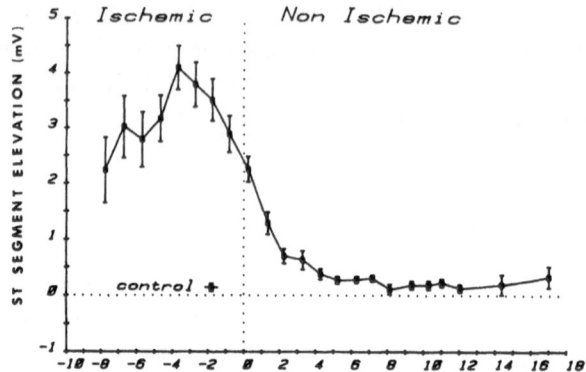

Figure 18. ST segment elevation as a function of the distance of the epicardial electrode from the boundary of fluorescence. In isolated perfused rabbit hearts, reduced nicotinamide adenine dinucleotide (NADH) fluorescence photography was used to map the epicardial topography of myocardial anoxia 10 min after occlusion of the left anterior descending coronary artery or a marginal branch of the left circumflex artery. The boundary between fluorescent and nonfluorescent tissue was defined by the border zone of NADH fluorescence. Simultaneous epicardial ST segment measurements were made at various distances from this boundary. (*Abscissa*) Epicardial electrode position from the boundary (mm). (*Ordinate*) Epicardial ST segment elevation (mV) above the PR segment 80 ms after the beginning of the QRS complex. Data points represent mean ± SEM. At 3.3 mm outside the boundary, the ST voltage rises significantly (p < 0.001) above that measured from sites more than 4.0 mm from the boundary and continues to rise as the boundary is approached. At 3.7 mm within the boundary, ST voltage peaks and then declines as the electrode moves further within the anoxic zone. The preocclusion control ST segment voltage was 0.16 mV. Adapted and reproduced with permission from Simson et al. [27].

of lactate and depletion of ATP and CP (Figure 20). Although the correspondence was not perfect, the electrophysiologic boundary appeared to be reasonably stable over the 2 h period of observation after occlusion. Much work needs to be done to develop quantitative predictions of the relationship of the electrophysiologic boundary to the underlying border zone of ischemia. More thorough definition of the perfusion and metabolic characteristics of the region and identification of those characteristics that predict irreversible injury will be of special importance if correlations with the electrophysiologic boundary are to have physiologic significance.

Finally most of the studies cited [23, 49, 50, 76] have related a 'lateral' border zone to electrophysiologic parameters. Undoubtedly the three-dimensional geometry of the transition zone between infarct and normal tissue is more complex, including not only 'lateral' but also 'epicardial' border zones [100]. Clearly more sophisticated electrophysiologic models will be required to make correlations between the boundary surrounding the evolving infarct and the extracellularly recorded potential.

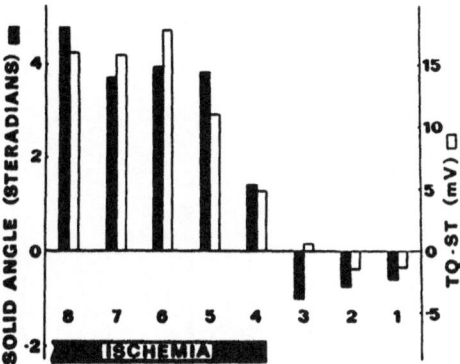

Figure 19. Calculated solid angle and epicardial TQ-ST segment change as a function of the distance from the ischemic boundary. After left anterior descending coronary artery ligation in a pig, epicardial electrograms were recorded at 2 mm intervals straddling the ischemic boundary. Sites with QRS duration greater than or equal to 80 ms were excluded. Subsequently, Thioflavin S, a fluorescent vital stain, was administered intravenously to demarcate the ischemic (nonfluorescent) tissue. The heart was frozen and serially sectioned. Fluorescence photography of the sections under ultraviolet illumination provided the templates for a wax reconstruction of the heart with ischemic zones removed. From this reconstruction, solid angles were calculated for electrode sites numbered 1–8. (*Abscissa*) Epicardial electrogram sites at 2 mm intervals with electrode 4 overlying the Thioflavin S boundary and electrode 7 located at the center of the zone of ischemia. (*Ordinate*) Solid bars: the calculated solid angle in steradians; open bars: the TQ-ST deflection (mV) measured as the vertical ST excursion from the TP segment 40 ms after the QRS. Note the transition in TQ-ST segment deflections across the ischemic boundary which parallels that predicted from solid angle calculations. The TQ-ST potential does not precisely follow the predicted pattern of negativity outside the boundary, however. Adapted with permission from Richeson et al. [23].

CLINICAL APPLICATION OF ELECTROPHYSIOLOGIC MAPPING AND VALIDATION TECHNIQUES

The feasibility of using epicardial potential distributions to delineate the borders of a region of myocardium in jeopardy has been discussed in the previous section. Further work must be directed toward developing quantitative predictions from these epicardial potential distributions. Clearly the limitations of this approach must be explored as well. As an example of such limitations, Holland and Brooks [22], using a model of anteroseptal infarct in the pig, found positive TQ-ST deflections from right ventricular epicardial sites lying outside the region of visible cyanosis. By contrast, equivalent left ventricular epicardial sites showed negative TQ-ST deflections. This apparent discrepancy in the relation between the TQ-ST deflection and the ischemic boundary at right as opposed to left ventricular sites could be explained by solid angle contributions from

94

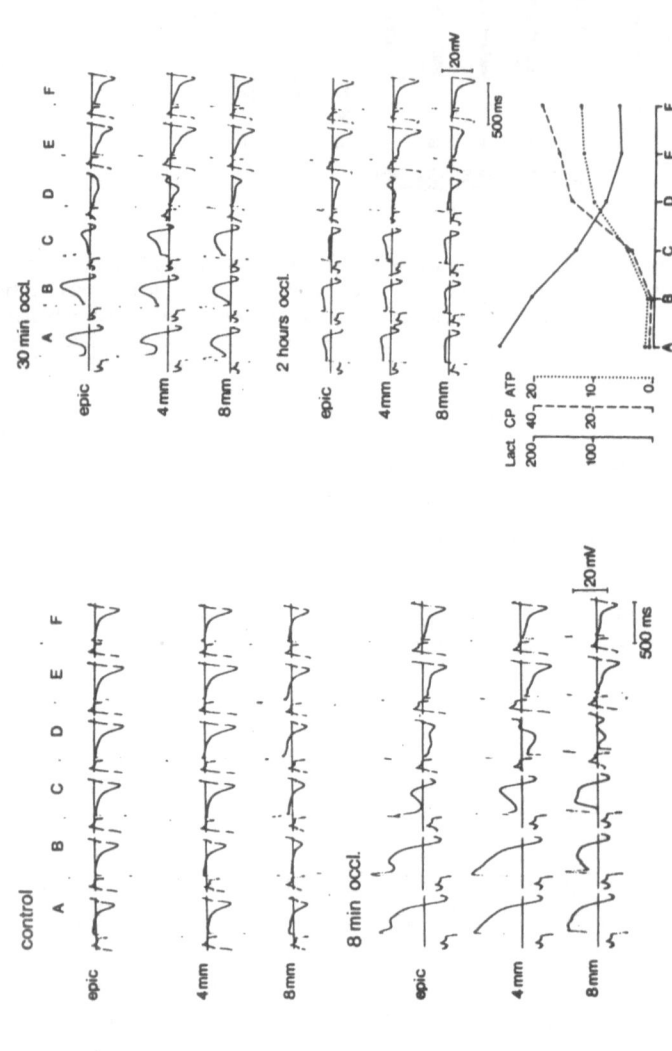

Figure 20. The effect of ischemia on epicardial (epi) and intramural (4 and 8 mm from the epicardial surface) d.c. electrograms and on lactate (lact), creatine phosphate (CP), and adenosine triphosphate (ATP) levels in the isolated perfused pig heart. The electrograms (zero reference is potential at aortic root) were recorded before and 8, 30, and 120 min after occlusion (occl) of the left anterior descending artery (LAD). Electrodes A to F were in a row separated by 4 mm. Electrode A was in the anterior wall of the left ventricle next to the LAD and electrode F was in the lateral wall. At 2 h after occlusion, transmural tissue biopsies were obtained with a 3 mm-diameter drill at the electrode sites and tissue levels of lactate, CP, and ATP were measured in μM/g dry tissue weight. Note the transition in TQ-ST deflections as the recording sites move across the biochemically defined boundary. Note also the relative constancy of the transition point between electrodes C and D at 2 hr after occlusion. Adapted with permission from Janse et al. [49].

ischemic septal tissue. These authors also demonstrated the influence of varying ventricular wall thickness on solid angle contributions to the measured extracellular potential. The function describing the position of the ischemic boundary from distributed epicardial potentials may have to incorporate corrections for such variables as infarct geometry and ventricular wall thickness. If these obstacles can be surmounted, the techniques of calculating epicardial potential distributions from body surface potentials introduced by Barr and Spach [39] may enable the noninvasive definition from precordial measurements of a region of myocardium at risk of infarct.

The problem of determining the ultimate fate of this region of risk remains. While pathologic evaluation offers the opportunity to accurately size infarcts, its clinical applicability is limited to patients who do not survive infarct. Furthermore, pathologic estimates of infarct volume or circumferential extent of infarct must be stratified for comparison as to age of infarct, since the geometry of the irreversibly damaged tissue evolves with time after onset of ischemia [91]. Histochemical analysis and tissue enzymatic analysis share similar limitations in clinical application. The development of radioactively labeled agents with relative affinity for infarcted myocardium [101] offer the potential for noninvasive detection, localization, and possibly sizing of infarcted myocardium (see Marcus, p. 325). The limitations imposed by the nonspecific localization of radionuclide, background radionuclide uptake, tissue attenuation factors, geometric arrangement of the region of interest, and constraints imposed by the resolution that can be achieved with current technology are amply discussed in other chapters (see Wackers, p. 199, and Okada, p. 295). Nonetheless, agents such as technetium pyrophosphate [102] or radiolabeled antimyosin FAB fragments [103], which localize to injured myocardial tissue, offer the prospect of noninvasively imaging infarcted myocardium. Detailed studies to define the specific properties of tissue that accumulates these and other agents will be required if these agents are to be used to determine the ultimate fate of the electrophysiologically defined myocardium at risk of infarct.

Other radiopharmaceuticals with high first-pass tissue extraction such as the potassium analogues, rubidium and thallium, are providing a qualitative noninvasive estimate of myocardial perfusion [104, 105]. Refinements of techniques such as these may ultimately provide a noninvasive validation technique for quantitating segmentally depressed regional myocardial blood flow that could be compared with electrocphysiologic indices of the extent of myocardium in jeopardy.

Tomographic representations of myocardial perfusion have been achieved by the coincidence detection of annihilation photons produced by positron-emitting radionuclides [106]. This technology may bring us closer to achieving clinically applicable noninvasive measurements of the anatomic extent of infarct or ischemia [107]. It has been suggested that we can take advantage of the differing myocardial extraction ratios among positron-emitting radionuclides. Whereas potassium analogues with relatively high myocardial extraction ratios would be expected to distribute to the myocardium initially in proportion to perfusion, other radionuclides (e.g., cesium or manganese) with lower extraction ratios might localize in tissue not only in proportion to flow but also in proportion to the ability of cells to extract the ion. Possibly the integrity of cellular ion pumps involved in extracting these cations might reflect the metabolic integrity of the cell. A comparison of the images created by these two types of agents might enable the identification of hypoperfused yet metabolically intact and hence potentially salvageable tissue (P. Harper, unpublished observations). [11]C palmitate may also serve as a metabolic probe, distinguishing cells capable of taking up this fatty acid from deranged cells that have lost this function.

As we come to understand the distinguishing metabolic and biophysical properties characterizing infarcted and reversibly ischemic myocardial tissue, perhaps new markers that can exploit these properties will be developed. Non-invasive imaging of the distribution of such agents offers a clinically applicable approach to the physiologic evaluation of the electrophysiologically defined region at risk of infarct.

CONCLUSIONS

Since the experimental observations of Smith in 1918 [108] and the clinical observations of Pardee [109] and others [110], physicians have looked to the electrocardiogram for aid in the diagnosis of acute myocardial infarct. Hellerstein and Kart [11] among others [110] described characteristic changes in specific leads that correlated with necrosis of portions of the myocardium. Even though these correlations are useful, we know that the specificity of the electrocardiographic information is rather poor [112, 113]. With our increasing awareness of the problem of 'pump failure' following myocardial infarct and subsequent hemodynamic performance [114, 115], it was not surprising that clinical investigators turned to the electrocardiogram to provide a simple noninvasive tool for 'sizing' myocardial infarct and assessing interventions designed to limit infarct size [116–121]. The surprise was that these studies lacked a strong biophysical foundation.

In this chapter, we have discussed the spatial and nonspatial determinants of the extracellularly recorded potential, the former relating the signal to the geometry of the boundary or boundaries and the position of the recording electrode and the latter relating the signal to the transmembrane voltage and ionic conductivities in various areas of the heart. We have reviewed the manner in which the spatial and nonspatial determinants could be affected by myocardial ischemia, injury, and infarct and by pharmacologic interventions. We concluded that clinical studies that lack a biophysical theoretical basis and that fail to consider the changes both in spatial and nonspatial determinants must be considered suspect.

Despite our rather pessimistic conclusions regarding much of the published literature, we postulated in this chapter that meaningful correspondence exists between the distributions of body surface potentials and the geography of ischemic, infarcted, and normal tissues. This postulate was based on four fundamental assumptions that were outlined in the introductory section and that were susceptible, in our view, to experimental testing. We outlined the need that due consideration be given to the variety of factors that may obfuscate the relation between the distributions of body surface potentials and the geometry of the normal, ischemic, and infarcted tissue. For example, the baseline 'normal' variations in potentials must be known for all points on the body surface if meaningful conclusions are to be drawn from measurements made during acute ischemia and infarct. Since the various potential measurements related to acute ischemia evolve with time after the onset of ischemia, standardization of the point in time at which data are acquired is mandatory if useful comparisons are to be made. Time may not necessarily be measured simply in hours and minutes, but perhaps in terms of metabolic markers as identified by radionuclides that are tracked in time. Clearly, exogenous factors that alter the extracellularly recorded potential such as electrolyte abnormalities and drug effects must be considered.

Even if such factors can be controlled or in some way estimated, the task remains of relating the extracellularly measured potential to underlying cellular electrophysiologic events. Research into the mechanisms by which cellular events shape the extracellularly recorded potential has increased our awareness of the limitations of electrocardiographic techniques. A major outgrowth of this work has been to direct attention away from overly simplistic attempts at relating magnitudes of 'injury currents' to underlying pathology and to focus instead on the definition of the electrophysiologic boundary or boundaries that are the sources of the TQ-ST potential. Efforts relating this *boundary* or series of boundaries to underlying pathologic events should be very fruitful endeavors in the next several years.

The requirements for developing electrocardiographic indices that are quantitative descriptors of pathologic change and perhaps are predictors of tissue viability are many. We require algorithms, instrumentation, and data processing that enable us to translate the electrical phenomena recorded at the body surface into electrophysiologic measurements that reflect underlying cellular events. We have reviewed several models of cardiac bioelectricity that are useful in conceptualizing the genesis of potentials measured at the body surface. Each of these models is overly simplified and has fundamental and important limitations. As these theories are refined, however, they will enable more accurate predictions, unveiling the inadequacies of previous theories and posing new hypotheses to be tested. We must retrieve or reconstruct the information that is lost from the signal as it is recorded from points progressively more remote from the primary events. Inverse mapping promises significant advances in this area. We must identify heretofore unidentified information in the extracellularly recorded signal. The surface electrogram contains a wealth of spatial detail and temporal information that we ordinarily do not use. Multiple recording sites, establishing patterns of body surface potential, and sampling at various moments during the cardiac cycle should uncover many spatial and temporal details that can be related to cardiac disease. We must pay attention to all parts of the electrocardiographic cardiac cycle and the interrelationship of all these parts, rather than narrowly focus on isolated portions of the electrocardiogram as has been the tendency in the past. Departure and QRST area mapping as well as other types of body surface recording have redirected our attention to these important details.

Even if we could predict electrophysiologic events in the heart from body surface potentials, the significance of these measurements depends on their relationship to the complex biochemical, biophysical, and metabolic events accompanying myocardial ischemia and infarct. Too often, attention has been directed at correlating the magnitude of ST potentials to the severity of a biologic derrangement in the subjacent myocardium. Only recently has work been directed toward defining an electrophysiologic boundary by examining transitions in TQ-ST deflections and relating the electrophysiologic boundary to a biologically relevant boundary zone as defined by measurements of regional myocardial blood flow, tissue metabolites concentrations, and histologic indices. The operational question that needs to be addressed is the following: 'How can we define the extent of myocardial tissue, that is reversibly injured, distinguishing it from normal and irreversibly injured tissue?' It follows that we need to better understand what the determinants are of irreversible injury. Only after we know how much reduction in regional myocardial blood flow results in cell death, how much lactate accumulation causes or reflects irreversible disruption of cellular metabolism, how much lysophosphoglyceride destroys cells, and the like, will we be able to give predictive physiologic meaning to the electrophysiologic boundary with such validation techniques.

Since therapeutic interventions can alter the extracellularly recorded potential by mechanisms other than direct effects on infarct size, it seems likely that other techniques will be required to define the ultimate fate of tissue identified as being at high risk by electrophysiologic techniques. Radionuclear techniques that reflect regional blood flow, metabolism, and necrosis hold the greatest promise in this regard.

The earliest electrophysiologists appreciated the fact that much information was hidden in the electrocardiographic signal. Only our ingenuity limits our ability to extract this information, appropriately interpret its biologic significance, and apply it profitably with the other tools of modern cardiology.

Acknowledgments. The time used in the preparation of this chapter was supported in part by a Research Development Award from the NHLBI 5-KO4-HL00196 to M.F.A., and by USPHS Multidisciplinary Sciences grant HL-07381 to E.K.L.

REFERENCES

1. Holland RP, Arnsdorf MF: Solid angle theory and the electrocardiogram: physiologic and quantitative interpretations. Prog Cardiovasc Dis 19:431–457, 1977.
2. Holland RP, Brooks H: TQ-ST segment mapping: critical review and analysis of current concepts. Am J Cardiol 40:110–128, 1977.
3. Fozzard HA, Das Gupta DS: ST-segment potentials and mapping. Theory Theory and experiments. Circulation 54:533–537, 1976.
4. Hillis LD, Askenazi J, Braunwald E, Radvany P, Muller JE, Fishbein MC, Maroko PR: Use of changes in the epicardial QRS complex to assess interventions which modify the extent of myocardial necrosis following coronary artery occlusion. Circulation 54:591, 1976.
5. Muller JE, Maroko PR, Braunwald E: Precordial electrocardiographic mapping. A technique to assess the efficacy of interventions designed to limit infarct size. Circulation 57:1–18, 1978.
6. Newton I: Philosophite Naturalis Principia Mathematica. Book I, Sect 12, Theorem 30. London: S Pepys (Cambridge: Harvard University Press,
7. Gauss CF: Carl Friedrich Gauss' Werke. Vol XI, Royal Society of Sciences, Tottingen, Berlin: Julius Springer, 1924, pp 148–150.
8. Maxwell JC: Electricity and magnetism, 2 vols. Oxford: Clarendon, 1891, pp 39–40. (New York: Dover).
9. Watson HW, Burbury SH: A mathematical theory of electricity and magnetism. Oxford: Clarendon, 1889, pp 2–3.
10. Masket AVH, Rodgers WD: Tables of solid angles. Washington DC: United States Atomic Energy Commission, 1962.
11. Wilson FN, Macleod AG, Barker PS: The distribution of the currents of action and of injury displayed by heart muscle and other excitable tissues. University of Michigan Studies, Scientific Series, vol 10. Ann Arbor: University of Michigan Press, 1933.
12. Bayley RH: An interpretation of the injury and the ischemic effects of myocardial infarction in accordance with the laws which determine the flow of electrical currents in homogeneous volume conductors, and in accordance with relevant pathological changes. Am Heart J 24:514–528, 1942.
13. Pruitt RD, Valencia F: The immediate electrocardiographic effects of circumscribed myocardial injuries: an experimental study. Am Heart J 35:161–197, 1948.
14. Hellerstein HK, Katz LN: The electrical effects of injury at various myocardial locations. Am Heart J 36:184–220, 1948.
15. Hecht HH: Some observations and theories concerning the electrical behaviour of heart muscle. Am J Med 30:720–746, 1961.
16. Bayley RH, Berry PM: The arbitrary electromotive double layer in the eccentri 'heart' of the nonhomogeneous circula lamina. IEEE Trans Biomed Eng 11:137, 1964.

17. Plonsey R: An evaluation of several cardiac activation models. J Electrocardiol 7:237, 1974.
18. Bayley RH: Biophysical principles of electrocardiography. New York: Heober, 1958, pp 19–34, 184–196, 207–222.
19. Plonsey R: Bioelectric phenomena. New York: McGraw-Hill, 1969, pp 202–275.
20. Holland RP, Arnsdorf MF: Nonspatial determinants of electrograms in guinea pig ventricle. Am J Physiol 240:C148–160, 1981.
21. Holland RP, Brooks H: Precordial and epicardial surface potentials during myocardial ischemia in the pig. A theoretical and experimental analysis of the TQ and ST segments. Circ Res 37:471, 1975.
22. Holland RP, Brooks H, Lidl B: Spatial and nonspatial influences on the TQ-ST segment deflection of ischemia. Theoretical and experimental analysis in the pig. J Clin Invest 60:197–214, 1977.
23. Richeson JF, Akiyama T, Schenk E: A solid angle analysis of the epicardial ischemic TQ-ST deflection in the pig. A thoeretical and experimental study. Circ Res 43:879–888, 1978.
24. Rudy Y, Plonsey R, Liebman J: The effects of variations in conductivity and geometrical parameters on the electrogardiogram using an eccentric sphere model. Circ Res 44:104–111, 1979.
25. Arnsdorf MF: Electrocardiography. I. Fundamental theory, parts 1 and 2. II. Applied theory, parts 1 and 2. In: Electrophysiology of the heart. Bethesda: Am Physiol Soc, 1978.
26. Spach MS, Barr RC, Benson DW, Walston A II, Warren RB, Edwards SB: Body surface low-level potentials during ventricular repolarization with analysis of the ST segment: variability in normal subjects. Circulation 59:822–836, 1979.
27. Simson MB, Harden WR III, Barlow CH, Harken AH: Epicardial ischemia as delineated with eipicardial S-T segment mapping and nicotinamide adenine dinucleotide (NADH) fluorescence photography. Am J Cardiol 44:263–269, 1979.
28. Taccardi B: La distribution spatiale des potentiels cardiaques. Acta Cardiol 13:173, 1958.
29. Schmitt OH, Levine RB, Simonson E: Electrocardiographic mirror pattern studies. I. Experimental validity tests of the dipole hypothesis and of the central terminal theory. Am Heart J 45:416, 1953.
   – Levine RB, Schmitt OH, Simonson E: II. The statistical and individual validity of the heart dipole concept as applied in electrocardiographic analysis. Am Heart J 45:500, 1953.
   – Simonson E, Schnmitt OH, Levine RB, Dahl J: III. Mirror pattern cancellation in normal and abnormal subjects. Am Heart J 45:655, 1953.
30. Frank E: Measurement and significance of cancellation potentials on the human subject. Circulation 11:937, 1955.
31. Morton RF, Romans WE, Brody DA: Cancellation of esophageal electrocardiograms. Circulation 15:897, 1957.
32. Brody DA, Copeland GD: Electrocardiographic cancellation: some observations concerning the 'nondipolar' fraction of precordial electrocardiograms. Am Heart J 56:381, 1958.
33. Pozzi L: Basic principles in vector electrocardiograph. Springfield IL: Charles C Thomas, 1961.
34. Holt JH Jr, Barnard ACL, Lynn MS, Svendsen P: A study of the human

heart as a multiple dipole electrical source. II. Diagnosis and quantitation of left ventricular hypertrophy. Circulation 40:697, 1969.

35. Holt JH Jr, Barnard ACL, Kramer JO Jr: Multiple dipole electrocardiography: a comparison of electrically and angiographically determined left ventricular masses. Circulation 57:1129, 1978.
36. Flowers NC, Horan LG, Sohi GS, Hand RC, Johnson JC: New evidence for inferoposterior myocardial infarction on surface potential maps. Am J Cardiol 38:576, 1976.
37. McLaughlin VW, Flowers NC, Horan LG, Killam HAW: Surface potential contribution from discrete elements of ventricular wall. Am J Cardiol 34:302–308, 1974.
38. McFee R, Baule GM: Research in electrocardiography and magnetocardiography. Proc IEEE 60:290–321, 1972.
39. Barr RC, Spach MS: Inverse calculation of QRS-T epicardial potentials from body surface potential distributions for normal and ectopic beats in the intact dog. Circ Res 42:661–675, 1978.
40. Barr RC, Spach MS: Inverse solutions directly in terms of potentials. In: Nelson CV, Geselowitz DB (eds) The theoretical basis of electrocardiology. Oxford: Clarendon Press, 1976, pp 294–304.
41. Barr BC, Ramsey M, Spach MS: Relating epicardial to body surface potential distributions by means of transfer coefficients based on geometry measurements. IEEE Trans Biomed Eng 24:1–11, 1977.
42. Spach MS, Barr RC, Lanning CF, Tucek PC: Origin of body surface QRS and T wave potentials from epicardial potential distributions in the intact chimpanzee. Circulation 55:268–278, 1977.
43. Spach MS, Barr RC, Warren RB, Benson DW, Walston A, Edwards SB: Isopotential body surface mapping in subjects of all ages: emphasis on low-level potentials with analysis of the method. Circulation 59:805–821, 1979.
44. Maroko PR, Libby P, Covell JW, Sobel BE, Ross J Jr, Braunwald E: Precordial S-T segment elevation mapping: an atraumatic method for assessing alterations in the extent of myocardial ischemic injury. The effects of pharmacologic and hemodynamic interventions. Am J Cardiol 29:223–230, 1972.
45. Mirvis DM: Body surface distributions of repolarization forces during acute myocardial infarction. Circulation 62:878–887, 1980.
46. Wilson FN, Macleod AG, Barker PS, Johnston FD: The determination and the significance of the areas of the ventricular deflections of the electrocardiogram. Am Heart J 10:46, 1934.
47. Abildskov JA, Burgess MJ, Urie PM, Lux RL, Wyatt RF: The unidentified information content of the electrocardiogram. Circ Res 40:3, 1977.
48. Abildskov JA, Evans AK, Lux RL, Burgess MJ: Direct evidence relating QRST deflection area and ventricular recovery properties [abstr]. Circulation 60 [Suppl 2]:11–110, 1979.
49. Janse MJ, Cinca J, Moréna H, Fiolet JWT, Kléber AG, de Vries GP, Becker AE, Durrer D: The 'border zone' in myocardial ischemia. An electrophysiological, metabolic, and histochemical correlation in the pig heart. Circ Res 44:576–588, 1979.
50. Hearse DJ, Opie LH, Katzeff IE, Lubbe WF, Van Der Werff TJ, Peisach M, Boulle G: Characterization of the 'border zone' in acute regional ischemia in the dog. Am J Cardiol 40:716–726, 1977.

102

51. Dunn RB, Griggs DM Jr: Transmural gradients in ventricular tissue metabolites produced by stopping coronary blood flow in the dog. Circ Res 37:438–445, 1975.
52. Harken AH, Barlow CH, Harden WR III, Chance B: Two and three dimensional display of myocardial ischemic 'border zone' in dogs. Am J Cardiol 42:954–969, 1978.
53. Simson MB, Harden W, Barlow C, Harken AH: Vizualization of the distance between perfusion and anoxia along an ischemic border. Circulation 60:1151–1155, 1979.
54. Hirzel HO, Sonnenblick EH, Kirk ES: Absence of a lateral border zone of intermediate creatine phosphokinase depletion surrounding a central infarct 24 hours after acute coronary occlusion in the dog. Circ Res 41:673–683, 1977.
55. Cox JL, McLaughlin VW, Flowers NC, Horan LG: The ischemic zone surrounding acute myocardial infarction. Its morphology as detected by dehydrogenase staining. Am Heart J 76:650, 1968.
56. Factor SM, Sonnenblick EH, Kirk ES: The histologic border zone of acute myocardial infarction – islands or peninsulas? Am J Pathol 92:111–120, 1978.
57. De Mello WC (ed): Intracellular communication. New York: Plenum, 1977.
58. Samson WE, Scher AM: Mechanism of S-T segment alteration during acute myocardial injury. Circ Res 8:780, 1960.
59. Cohen D, Kaufman LA: Magnetic determination of the relationship between the S-T segment shift and the injury current produced by coronary artery occlusion. Circ Res 36:414, 1975.
60. Downar E, Janse MJ, Durrer D: The effect of 'ischemic' blood as transmembrane potentials of normal porcine ventricular myocardium. Circulation 55:455, 1977.
61. Sobel BE, Corr PB, Robinson AK, Goldstein RA, Witkowski FX, Klein MS: Accumulation of lysophorphoglycerides with arrhythmogenic properties in ischemic myocardium. J Clin Invest 62:546–553, 1978.
62. Corr PB, Cain ME, Witkowski FX, Price DA, Sobel BE: Potential arrhythmogic electrophysiological derangements in canine Purkinje fibers induced by lysophosphoglycerides. Circ Res 44:822–832, 1979.
63. Arnsdorf MF, Sawicki GJ: The effects of lysophosphatidylcholine, a toxic metabolite of ischemia, on the components of cardiac excitability in sheep Purkinje fibers. Circ Res 49:16–30, 1981.
64. Snyder DW, Gross RW, Sobel BE, Corr PB: Comparable electrophysiological derangements induced by lysophosphoglycerides and acyl carnitine [abstr]. Circulation 60 [Suppl 2]:II–208, 1979.
65. Lazzara R, El-Sherif N, Hope RR, Scherlag BJ: Ventricular arrhythmias and electrophysiologocal consequences of myocardial ischemia and infarction. Circ Res 42:740–749, 1978.
66. Spear JF, Horowitz LN, Hodess AB, MacVaugh H III, Moore EN: Cellular electrophysiology of human myocardial infarction. 1. Abnormalities of cellular activation. Circulation 59:247–256, 1979.
67. Engelmann TW: Ueber die Leitung der Errung Im Herzmuskel. Pfluegers Arch Physiol 11:465–480, 1875 (Pfluegers Arch Gesamte Physiol Menschen Tiere).
68. Engelmann TW: Vergleichende Untersuchungen zur Lehre von der Muskelund Nervenelektricitat. Pfluegers Arch Physiol 15:116–148, 1877.

69. Anderson GJ, Reiser J, Gough WB: Intramyocardial current flow during acute coronary occlusion in the dog [abstr]. Circulation 60 [Suppl 2]:II–110, 1979.
70. Childers RW, Cope T, Lyon R, Holland R: Tissue resistance in ventricular ischemia [abstr]. Circulation 60:II–110, 1979.
71. Kléber AG, Janse MJ, van Capelle FJL, Durrer D: Mechanism and time course of S-T and T-Q segment changes during acute regional myocardial ischemia in the pig heart determined by extracellular and intracellular recordings. Circ Res 42:603–613, 1978.
72. Arnsdorf MF, Hsieh Y: Antiarrhythmic Agents. In: Hurst JW, Logue RB, Schlant RC, Wenger NK (eds) The heart, 4th edn. New York: McGraw-Hill, 1979, pp 1943–1963.
73. Hsieh Y, Goldberg L, Arnsdorf MF: Cardiac glycosides, theophylline, morphine, and vasodilators. In: Hurst JW, Logue RB, Schlant RC, Wenger NK (eds) The heart, edn. New York: McGraw-Hill, 1979, pp 1964–1980.
74. Maroko PR, Kjekshus JK, Sobel BE, Watanable T, Covell JW, Ross J Jr, Braunwald E: Factors influencing infarct size following experimental coronary artery occlusion. Circulation 43:67–82, 1971.
75. Sayen JJ, Peirce G, Katcher AH, Sheldon WF: Correlation of intramyocardial electrocardiograms with polarographic oxygen and contractility in the nonischemic and regionally ischemic left ventricle. Circ Res 9:1268–1279, 1961.
76. Ginks WR, Sybers HD, Maroko PR, Covell JW, Sobel BE, Ross J Jr: Coronary artery reperfusion. II. Reduction of myocardial infarct size at 1 week after the coronary occlusion. J Clin Invest 51:2717–2723, 1972.
77. Kjekshus JK, Maroko PR, Sobel BE: Distribution of myocardial injury and its relation to epicardial ST-segment changes after coronary artery occlusion in the dog. Cardiovasc Res 6:490–499, 1972.
78. Karlsson J, Templeton GH, Willerson JT: Relationship between epicardial S-T segment changes and myocardial metabolism during acute coronary insufficiency. Circ Res 32:725–730, 1973.
79. Timogiannakis G, Amende I, Martinez E, Thomas M: ST segment deviation and regional myocardial blood flow during experimental partial coronary artery occlusion. Cardiovasc Res 8:469–477, 1974.
80. Angell CS, Lakatta EG, Weisfeldt ML, Shock NW: Relationship of intramyocarrdial oxygen tension and epicardial ST segment changes following acute coronary artery ligation: effects of coronary perfusion pressure. Cardiovasc Res 9:12–18, 1975.
81. Khuri SF, Flaherty JT, O'Riordan JB, Pitt B, Brawley RK, Donahoo JS, Gotl VL: Changes in intramyocardial ST segment voltage and gas tensions with regional myocardial ischemia in the dog. Circ Res 37:455–463, 1975.
82. Smith HJ, Singh BN, Norris RM, John MB, Hurley PJ: Changes in myocardial blood flow and S-T segment elevation following coronary artery occlusion in dogs. Circ Res 36:697–705, 1975.
83. Heng MK, Singh BN, Norris RM, John MB, Elliott R: Relationship between epicardial ST-segment elevation and myocardial ischemic damage after experimental coronary artery occlusion in dogs. J Clin Invest 58:1317–1326, 1976.
84. Irvin RG, Cobb FR: Relationship between epicardial ST-segment elevation,

regional myocardial blood flow, and extent of myocardial infarction in awake dogs. Circulation 55:825–832, 1977.

85. Kléber AG, Janse MJ, van Capelle FJL, Durrer D: Mechanism and time course of S-T and T-Q segment changes during acute regional myocardial ischemia in the pig heart determined by extracellular and intracellular recordings. Circ Res 42:603–613, 1978.

86. Mallory GK, White PD, Salcedo-Salgar J: The speed of healing of myocardial infarction. A study of the pathologic anatomy in 72 cases. Am Heart J 18:647–671, 1939.

87. Reimer KA, Lowe JE, Rasmussen MM, Jennings RB: The wavefront phenomenon of ischemic cell death. I. Myocardial infarct size vs duration of coronary occlusion in dogs. Circulation 56:786–794, 1977.

88. Reimer KA, Jennings RB: The 'wavefront phenomenon' of myocardial ischemic cell death. II. Transmural progression of necrosis within the framework of ischemic bed size (myocardium at risk) and collateral flow. Lab Invest 40:633–644, 1979.

89. Reimer KA, Jennings RB: The changing anatomic reference base of evolving myocardial infarction. Underestimation of myocardial collateral blood flow and overestimation of experimental anatomic infarct size due to tissue edema, hemorrage and acute inflammation. Circulation 60:866–876, 1979.

90. Kjekshus JK, Sobel BE: Depressed myocardial creatine phosphokinase activity following experimental myocardial infarction in rabbit. Circ Res 27:403–414, 1970.

91. Fishbein MC, Maclean D, Maroko PR: Experimental myocardial infarction in the rat: qualitative and quantitative changes during pathologic evolution. Am J Pathol 90:57–70, 1978.

92. Rudolph AM, Heymann MA: The circulation of the fetus in utero. Methods for studying distribution of blood flow, cardiac output and organ blood flow. Circ Res 21:163–189, 1967.

93. Heymann MA, Payne BD, Hoffmann JIE, Rudolph AM: Blood flow measurements with radinuclide-labeled particles. Prog Cardiovasc Dis 20:55–79, 1977.

94. Fortuin NJ, Kaihara S, Becker LC, Pitt B: Regional myocardial blood flow in the dog studied with radioactive microspheres. Cardiovasc Res 5:331–336, 1971.

95. Utley J, Carlson EL, Hoffmann JIE, Martinez HM, Buckberg GD: Total and regional myocardial blood flow measurements with 25μ, 15μ, 9μ and filtered $1-10\mu$ diameter microspheres and antipyrine in dogs and sheep. Circ Res 34:391–405, 1974.

96. Buckberg GD, Luck JC, Payne DB, Hoffman JIE, Archie JP, Fixles DF: Some sources of error in measuring regional blood flow with radioactive microspheres. J Appl Physiol 31:598–609, 1971.

97. Marcus ML, Kerber RE, Ehrhardt J, Abboud FM, Schrader M, Panther D, Lim O: Three dimensional geometry of acutely ischemic myocardium. Circulation 52:254–263, 1975.

98. Jugdutt BI, Hutchins GM, Bulkley BH, Becker LC: The loss of radioactive microspheres from canine necrotic myocardium. Circ Res 45:746–756, 1979.

99. Rivas F, Cobb FR, Bache RJ, Greenfield JC Jr: Relationship between blood flow to ischemic regions and extent of myocardial infarction. Serial

measurement of blood flow to ischemic regions in dogs. Circ Res 38:439–447, 1976.

100. Darsee JR, Kloner RA, Braunwald E: Demonstration of lateral and epicardial border zone salvage by flurbiprofen using an in vivo method for assessing myocardium at risk. Calculation 63:29–35, 1981.

101. Wynne J, Holman BL, Lesch M: Myocardial scintigraphy by infarct-avid radiotracers. Prog Cardiovasc Dis 20:243–266, 1978.

102. Stokely EM, Buja LM, Lewis SE, Parkey RW, Bonte FJ, Harris RA Jr, Willerson JT: Measurement of acute myocardial infarcts in dogs with ^{99}mTc-stannous pyrophosphate scintigrams. J Nucl Med 17:1–5, 1976.

103. Khaw BA, Fallon JT, Beller GA, Haber E: Specificity of localization of myosin-specific antibody fragments in experimental myocardial infarction. Histologic, histochemical, autoradiographic and scintigraphic studies. Circulation 60:1527–1531, 1979.

104. Zaret BL: Myocardial imaging with radioactive potassium and its analogs. Prog Cardiovasc Dis 20:81–94, 1977.

105. DiCola VC, Downing SC, Donabedian RK, Zaret BL: Pathophysiological correlates of thallium-201 myocardial uptake in experimental infarction. Cardiovasc Res 11:141, 1977.

106. Weiss ES, Siegel BA, Sobel BE, Welch MJ, Ter-Pogossian MM: Evaluation of myocardial metabolism and perfusion with positron-emitting radionuclides. Prog Cardiovasc Dis 20:191–206, 1977.

107. Keyes JW, Leonard PF, Brody SL, Svetkoff DJ, Rogers WL, Lucchesi BR: Myocardial infarct quantication in the dog by single photon emission computed tomography. Circulation 58:227–232, 1978.

108. Smith FM: The ligation of coronary arteries with electrocardiographic study. Arch Intern Med 22:8–27, 1918.

109. Pardee HEB: An electrocardiographic sign of coronary artery obstruction. Arch Intern Med 26:244–257, 1920.

110. Burch GE, DePasquale NP: History of Electrocardiography. Chicago: Year Book Medical, 1964.

111. Hellerstein HK, Katz LN: The electrical effects of injury at various myocardial locations. Am Heart J 36:184–220, 1948.

112. Horan LG, Flowers NC, Johnson JC: Significance of the diagnostic Q wave of myocardial infarction. Circulation 43:428–436, 1971.

113. Horan LG, Flowers NC: Diagnostic power of the Q wave: critical assay of its significance in both detection and localization of myocardial deficit. In: Schlant RC, Hurst JW (eds) Advances in electrocardiography. Vol 1: Cardiovascular dieseases; current status and advances. New York: Grune and Stratton, 1972, pp 321–330.

114. Page DL, Caulfield JB, Kastor JA, DeSanctis RW, Sanders CA: Myocardial changes associated with cardiogenic shock. N Engl J Med 285:133–137, 1971.

115. Pfeffer MA, Pfeffer JM, Fishbein MC, Fletcher PJ, Spadaro J, Kloner RA, Braunwald E: Myocardial infarct size and ventricular function in rats. Circ Res 44:503–512, 1979.

116. Reid PR, Taylor DR, Kelly DT, Weisfeldt ML, Humphries JO, Ross RS, Pitt B: Myocardial-infarct extension detected by precordial ST-segment mapping. N Engl J Med 290: 123, 1974.

117. Maroko PR, Davidson DM, Libby P, Hagan AD, Braunwald E: Effects of hyaluronidase administration on myocardial ischemic injury in acute

infarction. A preliminary study in 24 patients. Ann Intern Med 82:516, 1975.

118. Come PC, Flaherty JT, Baird MG, Rouleau JR, Weisfeldt ML, Greene HL, Becker L, Pitt B: Reversal by phenylephrine of the beneficial effects of intravenous nitroglycerine in patients with acute myocardial infarction. N Engl J Med 293:1003, 1975.

119. Borer JS, Redwood DR, Levitt B, Cogin N, Bianchi C, Vallin H, Epstein SE: Reduction in myocardial ischemia with nitroglycerine or nitroglycerine plus phenylephrine administered during acute myocardial infarction. N Engl J Med 293:1008, 1975.

120. Maroko PR, Hillis LD, Muller JE, Tavazzi L, Hendrix GR, Ray M, Chiariello M, Distante A, Askenozi J, Salerno J, Carpentier J, Reshetnaya NI, Radvany P, Libby P, Raabe DS, Chazov EI, Babba P, Braunwald E: Favorable effects of hyaluronidase on electrocardiographic evidence of necrosis in patients with acute myocardial infarction. N Engl J Med 296:898, 1977.

121. Derrida JP, Sal R, Chiche P: Nitroglycerine infusion in acute myocardial infarction [lett]. N Engl J Med 297:336, 1977.

4. ENZYMATIC ESTIMATION: CREATINE KINASE

ROBERT ROBERTS

More than a decade has passed since the first enzymatic estimates of infarct size were performed based on creatine kinase [1]. During this time, many investigators have used the method, changing it significantly and making its clinical role more apparent. At the same time, intense research efforts have led to important observations applicable not only to infarct size but also to the diagnosis and assessment of ischemic heart disease and to enzymology in general.

Enzymatic estimation of infarct size is based on a simple concept, related to a well-known pathologic observation: when cells die, their contents are lost from an organ due to either destruction or release into the surrounding medium or both. The constituent of interest here is a protein with enzyme activity, creatine kinase (CK). Because creatine kinase activity is distributed uniformly throughout the myocardium, it was reasonable to hypothesize that the amount of CK lost from the heart subsequent to, say, 20 g necrosis would be twice that lost in association with 10 g necrosis. This hypothesis was tested and verified in the experimental animal by sacrificing the animal and determining directly the myocardial CK activity lost 24–48 h after inducing an infarct by acute coronary ligation. These observations set the stage for the next question, namely, how to assess myocardial CK depletion indirectly by in vivo techniques. This led to the development of a technique to estimate the total CK released into the blood, based on serial changes in plasma CK activity during the acute episode [2]. It remained to be determined whether a proportion or all of the CK lost from the heart would be released into the blood. Estimating the amount of CK released into the blood relies on several parameters among which are the plasma CK disappearance rate and the ratio of CK released into the blood to CK depleted from the heart. Interpretation of enzymatic estimates of infarct size by the plasma CK method depends on how well this approach reflects myocardial CK depletion. This chapter will discuss these processes and their limitations with the hope that it will lead to a better understanding of enzymatic estimation of infarct size and a better interpretation of the data resulting from clinical application of this method.

Wagner GS (ed): Myocardial Infarction: Measurement and Intervention, pp 107–142.
© *1982 Martinus Nijhoff Publishers, The Hague/Boston/London.*

ESTIMATION OF MYOCARDIAL CK DEPLETION

To appropriately apply and understand the inherent limitation of the in vivo enzymatic method of estimating infarct size from change in plasma CK activity, it is necessary to be acquainted with the experiment data relating myocardial CK depletion to morphologic estimates of infarct size. These data showed a quantitative relationship between the extent of myocardial damage as determined morphometrically and the loss of CK from the heart. This relationship has since been validated in several species of animals under a variety of experimental conditions.

Initially infarct was produced via coronary artery ligation in rabbits [1] and in dogs [2], with the animals sacrificed 24 h later. The heart was removed and weighed. The area of damage identified by gross morphology was dissected free of the normal tissue, weighed, and expressed as a percentage of the total weight of the heart. In the canine experiments, since only the left anterior descending coronary artery was ligated, the posterior ventricular wall was unaffected and thus would reflect normal myocardial CK activity. Biopsies were taken from the posterior ventricular wall of each animal and the CK activity was determined and expressed in international units per gram (IU/g) of myocardium, which represented normal myocardial CK activity (CK_n). The weight of the left ventricle times the normal CK activity represented the total activity expected in the left ventricle (CK_e). The remaining left ventricle was homogenized and the remaining actual CK activity was determined directly (CK_a). The difference between the CK expected (CK_e) and that actually present (CK_a) is the amount of CK activity depleted (CK_d) from the heart as a result of occlusion and represents an enzymatic estimate of infarct size. The total CK activity depleted from the heart correlated with the area of damage determined by gross morphology [1, 2]. Results of studies comparing morphologic estimates with those of CK depletion are illustrated in Figure 1 and show a correlation coefficient of 0.85 [3].

Direct assessment of CK activity in multiple transmural biopsies from the right and left ventricles of normal animals indicates CK activity per gram of myocardium is uniformly distributed with less than 6% variation [3]. This is also true for the transmural distribution from endo- to epicardium (Figure 2), a fact that has been confirmed by several investigators [4–8]. To convert total CK activity depleted from the heart into grams of myocardium undergoing necrosis, a second parameter was introduced, namely, the amount of CK activity lost per gram of homogeneous necrosis (CK_i). Biopsies were obtained from the center of the area of infarct which, on gross inspection, appeared to be uniformly damaged and was taken as representative of homogeneous necrosis. We found that one gram of homogeneous necrotic tissue lost about 75% ± 5% of its CK activity 24–48 h after infarct. This was further evaluated by Hirzel et al. [4], who dissected normal from abnormal tissue in the center of the area

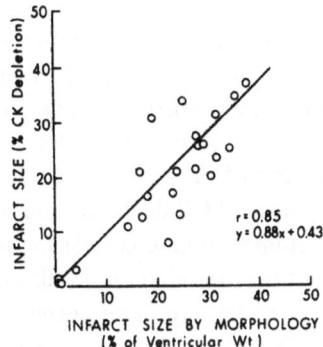

Figure 1. The close correlation between infarct size by morphology and that of myocardial CK depletion in untreated conscious dogs.

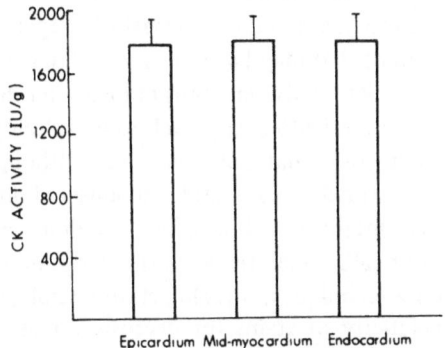

Figure 2. Creatine kinase activity per gram is uniformly distributed throughout the wall of the left ventricle, as determined by dividing the wall into three equal portions.

of infarct and confirmed that only about 75% of the CK was depleted. Other investigators confirmed these findings in several other animal models [3, 4, 6, 7, 9]. Total myocardial CK activity depleted can be converted into grams of myocardium undergoing necrosis, expressing infarct size in units of CK-gram-equivalence (CK-g-eq). The myocardial CK activity (25%) that remains despite homogeneous necrosis probably represents structural CK protein which has been shown to be a part of the myofibrils and forms a major portion of the so-called microscopically observed 'M' line [10].

Experimental studies in the rabbit and in the dog showed a quantitative relationship between infarct size detected by morphology and the total CK activity depleted from the myocardium [1–3]. The close correlation between myocardial CK depletion and morphologic estimates of necrosis has been demonstrated by several investigators after experimental infarct in several animals including the rat [11], rabbit [1], dog 2, 3], and baboon [6]. This correlation is maintained despite a variety of interventions including propranolol [12, 13], hyaluronidase [14], nitroglycerin [15], cobra venom factor [16], verapamil [17, 18], nifedipine [19], corticosteroids [20], and glucose, insulin and potassium [21]. Reperfusion, which alters coronary flow and might be expected to alter the proportion of CK released into the plasma, does not affect the relationship between myocardial CK depletion and morphologic estimates of infarct size [8, 22, 23]. All studies to date correlating myocardial CK depletion with morphologic evidence of necrosis either in localized biopsies or in the myocardium as a whole show a remarkably close correlation, reflecting a general agreement that myocardial CK depletion, when measured directly, accurately reflects infarct size. Furthermore, these experiments demonstrate that altering cardiac metabolism, increasing or decreasing myocardial oxygen consumption, modifying the immunologic response or inflammatory infiltrate, or altering coronary flow does not affect myocardial CK depletion. Thus, estimates of infarct size based on directly measured myocardial CK depletion are not affected by a variety of interventions that may be employed in the clinical setting.

The correlation coefficient between morphologic and enzymatic estimates may improve with a more meticulous approach to morphologic estimates. Since the area of infarction is somewhat heterogeneous, although less so in other animals than in man, difficulties are still encountered in providing precise morphologic estimates of infarct size. It is difficult, tedious, and time consuming to separate normal from abnormal tissue particularly in the border regions. Without special straining techniques, it is almost impossible, using such methods raises the issue of specificity of stains for necrosis versus reversible ischemia. Another problem related to morphologic methods is the interval between an infarct and its assessment. Reimer et al. [24] have shown that in the first few days after infarct, edema leads to overestimated infarct size; later, scar retraction leads to underestimated infarcts. The problems of heterogeneity, edematous expansion, and scar retraction are essentially eliminated by the CK method.

Direct assessment of myocardial CK depletion in the experimental animal is a more convenient and probably a more precise means of estimating infarct size than methods based on histologic approaches. Using the myocardial CK depletion method to estimate infarct size and normalizing for variation in heart size from animal to animal, it is possible to assess the effect of interventions in a small group of animals [18, 25, 26]. Using this new method, we have detected a reduction in infarct size of 17% or more in the treated groups versus controls with a sample size of 50 animals at an alpha level of 0.05 and a beta level of 0.20 [3]. Another approach recently introduced assesses the total area at risk by dye injection into the coronary vessels and expresses the area of infarct detected morphometrically as a percentage of the total area at risk [27]. This approach requires fewer animals, but has several drawbacks: (a) it must account for two variables, the area at risk and the actual amount of necrotic myocardium; (b) it does not eliminate the problem of border recognition and separation of normal from abnormal tissue; (c) there is considerable technical variation in the methods used to delineate the risk zone.

Myocardial CK depletion not only correlates well with morphologic estimates of myocardial damage but also with other parameters that reflect myocardial ischemia, including the distribution of reduced coronary blood flow as determined by the microsphere technique [1, 28], ST segment elevation [29], and histologically demonstrable necrosis [8, 30]. More recently, myocardial CK depletion after coronary occlusion has been shown to correlate with lack of uptake of ^{11}C-palmitate by the myocardium [31] and also with regional changes in the attenuation of transmitted ultrasound [32].

The observed quantitative relationship between myocardial CK depletion and morphologic estimates of infarct size provided a basis for the in vivo technique of estimating infarct size from plasma CK, the hypothesis being that total CK released into the plasma would reflect myocardial CK depletion. Estimation of the total CK activity released into the plasma is based on several parameters including: (a) the plasma CK disappearance rate (k_d), (b) the CK distribution volume (DV), (c) the ratio of CK released into the blood (CK_r) to that depleted from the myocardium (CK_d), and (d) the measurement of CK originating only from the heart. The accuracy of the in vivo method depends primarily on the precision with which these parameters can be estimated and characterized. Considerable strides have been made in attempting to determine myocardial CK depletion via plasma CK release despite the remaining inherent problems [33, 34].

ADVANTAGES OF CREATINE KINASE

Creatine kinase offers several advantages as a plasma marker for enzymatic estimation of infarct size. The myocardium is abundantly rich in CK activity and exhibits a very favorable gradient with respect to the blood since 1 g human myocardium has about 1600 IU versus the blood, which averages less than 0.050 IU/ml. Creatine kinase is rapidly released and has a rapid plasma turnover rate so that CK released into the blood can be estimated within 24–48 h (Figure 3). Even with minimal damage, the peak plasma CK activity after infarct is increased severalfold above baseline. Creatine kinase activity in the cellular components of the blood is negligible so that release from the heart as a result of the inflammatory infiltrate does not occur, unlike LDH or AST (SGOT) [28, 35]. Creatine kinase in the heart is essentially confined to the muscle and is negligible in connective and other tissues. Since creatine kinase has a molecular weight of 82,000 unlike low molecular weight markers such as myoglobin, its

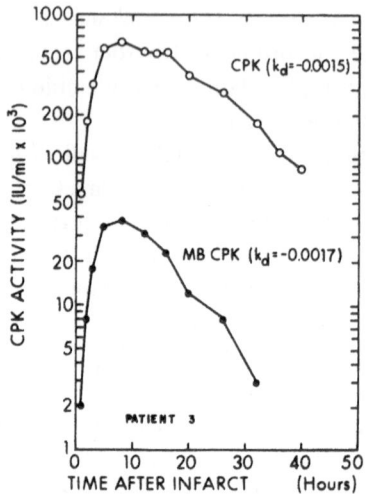

Figure 3. Serial changes in serum MB CK and total CK activity in a patient with acute myocardial infarction. As can be seen, MB CK activity declined somewhat more rapidly than total CK activity, although in this case the difference in disappearance rates (k_d) was small. In general, changes in total CK and MB CK followed the same pattern in patients with uncomplicated myocardial infarct.

clearance does not depend upon renal blood flow. The assay for total CK activity is rapid, convenient, and highly reproducible [36].

The diagnostic sensitivity of elevated plasma total CK activity for myocardial infarct exceeds that of other available conventional enzymes [37, 38]. Total CK lacks the necessary diagnostic specificity but its isoenzyme, MB CK, is virtually specific for the heart, having greater diagnostic specificity than SGOT, LDH, or LDH isoenzymes. The diagnostic specificity of plasma MB CK for myocardial infarct has been repeatedly demonstrated by utilizing qualitative and quantitative assays [39—42]. With the advent of quantitative assays [41] for MB CK and particularly the more rapid and convenient techniques [43—45], plasma MB CK can now be quantified on a routine basis. The distribution of MB CK activity in human tissues is shown in Figure 4; similar results have been observed by other investigators using quantitative assays [46, 47]. The myocardium is the only organ with more than trace amounts of MB CK [48]. We have observed trace amounts of MB CK in the gastrointestinal mucosa, the prostate, and the urethra. Several studies have documented plasma MB CK levels in the normal range (0.5—7.0 IU/l at 30°C despite elevated total CK activity after intramuscular injections, exercise, noncardiac surgery, trauma, cardiac catheterization, pericarditis, cardiac failure, tachyarrhythmias and lung disease [42, 49—53]. Myocardial infarct in man is consistently associated with elevated plasma MB CK [39, 40, 48] that remains elevated for 36—72h. Utilizing MB CK, it is possible to estimate infarct size in man despite concomitant release of MM CK

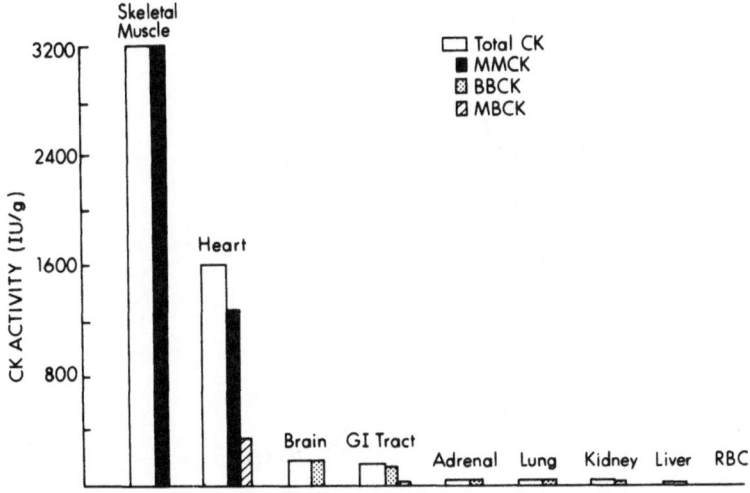

Figure 4. Shown here is the distribution of CK isoenzyme activity in human tissues. Samples of tissues were obtained during surgery and analyzed immediately. Results in each case represent averages based on analysis of tissue from at least four patients; GI, gastrointestinal; RBC, red blood cells.

from other organs even during complications such as cardiogenic shock [54]. If trace amounts of MB CK are present in skeletal muscles, they may detract from the diagnostic specificity, but such small amounts would not significantly affect estimates of infarct size based on plasma MB CK. In patients with concomitant congenital muscular dystrophy or acquired muscle disease, however, such as polymyositis, estimates of infarct size based on plasma MB CK may be artificially high. The advantage of plasma MB CK over total CK both as a diagnostic marker and as a means of assessing myocardial damage is illustrated in Figure 5. Creatine kinase activity, collected in EGTA (5 mM) and mercaptoethanol (10 mM) and stored at $-20°C$ or at $-70°C$ is extremely stable and activity can be preserved for years [55].

ESTIMATION OF INFARCT SIZE FROM PLASMA CK ACTIVITY

After establishing the quantitative relationship between myocardial CK depletion and infarct size, the relationship between plasma CK changes and myocardial CK depletion was assessed in the conscious dog after inducing an infarct by coronary occlusion. Conscious animals were used to avoid spurious estimates of myocardial CK release due to potential effects of anesthesia on CK kinetics. Blood samples were obtained every hour for 24 h, after which the animals were sacrificed. Each heart was removed and myocardial CK depletion, determined directly, was compared with the total CK released into the plasma [2].

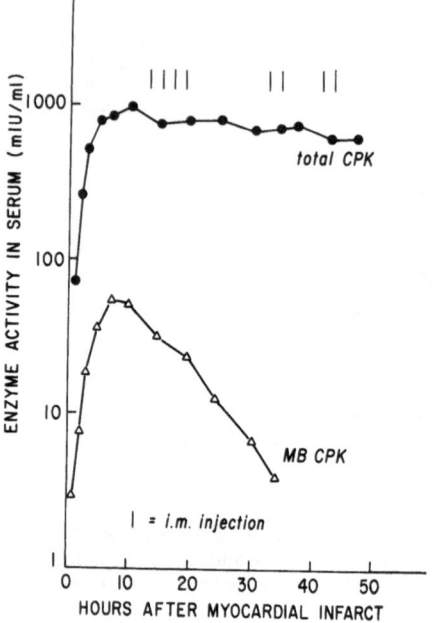

Figure 5. Serial changes in MB CK and total CK activity in samples from a patient with acute myocardial infarct complicated by frequent intramuscular injections. Required medication was administered by intramuscular injection at the times indicated by the arrows. This intervention persistently elevated total CK activity while MB CK activity declined in the pattern typical of patients with uncomplicated myocardial infarct.

In the initial formulation [2], serial changes in plasma CK activity were assumed to reflect release from irreversibly injured myocardium into the blood and simultaneous disappearance from the circulation. Thus, the rate of change of CK activity in the blood reflects two competing processes: the rate at which CK is released from the myocardium and the rate at which it disappears from the blood, which in mathematical terms may be stated as follows:

$$\frac{dE}{dt} = f(t) + k_d E$$

where E represents CK activity; t, time; and k_d the CK disappearance rate. Thus, dE/dt equals the rate of change of CK activity in the blood, and $f(t)$ equals the rate of release. The dE/dt can be determined from CK activity present in the blood samples. The k_d was determined in the experimental animal by bolus injections of purified CK, which was shown to disappear according to first-order kinetics, and the distribution volume was taken to be that of plasma. Knowing dE/dt and k_d, one can rearrange the equation to calculate $f(t)$, the rate of release. Knowing the total time during which CK is being released, it is possible to determine the total amount of CK released into the blood.

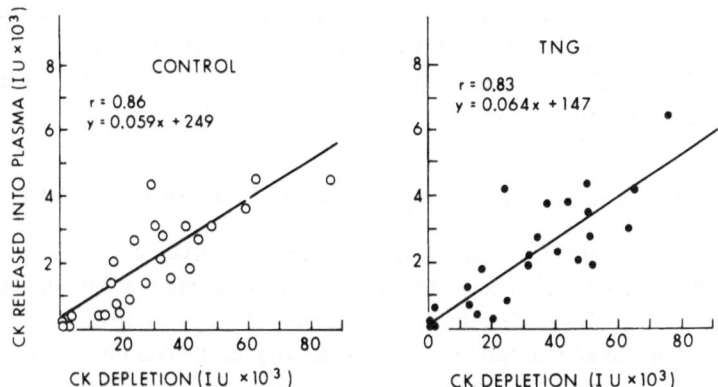

Figure 6. (*Left*) The close correlation between CK depletion and CK released into the plasma in untreated conscious animals. (*Right*) A similar close correlation was observed in nitroglycerin (TNG)-treated animals.

In animals with hemodynamically uncomplicated infarcts, CK depletion from the heart that was measured directly correlated well with CK released into the blood, which was estimated from analysis of serial changes in plasma CK activity ($r = 0.9$) [2]. These finding were not surprising in view of earlier observations by others [56–59] indicating that peak plasma enzyme levels correlated with the extent of infarction. Comparable correlations between estimates of infarct size based on plasma CK activity and those based on myocardial CK depletion have been observed in the baboon [9], in which the organ distribution of MB CK is similar to that in man, enabling improved estimates based on plasma MB CK rather than total CK activity. Even when a myocardial infarct is associated with experimentally induced reperfusion, the correlation between CK released into the blood and CK depleted from myocardium remains close ($r = 0.9$) although the slope of the function between the two appears to have changed [8]. A close correlation also was observed [3] between the CK released into the plasma and CK depleted from the myocardium in experimental infarcts in dogs treated with intravenous nitroglycerin ($r = 0.83$); a similar correlation was observed in controls ($r = 0.86$; Figure 6).

Failure by Swain et al. [60] to find a good correlation between histologic estimates of infarct size and infarct size estimated from plasma CK changes is due in part to several factors: (a) study of experimental animal preparations in a nonsteady state, reflected by the presence of high baseline CK values; (b) sampling by repetitive venipuncture, which is prone to release CK from the locally traumatized tissue; (c) the use of heavy sedation, which may alter the CK disappearance rate; and (d) the inability to establish appropriate baseline values for comparison because CK values were high before the study began. Furthermore, recent data by Reimer et al. [24] show that histologic techniques overestimate infarct size due to edema 4–5 days after occlusion. In the study by Swain et al., histologic estimates were performed 5–10 days after occlusion, which could explain why the estimates of infarct size from plasma CK and by histology do not correlate well.

COLLECTION, STORAGE, AND ANALYSIS OF PLASMA CK ACTIVITY

In assessing infarct size from plasma CK time activity curves, data of high quality can be obtained only if strict attention is paid to all steps from collection of blood to data analysis. One important source of error is in blood sampling, particularly in the animal model since CK activity in skeletal muscle 3000 IU/g, in contrast to plasma CK activity, which is in the range of 0.050–0.100 IU/ml. Even minor trauma to muscle near the sampling site can markedly distort results. Plasma CK time activity curves should not be assessed after surgery in experimental animals until values have returned to control levels. Repetitive venipuncture should be avoided. The samples, if not analyzed immediately, should be collected in EGTA (5 mM) and mercaptoethanol (10 mM). Animals should be in the conscious state since general anesthesia may delay the disappearance of CK from the circulation [61].

The assay for CK activity depends on temperature, pH, dilution, inhibitors, cofactors, and competing enzymes in the sample and, unless very rigid control is maintained, spurious results may occur. Dilution of samples should be sufficient to avoid saturation of coupling enzymes in the assay system and is preferably done with a Tris buffer. Standard curves are needed to avoid unrecognized error introduced by dilution because of the effects of inhibitors or conformational changes in the CK molecule. In the case of clinical studies, the assay for plasma MB CK must be quantitative and not based on electrophoresis with visual or fluorometric scanning that provides only semiquantitative information [41]. The plasma MB CK should be assessed by either the batch adsorption [43] or chromatographic technique [44,45]. The recently introduced immunoinhibition assay (Abbott) for MB CK may provide extremely erroneous results [62] and its use should be avoided.

Since enzymatic estimates of infarct size are expressed as CK-g-eq, that is, the amount of CK lost from one gram of myocardium undergoing homogeneous infarct, the value of 1 CK-g-eq should be appropriate for the CK values in the particular laboratory performing the study. In our initial studies, the value was 800 IU/g for dog and 500 IU/g for man in contrast to more recent values of 1500 and 1200 IU/g, respectively, with the currently available assay systems that are optimized for maximal CK activity. Obviously, gross overestimation of infarct size would occur if calculations based on parameters determined with the first assay system were utilized with results of determinations of plasma CK activity assayed with a system yielding substantially higher results [63].

Table 1. CK disappearance (k_d) in 30 conscious dogs

Exp. no.	Half-life (min)	k_d (min⁻¹)	SD of slope	r	Distribution vol (% body wt)
1	150	0.0046	9.2%	−0.97	5.3
2	178	0.0039	7.5%	−0.96	5.8
3	119	0.0058	6.0%	−0.92	5.9
4	144	0.0048	11.2%	−0.95	5.4
5	161	0.0043	16.4%	−0.99	5.0
6	131	0.0053	9.3%	−0.93	6.2
7	187	0.0037	8.7%	−0.96	4.9
8	100	0.0069	6.9%	−0.92	5.9
9	150	0.0046	10.5%	−0.95	5.5
10	178	0.0039	9.6%	−0.96	4.9
11	112	0.0062	6.2%	−0.94	5.2
12	161	0.0043	13.2%	−0.97	5.6
13	115	0.0060	14.3%	−0.95	5.2
14	154	0.0045	11.2%	−0.93	5.6
15	173	0.0040	9.1%	−0.95	5.4
16	88	0.0078	8.2%	−0.97	4.8
17	144	0.0048	7.5%	−0.96	5.2
18	100	0.0054	9.6%	−0.96	5.2
19	165	0.0042	10.2%	−0.98	5.7
20	105	0.0066	7.2%	−0.95	5.0
21	161	0.0043	6.2%	−0.95	5.2
22	133	0.0052	5.2%	−0.94	4.6
23	173	0.0040	7.5%	−0.96	5.7
24	131	0.0053	8.6%	−0.97	5.4
25	128	0.0054	10.9%	−0.93	5.2
26	157	0.0044	9.5%	−0.92	5.2
27	150	0.0046	7.8%	−0.99	4.9
28	178	0.0039	11.2%	−0.96	5.7
29	173	0.0040	9.6%	−0.95	5.2
30	110	0.0063	9.0%	−0.95	5.6
Mean	144.0	0.0048	9.2%	−0.95	5.4

FACTORS AFFECTING THE PLASMA CK DISAPPEARANCE RATE

The actual value used as an estimate of infarct size is directly related to the CK disappearance rate and thus significant error can be introduced if the CK disappearance rate is inaccurate. In the initial experimental studies, bolus injections of purified CK were performed and the disappearance rate was approximated by monoexponential fit [2]. It was clear at this time that the CK disappearance rate varied among animal species, but for the sake of convenience a mean CK disappearance rate was utilized. In a more extensive study since that time, we have shown that the CK disappearance rate varies markedly not only from species to species but also from animal to animal [32, 33] (Table 1). However, reapeated determinations of the CK disappearance rate in the same animal after inections of purified CK show it to be consistent from day to day [61] as illustrated in

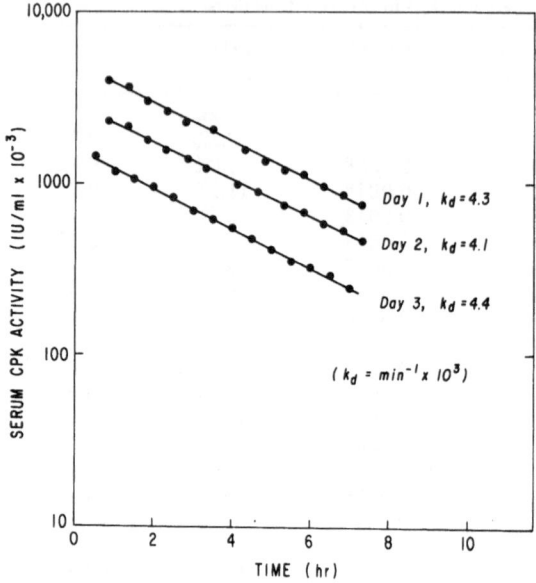

Figure 7. Serial changes in plasma CK activity after intravenous injection of canine myo-cardial CK on three successive days in the same conscious dog. Fractional rate of disap-pearance of CK activity was virtually constant on each of the three days in the same dog.

in Figure 7. For more precise estimates of infarct size it would clearly be necess-ary to obtain the individual k_d for each animal or patient. The individual k_d can be obtained in the animal by injections of purified CK. On the other hand, it is not possible to obtain the individual k_d from the downslope of the plasma CK time activity curve associated with an infarct, since release of even minimal amounts of CK will markedly disturb the disappearance rate [33]. Thus, the latter method offers very little advantage over a mean k_d. Consequently, we continue to use a mean k_d in patients [64].

Since a myocardial infarct may be associated with significant hemodynamic impairment and alterations in organ perfusion, it is reasonable to expect a resultant change in the CK disappearance rate. Multiple studies performed in the experimental animal have shown that the plasma CK disappearance rate is not affected by marked changes in heart rate, blood pressure, or cardiac output [32]. Furthermore, reduced hepatic flow or occlusion of the renal arteries did not affect CK disappearance (Figure 8). It is not surprising that renal blood failed to affect k_d since creatine kinase has a molecular weight of 82,000 and thus would not be expected to be filtered by the glomerulus. Furthermore, we have shown with ^{14}C-labeled CK that the intact molecule does not appear in the urine. Perhaps more important were the results of studies [6] showing that CK disap-pearance rates determined with ^{14}C-labeled CK before, during and after infarct

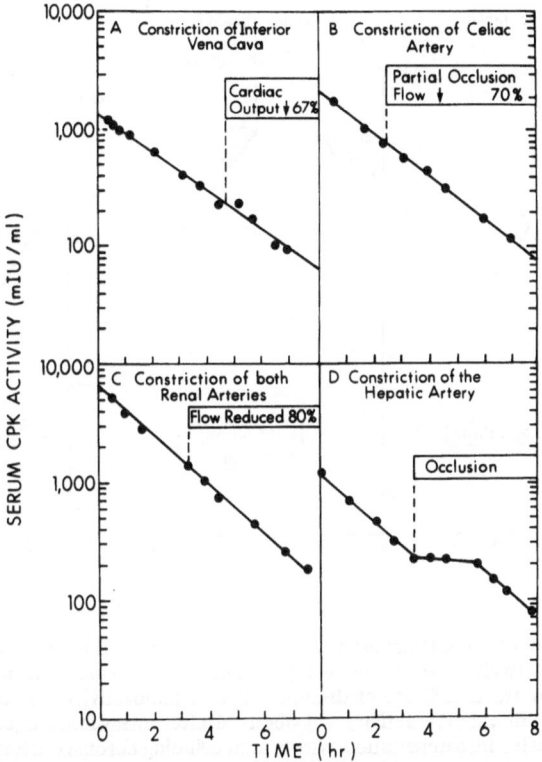

Figure 8. Myocardial CK was purified from dog hearts and injected intravenously into conscious dogs. The serum CK activity was determined serially to assess the CK disappearance rate. Following an inition control period of 3–4 h, the interventions were performed and the CK disappearance rates before and after the interventions were compared. At 5–10 days prior to the interventions, the animals had been instrumented and appropriate catheters exteriorized to the skin. Cardiac output was monitored with a flow meter on the aorta, and flow in the celiac, renal, and hepatic arteries was measured with flow meters distal to the balloon ligature, which was inflated while the dogs were conscious to reduce flow in the appropriate vessel.

in the experimental animal were virtually identical (Figure 9). We have also shown that therapeutic concentrations of commonly used drugs such as lidocaine, morphine, valium, and corticosteroids do not affect k_d but that high doses retard the disappearance rate [61]. Norris' parallel observations in patients [65] indicate that CK disappearance remains remarkably constant within the same patient in association with repeated infarcts. These data in experimental animals and patients support the view that the CK disappearance rate remains relatively constant during evolution of an infarct despite the variation in disappearance rates from animal to animal or patient to patient.

120

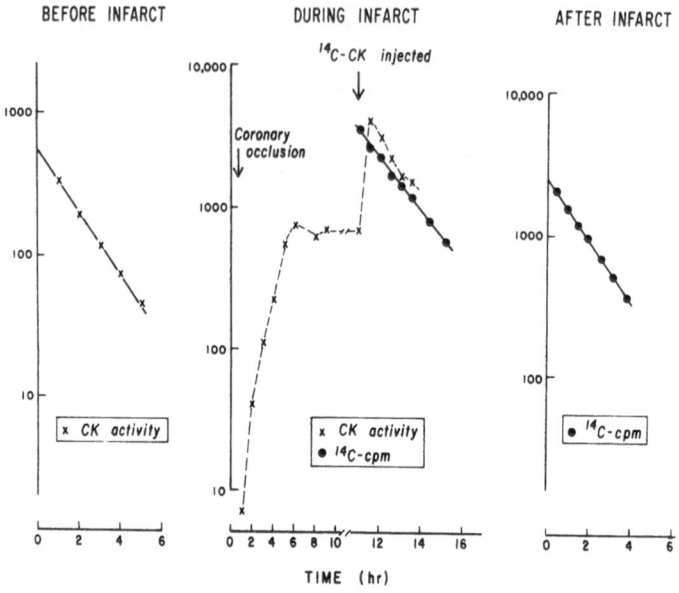

Figure 9. The effect of myocardial infarct on the disappearance rate of CK after intravenous injection of radioactively labeled canine myocardial CK in a conscious dog. In the experiment depicted, the fractional rate of disappearance of radioactivity remained constant for 5 h. (*Left*) Change in enzyme activity (*x*) observed after intravenous injection of CK in a conscious animal after instrumentation with a nonoccluding coronary artery snare. (*Center*) Serial changes in plasma CK activity (*x*) elicited by constriction of the snare in the same conscious animal. As can be seen, enzyme activity rose rapidly for approximately 6 h and then remained elevated as a result of the experimentally induced and evolving myocardial infarct. Approximately 11 h after the persistent coronary occlusion, exogenous ^{14}C-CK was injected intravenously during the continuing evolution of the infarct. The decline of radioactivity approximated a monoexponential function for 5 h with a slope similar to that observed with cold CK before infarct. (*Right*) A third study performed in the same dog after recovery from the experimentally induced myocardial infarct. Again, the fractional disappearance rate of radioactivity associated with ^{14}C-CK decline approximated first-order kinetics for 4 h with a similar fractional disappearance rate. Thus, the rate of disappearance of cold CK before infarct was similar to the rate of disappearance of radioactivity associated with ^{14}C-CK both during and after experimentally induced myocardial infarct. The calculated half-lives applicable to the three panels are 88, 84, and 80 min. This particular experiment was selected for purposes of illustration because the disappearance rate of counts approximated a first-order function for a relatively long interval. In other experiments (data not shown), deviation from first-order disappearance occurred as early as 3 h after injection, but the parallelism between k_d before, during, and after infarct was preserved.

DISTRIBUTION VOLUME AND THE RATIO OF CK_r/CK_d

Initially the distribution volume of CK was determined by the dilution principle after intravenous injection of partially purified canine myocardial CK in consious dogs. Using a one-compartment model and probably because of partial denaturation or the presence of other exogenous impurities, the initial distribution volume was found to be 11% of body weight [2]. With improved purification techniques for canine CK, based on first-order kinetics, the distribution volume was estimated to be approximately that of plasma volume, which in the dog is 5% of body weight. These revised estimates, however, of distribution volume do not necessitate alteration in estimates of infarct size published previously. This is the case because the proportionality constant comprises a derived value for CK_r/CK_d and therefore contains k_d in its denominator. On the other hand, calculations of infarct size include k_d in the numerator. Thus, a systematic error in the estimate of k_d appears in both terms and will offset for the value derived for infarct size [63]. Regardless of what method is used to estimate a parameter value for k_d, the same approach should be used in calculating infarct size and in determining the proportionality constant relating CK-g-eq calculated from plasma CK time activity curves to grams of infarct. However, it does change the ratio of CK_r/CK_d (P_k), which is delineated in the appendix and differs from that originally published in 1971 [2].

The term CK_r/CK_d, that is, the ratio of CK lost from the heart to that released into the blood, has been found experimentally to average 0.15 ± 0.016 (SEM) (based on a distribution volume equal to plasma volume). The relatively low proportion of CK reaching blood has not been well explained. Local inactivation of enzyme activity within the necrotic myocardium probably plays a major role. Another factor, cardiac lymph, may play a role in transporting CK from ischemic myocardium into the circulation. Since lymph flow is very slow, transport of the enzyme is likely to result in prolonged exposure. We have recently shown that CK, in contrast to several other enzymes, undergoes more rapid inactivation when exposed to lymph than when exposed to blood [66]. Although inactivation can be retarded by adding buffer, it appears to play a significant role in influencing plama CK time activity curves for myocardial infarcts. For example, the observed ratio of CK_r/CK_d in animals subjected to coronary occlusion followed by occlusion of the lymphatics draining the heart was substantially less than the ratio in animals with coronary occlusion alone, even though the disappearance rate of enzymes that reached the systemic circulation was comparable in the two groups and even though the amount of CK depleted from the heart was also comparable. Further studies are required to delineate the role of lymphatics since the lymphatic volume is extremely small and the evidence that lymphatic flow is a major carrier for enzymes from the heart is based on high activities observed in the lymph while simultaneously assessing CK activity in the blood. However, since the volume of lymph is so low and the flow is slow, CK accumulates; this may account in part for the high CK activity rather than the assumption that a higher proportion of the enzyme is being transported by the lymph [67]. Studies by Nordbeck et al. [68] indicate that the lymph is responsible for transporting only about 10%–15% of the CK activity released

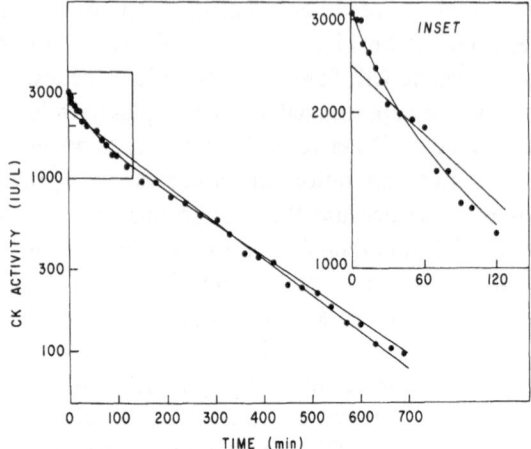

Figure 10. Single- and double-exponential fits to plasma creatine kinase (CK) activity after bolus injection of purified myocardial CK in a conscious dog, calculated by least-squares approximation.

from the myocardium. Despite the continuing controversy, alterations in lymph flow during infarction due to intramyocardial edema, changes in venous pressure, regional myocardial compliance, and heart rate may alter the duration of exposure of CK liberated from necrotic tissue to lymph in vivo and in turn affect the proportion of CK depleted to CK released into the blood. Characterization of lymphatic egress from the heart may therefore be useful in refining enzymatic estimates of infarct size.

MULTICOMPARTMENTAL VERSUS SINGLE-COMPARTMENTAL ANALYSIS

One other factor that may contribute to a low ratio of CK_r/CK_d is the probability that CK released from the heart is distributed in at least one extravascular compartment. The correct mathematical analysis of plasma fractional disappearance rates of enzymes and other proteins has been a source of considerable confusion among enzymologists, biochemists, and clinicians for several years. As can be observed from inspection of the CK disappearance curve in Figure 10, the decline of activity in the initial part of the curve is faster than the remaining portion. Interpretation of which portion of the curve, if either, reflects the true enzyme elimination rate varies. Some investigators have stated that the initial portion is a more appropriate disappearance rate; others have utilized the slow portion as a true elimination rate [33]. From work on several proteins, particularly albumin, and also other enzymes, it is clear that their behaviour is better

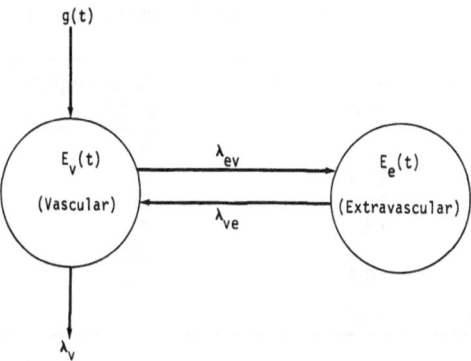

Figure 11. Diagrammatic illustration of the two-compartmenal model: $g(t)$ is any input function; $Ev(t)$ is enzyme activity in the vascular pool; $Ee(t)$ is enzyme activity in the extravascular pool; λev and λve are exchange rates from vascular to extravascular and extravascular to vascular pools; and λv is the true disappearance rate of CK from the blood pool. As indicated in the text, λv is not the same as the observed slope of the plasma CK time activity curve, which is influenced not only by disappearance but also by resupply of the vascular pool from an extravascular compartment. Although CK activity may be eliminated from the extravascular pool, we have assumed that elimination occurs from blood only for two reasons: (a) disappearance of activity in lymph in vitro is very slow compared with disappearance from blood in vivo, and (b) the assumption of elimination from both pools results in nonunique estimates for the two elimination rates.

described with multiple-compartment models, since these substances are distributed in extravascular as well as vascular pools [33]. Thus, the faster initial decline is probably due not only to removal of CK from the plasma compartment by metabolic pathways, also to diffusion into an extravascular compartment. The late slower decay may be due in part to back diffusion of the enzyme from extravascular to vascular pool. Extrapolation of the first portion of the curve to zero time provides a lower estimate of the volume of distribution that that obtained by extrapolation of the latter portion. Neither of these oversimplifications correctly approximates the true disappearance rate of the true distribution volume.

In a recent study [33], we compared fits of actual CK data to single- and double-exponential functions. The double-exponential function was used to obtain parameters for a two-compartment model assuming distribution of CK in an extravascular compartment, first-order transfer rates between blood and extravascular compartments, and a first-order elimination rate from blood (Figure 11). With this model, the amount of CK present in the vascular and extravascular compartments as a function of time can be described by the following system of differential equations in which $g(t)$ is an input function:

$$\frac{dEv(t)}{dt} = \lambda veEe(t) - (\lambda ev + \sigma v)\,Ev(t) + g(t)$$

Table 2. Overall standard deviation between data and fit curves[a]

Dog no.	Single-exponential fit (%)	Double-exponential fit (%)
1	20.8	3.6
2	10.4	6.7
3	15.9	5.6
4	18.2	7.3
5	15.4	10.0
6	10.3	5.2
Mean	15.2	6.4

[a]Expressed as the percentage of the data point values in each case.

$$\frac{dEe(t)}{dt} = \lambda evE(t) - \lambda veEc(t)$$

$Ev(t)$ and $Ee(t)$ represent enzyme activity in the vascular and extravascular compartments, respectively, and (t) equals time; λve and λev represent exchange rates from the vascular to the extravascular and from the extrascular to the vascular compartments, respectively. The two-compartment model provides an estimate of the true disappearance rate of CK from the circulation that is substantially greater than the observed elimination rate, that is, the rate of decline of activity from monoexponential fit. This is because the model takes into account a continuing supply of the vascular pool with enzyme from the extravascular compartment. The assumption that the disappearance rate obtained from a double-exponential fit approximates the true CK disappearance rate more closely than that obtained from a single-exponential fit is supported by the much smaller standard deviation of the data from the double-exponential than from the monoexponential fit as illustrated in Table 2. Since enzymatic estimates of infarct size are dependent on the true disappearance rate as one parameter, the two-compartment model accounts for more CK released from the heart, based on calculations with a given plasma curve, than the one-compartment model, as illustrated in Table 3.

To simplify the calculations, this model assumes no loss of CK from the extravascular compartment, since major assumptions would be required to account for, or solve for, loss of enzyme from the extravascular compartment and these assumptions themselves introduce a greater error. Although this model results in an apparent improvement in the estimation of CK disappearance rates, it does not take into account the observation that CK released from the heart enters the circulation at least in part via the lymph. It is also important to emphasize that although this mathematical analysis more closely reflects the experimental data, confirmation that the intercompartmental transfer rates are

Table 3. Calculated creatine kinase (CK) released (IU)

Dog no.	Two-compartment model (λv)	One-compartment model (k)
1	22,470	13,700
2	5,040	3,070
3	52,710	32,230

correct has not yet been obtained, nor has the nature of the extravascular compartment(s) been determined experimentally.

If CK disappearance is indeed multicompartmental, other influences must be accounted for in enzymatic estimates of infarct size. Changes in rates of exchange between compartments might be anticipated in association with hemodynamic compromise, hypovolemia, sepsis, or any other phenomenon altering permeability of vascular or lymphatic tissue. Improvement in enzymatic estimates of infarct size may be facilitated by development and application of direct means to assess distribution volumes and true enzyme disappearance rates in individual cases by using tracers. The two-compartment model is important for another reason as well. Because of resupply of the vascular space from an extravascular pool and from sustained release of enzyme from the heart relatively late after the onset of infarct, k_d cannot be estimated accurately in any individual case simply by analyzing the declining portion of the plasma time activity curve after infarct. If the k_d values are to be determined independently in individual cases, it will be necessary to perform analysis by tracer kinetics.

ENDOGENOUS VERSUS EXOGENOUS CK

The determination of CK disappearance is further complicated by the recent observation that purified myocardial CK injected as a bolus exhibited a different disappearance rate than CK-rich plasma that was collected from dogs subjected to infarct and that was then infused into a recipient animal. The CK disappearance from the CK-rich plasma was slower than that from the purified canine CK [33]. Despite this difference, purified canine myocardial CK based on electrophoresis and immunoelectrophoresis was similar to CK obtained from CK-rich plasma [33]. Similarly zymosan, which is known to inhibit the disappearance of purified myocardial CK, also inhibits the disappearance of endogenous-released CK. The estimates of the absolute amount of CK released utilizing values for k_d obtained from studies with purified myocardial CK would entail systematic errors, although estimates in infarct size would not, because they represent derived values. The difference in the disappearance rates of CK purified from plasma and CK from myocardium is illustrated in Figure 12. The reason for these observed differences is not clear, although it is anticipated that

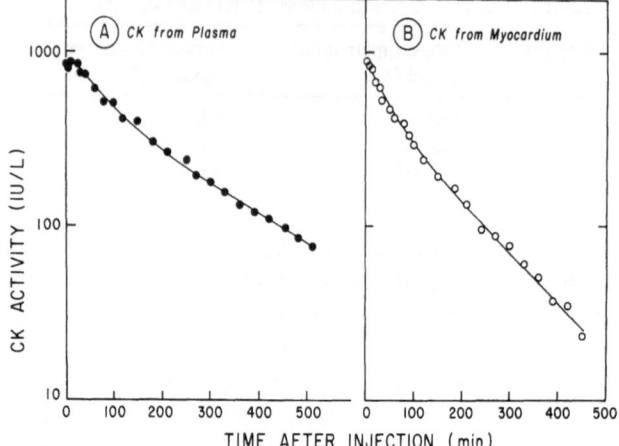

Figure 12. (*A*) The disappearance of purified myocardial CK injected in a conscious dog. (*B*) The disappearance of CK extracted from plasma injected intravenously in the same dog.

some conformational change is induced or a small carrier molecule is removed in the process of purification which alters its degradation or removal rate.

THE EFFECT OF CORONARY FLOW ON CK_r/CK_d

CK_r/CK_d may depend on coronary flow (see Cobb and Roe, p. 143). Cairns et al. [7] have shown in the dog that multiple small scattered areas of infarct induced by intracoronary glass beads were associated with a greater CK_r/CK_d than were transmural infarctions. In the animals with coronary artery ligation, CK released into the plasma correlated closely with that depleted from the myocardium, but a greater proportion of the CK depleted was released into the plasma after scattered small infarcts induced by glass beads. Swain et al. [60] observed in animals with myocardial damage secondary to coronary occlusion that infarct size as determined histologically was underestimated in large infarcts by the plasma CK method but the two methods correlated well in small and medium-sized infarcts. Regional myocardial blood flow estimated with the microsphere technique showed less coronary flow to the center of large infarct than to small areas of damage. The explanation put forward by Swain et al. [60] and Cairns et al. [7] was similar, namely that with less flow to the center of a large area of damage, there was less CK transported into the blood. As a result, more CK was degraded locally, which would tend to decrease the ratio of CK released to that depleted. In small areas of necrosis, where access of CK to coronary flow would be greater, the reverse effect on the ratio would occur. The disparity between enzymatic estimates of infarct size and those of histology performed 4—5 days after coronary occlusion as observed by Swain et al. may be due in part to overestimates of infarct size by histology that is known to occur because of edematous expansion [24]. Results of the study by Cairns et al. [7] may not be relevant to man since infarcts induced by glass beads are unlikely to simulate infarcts in man. Nevertheless, results of both studies indicate that the ratio of CK released to that depleted is indeed influenced by coronary flow. Until precise estimates of the CK disappearance rate and distribution volume can be determined, however, it is not feasible to assess quantitatively the effect of coronary flow versus other parameters on CK_r/CK_d since this ratio is derived from the plasma CK disappearance rate and distribution volume. There is increasing evidence that myocardial infarct in man is frequently associated with less than complete coronary occlusion and is not represented by the model of infarcts induced experimentally by complete coronary ligation or by the insertion of intracoronary glass beads, which tends not only to cause complete obstruction but also to inhibit collateral flow. Despite these imperfections, the correlations in man are remarkably good between enzymatic estimates of infarct size and other clinical parameters known to reflect morbidity and mortality.

CK AS A MARKER OF IRREVERSIBLE INJURY

It remains to be determined whether release of CK from the myocardium reflects irreversible injury. This is in part related to the fact that there is no available proven in vivo indicator for irreversible myocardial injury. Based on results of experimental and clinical studies to date, however, it is perhaps reasonable to assume that release of CK from the myocardium reflects irreversible injury. Hirzel et al. [4] showed in a histologic study that myocardial CK depletion was an all or none phenomenon. At 24 h after occlusion, myocardial cells in the dog exhibited either complete depletion of CK activity or normal CK activity. There was no border zone with partial depletion as might be expected if release occurred as a result of ischemia. In a series of experiments in which coronary occlusion was performed for durations of 10 min to 48 h, release of CK corresponded to morphologic evidence of necrosis as assessed by histology 48 h after occlusion [69]. Less than 30 min of coronary occlusion was not associated with release of CK or histologic evidence of infarct.

Clinical studies in patients with prolonged chest pain and unstable angina have shown that plasma MB CK remains in the normal range [70]. We have documented in patients with coronary artery disease (documented by coronary antiograms) and exercise-induced ischemia (detected by ECG) that total plasma CK is significantly elevated due to release of MM from sketal muscle, but plasma MB CK remains normal [71]. Release of CK from the myocardium has been shown to correlate closely with many conventional parameters that reflect myocardial injury, as previously discussed.

Results of studies with isolated perfused hearts have shown that transient anoxia or hypoxia is associated with release of CK, but in none of these experiments has histologic assessment been performed to exclude myocardial necrosis [72]. Perfusion of isolated hearts with calcium free media is also known to be associated with release of CK but this is not a physiologic condition or one simulated by clinical ischemic states. Exercise is known to cause release of CK from sketal muscles particularly in the nonconditioned individual, but cellular damage, which may be only minimal and may significantly elevate plasma CK in view of the abundance of CK in skeletal muscle, has not been excluded. Cellular damage may account for the severe muscle aches that accompany exercise. Even if release of CK occurs from skeletal muscle without irreversible injury, the myocardium may respond differently, particularly since cardiac muscle has a different outer calyx and also a somewhat different plasma membrane.

CLINICAL APPLICATION OF ENZYMATIC ESTIMATES OF INFARCT SIZE

Enzymatic estimates of infarct size in patients are based on a similar approach to that in the animal [32, 64]. Blood samples are collected serially every 4 h from an indwelling catheter for a minimum of 72 h, are assayed for plasma total and MB CK activity, and analyzed as previously discussed to obtain estimates of infarct size expressed as CK-g-eq. CK activitiy in human myocardium obtained within 1 h of death showed a normal average of 1600 IU/g [63]. The distribution of myocardial CK activity in the myocardium has not been adequately determined for humans due to the lack of fresh material and hearts that are free of previous or new myocardial damage. However, based on the uniform distribution of CK activity in the dog and observations in a limited number of samples from normal human myocardium, a uniform distribution is assumed throughout the human myocardium. The CK disappearance rate in man is derived from the downslope of the plasma CK time activity curve utilizing the portion that closely approximates monoexponential decay. A mean fractional disappearance rate of $0.001 \, min^{-1}$ is utilized routinely rather than the individual CK disappearance rate. This number was obtained from data in 80 patients with uncomplicated myocardial infarcts in whom plasma CK time activity curves exhibited a monoexponential downslope. It is assumed that 1 g homogeneous necrosis loses 75% of its CK activity as observed in the experimental animal. The CK_r/CK_d is assumed to be 0.15, an assumption also based on data observed in the experimental animal. The distribution volume is assumed to be that of plasma, which in man is equal to 4.5% of body weight. The values included in the appendix for estimating infarct size from total plasma CK have been revised from those originally published [64], which assumed from papillary muscle biopsies that human myocardium contained about 900 IU/g; this Figure has been increased to 1600 IU/g. Estimates of infarct size based on plasma MB CK also have been included; the constant differs from that of total CK since only 15% of myocardial CK activity is MB CK and its disappearance rate is faster than that of MM.

Enzymatic estimates of infarct size have now been utilized by numerous investigators in patients with acute myocardial infarcts. Utilizing plasma MB CK, it is possible to estimate infarct size despite complications such as intramuscular injections, cardiac failure, cardiogenic shock, and noncardiac surgery. Studies have been performed to examine the relationship between infarct size and ventricular performance, electrical instability of the heart, altered venticular compliance, morbidity, and mortality after the onset of myocardial infarct as well as exercise tolerance during the late recovery period [64, 65, 73–77].

Impairment of left ventricular performance assessed with [99m]TC-labeled albumin in patients 24–48 h after hospital admission correlated with enzymatically estimated infarct size [78], as did a reduction in ejection fraction assessed by contrast ventricular angiography in studies by Rogers and his associates [77]. Mathey et al. [79] have observed a close correlation between impairment of hemodynamic performance and infarct size. Patients with small infarcts (averaging 17 CK-g-eq) and without hemodynamic dysfunction had a mortality in the hospital of only 5%. In contrast, patients with moderate increases in left ventricular filling pressure and larger infarcts (averaging 42 CK-g-eq) had a mortality of 21%. Among those patients with marked impairment of left ventricular function and a high pulmonary artery end-diastolic pressure (exceeding 20 mmHg), infarct size averaged 99 CK-g-eq and mortality was 60% [73, 79]. Studies by Kahn et al. [80] showed that left ventricular failure occurred in about 5% of patients with infarcts less than 20 CK-g-eq, in one-third of patients with infarcts of 30–50 CK-g-eq, and in two-thirds of patients with infarcts greater than 50 CK-g-eq. Norris et al. [81] have demonstrated that the presence or absence of pulmonary venous congestion is a powerful clinical discriminator in distinguishing survivors from nonsurvivors after infarct. Other studies by Norris et al. [65] showed a good correlation between pulmonary venous hypertension detected radiographically and infarct size estimated enzymatically.

Recently, Rogers et al. [77] have observed a close correlation between enzymatically estimated infarct size and the mass of the left ventricle exhibiting dyskinesis as detected by left ventricular angiography in patients with acute myocardial infarct. This correlation coefficient exceeded 0.9 as did the correlation coefficient for the relationship between decreased ventricular compliance or increased pulmonary artery end-diastolic pressure and enzymatically estimated infarct size [79]. (see Rogers, p. 164). However, in patients with a previous myocardial infarct, the correlation was less close, reflecting a cumulative effect of myocardial damage on ventricular dyskinesis. Bleifeld and his associates have observed similar correlations between hemodynamic impairment and enzymatic estimates of infarct size in patients with initial infarction [73]. They found that infarct size estimated in patients by the CK method correlated closely with morphologic estimates of infarct size obtained at postmortem examination in patients who succumbed.

In the initial study correlating enzymatically estimated infarct size and prognosis of 12 patients with infarcts larger than 65 CK-g-eq, eight died within six months of infarction [64] and the four survivors manifested marked functional impairment. Only one of 21 patients with small infarcts died within six months. The average infarct size in survivors in class I and class II (New York Heart Association Clinical Classification) was 50% less than in the other patients studied. In a later series of 69 consecutively admitted patients whose plasma CK values were increasing at the time of admission and in whom a myocardial infarct was documented conventionally, mean infarct size among survivors was significantly less than among nonsurvivors (22 ± 2.5 vs 66 ± 6.9 CK-g-eq; mean $\pm$ SEM). These observations indicate that enzymatic estimates of infarct size represent a major determinant of acute mortality. In a recent report by Carter and Amundsen [74], recovery of exercise tolerence at three and six months after infarct appeared to be directly related to enzymatically estimated infarct size.

We have recently completed a study in 173 patients who survived their initial infarct and to our knowledge did not have a previous infarct [82]. Infarct size was estimated enzymatically and ventricular dysrhythmias were quantified by Holter monitor at the time of infarct and repeated every three months for the first year and yearly thereafter. The minimum follow-up was three months and the mean follow-up of the group was 21.7 months and ranged from three to 38 months. The mean infarct size of those patients who died was significantly larger than that of survivors (46.5 ± 5.8 vs 21.1 ± 1.4 CK-g-eq/m^2, $p < 0.001$). Overall survival was significantly better after small (less than 15 CK-g-eq/m^2) or moderate-sized infarcts (15–30) than after large infarcts (greater than 30) and the differences were significant ($p = 0.01$). Regardless of the locus of the infarct, patients with small infarcts had a better prognosis than those with larger infarcts. Late mortality was comparable after transmural and subendocardial infarcts but higher after anterior than after inferior infarcts (15% vs 6%; $p < 0.05$) [83]. Premature ventricular complexes were more frequent among patients with moderate-sized or large infarcts throughout the follow-up regardless of infarct locus. Similar results were obtained by Thompson et al. [84], who correlated peak plasma CK activity with long-term mortality and morbidity. Thus, the extent of infarct is a strong determinant of both ventricular dysrhythmia and mortality late as well as early after acute myocardial infarct.

Enzymatic estimates of infarct size have been used widely by numerous investigators to evaluate the effect of various interventions on ischemic myocardium. The interventions evaluated have included afterload reduction [85],

Table 4. Sample size required for mortality versus infarct size as an end point

Power	Mortality	Infarct size
	Sample size per group (to detect 20% difference)	
0.5	1105	113
0.667	1761	179
0.75	2197	223
0.8	2525	257
0.9	3497	355
0.95	4419	448
	Sample size per group (to detect 30% difference)	
0.5	465	41
0.667	740	65
0.75	923	81
0.8	1061	93
0.9	1470	128
0.95	1857	162

Each experiment was performed by injecting approx. 3000–5000 IU canine myocardial CK dissolved in saline intravenously in conscious dogs. The fractional disappearance rate of CK (k_d) was estimated from the slope of the best fit regression line (least-squares method) characterizing the decline of CK activity as a function of time after injection. It clearly shows the marked variation in disappearance rates from animal to animal.

methylprednisolone [86], acebutolol [87], external counterpulsation [88], nifedipine [89], propranolol [90, 91], aprindine [92], dobutamine [93], digitalis [94], and nitroglycerin [95]. In the initial studies to assess interventions, the CK prediction method was used. Based on a lognormal function fit to the plasma CK values of the first 7 h, we projected the remainder of the plasma CK curve, from which infarct size was calculated [85]. The intervention was then initiated and its effect assessed by comparing the actual infarct size estimated from all the CK values (96 h) with that of infarct size projected prior to the intervention. The correlation between predicted and actual infarct size was close, provided certain limitations were met: an initial baseline plasma CK value was obtained, the upslope of the curve was smooth with small standard deviation of the CK values, and the patient did not develop an extension. However, as more information was accrued on protection of ischemic myocardium, the long interval required to obtain adequate CK values for prediction precluded use of the method since the potential for salvage of ischemic myocardium is probably maximal in the first 6–12 h. At present, interventions are assessed by comparing infarct size in treated and placebo groups when therapy is initiated immediately after admission. The impact of enzymatic estimates of infarct size as an end point using this approach is illustrated in Table 4, which shows a marked reduction in the number of patients required to evaluate an intervention by using infarct size rather than mortality as an end-point. To demonstrate a 30% reduction in mortality, 1857 patients were needed as opposed to 162 patients needed for a 30% reduction in infarct size at an alpha level of 0.05 and a beta level of 0.20. Investigators have shown a close correlation between peak plasma CK and infarct size or total CK released [84]. The correlation between peak plasma CK and enzymatic estimates of infarct size is good if the upslope and downslope are fast with a sharp peak, but often there is a plateau peak in which case peak CK would underestimated infarct size. Frequently the plasma CK time activity curve is skewed and the correlation may be poor in such cases.

Adequate interpretation of qualitative and quantitative changes in infarct size induced by interventions requires delineation of the sensitivity, precision, and limitation of methods utilized. It is important before assessing the effect of a particular intervention on infarct size estimated by the CK method that the particular drug or agent be assessed for any potential influence it may have per se on CK disappearance, the CK assay, or the plasma CK release ratio. At the present time, the plasma CK method provides a reasonably objective quantitative approach for assessing infarct size. With the present intense interest and focus on infarct size, estimations of infarct size should improve.

CURRENT AND FUTURE STUDIES

Mitochondrial creatine kinase

Creatine kinase isoenzymes MM, MB, and BB are present in the cytosol, and a significant proportion of MM CK is bound to myosin and forms the so-called 'M' line of muscle [10]. Jacobs et al. [96] showed that mitochondria were also rich in CK activity and postulated that they contained a CK isoenzyme different from the cytosolic isoenzymes. Subsequently, CK activity associated with rat and dog heart mitochondria has been shown to exhibit several distinctive properties [97, 98] including a different k_m with a preference for ATP as substrate. Further characterization of mitochondrial CK has been difficult because of its lability and the difficulty of isolating it is pure form. Furthermore, it was argued on theoretical grounds that because there were only two subunits, a fourth isoenzyme would imply a different subunit. Recently, we have developed a method for purifying mitochondrial CK from dog hearts that results in a preparation that is devoid of other isoenzymes [99]. It remains to be determined whether mitochondria synthesizes its own creatine kinase or whether it is made in the nucleus and altered in some way during transport into the mitochondria. Synthesis by the mitochondria is possible since it does possess its own DNA and

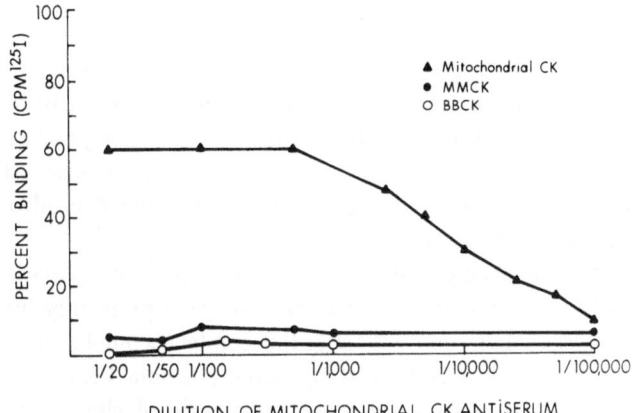

Figure 13. The specificity of mitochondrial CK antiserum. Maximum binding of mitochondrial CK occurs in a dilution of about 1:1,000 and decreases to about 10% at a titer of 1:100,000, indicating that binding depends on antibody concentration. In contrast, no binding above background is observed between MM or BB CK and that of mitochondrial CK antiserum, indicating no cross-reactivity between mitochondrial CK antiserum and that of the B or M subunits.

RNA apparatus. Furthermore, we have obtained an antibody to mitochondrial CK that appears to be specific since it exhibits no cross-reactivity with MM, MB, or BB even when the latter are present in 20,000-fold excess [100] (Figure 13). In view of these and other properties of mitochondrial CK (lability, rapid disappearance rate, and intracellular location), the use of mitochondrial CK in estimating infarct size may offer several potential advantages. Release of miotchondrial CK into the plasma almost certainly would reflect irreversible myocardial damage. Thus, comparative analysis would help to determine whether cytosolic isoenzymes are released under conditions other than those entailing cell death. Since mitochondrial CK disappears rapidly, diffusion into the extravascular compartment may be negligible due to the rapid removal within the vascular compartment is likely to be minimal compared with that observed with cytosolic CK isoenzymes. Accordingly, the plasma mitochondrial CK time activity curve should more closely reflect true enzyme disappearance rate, and may provide an approach to clinical estimation of individual values of k_d. Since mitochondrial CK is labile, local degradation is likely to be rapid, and washout or late release from zones of previous damage is unlikely. Accordingly, the declining portion of the curve is unlikely to be influenced by late release. If a radioimmunoassay could be developed for mitochondrial CK isoenzyme, it might provide not only a valuable diagnostic method for myocardial infarcts but also a more precise assessment of the extent of myocardial damage than that obtainable with the cytosolic CK isoenzymes.

Problems for future investigation

The estimation of CK release as a quantitative index of myocardial infarct has yielded important information and stimulated the development of new and improved techniques for the diagnosis and the assessment of patients with myocardial infarcts, but the data obtained thus far clearly indicate that further studies are necessary to characterize and refine the parameters needed for a more precise estimation of infarct size:

(1) The fractional disappearance rate of CK from the circulation must be individualized in each patient or animal, and analyzed preferably by multicompartmental analysis. At the present time, this can be accomplished in the experimental animal following injections of purified myocardial CK or of endogenous plasma CK obtained from an infarcted donor animal. A clinical application of this approach, however, is not possible. In the patient, the disappearance rate must be obtained from the plasma CK time activity curve and the possibility of continuing release, together with the lack of knowledge of the input, make further investigation necessary in order to obtain the most appropriate approximation of this mathematical analysis.

(2) With the present approach, only a small proportion of the CK depleted from the myocardium can be accounted for in the circulation. Further work is needed to assess whether this CK is really released or is degraded locally, and to characterize the factors involved in this process.

(3) Since only a portion of CK is released, it will be important to determine the factor(s) that may influence release and could potentially alter the ratio of CK released to CK depleted from the myocardium.

(4) Characterization of the mechanisms of CK disappearance from plasma and of the possible role of cell receptors is also needed.

(5) A complete characterization of mitochondrial CK isoenzyme is highly desirable in view of its potential as a marker of irreversible injury.

(6) An assessment of the role of lymph in enzyme release, transport, and removal also seems important, as it may contribute significantly to a more precise estimate of infarct size.

APPENDIX

CALCULATIONS OF INFARCT SIZE FROM SERIAL CHANGES IN MB OR TOTAL CK (EXPRESSED AS CK-G-EQ)

(1) $E(t)$ — activity of CK in blood (IU/ml^{-1})
          $f(t)$ — rate of change of CK activity due to enzyme being released by heart $(IU/min^{-1}/ml^{-1})$

k_d – fractional rate of disappearance of CK from blood (min^{-1})

$$\frac{dE}{dt} = f(t) - k_d e$$

(2) CK_r – cumulative activity of CK released by heart up to time T (IU/ml^{-1})

$$CK_r = \int_0^T f(t)\,dt = E(T) + k_d \int_0^T E(t)\,dt$$

(Note that CK_r is a function of T).

(3) K – proportionality constant $(\text{ml CK-g-eq/kg}^{-1}/\text{IU}^{-1})$

DV – distribution volume/unit body weight (ml/kg^{-1})

P_{ck} – proportion of CK released into blood compared to Ck depleted from the heart $(\text{IU/CK-g-eq}^{-1})/(\text{IU/g}^{-1})$

CK_n – CK activity in a homogeneous section of normal myocardial (IU/g^{-1})

CK_i – CK activity in a homogeneous section of infarcted myocardium (IU/g^{-1})

$$K = \frac{DV}{P_{ck}(CK_n - CK_i)}$$

(4)   IS   – infarct size (CK-g-eq)

BW – body weight (kg)

$$IS = (K)(BW)(CK_r)$$

(5)   Given N observed values of CK activity, $E(t_i), i = 1, 2, \ldots, N$, CK_r can be estimated from (see 2)

$$CK_r \approx \sum_{i=1}^{n-1} \bar{f}_i \Delta t_i = \sum_{i=1}^{n-1} \left(\frac{\Delta E_i}{\Delta t_i} + k_d \bar{E}_i \right) \Delta t_i = E(t_n) + k_d \sum_{i=1}^{n-1} \bar{E}_i \Delta t_i,$$

where

$$\Delta t_i = t_{i+1} - t_i,$$

$$\Delta E_i = E(t_{i+1}) - E(t_i),$$

$$E_i = \frac{E(t_{i+1}) + E(t_i)}{2}$$

and

$$\bar{f}_i = \frac{f(t_{i+1}) + E(t_i)}{2}$$

(Note that $E(t_1) = 0$ is assumed.)

VALUES CURRENTLY USED FOR CONSTANTS (BODY WEIGHT EXPRESSED IN KG)

Infarct size based on CK-MB	*Infarct size based on total CK*

$$k_d(CK - MB) = 0.0015 \qquad k_d(CK) = 0.001$$
$$DV^a = 44 \, ml \, kg^{-1} \qquad DV^a = 44 \, ml \, kg^{-1}$$
$$P_{CK-MB}{}^d = 0.15 \qquad P_{CK}{}^d = 0.15$$
$$CK_n - MB = 224 \, IU \, g^{-1\,b} \qquad CK_n = 1500 \, IU \, g^{-1\,b}$$
$$CK_i - MB = 44 \, IU \, g^{-1\,c} \qquad CK_i = 315 \, IU \, g^{-1\,c}$$
$$K = 1.6 \qquad K = 2.5 \times 10^{-1}$$

[a]Estimated as plasma volume for man (Nachman HM, James GW III, Moore JW, Evans EI: Comparative study of red cell volumes in human subjects with radioactive phosphorus tagged red cells and T-1824 dye. J Clin Invest 29:258, 1950).

[b]Measured directly.

[c]Calculated from percentage of myocardial CK depleted measured directly in conscious dogs 48 h after coronary occlusion.

[d] Calculated by analogy based on the empirical relation between CK release calculated from serum changes, and myocardial CK depletion measured directly in conscious dogs with coronary occlusion.

REFERENCES

1. Kjekshus JK, Sobel BE: Depressed myocardial creatine phosphokinase activity following experimental myocardial infarction in rabbit. Circ Res 27:403, 1970.
2. Shell WE, Kjekshus JK, Sobel BE: Quantitative assessment of the extent of myocardial infarction in the conscious dog by means of analysis of serial changes in serum creatine phosphokinase (CPK) activity. J Clin Invest 50:2614, 1971.
3. Fukuyama T, Roberts R: The effect of intravenous nitroglycerin on coronary blood flow and infarct size during myocardial infarction in conscious dogs. In: Nitrate I. Rudolph W, Schrey A (eds). Munchen—Wien—Baltimore: Urban and Schwarzenberg, 1980, p 342.
4. Hirzel HO, Sonnenblick EH, Kirk ES: Absence of a lateral border zone of intermediate creatine phosphokinase depletion surrounding a central infarct 24 hours after acute coronary occlusion in the dog. Circ Res 41:673, 1977.
5. Kjekshus JK: Assessment of myocardial injury with creatine phosphokinase (CPK). Circulation [Suppl 1] 53:106, 1976.
6. Kjekshus JK, Maroko PR, Sobel BE: Distribution of myocardial injury and its relation to epicardial ST-segment changes after coronary artery occlusion in the dog. Cardiovasc Res 6:490, 1972.
7. Cairns JA, Missirlis E, Fallen EL: Myocardial infarction size from serial

CPK: variability of CPK serum entry ratio with size and model of infarction. Circulation 58:1143, 1978.

8. Manders T, Vatner S, Millard R, Heyndrickx G, Maroko PR: Altered relationship between creatine phosphokinase release and infarct size with reperfusion in conscious dogs [abstr]. Circulation [Suppl] 52:II-5, 1975.

9. Yasmineh WG, Pyle RB, Cohn JN, Nicoloff DM, Hanson NQ, Steele BW: Serial serum creatine phosphokinase MB isoenzyme activity after myocardial infaction. Studies in the baboon and man. Circulation 55:733, 1977.

10. Wallimann T, Turner DC, Eppenberger HM: Localization of creatine kinase isoenzymes in myofibrils. I. Chicken skeletal muscle. J Cell Biol 75:297, 1977.

11. Maclean D, Fishbein MC, Maroko PR, Braunwald E: Hyaluronidase-induced reductions in myocardial infarct size. Science 194:199, 1976.

12. Kloner RA, Fishbein MC, Maroko PR, Braunwald E: The effect of propranolol on the ultra-structure of the myocardium following an experimental coronary artery occlusion [abstr]. Circulation [Suppl] 55 and 56:III-205, 1977.

13. Heng MK, Peter T, Norris RM, Nisbet H, Howell D, Ambler P: Failure of high doses of propranolol to reduce experimental infarct size in dogs [abstr]. Circulation 53 and 54:II-159, 1976.

14. Maroko PR, Libby P, Bloor CM, Sobel BE, Braunwald E: Reduction by hyaluronidase of myocardial necrosis following coronary artery occlusion. Circulation 46:430, 1972.

15. Fukuyama T, Roberts R: The effect of intravenous nitroglycerin on coronary blood flow and infarct size during myocardial infarction in conscious dogs. Clin Cardiol 3:317, 1980.

16. Muller JE, Maroko PR, Braunwald E: Evaluation of precordial electrocardiographic mapping as a means of assessing changes in myocardial ischemic injury. Circulation 52:16, 1975.

17. Smith HJ, Singh BN, Nisbet HD, Norris RM: Effects of verapamil on infarct size following experimental coronary occlusion. Cardiovasc Res 9:569, 1975.

18. Karlsberg RP, Henry PD, Ahmed SA, Sobel BE, Roberts R: Lack of protection of ischemic myocardium by verapamil in conscious dogs. Eur J Pharmacol 42:339, 1977.

19. Henry PD, Shuchleib R, Borda LJ, Roberts R, Williamson JR, Sobel BE: Effects of nifedipine on myocardial perfusion and ischemic injury in dogs. Circ Res 43:372, 1978.

20. Libby P, Maroko PR, Bloor CM, Sobel BE, Braunwald E: Reduction of experimental myocardial infarct size by corticosteroid administration. J Clin Invest 52:599, 1973.

21. Henry PD, Sobel BE, Braunwald E: Protection of hypoxic guinea pig hearts with glucose and insulin. Am J Physiol 226:309, 1974.

22. Jarmakani JM, Limbird L, Graham TC, Marks RA: Effect of reperfusion on myocardial infarct and the accuracy of estimating infarct size from serum creatine phosphokinase in the dog. Cardiovasc Res 10:245, 1976.

23. Bresnahan GF, Roberts R, Shell WE, Ross J Jr, Sobel BE: Deleterious effects due to hemorrhage after myocardial reperfusion. Am J Cardiol 33:82, 1974.

24. Reimer KA, Jennings RB: The changing anatomic reference base of evolving myocardial infarction. Underestimation of myocardial collateral blood flow and overestimation of experimental anatomic infarct size due

138

to tissue edema, hemorrhage and acute inflammation. Circulation 60:866, 1979.

25. Penkoske PA, Karlsberg RP, Roberts R: Salutary effects of anesthesia on myocardial infarction [abstr]. Clin Res 26:10A, 1978.

26. Karlsberg RP, Sobel BE, Roberts R: A standardized model for assessment of early interventions designed to protect ischemic myocardium [abstr]. Physiologist 19:249, 1976.

27. Lowe JE, Reimer KA, Jennings RB: Experimental infarct size as a function of the amount of myocardium at risk. Am J Pathol 90:363, 1978.

28. Roman W: Quantitative estimation of lactate dehyrogenase isoenzymes in serum. I. Review of methods and distribution in human tissues. Enzymologia 36:189, 1969.

29. Maroko PR, Kjekshus JK, Sobel BE, Watanbe T, Covell JW, Ross J Jr, Braunwald E: Factors influencing infarct size following experimental coronary artery occlusions. Circulation 43:67, 1971.

30. Maclean D, Fishbein MC, Maroko PR, Braunwald E: Hyaluronidase-induced reductions in myocardial infarct size. Science 194:199, 1976.

31. Weiss ES, Ahmed SA, Welch MJ, Williamson JR, Ter-Pogossian MM, Sobel BE: Quantification of infarction in cross sections of canine myocardium in vivo with positron emission transaxial tomography and ^{11}C-palmitate. Circulation 55:66, 1977.

32. Mimbs JW, Yuhas DE, Miller JG, Weiss AN, Sobel BE: Detection of myocardial infarction in vitro based on altered attenuation of ultrasound. Circ Res 41:192, 1977.

33. Roberts R, Henry PD, Sobel BE: An improved basis for enzymatic estimation of infarct size. Circulation 52:743, 1975.

34. Sobel BE, Markham J, Karlsberg RP, Roberts R: The nature of disappearance of creatine kinase from the circulation and its influence on enzymatic estimation of infarct size. Circ Res 41:836, 1977.

35. Batsakis JG, Briere RO: Interpretive enzymology. Springfield IL: Charles C Thomas, 1967.

36. Rosalki SB: Methods in the study of isoenzymes. Histochem J 6:361, 1974.

37. Goldberg DM, Winfield DA: Diagnostic accuracy of serum enzyme assays for myocardial infarction in a general hospital population. Br Heart J 34:597, 1972.

38. Smith AF: Diagnostic value of serum-creatine-kinase in coronary-care unit. Lancet 2:178, 1967.

39. Roe CR, Limbird LE, Wagner GS, Nerenberg ST: Combined isoenzyme analysis in the diagnosis of myocardial injury: application of electrophoretic methods for the detection and quantitation of the creatine phosphokinase MB isoenzyme. J Lab Clin Med 80:577, 1972.

40. Konttinen A, Sommer H: Determination of serum creatine kinase isoenzymes in myocardial infarction. Am J Cardiol 29:817, 1972.

41. Roberts R, Henry PD, Witteeveen SA, Sobel BE: Quantification of serum creatine phosphokinase (CPK) isoenzyme activity. Am J Cardiol 33:650, 1974.

42. Roberts R, Sobel BE: Creatine kinase isoenzymes in the assessment of heart disease. Am Heart J 95:521, 1978.

43. Henry PD, Roberts R, Sobel BE: Rapid separation of plasma creatine kinase isoenzymes by batch adsorption with glass beads. Clin Chem 21:844, 1975.

44. Mercer DW: Separation of tissue and serum creatine kinase isoenzymes by ion-exchange column chromatography. Clin Chem 29:36, 1974.
45. Yasmineh WG, Hanson NQ: Electrophoresis on cellulose acetate and chromatography on DEAE-sephadex A-50 compared in the estimation of creatine kinase isoenzymes. Clin Chem 21:381, 1975.
46. Tsung SH: Creatine kinase isoenzyme patterns in human tissues obtained at surgery. Clin Chem 22:173, 1976.
47. Ogunro EA, Hearse DJ, Shillingford JP: Creatine kinase isoenzymes: their separation and quantitation. Cardiovasc Res 11:94, 1977.
48. Roberts R, Gowda KS, Ludbrook PA, Sobel BE: Specificity of elevated serum MB creatine phosphokinase activity in the diagnosis of acute myocardial infarction. Am J Cardiol 36:433, 1975.
49. Strauss HD, Roberts R: Plasma MB creatine kinase activity and other conventional enzymes. Comparison in patients with chest pain and tachyarrhythmias. Arch Intern Med 140:336, 1980.
50. Roberts R, Ludbrook PA, Weiss ES, Sobel BE: Serum CPK isoenzymes after cardiac catheterization. Br Heart J 37:1144, 1975.
51. Smith AF, Radford D, Wong CP, Oliver MF: Creatine kinase MB isoenzyme studies in diagnosis of myocardial infarction. Br Heart J 38:225, 1976.
52. Veen KJ van der, Willebrands AF: Isoenzymes of creatine phosphokinase in tissue extracts and in normal and pathological sera. Clin Chim Acta 13:312, 1966.
53. Roberts R, Sobel BE: Elevated plasma MB creatine phosphokinase activity. A specific marker for myocardial infarction in perioperative patients. Arch Intern Med 136:421, 1976.
54. Gutovitz AL, Sobel BE, Roberts R: Progressive nature of myocardial injury in selected patients with cardiogenic shock. Am J Cardiol 41:469, 1978.
55. Marmor A, Fukuyama T, Roberts R: Integrity of creatine kinase isoenzymes maintained in a frozen state for up to three years [abstr]. Clin Res 27:617A, 1979.
56. Lemley-Stone J, Merrill JM, Grace JT, Meneely GR: Transaminase in experimental myocardial infarction. Am J Physiol 183:555, 1955.
57. Nydick I, Wroblewski F, LaDue JS: Evidence for increased serum glutamic oxalacetic transaminase (SGOT) activity following graded myocardial infarcts in dogs. Circulation 12:161, 1955.
58. Agress CM, Jacobs HI, Glassner HF, Lederer MA, Clark WG, Wroblewski F, Karman A, LaDue JS: Serum transaminase layers in experimental myocardial infarction. Circulation 11:711, 1955.
59. Nachlas MM, Friedman MM, Cohen SP: A method for the quantitation of myocardial infarcts and the relation of serum enzyme levels to infarct size. Surgery 55:700, 1964.
60. Swain JL, Cobb FR, McHale PA, Roe CR: Nonlinear relationship between creatine kinase estimates and histological extent of infarction in conscious dogs: effects of regional myocardial blood flow. Circulation 62:1239, 1981.
61. Roberts R, Sobel BE: Effect of selected drugs and myocardial infarction on the disappearance of creatine kinase from the circulation in conscious dogs. Cardiovasc Res 11:103, 1977.
62. Foo Y, Rosalki SB: Creatine kinase isoenzyme MB: discrepancy between

immuno-inhibition and electrophoretic measurement in lyophilized proficiency samples [lett]. Clin Chem 25:1341, 1979.

63. Sobel BE, Markham J, Roberts R: Factors influencing enzymatic estimates of infarct size. Am J Cardiol 39:130, 1977.

64. Sobel BE, Bresnahan GF, Shell WE, Yoder RD: Estimation of infarct size in man and its relation to prognosis. Circulation 46:640, 1972.

65. Norris RM, Whitlock RM, Barratt-Boyes C, Small CW: Clinical measurement of myocardial infarct size. Modification of a method for the estimation of total creatine phosphokinase release after myocardial infarction. Circulation 51:614, 1975.

66. Clark GL, Robison AK, Gnepp DR, Roberts R, Sobel BE: Effects of lymphatic transport of enzyme on plasma creatine kinase time-activity curves after myocardial infarction in dogs. Circ Res 43:162, 1978.

67. Gervin CA, Hackel DB, Roe CR: Enzyme content of canine cardiac lymph during acute myocardial infarction. Surg Forum 25:175, 1974.

68. Nordbeck H, Kahles H, Preusse CJ, Spieckermann PG: Enzymes in cardiac lymph and coronary blood under normal and pathophysiological conditions. J Mol Med 2:255, 1977.

69. Ahmed SA, Williamson JR, Roberts R, Clark RE, Sobel BE: The association of increased plasma MB CPK activity and irreversible ischemic myocardial injury in the dog. Circulation 54:187, 1976.

70. Klein MS, Ludbrook PA, Mimbs JW, Gafford FH, Gillespie TA, Weldon CS, Sobel BE, Roberts R: Perioperative mortality rate in patients with unstable angina selected by exclusion of myocardial infarction. J Thorac Cardiovasc Surg 73:253, 1977.

71. Klein MS, Weiss AN, Roberts R, Coleman RE: Technetium-99m stannous pyrophosphate scintigrams in normal subjects, patients with exercise-induced ischemia and patients with a calcified valve. Am J Cardiol 39:360, 1977.

72. Sakai K, Gebhard MM, Spieckermann PG, Bretschneider HJ: Enzyme release resulting from total ischemia and reperfusion in the isolated, perfused guinea pig heart. J Mol Cell Cardiol 7:827, 1975.

73. Bleifeld W, Mathey D, Hanrath P, Buss H, Effert S: Infarct size estimated from serial serum creatine phosphokinase in relation to left ventricular hemodynamics. Circulation 55:303, 1977.

74. Carter CL, Amundsen LR: Infarct size and exercise capacity after myocardial infarction. J Appl Physiol 42:782, 1977.

75. Roberts R, Husain A, Ambos HD, Oliver GC, Cox J Jr, Sobel BE: Relation between infarct size and ventricular arrhythmia. Br Heart J 37:1169, 1975.

76. Cox JR Jr, Roberts R, Ambos HD, Oliver GC, Sobel BE: Relations between enzymatically estimated myocardial infarct size and early ventricular dysrhythmia. Circulation [Suppl] 53:I-150, 1976.

77. Rogers WI, McDaniel HG, Smith LR, Mantle JA, Russell RO Jr, Rackley CE: Correlation of angiographic estimates of myocardial infarct size and accumulated release of creatine kinase MB isoenzyme in man. Circulation 56:199, 1977.

78. Kostuk WJ, Ehsani AA, Karliner JS, Ashburn WL, Peterson KL, Ross J Jr, Sobel BE: Left ventricular performance after myocardial infarction assessed by radioisotope angiocardiography. Circulation 47:242, 1973.

79. Mathey D, Bleifeld W, Hanrath P, Effert S: Attempt to quantitate relation

between cardiac function and infarct size in acute myocardial infarction. Br Heart J 36:271, 1974.

80. Kahn JC, Gueret P, Menier R, Giraudet P, Farhat MB, Bourdarias JP: Prognostic values of enzymatic (CPK) estimation of infarct size. J Mol Med 2:223, 1977.

81. Norris RM, Brandt PWT, Caughey DE, Lee AJ, Scott PJ: A new coronary prognostic index. Lancet 1:274, 1969.

82. Geltman EM, Ehsani AA, Campbell MK, Schechtman K, Roberts R, Sobel BE: The influence of location and extent of myocardial infarction on long-term ventricular dysrhythmia and mortality. Circulation 60:805, 1979.

83. Strauss HD, Sobel BE, Roberts R: The influence of occult right ventricular infarction on enzymatically estimated infarct size, hemodynamics and prognosis. Circulation 62:503, 1980.

84. Thompson PL, Fletcher EE, Katavatis V: Enzymatic indices of myocardial necrosis: influence on short- and long-term prognosis after myocardial infarction. Circulation 59:113, 1979.

85. Shell WE, Sobel BE: Protection of jeopardized ischemic myocardium by reduction of ventricular afterload. N Engl J Med 291:481, 1974.

86. Roberts R, DeMello V, Sobel BE: Deleterious effects of methylprednisolone in patients with myocardial infarction. Circulation [Suppl] 53:I-204, 1976.

87. Ahumada GG, Karlsberg RP, Jaffe AS, Ambos HD, Sobel BE, Roberts R: Reduction of early ventricular arrhythmia by acebutolol in patients with acute myocardial infarction. Br Heart J 41:65, 1979.

88. Gowda SK, Gillespie TA, Byrne JD, Ambos HD, Sobel BE, Roberts R: Effects of external counterpulsation on enzymatically estimated infarct size and ventricular arrhythmia. Br Heart J 40:308, 1978.

89. Henry PD, Shuchleib R, Borda LJ, Roberts R, Williamson JR, Sobel BE: Effects of nifedipine on myocardial perfusion and ischemic injury in dogs. Circ Res 43:372, 1978.

90. Peter T, Norris RM, Clark ED, Heng MK, Singh BN, Williams B, Howell DR, Ambler PK: Reduction of enzyme levels of propranolol after acute myocardial infarction. Circulation 57:1091, 1978.

91. Mueller H, Rao P, Evans R, Hamilton W, Ayres S: Propranolol reduces sympathetic activity during evolving myocardial infarction [abstr]. Circulation [Suppl] 58:II-60, 1978.

92. Geltman EM, Nordlicht SM, Gwinn JS Jr, Ambos HD, Roberts R: Effects of aprindine in patients with acute myocardial infarction [abstr]. Circulation [Suppl] 55 and 56:III-176, 1977.

93. Gillespie TA, Ambos HD, Sobel BE, Roberts R: Effects of dobutamine in patients with acute myocardial infarction [abstr]. Am J Cardiol 39:588, 1977.

94. Varonkov Y, Shell WE, Smirnow V, Gukovsky D, Chazov EI: Augmentation of serum CPK activity by digitalis in patients with acute myocardial infarction. Circulation 55:719, 1977.

95. Bowen WG, Branconi JM, Goldstein RA, Cain ME, Brodarick SM, Geltman EM, Jaffe AS, Ambos HD, Roberts R: A randomized prospective study of the effects of intravenous nitroglycerin in patients during myocardial infarction. Circulation 60:II-70, 1979.

96. Jacobs H, Heldt HW, Klingenberg M: High activitiy of creatine kinase in

mitochondrial from muscle to brain and evidence for a separate mitochondrial isoenzyme of creatine kinase. Biochem Biophys Res Commun 16:516, 1966.

97. Jacobus WE, Lehninger AL: Creatine kinase of rat heart mitochondrial. Coupling of creatine phosphorylation to electron transport. J Biol Chem 248:4803, 1973.

98. Sobel BE, Shell WE, Klein MS: An isoenzyme of creatine phosphokinase associated with rabbit heart mitochondria. J Mol Cell Cardiol 4:367, 1972.

99. Roberts R, Grace AM: Purification of mitochondrial creatine kinase: biochemical and immunological characterization. J Biol Chem 255:2870, 1980.

100. Grace A, Fukuyama T, Roberts R: Detection of elevated mitochondrial CK in plasma after infarction by a specific radioimmunoassay [abstr]. Am J Cardiol 45:414, 1980.

5. ENZYMATIC ESTIMATION: CONFOUNDING EFFECTS OF BLOOD FLOW TO INFARCTED MYOCARDIUM

FREDERICK R. COBB and CHARLES R. ROE

Studies from our laboratory [1–3] and others [4] have not demonstrated a close linear relationship between CK estimates and the histologic extent of myocardial infarction over the entire range of infarct sizes in experimental animals. The leading cause of this poor correlation is that CK appearance in the blood is disproportionately less and exhibits wide variation in animals that experience large as compared with small histologic infarcts. When myocardial tissue becomes totally necrotic, CK activity in the infarcted myocardium has been reported to decrease to approximately 25% [5, 6]. Only a small fraction of the depleted CK activity, approximately 15%–30% [5] (see Roberts, p. 115), has been reported to reach the circulating blood. The major fraction of depleted cellular CK activity is inactivated within the infarcted tissue and/or in lymph vessels which drain the infarcted myocardium [5, 7–9]. Quantitation of the extent of myocardial necrosis from analysis of serial measurements of CK activity in the blood requires that the fraction of CK activity per gram of infarcted myocardium that eventually appears in the blood is constant over the entire range of possible clinical infarcts. Additional parameters, which must be constants, include the body distribution space for CK enzyme and the rate at which CK disappears from the blood [5] (see Roberts, p. 114). This report will present studies from our laboratory [1–3] and others [4, 7, 8] which support the hypothesis that myocardial blood flow to regions of acutely infarcted myocardium is a variable that has a confounding influence on the appearance of CK activity in the blood. These studies have been performed in chronically instrumented, awake animals subjected to (a) permanent complete coronary artery occlusion [3], (b) extension of acute myocardial infarction effected by reduction of blood flow to the ischemic region [2], and (c) increases in blood flow to an acutely ischemic region by reperfusion at intervals after coronary occlusion.

RELATIONSHIP BETWEEN ENZYME ESTIMATES AND HISTOLOGIC EXTENT OF MYOCARDIAL INFARCTION FOLLOWING PERMANENT CORONARY ARTERY OCCLUSION

Studies were carried out in 23 healthy adult mongrel dogs, chronically prepared with catheters in the aorta and left atrium and adjustable snare type occluders

Wagner GS (ed): Myocardial Infarction: Measurement and Intervention, pp 143–158.
© *1982 Martinus Nijhoff Publishers, The Hague/Boston/London.*

on the distal or proximal left anterior descending coronary artery [3]. Studies were performed when the animals were in the awake resting state after complete recovery from surgery and free of anemia or signs of infection. Infarction was initiated by complete permanent coronary artery occlusion. Serial blood samples were obtained over a 72 h period for enzyme analysis. Enzyme estimates of infarction were calculated using the Shell formula [5], which assumes a constant serum CK appearance ratio K_r from infarcted myocardium. Regional myocardial blood flow was measured before coronary artery occlusion and at 15 min, and 2, 6, and 24 h after occlusion by using $9 \pm 1\,\mu$ microspheres. We then waited 5–6 days so that infarcted and noninfarcted myocardium would become sharply delineated and thus easily quantitated from routine histologic section. The left ventricle was sectioned into transverse rings, circumferential regions, and finally into four transmural layers; each sample size was 1–2 g. Regional blood flow and the extent of histologic infarction in each sample were quantitated. Special care was taken to ensure that all animals were studied in a steady, quiet, resting state and that all were treated identically. Each animal was sedated lightly with morphine sulphate at the initiation of coronary artery occlusion to minimize pain. Lidocaine, 2 mg/kg, was administered during the first hour of the occlusion. Analgesics and antiarrhythmic agents were not given after the first hour. To avoid repeated venipunctures, serial blood samples for CK analysis were obtained from a chronically implanted catheter in the superior vena cava. All animals that developed ventricular fibrillation were excluded; no animal was subjected to DC cardioversion; intramuscular injections were not used.

Occlusion of the left anterior descending coronary artery at various distances from the origin resulted in a wide range of histologic infarct size, i.e. 0.7–54.0 g or 0.7%–44.0% of the left ventricular weight. Figure 1 illustrates serial measurements of CK activity in six animals from this group; histologic infarct sizes were 10.0, 15.9, 18.2, 32.4, 38.8, and 40.5 g, and corresponding enzyme estimates were 50.5, 100.3, 77.8, 79.4, 76.9, and 113.2 g-eq, respectively. CK activity increased in the blood 2–3 h postocclusion and reached peak values 12–14 h after occlusion. These serial changes in CK activity in the blood are similar to those described by Shell et al. [9]. Figure 2 demonstrates the relationship between CK enzyme estimates in g-eq and histologic infarct size in grams in the total group of animals. In contrast to the linear relationship between infarct size and enzyme estimates described by Shell et al. [5], the equation that best described this relationship was a power function:

$$EE = 18.6 \times HI^{0.4} \qquad r = 0.91$$

Considering the entire range of infarcts, linear regression analysis between CK estimates and histologic extent of infarction demonstrated a poor correlation coefficient, 0.75, and a large SEE, ± 23 g. As the histologic infarct size increased above 20 g, CK appearance in the blood was variable and disproportionately

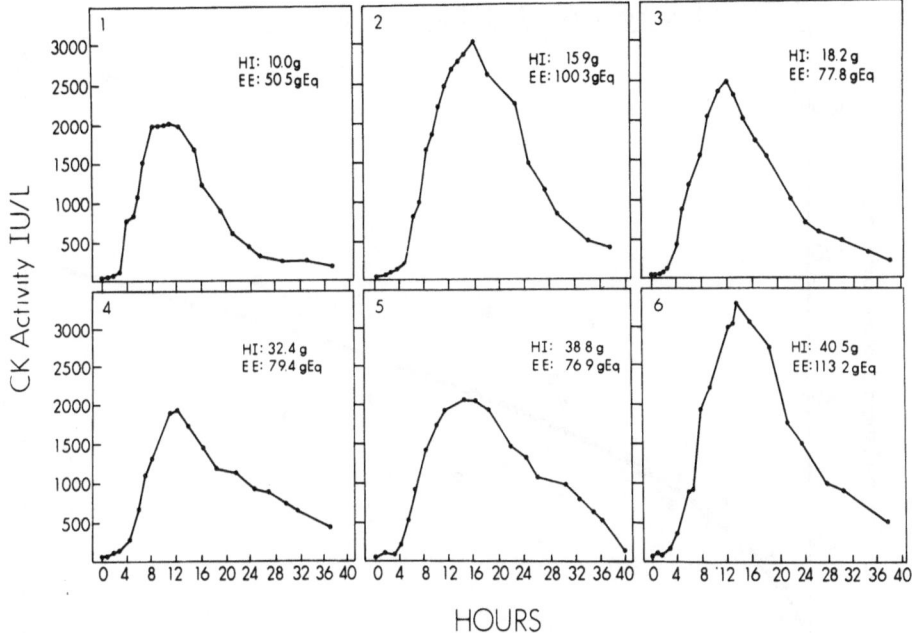

Figure 1. Serial measurements of CK activity (IU/L) following permanent occlusion of the left anterior descending coronary artery: HI, histologic infarct; EE, enzyme estimates of infarct in g-eq.

less. Consequently enzyme estimates did not differentiate infarct sizes above 20 g. If the upper range of infarcts in the present study had not exceeded 20 g, an excellent linear relationship between enzyme estimates and histologic infarcts would have been observed, $r = 0.94$.

K_r, the ratio of CK entering the serum to that released from infarcted tissue, was calculated using the Shell equation, the histologic extent of infarcts, and the serum CK appearance function:

$$K_r = \frac{\int_0^T f(t)\,dt \cdot K_w \cdot BW}{CK_D \cdot HI}$$

Figure 3 illustrates the relationship between the calculated K_r and the histologic infarct size. The equation that best described the relationship between K_r and histologic infarction was:

$$K_r = 5.53\,HI^{0.54} \qquad r = 0.93$$

As the histologic infarct size increased, the calculated K_r decreased as a power function. These data indicate a relative decrease in the appearance of enzyme activity in the serum as the infarct size increased.

Serial regional blood flow measurements demonstrated that as the extent of

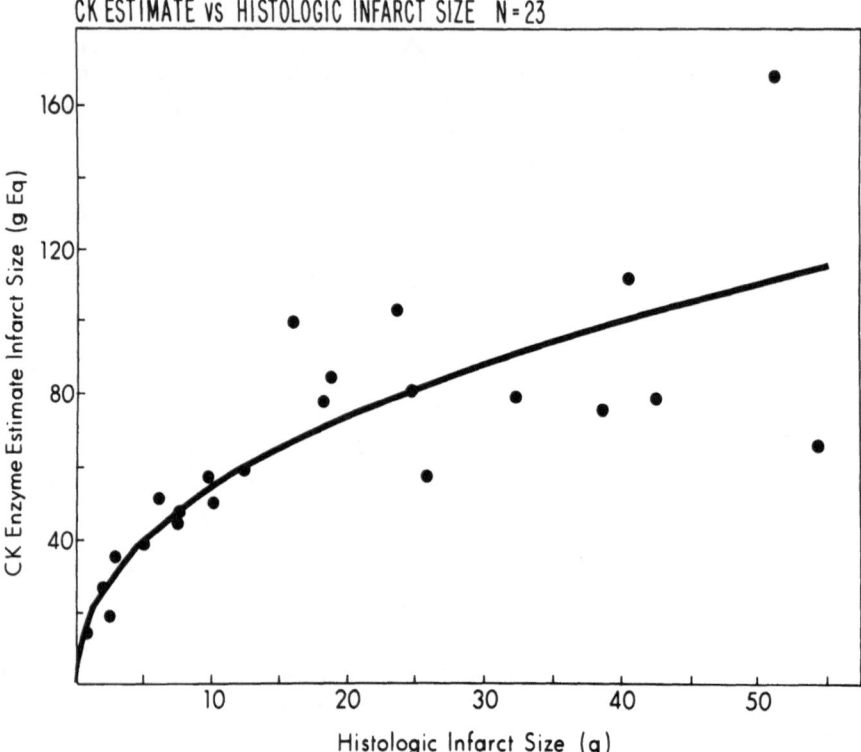

CK ESTIMATE vs HISTOLOGIC INFARCT SIZE   N = 23

Figure 2. Relationship between CK estimates of infarction and histologic extent of infarction. The equation that best describes the realtionship is a power function:

$$EE = 18.6 \ HI^{0.45} \qquad r = 0.91$$

Reprinted by permission of the American Heart Association [3].

infarction increased, the myocardial regions which remained severely ischemic
during the interval of greatest CK appearance in the blood also progressively
increased. Since most CK activity from infarcted myocardium is degraded within
the infarcted myocardium and does not appear in the blood [5] (see Roberts,
p. 115), we reasoned that areas that were severely ischemic during the interval
of CK appearance may release disproportionately smaller amounts of CK. In
an attempt to test this hypothesis, the tissue samples from the ischemic zone
were grouped according to the degree of severe ischemia, i.e., 0–0.05, 0–0.10,
0–0.15, 0–0.20 ml/min/g at each interval after occlusion, and the weight of
tissue perfused by each range of blood flow was calculated for each interval.
The total histologic infarct size was modified by subtracting the weight of
infarcted tissue in each blood flow range from the total weight of infarcted
tissue. This procedure resulted in a series of modifications of the original infarct

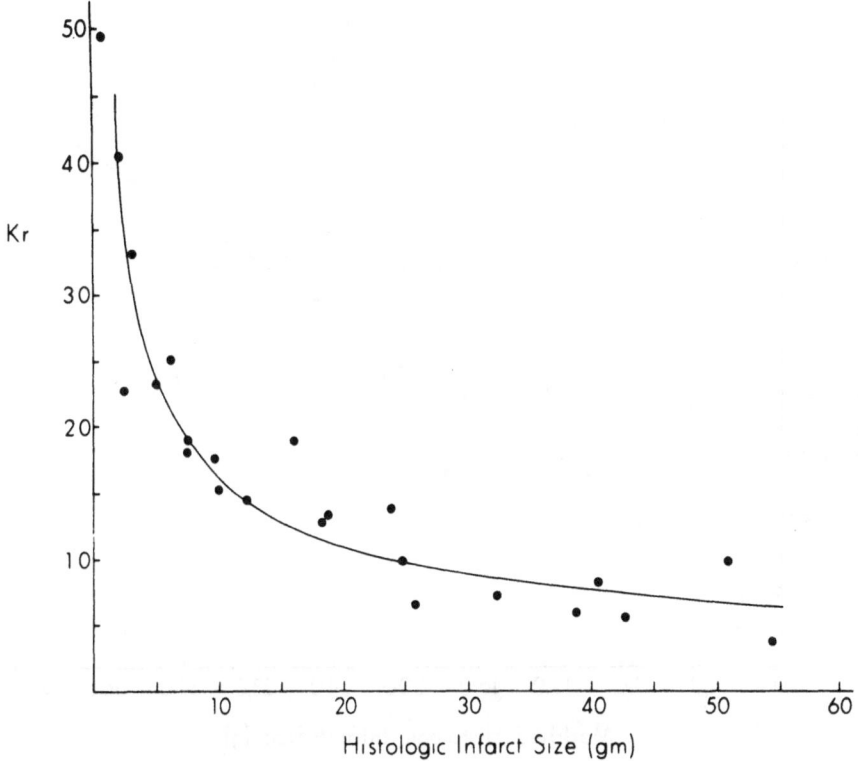

Figure 3. Relationship between the calculated K_r and the histologic extent of infarction:

$$K_r = 5.53 \, HI^{-0.54} \qquad r = 0.93$$

Reprinted by permission of the American Heart Association [3].

size. Linear regression analyses between CK estimates and each modification of histologic infarct size were carried out. The best linear correlation between CK estimates and a modified histologic infarct resulted from subtracting the tissue weight of samples in which blood flow 24 h after occlusion was in the 0–0.10 ml/min/g flow range, $r = 0.81 \pm 20$ SEM, Figure 4. None of the animals with less than 10 g of histologic infarction had tissue samples with less than 0.10 ml/min/g at 24 h and consequently no corrections were made. Although this modification resulted in a modest improvement in the linear correlation coefficient, significant variability in the relationship still remained, indicating an imprecise relationship between reduced blood flow and reduced CK appearance. As will be discussed in the final section of this report, increases in blood flow to regions containing infarcted myocardium may effect increases in CK appearance. Serial measurements of blood flow following permanent coronary

148

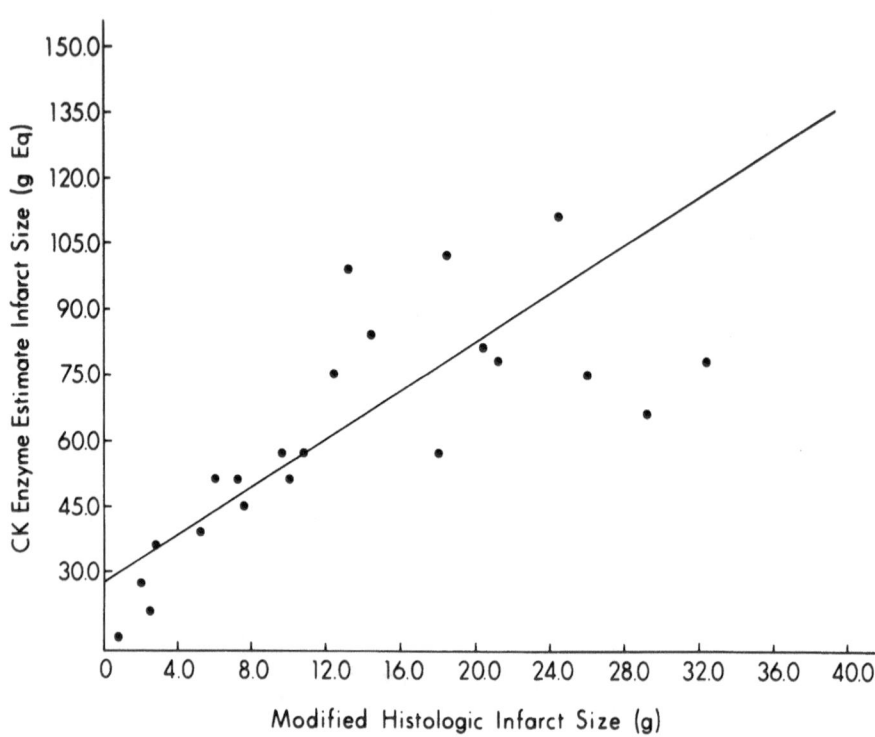

Figure 4. Relationship between CK estimate of infarction and the histologic infarct size modified by subtraction of tissue perfused by blood flow less than 0.10 ml/min/g at 24 h. Reprinted by permission of the American Heart Association [3].

occlusion have demonstrated significant but variable increases in collateral blood during the first 24 h post occlusion; this collateral flow is preferentially delivered to the periphery of the ischemic zone [10]. It is thus possible that CK appearance in the blood is influenced by complex interactions between regional necrosis and regional blood flow; this interaction may be different in different regions of the infarcted zone as well as in different-sized infarcts.

Certain anatomic characteristics of the acutely injured region may have contributed to disproportionate release of CK. The infarcted region in the small infarcts tends to be patchy with considerable interdigiting of normal and infarcted tissue; the large infarcts are characterized by extensive areas of confluent necrosis. The interface between noninfarcted and infarcted tissue would be relatively larger in the small infarcts. It is possible that the infarct pattern affects the diffusion distance of CK enzymes and consequently influences the time that the enzyme is exposed to factors that bring about enzyme degradation before release from the heart. Finally, previous studies have reported that cardiac lymphatics transport a major portion of the released myocardial CK to the blood [11, 12]. The K_d of the CK in lymphatic fluid is much higher than the K_d in serum. The time that CK remains in the lymph vessels may influence the net appearance of CK acitivty in the blood. Clark et al. [13] reported that interruption of cardiac lymph flow by occlusive snares 5 h after coronary occlusion reduced the total CK activity released into the blood. Effects of the extent of infarction and/or degree of ischemia on cardiac lymph flow are not known. A variable and/or reduced lymph flow in large infarcts could contribute to variable and disproportionate appearance of CK in the peripheral blood.

These studies indicate that over the entire range of myocardial infarcts produced by permanent coronary occlusion that the relationship between enzyme estimates and histologic extent of infarction is best described by a power function rather than a linear function. This relationship may be caused by progressive reductions of CK activity released from regions of severely reduced blood flow. Estimates of infarct size from serum CK measurements using a constant K_r introduced an error that increased as infarct size increased. This conclusion is consistent with the observation made by Cairns et al. [4], who observed an inverse linear relationship between the serum entry ratio and the extent of infarction in nine dogs after total coronary artery occlusion. Consequently there was disproportionately less CK appearance in the blood in the larger infarcts.

Studies by Reimer et al. [14] and Jugdutt et al. [15] have reported significant tissue edema occurring after myocardial infarction. Tissue edema would tend to increase the weight of the infarcted tissue preferentially. It has been reasoned that edema of infarcted myocardium accounts for a portion of the apparent microsphere loss that has been observed after myocardial infarction [14–17]. Tissue edema would also tend to dilute the content of radioactive microspheres present in the tissue prior to infarction, resulting in a calculated apparent microsphere loss. Studies have demonstrated that apparent microsphere loss in infarcted myocardium is near maximum 24 h after coronary occlusion [15–17]. It follows that tissue edema would also be near maximum approximately 24 h after coronary occlusion. Tissue edema would also dilute the content of enzyme activity present in the infarcted myocardium, which would influence calculations of infarct size based on analysis of tissue enzymes as well as from histologic sections. It is thus unlikely that tissue edema accounts for the differences observed in the present study which utilized histologic quantitation and previous studies which utilized depletion of myocardial enzymes to quantitate infarction. This view is supported by the studies by Kjekshus et al. [18], Shell et al. [5], and Fukuyama [6] (see Roberts, p. 109), which indicate a close linear correlation between myocardial infarction quantitated from myocardial CK depletion and histologic sections. As noted above,

Cairns et al. [4] quantitated the extent of infarction at 48 h by analysis of myocardial CK depletion and observed disproportionately less CK appearance when the infarction exceeded approximately 20% of the left ventricle.

THE EFFECTS OF EXTENSION OF INFARCTION ON SERUM CK ACTIVITY

We have also performed studies to examine the effects of extension of myocardial infarction produced by reduction of regional blood flow to an ischemic region on serum CK activity [2]. The animals were chronically prepared and studied as described in the previous section. However, two adjustable snare type occluders were positioned on the coronary artery: one was placed on the distal and the other on the proximal left circumflex coronary artery. Initial infarction was effected by occlusion of the distal left circumflex coronary artery; subsequent extension was produced by occlusion of the proximal circumflex coronary artery 6, 12, or 18 h after the distal occlusion. The extension was verified by serial measurements of regional myocardial blood flow by using $9 \pm 1 \mu$ microspheres which were injected before and after proximal occlusion. Figures 5–7 illustrate the effects of the initial coronary occlusion and subsequent infarct extension at 18, 12, and 6 h, respectively, on serial CK activity. Serum CK activity increased approximately 2–4 h after occlusion. As illustrated in Figure 5, after the initial increase, CK values increased rapidly and reached peak values approximately 12 h after the initial occlusion. Thus, extending the infarct at 6, 12, or 18 h after initiation of infarction coincided respectively with the period of rapidly increasing CK activity, peak CK activity, or after approximately 6 h of decreasing CK activity. Extension of infarction 18 h after the initial occlusion (Figure 5) effected no immediate change in CK activity that could be differentiated from endogenous clearance; CK levels continued to decrease for 2–5 h and then increased to reach a secondary peak value approximately 12 h after extension. Extension of infarction 12 h after the initial occlusion (Figure 6) resulted in an immediate decrease in CK activity; CK activity continued to decrease for at least 3 h before increasing to reach secondary peak values approximately 12 h after extension. Extension of infarction at 6 h (Figure 7) effected an immediate decrease in the rate of CK appearance and prolonged the time from the initial occlusion to peak CK activity; peak CK activity occurred 12 h after extension or 18 h after the initial occlusion. Proximal occlusion in animal 4 resulted in only a slight additional reduction in regional blood flow and no significant change in CK appearance.

These data demonstrate that reduction in blood flow to a region containing

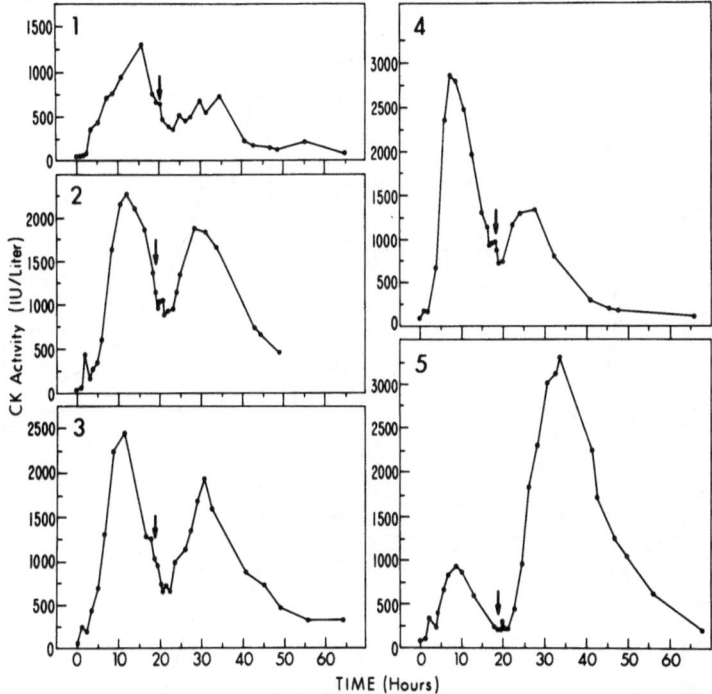

Figure 5. Effects of extension of infarction by occlusion of the proximal circumflex coronary artery 18 h after distal occlusion on serial CK activity (IU/L) in five dogs. The arrows indicate the time of proximal occlusion. Reprinted by permission of the American Heart Association [2].

ischemic myocardium is characterized by (a) an immediate decrease or no change in the appearance of CK which was a function of the time interval between the initial occlusion and extension, (b) subsequent increases in CK beginning 2–5 h after reduction in blood flow, and (c) secondary peak levels approximately 12 h after the second occlusion. It is likely that the immediate effects of reducing blood flow reflect effects of decreased myocardial perfusion on release of CK from myocardium which is infarcted whereas delayed increases in CK reflect additional myocardial necrosis. Immediate effects of decreasing blood flow to an area containing infarcted myocardium will depend on whether the infarcted myocardium is releasing CK, i.e., 6 and 12 h after coronary occlusion. If the infarcted myocardium is no longer releasing CK, i.e., 18 h post occlusion, reducing blood flow will not influence serum CK levels immediately, but may delay increases as a result of additional myocardial infarction. The immediate effects of reducing blood flow were also a function of the magnitude of the blood flow reduction; a large reduction in blood flow effected larger alterations in CK appearance.

152

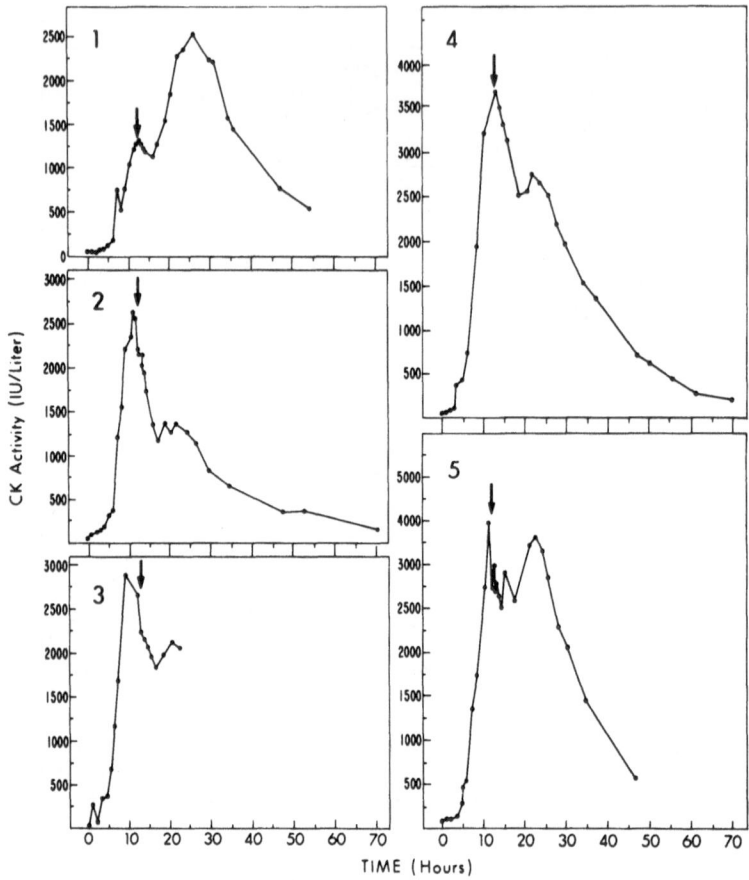

Figure 6. Effects of extension of infarction by occlusion of the proximal circumflex coronary artery 12 h after distal occlusion on serial CK activity (IU/L) in five dogs. The arrows indicate the time of proximal occlusion. Reprinted by permission of the American Heart Association [2].

The results of the present study are pertinent to the use of serial changes in CK activity as indices of the effects of intervention therapy on the course of acute myocardial infarction. Shell et al. [10, 19, 20] have described serial changes in serum CK during the course of acute myocardial infarction in experimental animals and patients. Enzyme values during early increases in CK were used to predict the subsequent CK curves based on nonlinear curve fitting techniques [19]. Certain deviations from the projected curves were interpreted as extension of infarction and others as salvage of ischemic myocardium [9, 19]. When propranolol was administered 5 h after coronary occlusion, i.e., during the rapid rise phase of CK, CK activity in the blood immediately

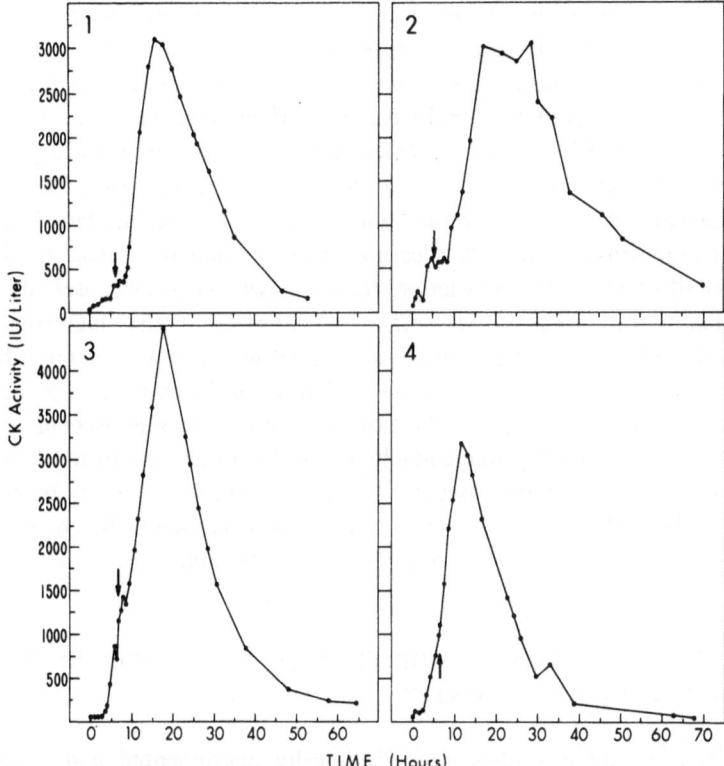

Figure 7. Effects of extension of infarction by occlusion of the proximal circumflex coronary artery 6 h after distal occlusion on serial CK activity (IU/L) in five dogs. The arrows indicate the time of proximal occlusion. Reprinted by permission of the American Heart Association [2].

fell below the projected enzyme curves; there were delayed increases in CK with peak levels occurring approximately 10 h later [19]. The immediate reduction of CK activity was interpreted as salvage of myocardium and the delayed peak as extension of infarction. The investigators concluded that propranolol resulted in salvage of myocardium in 50% of the animals studied. In another study, reductions in blood flow with trimethaphan in hypertensive patients with acute myocardial infarction was accompanied by an initial rapid decrease in serum CK to values below those predicted from the initial CK curve [20]. CK values then remained on a plateau for approximately 10 h before decreasing. These investigators concluded that trimethaphan reduced infarct size approximately 24% as compared with the predicted size. Since blood flow via the collateral vasculature is pressure dependent [21], an alternative hypothesis is that reduction in perfusion pressure may have reduced collateral flow and consequently CK appearance from the infarcted myocardium. Other studies have indicated that increasing heart rate by pacing or an isoproterenol infusion effects an increase in CK activity above the projected enzyme curves [9]. As will be discussed in the next section, increasing blood flow to a myocardial region subjected to prolonged ischemia may effect immediate and very rapid increases in serum CK activity. Interventions that affect myocardial perfusion thus may cause an immediate and/or delayed change in serum CK activity. The immediate changes may reflect increases or decreases in blood flow to infarcted myocardium which is releasing CK. Development of delayed changes in CK activity will depend on whether the decreased perfusion causes additional myocardial necrosis. The CK pattern of an intervention that increases blood flow to an ischemic area but extends an infarction i.e., isoproterenol infusion, may be a combination of immediate and delayed increases in CK activity. Interventions that decrease blood flow without increasing ischemic injury may decrease CK activity immediately without producing a delayed increase in CK. Thus, immediate increases in CK activity cannot necessarily be equated with extending infarction and decreases in CK activity cannot be equated with reduction of infarction or salvage of ischemic myocardium.

EFFECTS OF INCREASING BLOOD FLOW TO AN ACUTELY INFARCTED REGION ON SERUM CK ACTIVITY

The animals in these studies were chronically instrumented and studied as described in the previous section. However, in these animals an inflatable pneumatic occluder was positioned on the proximal circumflex coronary artery. Acute infarction was initiated by inflation of the pneumatic occluder; 2 h later the occluder was deflated to reestablish blood flow to the area subjected to ischemia. Regional blood flow measurements immediately after reperfusion in this model demonstrate an attenuated reactive hyperemia response in each region of the infarct zone [22]. Serial blood samples were obtained and analyzed for CK activity as previously described; samples were also obtained at 15 min intervals after reperfusion for a 1 h period. Histologic infarction was quantitated from multiple sections of the entire left ventricle. Figure 8 illustrates the effects of reperfusion or increasing blood flow 2 h after occlusion on serum CK activity in four representative animals. CK activity increased immediately after restoring blood flow to the ischemic region. In contrast to the animals subjected to permanent occlusion in which CK activity reached peak values 12–14 h after occlusion (Figure 1), CK activity increased rapidly after reperfusion to reach peak values 1–4 h after reperfusion or 3–6 h after initial occlusion. After reaching peak values, CK activity decreased rapidly. Figure 8 also illustrates the extremely variable relationship between enzyme estimates and histologic extent of infarction that was observed in these animals; animals

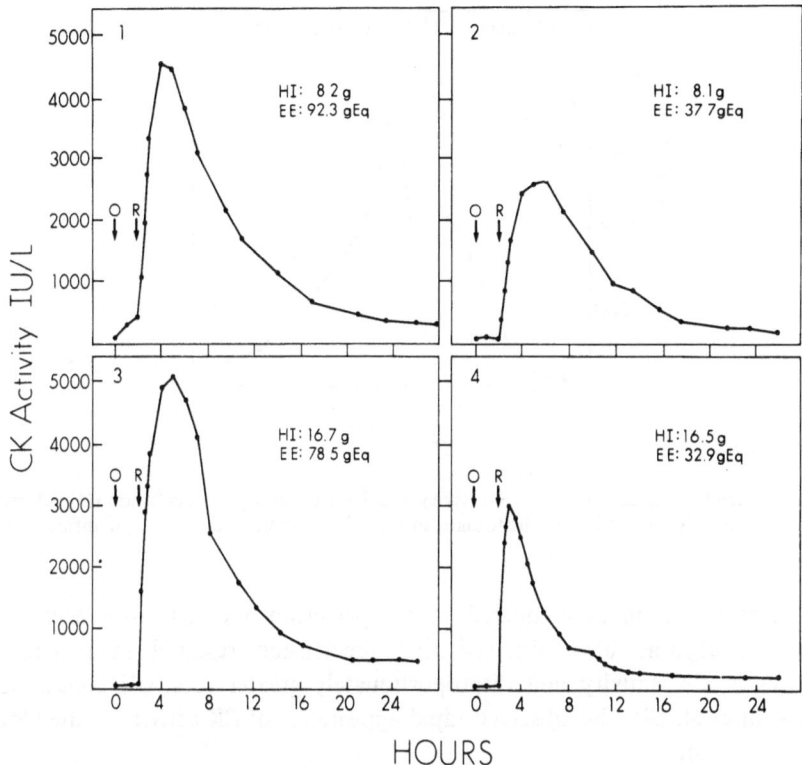

Figure 8. Serial measurements of CK activity (IU/L) after complete occlusion (0) followed by reperfusion (R) at 2 h: HI, histologic infarct; EE, enzyme estimates of infarction in g-eq.

1 and 2 had histologic infarcts of 8.2 and 8.1 g enzyme estimates of 92.3 and 37.7 g-eq, respectively; animals 3 and 4 had histologic infarcts of 16.7 and 16.5 g and enzyme estimates of 78.5 and 33.9 g-eq, respectively.

Figure 9 illustrates the effects of reperfusion 11 h after occlusion on serial measurements of CK activity. In this study, reperfusion was initiated when CK activity had peaked and was decreasing in the blood. Increasing blood flow to the infarcted region resulted in an immediate increase in CK activity; a secondary peak in CK activity occurred 2 h later followed by rapid decline. Thus, increasing blood flow when CK activity was decreasing resulted in the immediate appearance of additional CK activity in the blood. There was no delayed increase in CK activity, indicating that reestablishing blood flow at this interval washed out additional CK activity present in the infarcted zone rather than initiating additional myocardial necrosis.

Vatner et al. [7] reported different linear relationships between CK estimates of infarction and pathologic infarct size in experimental animals subjected to

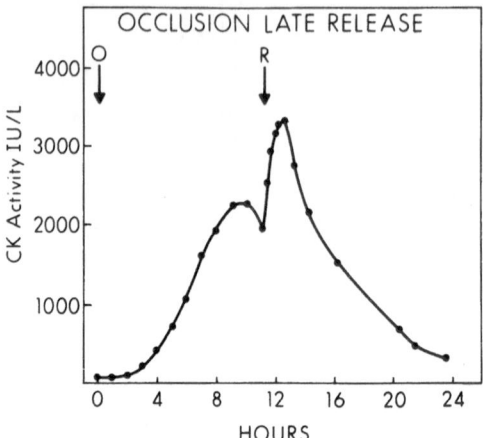

Figure 9. Serial measurements of CK activity (IU/L) after complete occlusion (O) followed by reperfusion (R) at 11 h: HI, histologic infarct; EE, enzyme estimates of infarction in g-eq.

permanent occlusion as compared with reperfusion 1 or 3 h after occlusion. These investigators also observed that reperfusion resulted in immediate increases in CK activity and disproportionately greater total CK appearance. Jarmakani et al. [8] also observed rapid appearance of CK activity in the blood after reperfusion.

CONCLUSION

In the animals subjected to permanent coronary occlusion, the relationship between enzyme estimates and the histologic extent of infarcts is best described by a power function indicating a disproportionate decrease in CK appearance in the blood as infarct size increased. Calculation of the fraction of CK activity released from infarcted myocardium, K_r, using the appearance function of CK and the extent of histologic infarction demonstrated that K_r decreased as a power function as histologic infarct size increased. The use of a constant K_r as recommended by the Shell equation introduced an error that increased as infarct size increased. Regional blood flow measurements demonstrated that the fraction of the infarct zone that remained severely ischemic during the period of CK appearance in the blood increased progressively as infarct size increased. Consequently, it is likely that the diffusion distance from the central core of the infarct zone and the time that CK is exposed to factors that inactivate enzyme activity increased as infarct size increased. Since only a small fraction of the depleted CK activity eventually appears in the circulating blood, it is reasonable to hypothesize that the fraction of CK appearing from cells in the center versus the periphery of a given infarct or from the center of small versus large infarcts will be different. A linear correlation between enzyme estimates and histologic extent of infarcts could be achieved by eliminating infarct sizes above 20 g from the analysis; the linear correlation was improved by modifying the histologic infarct size by subtracting tissue samples that remained severely ischemic during the period of CK release. The view that blood flow to the infarcted myocardium is an important variable that influences the appearance of CK activity in the blood is supported by studies that demonstrated the profound effects that changing blood flow to an ischemic region may have on CK activity in the blood. Decreasing blood flow to an acutely infarcted region at the time that CK activity was increasing in the blood resulted in an immediate decrease in enzyme appearance. Increasing regional blood flow as early as 2 h or as late as 11 h after coronary occlusion effected a rapid, marked increase in CK activity in the blood. These studies support the view that regional blood flow is a variable that has a confounding effect on the appearance of CK activity in the blood and thus on the relationship between enzyme estimates and histologic extent of myocardial infarcts.

Acknowledgments. The following persons have been collaborating investigators in these studies, Dr. Robert G. Irvin, Dr. Richard C. Hagerty, Dr. C.F. Starmer, Dr. Philip A. McHale, and Dr. Judith L. Swain. This work is supported in part by NIH grant HL 18537 and by the Medical Research Service of the Veterans Administration. Dr. Frederick R. Cobb received support as an Established Investigator of the American Heart Association.

REFERENCES

1. Roe CR, Cobb FR, Starmer CF: The relationship between enzymatic and histologic estimates of the extent of myocardial infarction in conscious dogs with permanent coronary occlusion. Circulation 55:438, 1977.
2. Cobb FR, Irvin R, Hagerty P, Roe CR: Effect of extension of infarction on serial CK activity. Circulation 60:145, 1979.
3. Swain JL, Cobb FR, McHale PA, Roe CR: Nonlinear relationship between creatine kinase estimates and histologic extent of infarction in conscious dogs: effects of regional myocardial blood flow. Circulation 62:1239, 1980.
4. Cairns JA, Missirlis E, Fallen EL: Myocardial infarction size from serial CPK: variability of CPK serum entry ratio with size and model of infarction. Circulation 58:1143, 1978.
5. Shell WE, Kjekshus JK, Sobel BE: Quantitative assessment of the extent of myocardial infarction in the conscious dog by means of analysis of serial changes in serum creatine phosphokinase activity. J Clin Invest 50:2614, 1971.

6. Fukuyama T, Robert R: The effect of intravenous nitroglycerin on coronary blood flow and infarct size during myocardial infarction in conscious dogs. In: Rudolph W, Schrey A (eds) Nitrate II. München–Wein–Baltimore: Urban and Schwarzenberg, 1980, p. 342.
7. Vatner SF, Baig H, Manders WT, Maroko PR: Effects of coronary artery reperfusion on myocardial infarct size calculated from creatine kinase. J Clin Invest 61:1048, 1978.
8. Jarmakani JM, Limbird L, Graham RC, Marks RA: Effect of reperfusion on myocardial infarct, and the accuracy of estimating infarct size from serum creatine phosphokinase in the dog. Cardiovasc Res 10:245, 1976.
9. Shell WE, Sobel BE: Deleterious effects of increased heart rate on infarct size in the conscious dog. Am J Cardiol 31:474, 1973.
10. Rivas F, Cobb FR, Bache RJ, Greenfield JC Jr: Relationship between blood flow to ischemic regions and extent of myocardial infarction. Circ Res 38:439, 1976.
11. Gervin CA, Hackel DB, Roe CR: Enzyme content of canine cardiac lymph during acute myocardial infarction. Surg Forum 25:175, 1974.
12. Malmberg P: Time course of enzyme escape via heart lymph following myocardial infarction in the dog. Scand J Clin Lab Invest 30:405, 1972.
13. Clark GL, Robinson AK, Gnepp DR, Roberts R, Sobel BE: Effects of lymphatic transport of enzyme on plasma creatine kinase time-activity curves after myocardial infarction in dogs. Circ Res 43:162, 1978.
14. Reimer KA, Jennings RB: The changing anatomic reference base of evolving myocardial infarction. Under estimation of myocardial collateral flow and over estimation of experimental anatomic infarct size due to tissue edema, hemorrage and acute inflammation. Circulation 60:866, 1979.
15. Jugdutt MI, Hutchins GM, Bulkley BH, Becker LC: The loss of radioactive microspheres from canine necrotic myocardium. Circ Res 45:746, 1979.
16. Capurro NL, Goldstein RE, Aamodt R, Smith HJ, Epstein SE: Loss of microspheres from ischemic canine cardiac tissue: an important technical limitation. Circ Res 44:223, 1979.
17. Murdock RH Jr, Cobb FR: Effects of infarcted myocardium on regional blood flow measurements to ischemic regions in canine hearts. Circ Res 47:701, 1980.
18. Kjekshus JK, Sobel BE: Depressed myocardial creatine phosphokinase activity following experimental myocardial infarction in rabbit. Circ Res 27:403, 1970.
19. Shell WE, Lavelle JF, Covell JW, Sobel BE: Early estimation of myocardial damage in conscious dogs and patients with evolving acute myocardial infarction. J Clin Invest 52:2579, 1973.
20. Shell WE, Sobel BE: Protection of jeopardized ischemic myocardium by reduction of ventricular afterload. N Engl J Med 291:481, 1974.
21. Gregg DE, Mautz FR: Dynamics of collateral circulation following chronic occlusion of coronary arteries. Am J Physiol 123:84, 1938.
22. Cobb FR, McHale PA, Rembert JC: Effects of acute cellular injury on coronary vascular reactivity in awake dogs. Circulation 57:962, 1978.

6. HEMODYNAMIC MEASUREMENTS

WILLIAM J. ROGERS, HUEY G. McDANIEL, JOHN A. MANTLE, SILVIO E.
PAPAPIETRO, RICHARD O. RUSSELL, JR., and CHARLES E. RACKLEY

Perhaps the most striking feature of the clinical syndrome of acute myocardial infarction is the propensity toward hemodynamic alterations, ranging from the subtle to the catastrophic. With few exceptions, these hemodynamic changes directly reflect the extent of myocardial necrosis and thus provide a readily available clinical tool for estimating infarct size. This chapter will examine how certain common hemodynamic parameters obtained during the early or late convalescent phase following a myocardial infarct can be utilized to assess infarct size indirectly.

ALTERED HEMODYNAMICS IN ACUTE MYOCARDIAL INFARCT

When part of the myocardium dies, cardiac pump performance diminishes, left ventricular compliance or distensibility changes, and dysrhythmias appear, including both supraventricular and ventricular brady- and tachyarrhythmias and conduction disturbances (Figure 1). All hemodynamic sequelae of a myocardial

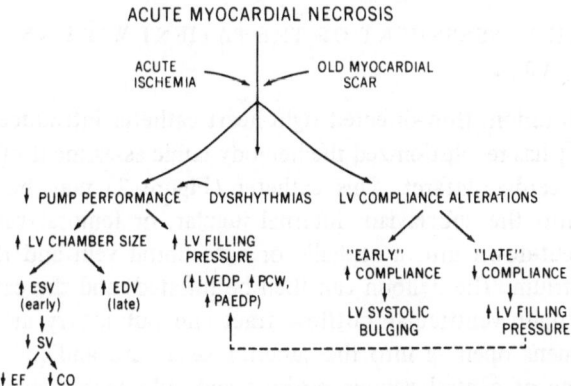

Figure 1. Sequelae of acute myocardial necrosis: LV, left ventricular; ESV, end-systolic volume; EDV, end-diastolic volume; SV, stroke volume; CO, cardiac output; LVEDP, left ventricular end-diastolic pressure; PCW, pulmonary capillary wedge pressure; PAEDP, pulmonary arterial end-diastolic pressure.

Wagner GS (ed): Myocardial Infarction: Measurement and Intervention, pp 159–172.
© *1982 Martinus Nijhoff Publishers, The Hague/Boston/London.*

infarct, including alterations in both pump performance and compliance, depend on not only the extent of acute myocardial necrosis but also the magnitude of acute ischemia and the size of old myocardial scar. Hemodynamic measurements alone cannot separate the individual contributions of acute necrosis, acute ischemia, and old scar.

The damaged left ventricle, unable to achieve proper systolic emptying, has an increased end-systolic volume and a diminished stroke volume [1]. Unless there is compensatory tachycardia, diminished compliance, or increased contractility of the noninfarcted area, there will also be a reduction in cardiac output (the product of stroke volume and heart rate). Later, the end-diastolic volume will begin to increase and may partially compensate for the reduced stroke volume via the Starling mechanism. Left ventricular ejection fraction — the stroke volume normalized for end-diastolic volume — also decreases [2].

Left venticular compliance is initially increased with an acute myocardial infarct, the acutely ischemic zone bulging outward with systole. As edema accumulates, and subsequently as fibrosis ensues, the infarcted ventricle becomes markedly noncompliant [3—6].

As a result of both inadequate pump performance and diminished compliance, the filling pressure of the left ventricle (the left atrial or left ventricular end-diastolic pressure) increases. In patients without mitral valve stenosis, left ventricular filling pressure can be conveniently assessed by measuring pulmonary capillary wedge pressure, or even more conveniently, by measuring pulmonary arterial end-diastolic pressure, provided there is no significant pulmonary vascular disease [7,8].

HEMODYNAMIC ASSESSMENT OF THE PATIENT WITH AN ACUTE MYOCARDIAL INFARCT

The balloon flotation, flow-directed right-heart catheter introduced in 1970 by Swan et al. [9] has revolutionized the hemodynamic assessment of patients with an acute myocardial infarct. This catheter (Figure 2) may be inserted percutaneously into the subclavian, internal jugular, or femoral vein or inserted by a venous cut-down into a cephalic or antecubital vein and then advanced to the right atrium. The balloon can then be inflated, and the catheter floated out into the right ventricular outflow tract and pulmonary artery. Proximal and distal lumens opening into the superior vena cava and pulmonary artery enable sampling of central venous pressure and pulmonary arterial pressure. A thermistor, located near the distal catheter tip, can be utilized for cardiac output determinations by the thermodilution technique. Optional electrodes mounted along the catheter shaft facilitate the recording of atrial and/or ventricular electrograms and, in many instances, enable atrial and/or ventricular pacing when necessary [10, 11].

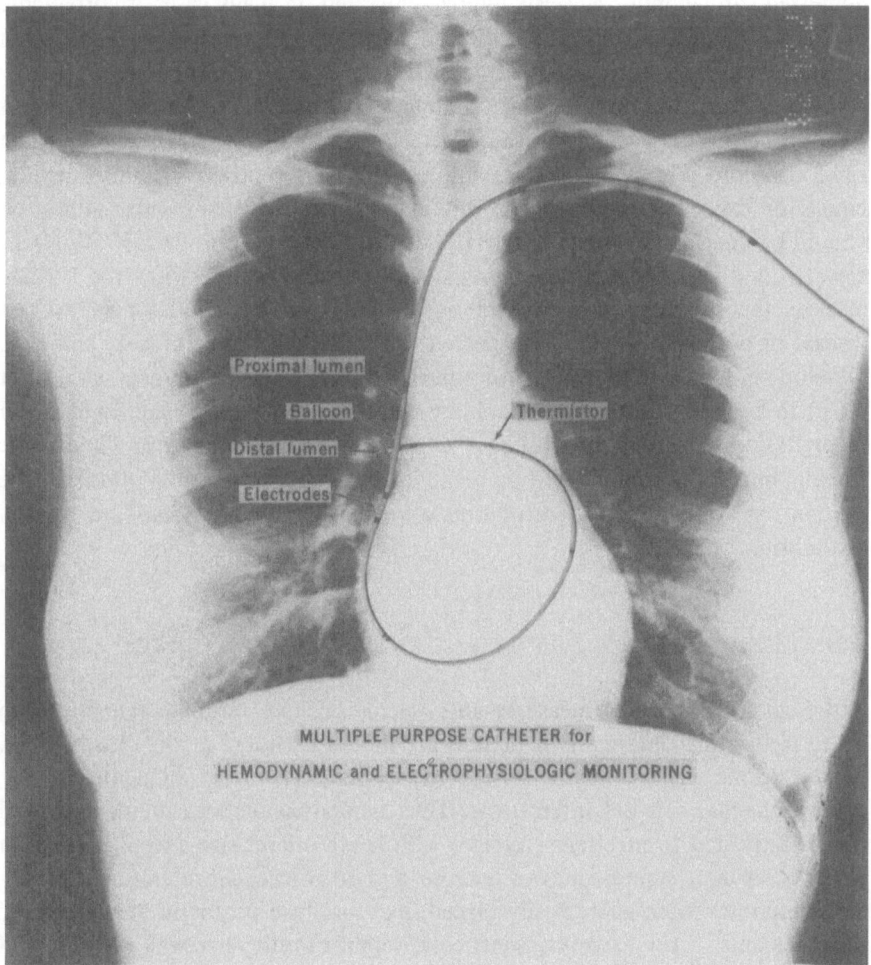

Figure 2. Multiple-purpose catheter for hemodynamic and electrophysiologic monitoring. In addition to proximal and distal lumens, this balloon flow-directed catheter has a thermistor near its tip and a pair of electrodes along the shaft at the high right atrial level. Reprinted with permission from Mantle et al. [11].

Although many patients with an acute myocardial infarct may have an adequate cardiac index with a normal or subnormal left ventricular filling pressure, studies have demonstrated that when the pulmonary aterial end-diastolic pressure is 18–24 mmHg, cardiac index is maximal in patients with acute myocardial infarct [12]. When pulmonary arterial end-diastolic pressure exceeds 24 mmHg, pulmonary edema occurs in most patients.

Data obtained from the catheter enable the diagnosis of a wide variety of clinical disorders. Depressed left ventricular filling pressure along with a depressed cardiac index suggests hypovolemia and, in many cases, is correctable by simple volume expansion. On the other hand, a reduced cardiac index when accompanied by an elevated left ventricular filling pressure suggests a low cardiac output syndrome in which volume expansion would be hazardous, but diuretics, inotropic agents, and vasodilators occasionally prove efficacious. When right atrial pressure, which is normally less than left ventricular filling pressure, equals or exceeds left ventricular filling pressure, right ventricular infarction should be considered [13–15]. If all diastolic pressures (RA, PAEDP, PCW) are elevated and equal, cardiac tamponade should be suspected. When the PAEDP exceeds the PCW by more than about 5 mmHg, intrinsic pulmonary arterial disease or occlusion should be suspected, particularly acute pulmonary embolus. Development of a loud systolic murmur following an acute myocardial infarct is apt to be secondary to acute papillary muscle rupture with severe acute mitral regurgitation in a patient with large 'V waves' in the pulmonary capillary wedge tracing, but the murmur might be secondary to ventricular septal rupture if the pulmonary arterial oxygen saturation exceeds the superior vena cava oxygen saturation.

USING HEMODYNAMIC DATA TO QUANTIFY ACUTE INFARCT

Although hemodynamic measurements can be used to estimate the size of an acute myocardial infarct, two limitations should be noted at the outset. First, hemodynamic measurements reflect the *cumulative* effect of acute infarct, acute ischemia, and old infarct/scar. Thus hemodynamic measurements would not be expected to precisely correlate with acute infarct size except perhaps in patients having discrete zones of necrosis and no antecedent infarction. Second, small infarcts, when strategically placed, may produce profound hemodynamic derangements — for example, ventricular septal rupture, free-wall rupture, and ruptured papillary muscle. Fortunately these sequelae of acute myocardial infarct are rare and usually identifiable. In spite of these limitations, hemodynamic measurements are often very useful clinically because they reflect the cumulative insult to cardiac performance with which the patient and physician must now cope.

To investigate the relation of initial hemodynamic findings to infarct size, we have correlated myocardial infarct size estimated by enzyme analysis (see Roberts, p. 129) with initial hemodynamic findings in 21 patients admitted to our coronary care unit with their first myocardial infarct and no evidence of con-comitant RV infarct, papillary muscle rupture, or ventricular septal rupture [16]. All patients had a Swan–Ganz catheter inserted within 18 h of first symptom of infarct (mean 7 h), and heart rate, arterial pressure, pulmonary arterial end-diastolic pressure, cardiac index, and stroke index were measured. Blood samples obtained at 3-h intervals for 96 h were utilized to determine creatine kinase MB isoenzymes and to calculate enzymatic infarct size. Left ventricular mass was measured in each patient, either by subsequent left ventricular angiography or from autopsy. Each patient's estimated infarct size was *normalized* for his left ventricular mass, giving an index of the *proportion* of the left ventricle that had undergone acute necrosis.

The results of our study showed that systolic blood pressure and heart rate on admission were of no use in estimating infarct size, and cardiac index showed a weak inverse correlation with infarct size. When cardiac index was normalized for heart rate, yielding stroke index, a much better inverse relationship, $r = -0.74$, was found (Figure 3). The strongest correlation observed was that between admission PAEDP and CK-infarct size ($r = 0.91$) (Figure 4). As noted in the preceding pathophysiology discussion, alterations in left ventricular filling pressure in the setting of acute myocardial infarct reflect both diminished pump performance and reduced LV compliance (Figure 1).

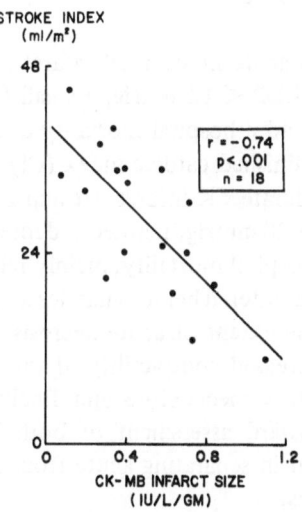

Figure 3. Relation of enzymatic infarct size to stroke index in patients with a first myocardial infarct.

Our results showing that left ventricular filling pressure is directly proportional and cardiac index is inversely proportional to CK infarct size agree with data of Mathey et al. [17], who found that a decrease in cardiac function acutely post infarct was usually a function of the extent of myocardial necrosis. These investigators studied the hemodynamics and creatine kinase enzyme

164

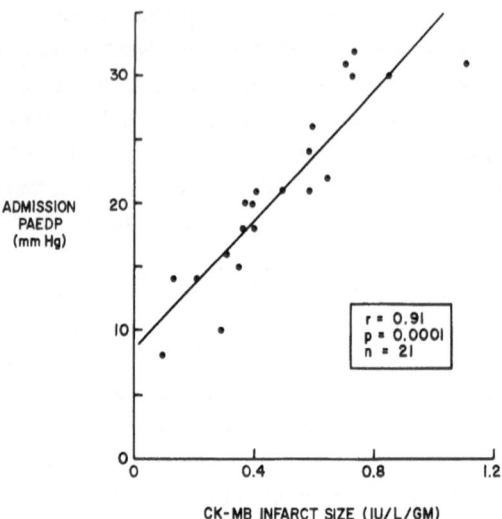

$$r = 0.91$$
$$p = 0.0001$$
$$n = 21$$

CK-MB INFARCT SIZE (IU/L/GM)

Figure 4. Relation of enzymatic infarct size to admission pulmonary arterial end-diastolic pressure (PAEDP) in patients with a first myocardial infarct. An excellent correlation over a wide range of infarct sizes was found.

release of patients with an acute myocardial infarct and identified three patient groups: (a) group I – PAEDP < 12 mmHg, a small CK infarct size, no impairment of cardiac function and a hospital mortality of 5%; (b) group II – PAEDP 12–20 mmHg, slightly diminished cardiac index (CI) and left ventricular stroke work index (LVSWI), moderate CK infarct size and 21% hospital mortality; and (c) group III – PAEDP > 20 mmHg, markedly depressed CI and LVSWI, large CK infarct size and 60% hospital mortality, mainly related to cardiogenic shock. Mathey et al. concluded that altered hemodynamics acutely following myocardial infarct usually reflected the extent of acute necrosis, that increased stiffness in the infarcted zone and increased contractility of the noninfarcted myocardium were important compensatory mechanisms and, finally, that a combined investigative approach aimed toward assessment of both hemodynamics and serial enzyme changes was useful in separating acute from remote myocardial infarct and for predicting prognosis.

Another technique for assessing left ventricular infarct size by hemodynamics compares the left ventricular forward stroke volume determined by either thermodilution, green dye, or the Fick technique with left ventricular stroke volume determined independently by M-mode echocardiography (see Stack and Kisslo, p. 235). The M-mode echocardiogram often underestimates end-systolic left ventricular volume because of regional wall motion abnormalities that are outside the path of the echobeam (Figure 5); as a result, the echocardiographically determined stroke volume is also underestimated. Sweet et al. [18]

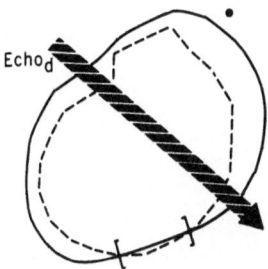

Figure 5. Position of M-mode electrocardiographic beam for assessing left ventricular dimension (Echo$_d$) in left ventricular volume determination. Shown in brackets in a region of abnormally contracting (akinetic or dyskinetic) myocardium which lies outside the zone of the echo beam. Reprinted with permission from Sweet et al. [18].

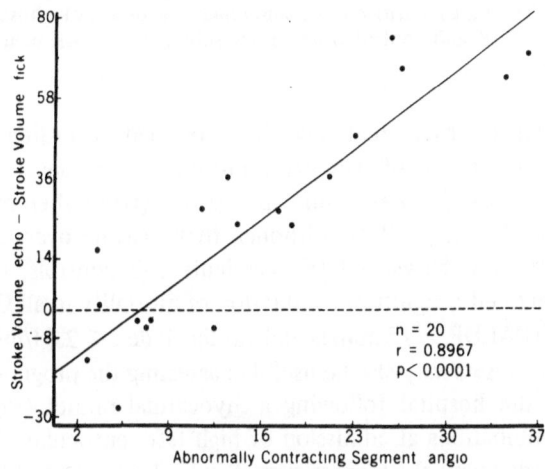

Figure 6. Relationship of the difference in stroke volume between echocardiographic and Fick techniques to the magnitude of the angiographic abnormally contracting segment in patients following myocardial infarct. Reprinted with permission from Sweet et al. [18].

showed that the extent of this underestimation was actually proportional to the left ventricular scar size estimated angiographically (Figure 6).

HEMODYNAMIC SUBSET ANALYSIS

Apart from their ability to quantify the extent of myocardial necrosis, an approximate estimation at best, hemodynamic measurements are also useful in stratifying groups of patients with homogeneous risks. Such stratification may be useful in determining which subsets benefit from interventions designed to limit infarct size.

166

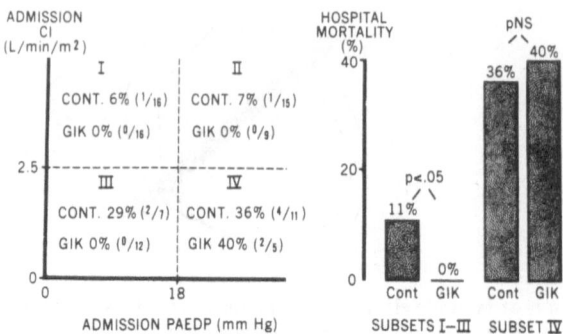

Figure 7. Use of admission hemodynamics to subdivide patients in a study of the effects of glucose–insulin–potassium (GIK) versus control (CONT) on hospital mortality of acute myocardial infarct. The plot identified one hemodynamic subset (IV) whose mortality rates were similar between GIK and control; otherwise in subsets I–III, GIK recipients had lower hospital mortality rates.

Figure 7 contains subsets that have been defined according to admission PAEDP and CI for a group of patients admitted to a coronary care unit and randomly allocated to glucose–insulin–potassium (GIK) therapy or placebo control [19] (see Swain, p. 488). Although there was no overall difference in hospital mortality rate between GIK recipients and controls, hemodynamic subset analysis revealed a significant reduction of mortality in all GIK recipients except subset IV (PAEDP > 18 mmHg and cardiac index $\leqslant$ 2.5 l/min/m²).

Hemodynamic subsets may also be useful in assessing the prognosis of patients discharged from the hospital following a myocardial infarct (Figure 8) [20]. Patients with combinations at admission of high left ventricular filling pressure and low cardiac index have the highest mortality both acutely and long-term.

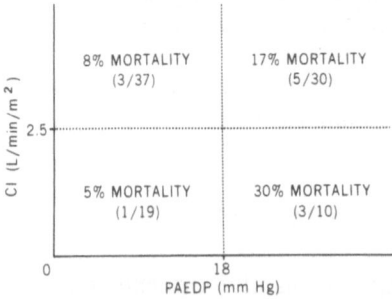

Figure 8. Use of admission hemodynamics to subdivide patients according to mortality following hospital discharge: CI, cardiac index; PAEDP, pulmonary arterial end-diastolic pressure.

LEFT VENTRICULAR FUNCTION CURVES

Another hemodynamic approach to quantify left ventricular damage utilizes the concept of left ventricular function curves [21]. To construct these curves, baseline measurements of PAEDP and CI are made, increments of low molecular weight dextran are infused sufficient to increase the PAEDP by $\geq 4\,mmHg$, and PAEDP and CI are again measured. These two sets of measurements are plotted on a graph of CI versus PAEDP and connected with a straight line (Figure 9). The lines obtained are termed left ventricular function curves and have a slope ($\Delta CI/\Delta PAEDP$) that has been shown to correlate with LV ejection fraction determined angiographically (Figure 10). In constructing these curves, care should be taken to wait at least 48 h after an infarct so that left ventricular compliance has presumably begun to stabilize. Dextran should not be infused in patients having $PAEDP \geq 22\,mmHg$, lest pulmonary edema be precipitated.

Since there is a natural tendency for the left ventricular filling pressure to fall and the cardiac index to rise as a patient recovers from a myocardial infarct, these changes can be analyzed in terms of a 'shift' from one ventricular function

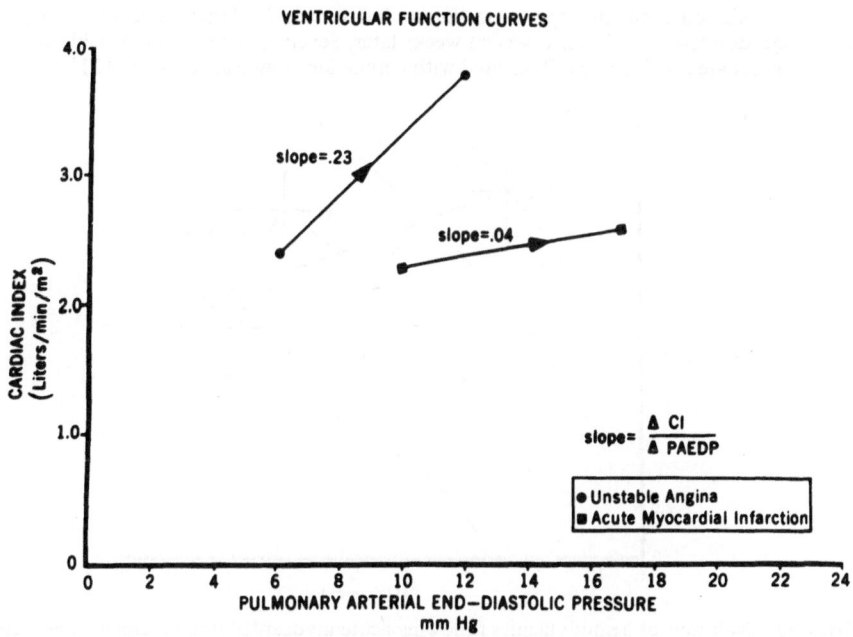

Figure 9. Construction of left ventricular function curves by obtaining measurements of cardiac index and pulmonary arterial end-diastolic pressure before and after infusion of low molecular weight dextran. Note that the slope of the curve from the patient with unstable angina and good left ventricular function is greater than that of the patient with acute myocardial infarct. Reprinted with permission from Raphael et al. [21].

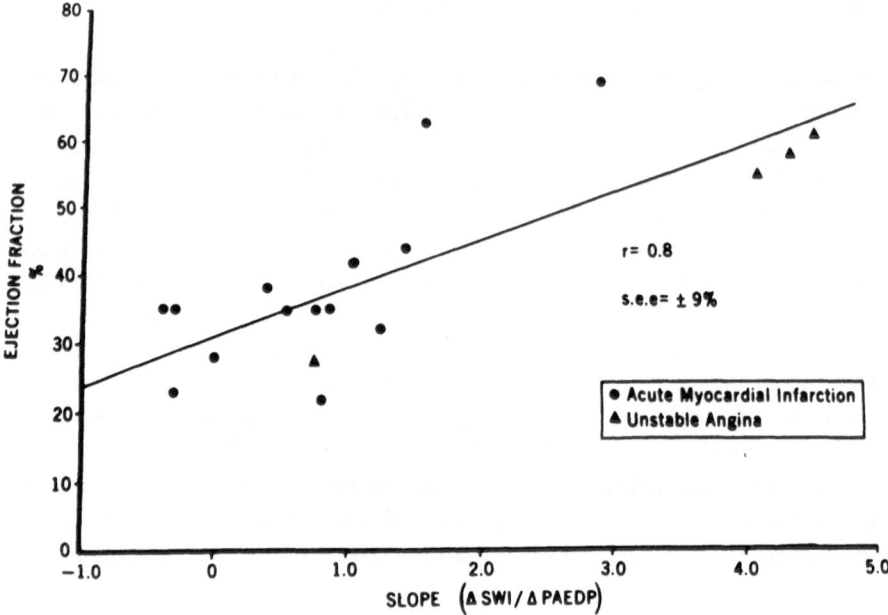

Figure 10. Relation between slope of postinfarct left ventricular function curve and angiographic ejection fraction obtained several weeks later. Several patients with unstable angina and no infarct are also included. Reprinted with permission from Raphael et al. [21].

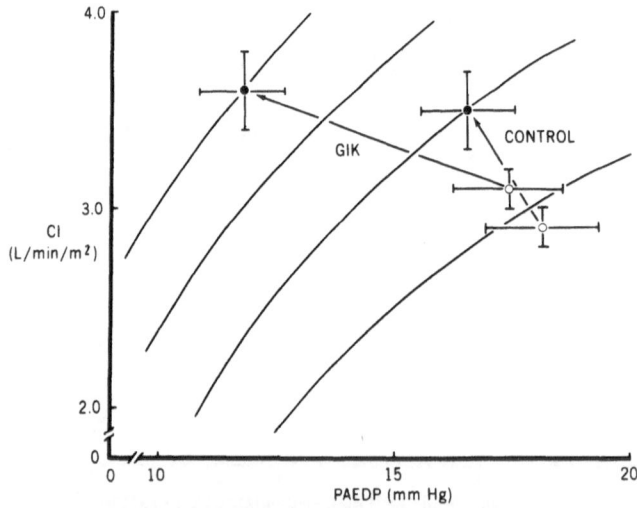

Figure 11. Evolution of hemodynamics following acute myocardial infarct. Open circles represent baseline hemodynamics obtained within 12 h of first symptoms. Closed circles represent hemodynamics obtained 3–4 days post infarct. In general, a fall in pulmonary arterial end-diastolic pressure (PAEDP) and a rise in cardiac index (CI) is observed. In this example, glucose–insulin–potassium (GIK) recipients had a more profound fall in PAEDP than the control patients. The data may be interpreted as a shift to another ventricular function curve secondary to improved contractility, or as an increase in left ventricular compliance.

curve to another (Figure 11). Such hemodynamic changes over time also enable comparison of groups receiving interventions designed to limit infarct size [19]. Though it is impossible in such cases to ascertain whether the hemodynamic improvement represents increased contractility or increased compliance, either of these factors represents clinical improvement.

HEMODYNAMIC PARAMETERS DERIVED FROM CARDIAC CATHETERIZATION FOLLOWING MYOCARDIAL INFARCT

Diagnostic cardiac catheterization following myocardial infarction is being utilized increasingly in order to ascertain coronary anatomy and left ventricular function and also to select certain patients for coronary revascularization surgery [22]. From left ventriculography (see Behar, p. 179), quantitative measurements allow calculation of several indices that relate to myocardial infarct size (Figure 12): (a) the percent of abnormally contracting segment, that is, the percentage of the end-diastolic circumference found to be akinetic or dyskinetic when end-diastolic and end-systolic silhouettes are superimposed; (b) the left ventricular ejection fraction [(end-diastolic volume − end-systolic volume)/(end-diastolic volume)] ; and (c) the left ventricular diastolic specific compliance (angiographic stroke volume/end-diastolic volume/ΔP where ΔP = LV diastolic pressure change) [23].

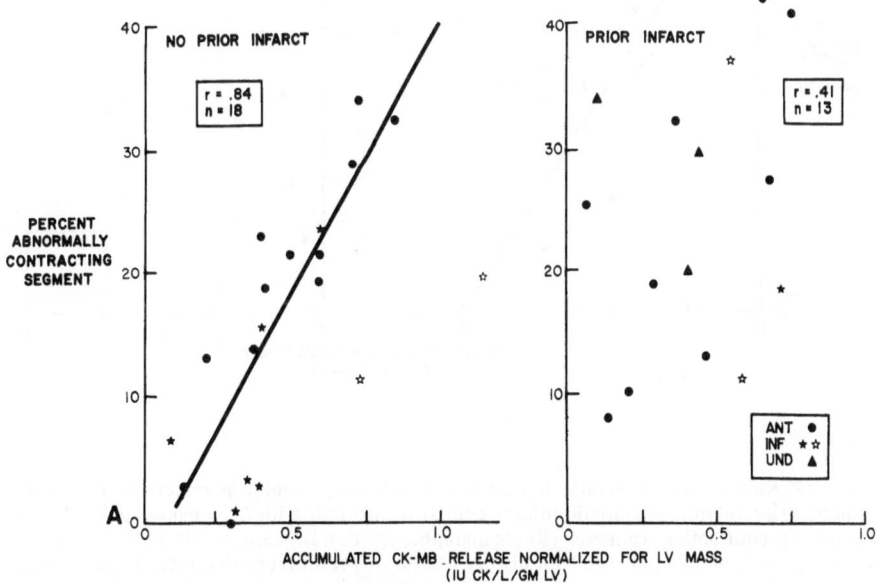

Figure 12A. See the legend on the next page.

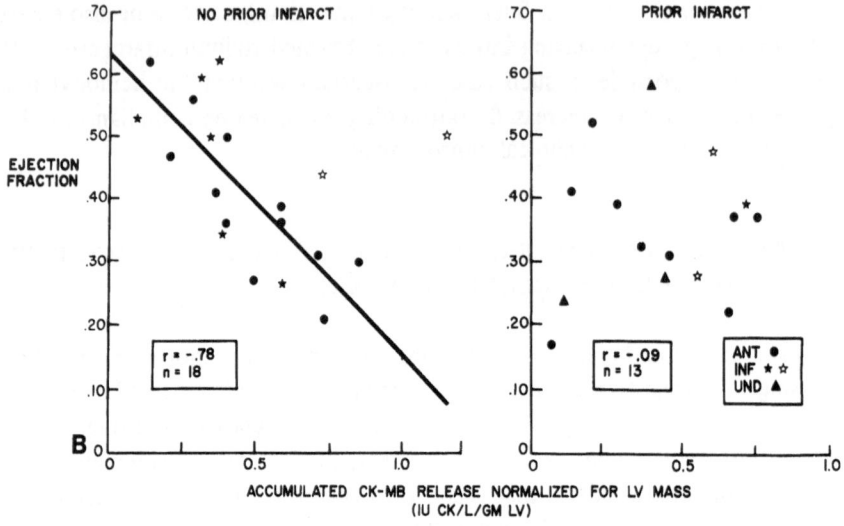

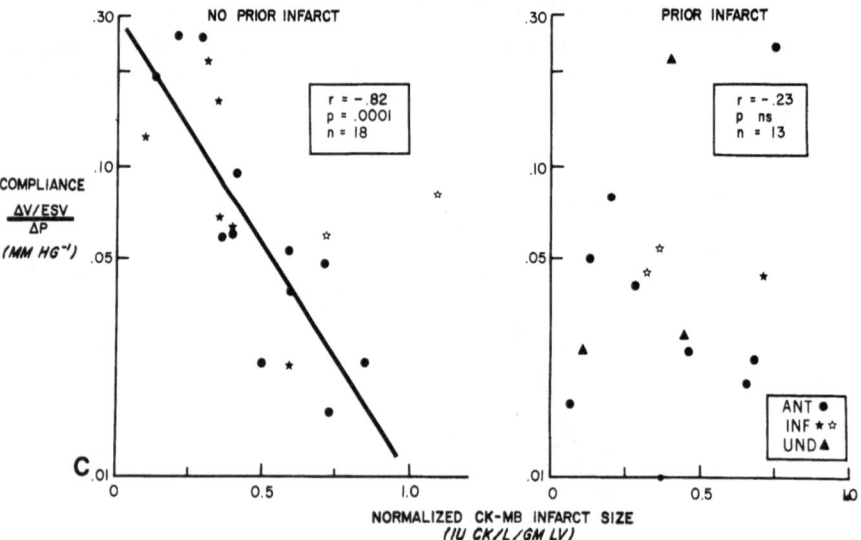

Figure 12. Relation of enzymatic infarct size to late angiographic parameters. In patients without prior infarct, enzymatic infarct size correlates well with (*A*) angiographic percent abnormally contracting segments; (*B*) angiographic ejection fraction, and (*C*) left ventricular specific compliance. In patients with history of remote prior myocardial infarct, these correlations are not found, because the enzymatic infarct size measurement assesses only the acute event. *A* and *B* reprinted from Rogers et al. [23] with permission.

Acknowledgments. This work was supported in part by the National Heart, Lung, and Blood Institute (Specialized Center of Research for Ischemic Heart Disease, contract 5P50HL17667-05, Program Project grant HL11310 and the General Research Unit grant MORR00013, General Clinical Research Centers Program Division of Research Resources) of the National Institutes of Health. The authors appreciate the assistance of Mrs. Dot Green in preparation of this chapter.

REFERENCES

1. Swan HJC, Forrester JS, Diamond G, Chatterjee K, Parmley WW: Hemodynamic spectrum of myocardial infarction and cardiogenic shock. A conceptual model. Circulation 45:1097–1110, 1972.
2. Kostuk WJ, Ehsani AA, Karliner JS, Ashburn WL, Peterson KL, Ross J Jr, Sobel BE: Left ventricular performance after myocardial infarction assessed by radioisotope angiocardiography. Circulation 47:242–249, 1973.
3. Tennant R, Wiggers CJ: The effect of coronary occlusion on myocardial contraction. Am J Physiol 112:351–361, 1935.
4. Ekong EA, Pirzada, FA, Vokonas PS, Hood WB Jr: Changes in ventricular compliance during experimental myocardial infarction [abstr]. Circulation 46:II-148, 1972.
5. Hood WB, Bianco JA, Kumar R, Whiting RB: Experimental myocardial infarction. IV. Reduction of left ventricular compliance in the healing phase. J Clin Invest 49:1316–1322, 1970.
6. Diamond G, Forrester JS: Effect of coronary artery disease and acute myocardial infarction on left ventricular compliance in man. Circulation 45:11–19, 1972.
7. Jenkins BS, Bradley RD, Branthwaite MA: Evaluation of pulmonary arterial end-diastolic pressure as an indirect estimate of left atrial mean pressure. Circulation 42:75–78, 1970.
8. Falicov RE, Resnekov L: Relationship of the pulmonary artery end-diastolic pressure to the left ventricular end-diastolic and mean filling pressures in patients with and without left ventricular dysfunction. Circulation 42:65–73, 1970.
9. Swan HJC, Ganz W, Forrester J, Marcus H, Diamond G, Chonette D:Catheterization of the heart in man with use of a flow-directed balloon-tipped catheter. N Eng J Med 283:447–451, 1970.
10. Chatterjee K, Swan HJC, Ganz W, Gray R, Loebel H, Forrester JS, Chonette D: Use of a balloon-tipped flotation electrode catheter for cardiac monitoring. Am J Cardiol 36:56–61, 1975.
11. Mantle JA, Massing GK, James TN, Russell RO Jr, Rackley CE: A multipurpose catheter for electrophysiologic and hemodynamic monitoring plus atrial pacing. Chest 72:285–290, 1977.
12. Russell RO Jr, Rackley CE, Pombo J, Hunt D, Potanin C, Dodge HT: Effects of increasing left ventricular filling pressure in patients with acute myocardial infarction. J Clin Invest 49: 1539–1550, 1970.

13. Rotman M, Ratliff NB, Hawley J: Right ventricular infarction: a haemo-dynamic diagnosis. Br Heart J 36:941—944, 1974.
14. Sharpe DN, Botvinick EH, Shames DM, Schiller NB, Massie BM, Chatterjee K, Parmley WW: The noninvasive diagnosis of right ventricular infarction. Circulation 57:483—490, 1978.
15. Lorell B, Leinbach RC, Pohost GM, Gold HK, Dinsmore RE, Hutter AM, Pastore JO, DeSanctis RW: Right ventricular infarction: clinical diagnosis and differentiation from cardiac tamponade and pericardial constriction. Am J Cardiol 43:465—471, 1979.
16. Rogers WJ, McDaniel HG, Smith LR, Mantle JA, Russell RO Jr, Rackley CE: Prediction of myocardial infarct size from admission clinical and hemodynamic data in patients with first infarct. Clin Res 25:7A, 1977.
17. Mathey D, Bleifeld W, Hanrath P, Effert S: Attempt to quantitate relation between cardiac function and infarct size in acute myocardial infarction. Br Heart J 36:271—279, 1974.
18. Sweet RL, Moraski RE, Russell RO Jr, Rackley CE: Relationship between echocardiography, cardiac output, and abnormally contracting segments in patients with ischemic heart disease. Circulation 52:634—641, 1975.
19. Rogers WJ, Mantle JA, McDaniel HG, Russell RO Jr, Rackley CE: Prospective randomized trial of glucose—insulin—potassium in acute myocardial infarction. Circulation 60:II-165, 1979.
20. Rogers WJ, Smith LR, Oberman A, Mantle JA, Russell RO Jr, Rackley CE: Invasive measurements relating to long-term survival post-myocardial infarction. Circulation 60:II-232, 1979.
21. Raphael LD, Mantle JA, Moraski RE, Rogers WJ, Russell RO Jr, Rackley CE: Quantitative assessment of ventricular performance in unstable ischemic heart disease by dextran function curves. Circulation 55:858—863, 1977.
22. Turner JD, Rogers WJ, Mantle JA, Rackley CE, Russell RO Jr: Coronary arteriography soon after myocardial infarction. Chest 77:58—64, 1980.
23. Rogers WJ, McDaniel HG, Smith LR, Mantle JA, Russell RO Jr, Rackley CE: Correlation of angiographic estimates of myocardial infarct size and accumulated release of creatine kinase MB isoenzyme in man. Circulation 56:199, 1977.

7. CONTRAST VENTRICULOGRAPHY

VICTOR S. BEHAR

Global as well as regional ventricular function may be altered as a result of obstructive coronary artery disease. These changes may be caused by myocardial ischemia or as a result of a healed transmural myocardial infarct. Contrast ventriculography is a useful technique by which both global and regional abnormalities of left ventricular function may be clinically demonstrated.

The first measurements of intracardiac volumes in patients were reported by Arvidsson in 1958 [1]. The biplane radiographic technique that he used employed a filming speed of six film pairs per second. A similar method was used by Dodge and co-workers to derive pressure—volume curves in patients with valvular heart disease [2]. Because of the relatively slow film speed, several consecutive cardiac cycles had to be used to construct a single composite ventricular volume curve. End-diastolic and end-systolic volumes could then be obtained directly from these curves. In order to obviate the use of multiple cardiac cycles, faster filming speeds were needed. Initially, speeds of 15 or 30 frames per second were used [3], but because of the excessive radiation necessary with early cineradiographic equipment, the technique was applicable primarily for animal studies [3] and selective studies of patients [3–5]. With the introduction of image intensification and higher film speeds, pressure—volume observations from single cardiac cycles became readily available in patients [6]. With a film speed of 60 frames per second, it became relatively simple to identify biplane film pairs at end-diastole and end-systole for calculating end-diastolic and end-systolic ventricular volumes without constructing complete volume curves. These measurements can now be routinely obtained in over 90% of patients undergoing diagnostic cardiac catheterization [7]. They provide useful information to the clinician concerning ventricular function and the natural history of coronary artery disease, and they can be used to predict treatment outcomes [7–9].

The contrast material used for cineventriculography has been shown to produce peripheral hemodynamic changes [10, 11] as well as to directly depress myocardial contractility [12, 13]. For these reasons, the cardiac cycle selected for analysis should be: (a) the earliest opacified cycle suitable for accurate tracing and within the first five opacified beats in order to avoid the negative inotropic effect of the contrast agent, and (b) remote from premature ventricular

Wagner GS (ed): Myocardial Infarction: Measurement and Intervention, pp 173–197.
© *1982 Martinus Nijhoff Publishers, The Hague/Boston/London.*

contractions in order to avoid the postextrasystolic potentiation of the cardiac cycle immediately following a premature beat [12].

VENTRICULAR VOLUME CALCULATIONS

Although the original method described for the calculation of ventricular volume employed a biplane radiographic technique with strict anteroposterior and lateral views of the heart, most laboratories currently using biplane cine equipment find it necessary to position the patient in a slight right anterior oblique position in order to provide the sharpest detail and to avoid the superimposition of cardiac chambers upon the spinal column. Wynne and co-workers [14] and more recently Rogers and co-workers [15] have validated the accuracy of the area—length method of Dodge et al. [16] for calculating ventricular volumes with the patient in the right anterior oblique position as compared with the strict anteroposterior position.

Many laboratories, however, by virtue of their use of a single-plane filming technique, have introduced still another variable into the calculation of venticular volume. Although single-plane estimates of ventricular volume had been shown to compare favorably with biplane estimates in normals and patients with valvular heart disease [17–20], more recent studies have shown that the single-plane angiogram consistently overestimates the data. Studies of 100 normal patients showed a slight overestimation of end-diastolic volume and ejection fraction and an underestimation of end-systolic volume when single-plane data were compared with biplane data [21]. This discrepancy was due primarily to differences between the right anterior oblique and left anterior oblique minor axes. The high degree of correlation between single- and biplane end-diastolic ($r = 0.92$) and end-systolic ($r = 0.93$) volume data depends upon the relatively symmetrical contraction of the ventricle during systole so that dimensions used in one plane are representative of the dimensions not viewed in the perpendicular plane. A problem would therefore seem evident in patients with coronary artery disease in whom there is asynergy, or an asymmetry in the contraction pattern, secondary to acute or chronic ischemia or a previous transmural myocardial infarct. Studies by Vogel et al. [22] and by Walsh et al. [23] demonstrated that, in patients with coronary artery disease, the single-plane ejection fraction underestimated the biplane data. Gentzler and co-workers [24] compared single-plane frontal and single-plane lateral ventricular volume data and demonstrated that the lateral ejection fraction was considerably less than that obtained from the frontal view. In comparing single-plane frontal and biplane data, there was good correlation for end-diastolic volume but marked differences in stroke volume and ejection fraction. These differences were due to a disparity in the extent of minor axis shortening measured in the anteroposterior and lateral views. Cohn and co-workers [25] also addressed this problem and substantiated the previously reported good correlation in normal patients. Although they found a reasonable correlation between single-plane and biplane end-diastolic volume, end-systolic volume, and ejection fraction in patients with coronary artery disease, the scatter was greater than found in the normals, especially in the presence of regional wall motion abnormalities. As shown in Figures 1–3, studies in our own laboratory showed excellent correlation between single-plane and biplane end-diastolic volumes ($r = 0.969$ in those with asynergy and 0.951 in those without asynergy), end-systolic volume ($r = 0.984$ in those with asynergy and 0.965 in those without asynergy), and ejection fraction ($r = 0.942$ in those with asynergy and 0.889 in those without asynergy). When the slopes of the regression lines expressing these relationships were tested, no significant differences were observed between patients with asynergy and those without asynergy for end-diastolic volume and ejection fraction. The slopes for end-systolic volume were found to differ significantly ($p < 0.0001$), but it is apparent from direct observation of the data points (Figure 2) that this difference is of no practical importance and probably reflects the large amount of data being analyzed as much as anything

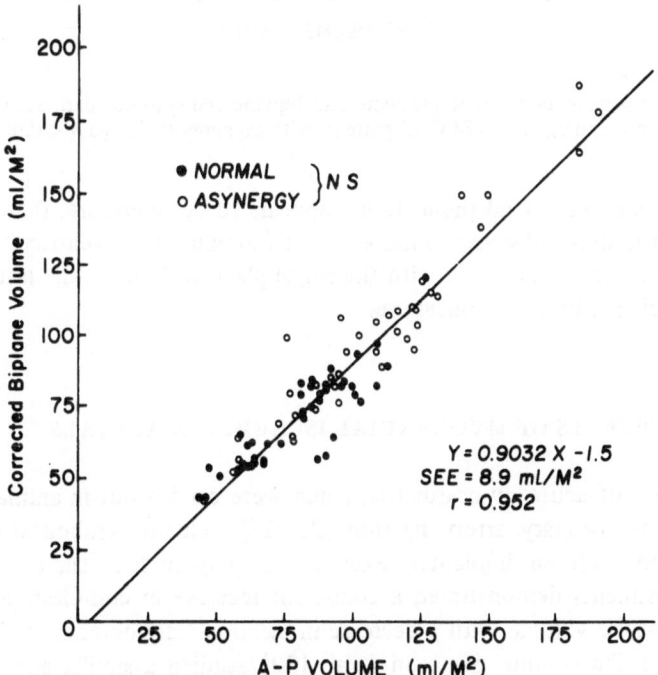

Figure 1. Comparison between single-plane and biplane end-diastolic volumes in 248 patients with coronary artery disease (CAD) and no asynergy and 474 CAD patients with asynergy ($p = $ NS).

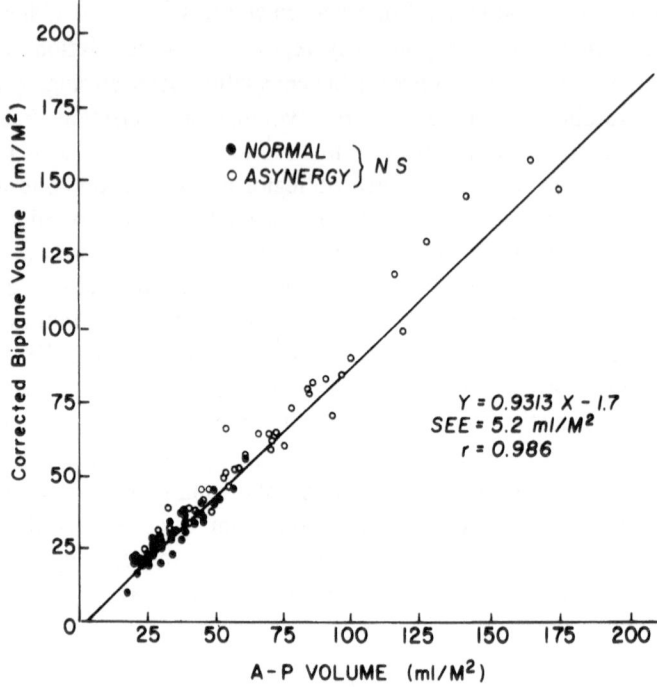

Figure 2. Comparison between single-plane and biplane end-systolic volumes in 248 CAD patients with no asynergy and 474 CAD patients with asynergy (adjusted *p* < 0.0001).

else. The consensus of all these studies appears to be, therefore, that although biplane ventriculography gives a more precise estimate of left ventricular volume and function when compared with the single-plane technique, the latter is still an acceptable method for clinical use.

GLOBAL EFFECTS OF MYOCARDIAL ISCHEMIA IN ANIMALS

Early studies of acute myocardial ischemia were carried out in animal models by means of coronary artery ligation [26, 27], selective embolization [28], or occlusion with an implanted exteriorized polyethylene snare [29]. The latter experiments demonstrated a consistent increase in end-diastolic volume and end-systolic volume with a decrease in ejection fraction and no significant change in stroke volume. Simpson et al. [30] studied a similar animal model in an attempt to determine how long a complete coronary artery occlusion could be tolerated by the animal without changing ventricular function irreversibly or producing a transmural myocardial infarct. Animals were studied

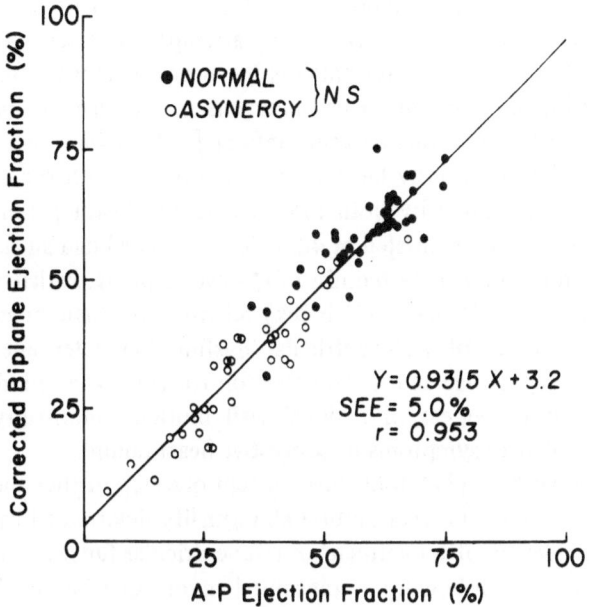

Figure 3. Comparison between single-plane and biplane ejection fractions in 248 CAD patients with no asynergy and 474 CAD patients with asynergy (*p* = NS).

near the end of a 30-, 45-, or 60-min snare occlusion of the left anterior descending coronary artery. Repeat ventriculography was performed 30 min and 90 min following release and at four days, prior to sacrifice. All animals showed an increase in end-diastolic and end-systolic volumes with a decrease in ejection fraction during occlusion. In the animals subjected to the 30-min occlusion, full return of function was observed within 90 min of snare release. The animals subjected to 60 min of occlusion retained abnormal ventricular function throughout the study period although improvement was observed at four days. The changes in the animals with 45-min occlusions were quite variable, with normal function returning in only a single animal. At postmortem examination four days after the transient occlusion, there was both gross and histologic evidence of myocardial necrosis in all of the animals in the 45- and 60-min occlusion groups, with no demonstrable changes in the 30-min group.

GLOBAL EFFECTS OF MYOCARDIAL ISCHEMIA IN HUMANS

Studies of patients following a documented transmural myocardial infarct have demonstrated similar changes in ventricular volume and ejection fraction [31, 32]. Based upon the observation that pathologic Q waves on the electrocardiogram, indicative of a myocardial infarct, correlate strongly with the presence of significant coronary artery stenosis as well as an abnormality of regional wall motion [33–35], Awan and co-workers [36] attempted to assess left ventricular function in postmyocardial infarct patients by means of Q wave mapping. This noninvasive technique was felt to be analogous to ST segment maps used to estimate ischemic zones during an acute infarct [37]. Q wave mapping studies in a dog model had previously been shown to correlate with the area of myocardial necrosis determined by both biochemical and histologic criteria [38]. Awan's study population consisted of 48 patients who had had an acute anterior myocardial infarct within three months of Q wave mapping. Patient groups with increasing numbers of Q waves (Q index) recorded on their precordial maps had increasing degrees of left ventricular dysfunction determined from the stroke work index, cardiac index, and ejection fraction. The Q index was also related to increasing degrees of regional wall motion abnormality on ventriculography as well as to symptoms of congestive heart failure.

Feild and co-workers [31] took this concept one step further and attempted to relate the extent of the wall motion abnormality determined by the ventriculogram to the degree of impairment of left ventricular function. They studied 25 patients one year following a transmural myocardial infarct. The relative extent of the infarct characterized on the ventriculogram as either a localized lack of motion of a ventricular wall (akinesis) or paradoxical expansion of a ventricular wall (dyskinesis) was quantitated and expressed as a percent of the total diastolic ventricular circumference. The percent abnormally contracting segment (% ACS) was found to be negatively correlated with the ejection fraction. This was the first time that an abnormality in regional myocardial function was quantitatively related to depressed global ventricular function. In addition, the % ACS was positively related to left ventricular end-diastolic pressure and end-diastolic volume. Regression lines developed in this study showed that when ACS exceeded 15% the left ventricular end-diastolic pressure was increased above 12 mmHg, and when the ACS exceeded 17% the end-diastolic volume was increased above 110 ml/m^2.

These findings supported the observations reported by Klein and co-workers [39] who described a theoretical spherical model relating the fiber-shortening requirements of myocardium to nonfunctioning or inactive muscle, expressed as a percent of the total left ventricular surface area. In that study, it was estimated that with the loss of approximately 20% of ventricular surface, the heart must undergo compensatory dilatation in order to maintain adequate pump function. Data reported by Klein and co-workers in patients with ventricular aneurysms substantiated their theoretical data by showing that when nonfunctioning myocardium exceeded 20% of the total left ventricular surface area, the ability of the remaining myocardium to maintain stroke volume was compromised. Cardiac enlargement must then ensue as a compensatory mechanism according to the Frank–Starling principle. Field et al. [31] found that, in patients with clinical evidence of congestive heart failure, the ACS was greater than 23% and the ejection fraction was less than 30%. In a subsequent study, the same investigators [32] found a hyperbolic relation between ejection fraction and end-diastolic volume. Because of the hyperbolic shape of the curve, when the end-diastolic volume was normal ($< 110\,\mathrm{ml/m^2}$) small increases in end-diastolic volume were associated with large decreases in ejection fraction. At the other end of the hyperbolic regression curve where end-diastolic volume exceeded $150\,\mathrm{ml/m^2}$, large increases in end-diastolic volume were associated with a small decrease in ejection fraction. The following conclusions were drawn from their observations: (a) when the end-diastolic volume was more than $70\,\mathrm{ml/m^2}$, the ejection fraction was decreased ($< 50\%$); (b) when the end-diastolic volume exceeded the upper limit of normal ($> 110\,\mathrm{ml/m^2}$), the ejection fraction was less than 35%; and (c) when the end-diastolic volume was greater than $150\,\mathrm{ml/m^2}$, the ejection fraction was less than 25%.

ANGIOGRAPHIC CORRELATES OF MYOCARDIAL INFARCT SIZE

Although there are major assumptions involved with all current techniques to estimate infarct size, both the accumulated release of creatine kinase MB isoenzymes (see Roberts, p. 114) and the % ACS have received much clinical use. Rogers et al. [40] correlated these two independent techniques in a series of patients studied during the postmyocardial infarct convalescent period. They found that, in the absence of a preceding myocardial infarct, there was excellent correlation between % ACS and the normalized Σ CK-MB ($r = 0.84$). This relationship was further improved when only patients with anterior infarction were considered ($r = 0.88$). An excellent negative correlation was found between ejection fraction and normalized Σ CK-MB; the intercept of the least-squares regression line relating these two variables was an ejection fraction of 63%. This theoretical value representing the ejection fraction for a zero enzymatic infarct compares favorably with a normal mean value for this descriptor of pump function. In patients with a previous myocardial infarct, there was no correlation between the normalized Σ CK-MB and either % ACS or ejection fraction. This was felt to be the consequence of preexisting ventricular dysfunction.

Rigaud and co-workers [41] have recently reported their findings in a group of patients who underwent contrast ventriculography 2–6 days following an acute myocardial infarct. The end-diastolic volume was increased only in patients with overt pulmonary edema or cardiogenic shock, while end-systolic volume was increased in patients with lesser degrees of heart failure. The ejection fraction was reduced in all patients, with more dysfunction observed in patients with increasing clinical findings of congestive heart failure. In addition, there was an inverse linear relation between ejection fraction and % ACS ($r = -0.97$). Although patients with an anterior infarct had a greater % ACS than patients with an inferior infarct, when comparable subgroups of % ACS were analyzed, there were no significant differences in left ventricular function. If one compares the relationship of % ACS and ejection fractions in these patients with the theoretical spherical model reported by Swan and co-workers [42], some differences are noted. The theoretical model assumes a negative linear correlation between ejection fraction and the relative area of inert or non-contractile myocardium. The slope of the regression line for the patients reported by Rigaud et al. [41] was significantly higher than the line for the theoretical spherical model of Swan and co-workers. This results in a greater than predicted ejection fraction for patients with an ACS < 25% and a lower than predicted ejection fraction for patients with an ACS > 25%. This may be restated to imply that, in patients with smaller infarcts, the noninfarcted myocardium functioned at a supernormal level. Since the end-diastolic volume in these patients was normal, the hypercontractile response cannot be explained by the Frank–Starling mechanism and must be related to an increased endogenous sympathetic drive. Conversely, although the end-diastolic volume was increased in the patients with an ACS > 25%, the compensatory response with respect to preload was inadequate and the hypocontractile response of the noninfarcted muscle resulted in ventricular dysfunction and pump failure. The authors postulated that the hypocontractile response could be due to preexisting but unrecognized myocardial damage or to reduced coronary blood flow to the noninvolved myocardium.

Rigaud et al. [41] also demonstrated that patients with cardiogenic shock had a higher % ACS than those without cardiogenic shock, and that death occurred consistently in patients with an ACS in excess of 40%–50%. Studies in our own laboratory comparing angiographic and postmortem data demonstrated that the ejection fraction was inversely related to the extent of myocardial fibrosis found at autopsy [43].

THE CHARACTERIZATION OF WALL MOTION ABNORMALITIES

Global ventricular function is depressed following a transmural myocardial infarct; the increase in ventricular volumes and the decrease in ejection fraction are related to the amount of inactive muscle comprising the ventricular surface as viewed on the ventriculogram. Studies relating % ACS to ventricular function are based upon severe changes in regional ventricular performance, i.e., akinesis or dyskinesis.

Regional wall motion abnormalities were classically described by Herman and co-workers [44, 45]. The normal pattern of ventricular contraction is a uniform, almost concentric, inward movement of the ventricular wall during systolic ejection. The aortic–apical axis shortens approximately 20% while hemiaxes perpendicular to this long axis shorten as much as 50% along the anterior wall and the periapical region of the ventricle. This normal or uniform pattern of contraction is termed synergy. Four abnormal patterns of contraction were also described: akinesis, total absence of movement of a wall segment; dyskinesis, paradoxical expansion of a wall segment; asyneresis, decreased inward movement of a wall segment; and asynchrony, a disturbance in the temporal relationship of movement in one area of the wall in relation to the other wall segments (Figure 4). Asyneresis is used synonymously with hypokinesis by many investigators, and few use the term asynchrony.

Ideker et al. [43] studied the relationship of the classifications of asynergy to the extent of fibrosis quantitatively determined at postmortem examination. Of the ventricular walls with significant fibrosis, 95% exhibited asynergy determined by an automated quantitative technique. The amount of fibrosis increased progressively with the increasing severity of asynergy: normal wall motion, 0.4% fibrosis; hypokinesis, 6.3% fibrosis; akinesis, 14.3%; and dyskinesis, 30.1%. Therefore, although the classification of asynergy was based upon both gross inspection of the ventriculogram as well as an empirically defined mathematical model, it can provide us with important pathophysiologic information.

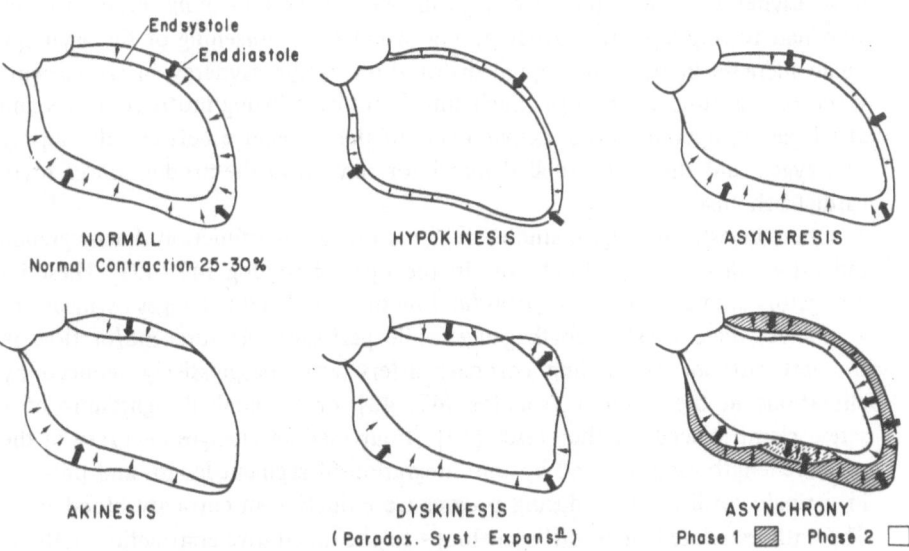

Figure 4. Left ventricular contraction patterns viewed in the right anterior oblique projection. Arrows indicate direction of movement during systole. Reprinted with permission of Herman MV, et al., *New England Journal of Medicine* 277:222, 1967.

Herman et al. demonstrated a high degree of correlation between areas of asynergy and significant obstructive coronary artery disease, electrocardiographic abnormalities, and abnormal regional lactate metabolism [44, 45]. Hemodynamic compromise was found in those patients with asynergy manifest by a decrease in cardiac index and an increase in left ventricular end-diastolic pressure and end-diastolic volume, especially in those patients with fibrotic ventricular aneurysms. However, equivalent degrees of coronary obstruction were present in patients without asynergy, and other patients had evidence of myocardial ischemia manifest by abnormal regional lactate metabolism or electrocardiographic changes without asynergy being observed. Upon direct observation at surgery or at postmortem examination, most asynergic zones were found to contain fibrotic scar although five of 22 of these areas were composed of full-thickness myocardium. Ventriculography performed in two patients with asynergy demonstrated improvement in the asynergic zone during epinephrine infusion and marked worsening following intravenous beta-adrenergic blockade. Thus, asynergic zones of myocardium may not necessarily be permanent fibrotic changes but may represent a dynamic phenomenon that may change with the changing metabolic demands of the regional myocardium. Pasternac and co-workers [46] addressed this question by using pacing-induced ischemia during cineventriculography. Of their ten patients with arteriographically proven coronary artery disease, three had normal ventriculograms at rest. Repeat ventriculography during atrial pacing in these three patients demonstrated de novo asynergy in two and no change in one. In the remaining seven patients, who had resting asynergy, atrial pacing produced a worsening of the asynergy or an increase in the topographic distribution of the asynergy in six patients while one showed no change. Such interventions utilizing inotropic drugs and atrial pacing operate on the demand side of the imbalance between the supply of oxygen and the myocardial demand for oxygen in the production of myocardial ischemia.

Other investigators have studied regional myocardial function during graded reductions in coronary blood flow in the open-chest dog [47–49]. These investigators studied regional myocardial function and length changes by means of a mercury-filled silastic length gauge while perfusion pressure and/or flow in the left anterior descending coronary artery were progressively reduced by alterations in the pump-oxygenator [47, 48] or by gradual tightening of a screw clamp placed on the vessel [49]. Four distinct changes occurred in the pressure-length loop, derived by the integration of segment length and pressure in a single cardiac cycle, during progressive reduction in coronary blood flow. The authors related these different loops to the qualitative contraction patterns observed by Herman et al. on the ventriculograms of patients with coronary artery disease [44, 45]. These changes coincided with regional lactate production indicating myocardial ischemia [49] and were reversible upon reoxygenation

[48]. Each of these studies suffers from the inherent effects of an open-chest preparation on ventricular function.

Tzivoni et al. [50] studied the effects of balloon occlusion of the left anterior descending artery and its attendant ischemia of the anterior ventricular wall in the closed-chest dog. Regional ventricular wall motion was assessed by means of quantitative left ventricular cineangiography. These studies demonstrated a rapid decrease in systolic shortening, leading ultimately to complete absence of inward movement in the anterior wall and outward systolic movement of the ventricular apex. This was accompanied by an increase in the inward movement of the inferior ventricular wall. These quantitative changes were comparable to the changes observed by means of directly implanted length gauges [47–49] as well as the subjective ventriculographic changes observed following snare occlusion of the left circumflex artery [29].

There is little doubt that ventricular asynergy may be produced by a fibrotic scar secondary to a transmural infarct as well as by acute myocardial ischemia. Furthermore, there is reason to believe that asynergy may be produced by subacute or chronic myocardial ischemia in the absence of a transmural infarct. For instance, in the patients reported by Herman et al. [44, 45], the observation was made both at postmortem examination and at surgery that the asynergic zone was not infrequently composed of muscle and not scar tissue and that such areas were producing lactate. Chatterjee and co-workers [51] studied a group of patients with preinfarct angina before and after aortocoronary bypass surgery. Five of their six patients had depressed ventricular function and localized asynergy preoperatively that returned to normal following the restoration of coronary blood flow by surgery. While patients with preinfarct or unstable angina probably represent a subacute stage of myocardial ischemia, the literature is replete with reports of ventricular asynergy in the absence of electrocardiographic evidence of an infarct [34, 35, 52–56], as well as asynergy that normalizes following revascularization [52, 55–57].

INTERVENTION VENTRICULOGRAPHY

It would seem imperative that the clinical investigator have available a means of separating patients with asynergy into those with permanent fibrotic scars and those with potentially reversible myocardial ischemia. The dynamic nature of the asynergy observed in some patients by Herman et al. [44, 45] led Helfant and co-workers [57] to study the effects of sublingual nitroglycerin on the ventriculogram of 35 patients with asynergy, 12 of whom were restudied following aortocoronary bypass surgery. They found improved wall motion in 73% of the hypokinetic zones and 57% of the akinetic zones (44% returning to normal), while none of the dyskinetic segments showed any significant change.

In the patients who were restudied following aortocoronary bypass surgery, 91% of the hypokinetic segments that responded preoperatively to nitroglycerin were improved and 71% of the preoperatively responsive akinetic segments showed improvement. Patients who were nonresponders preoperatively showed no improvement postoperatively despite the presence of patent grafts, while all segments showing deterioration in the postoperative ventriculogram had evidence of a perioperative infarct. Fibrous scar tissue was observed frequently at surgery in the nonresponsive hypokinetic zones, more frequently in the nonresponsive akinetic zones, and invariably in areas of dyskinesis. These data provided the first evidence that nitroglycerin intervention ventriculography may be useful in determining the extent of residual contractile ability in asynergic regions of the myocardium as well as in predicting optimum candidates for bypass surgery. Similar improvement in regional asynergy was observed by Sniderman et al. [58] and McAnulty et al. [59] following the administration of sublingual nitroglycerin. In addition, McAnulty and co-workers noted an improvement in ejection fraction from 47% to 62% in the nitroglycerin responders while there was no significant change in the nonresponders.

Banka et al. [53] correlated the presence of Q waves on the electrocardiogram and collaterals on the coronary arteriogram to the responsiveness of asynergy to nitroglycerin in 36 patients. In the absence of Q waves, 83% of the segments showed improvement while 16% had no change. When pathologic Q waves were present, on the other hand, only 44% improved following nitroglycerin while 56% were unchanged. The severity of the asynergy was further analyzed and demonstrated no independent effect of the presence of Q waves in the presence of hypokinesis. However, in the presence of akinesis, only 28% of patients with Q waves were responders in contrast to 80% of those without Q waves. Collaterals were an important predictor of responsiveness in that 84% of segments associated with collateral vessels showed improvement following nitroglycerin as opposed to only 15% without collaterals. In the absence of collaterals, approximately half were responders and half nonresponders. The presence of collaterals did not appear to influence the response to nitroglycerin for hypokinetic segments, although in patients with collaterals there was a higher response rate for akinetic segments.

This improvement in regional myocardial performance following sublingual nitroglycerin may be due to improvement in collateral blood flow, to reflex release of catecholamines secondary to vasodilation and hypotension, or to a reduction in wall stress. The latter is produced by a reduction in ventricular volume and systolic pressure. These changes would serve to decrease the metabolic requirements of the myocardium for oxygen and therefore to improve the balance between myocardial oxygen supply and demand. Banka et al. evaluated the influence of the severity of the coronary artery stenotic lesion and the caliber of the distal vessels on the reversibility of asynergy [54]. They found that in patients with coronary lesions ≥ 90%, akinesis/dyskinesis was present in 64% and hypokinesis in 36%. When the stenotic lesion was estimated to be < 90%, akinesis/dyskinesis was present in only 29% and hypokinesis in 71%. This finding was of significance in view of the previous observations that reversibility of an asynergic zone depends partly on the absence of fibrotic scar. Since the more severe forms of asynergy have previously been shown to have a greater likelihood of being fibrotic, it was not surprising that Banka et al. found that 69% of asynergic zones with < 90% stenosis were reversible and only 45% with ≥ 90% lesions were reversible. They further observed that in the presence of ≥ 90% stenosis there was a higher incidence of reversible asynergy when collateral vessels were present, suggesting that they served a protective function. When similar comparisons were made concerning the caliber of distal vessels, no significant differences were found.

Postextrasystolic potentiation (PESP) has also been used to demonstrate the reversibility of ventricular asynergy. The increase in contractile force of the sinus beat following a premature ventricular contraction may reflect a Frank–Starling mechanism or may occur in the absence of any increase in preload, indicating a positive inotropic response. Hamby and co-workers [55] reported findings similar to those observed with sublingual nitroglycerin: asynergic zones were more likely to revert to normal in patients without a preceding myocardial infarct. Furthermore, patients with hypokinesis were more likely to show improved regional function than those with akinesis. The ejection fraction of the sinus beat following the premature ventricular contraction improved in all patients in their study including normals, patients with coronary artery disease and normal ventricles, patients with asynergy and no previous infarct, and patients with asynergy and a previous infarct. The greatest degree of improvement in the ejection fraction was observed in the patients with asynergy, either with or without Q waves. In a subgroup of patients undergoing aortocoronary bypass surgery and repeat left ventriculography, there was excellent agreement between the response of the asynergic zone to PESP and revascularization. Similar observations before and after bypass surgery were reported by Popio et al. [56], who also demonstrated that the improvement in ejection fraction in the potentiated beat correlated with the improved ventricular function observed in patients following bypass surgery.

These studies demonstrated, therefore, that postnitroglycerin and PESP ventriculography are useful adjuncts to investigate the potential usefulness of bypass surgery upon both regional and global ventricular function. From a practical standpoint, PESP is simpler to use as it does not require a second ventriculogram. Banka et al. [60] and Klausner et al. [61] studied the separate and the combined effects of nitroglycerin and PESP. Both studies demonstrated a similar ability of all three modalities to unmask asynergy without any particular advantage of one over another. Thus, the specific intervention used in any given clinical situation should be individualized for the particular patient.

As described earlier in this chapter, Herman and co-workers [44, 45] made the observation at surgery and at postmortem examination that asynergic zones were not invariably composed of fibrotic scar but frequently had the appearance of full-thickness myocardium. Similar observations were reported by Helfant et al. [57] in their study of nitroglycerin-reversible asynergy. They found by direct observation at surgery that scar tissue was frequently present in unresponsive hypokinetic zones, more commonly present in unresponsive akinetic zones, and always present in dyskinetic zones. Since nitroglycerin-induced reversible asynergy is less likely to occur in the presence of Q waves, severely stenotic coronary artery lesions ($\geqslant 90\%$ obstruction), and the more severe forms of asynergy (akinesis/dyskinesis), it is likely, in light of the findings of Helfant et al. [57] and Herman et al. [44, 45] that these conditions are all associated histologically with transmural infarcts. Bodenheimer et al. [62, 63] studied precisely this relationship in patients with coronary artery disease undergoing aortocoronary bypass and/or left ventricular aneurysmectomy. Epicardial electrograms were recorded during surgery from multiple sites on the right ventricle, septal area, anteroapical area, and the lateral and inferior walls of the left ventricle. Punch biopsies were obtained from the anteroapical and inferior regions of the left ventricle. Each tissue specimen was graded for the degree of muscle loss and the percent replacement by fibrosis. Particular care was taken so that biopsy and electrogram data could be correlated with the ventriculographic findings obtained prior to surgery. The presence of pathologic Q waves on the surface electrogram correlated best with the more severe forms of asynergy (akinesis/dyskinesis) on the control ventriculogram and with the failure to show improvement of the asynergy on the nitroglycerin ventriculogram. Conversely, almost two-thirds of those with an initial R wave on the surface electrogram had hypokinesis on the control ventriculogram and about 90% of these showed improvement following nitroglycerin. The biopsy data showed that of the 17 akinetic/dyskinetic zones that did not respond to nitroglycerin, 11 demonstrated more than 75% fibrosis and two had more than 50% fibrosis. In contrast, all 12 of the patients who responded to nitroglycerin (11 with hypokinesis and one with dyskinesis) had less than 10% replacement by fibrosis. Generally speaking, the more severe forms of asynergy were more likely to have the greatest amount of muscle loss. However, a significant number of patients with severe asynergy (akinesis/dyskinesis) were found to have minimal fibrosis and a structurally intact myocardium. A reasonable conclusion would be that such zones are rendered asynergic by ischemia rather than by muscle loss and should therefore demonstrate improved performance following myocardial revascularization.

OBSERVER VARIABILITY OF VENTRICULAR ASYNERGY

There seems to be little doubt that the characterization of regional myocardial performance according to the criteria of Herman et al. [44, 45] and the response of asynergic zones to inotropic interventions and changes in the loading conditions of the heart provide useful pathophysiologic information. One must raise the question, however, as to the reproducibility of these observations in terms of both intraobserver and interobserver variability Chaitman et al. [64] demonstrated excellent intraobserver and interobserver agreement for quantitatively analyzed asynergy, while there was considerable disagreement when similar comparisons were made using a subjective assessment of asynergy. Zir et al. [65] divided the ventricle into five segments and classified the wall motion into six grades: normal, mild hypokinesis, moderate hypokinesis, severe hypokinesis, akinesis, and dyskinesis. They found a mean rate of disagreement of 42% between the observers with the least disagreement in the anterobasal region of the ventricle. When disagreement was defined as a difference of more than one class, the mean rate of disagreement decreased to 16%. Tzivoni et al. [50] had a similar degree of interobserver disagreement in the reading of wall motion in an animal model for the study of acute myocardial ischemia. Of 540 total readings, there was disagreement between three observers 22% of the time. Ideker et al. [43] compared qualitatively and quantitatively determined wall motion with each other as well as with the presence of myocardial fibrosis found at postmortem examination. The quantitative method demonstrated the presence of asynergy more often than the qualitative method. Of the walls identified as quantitatively abnormal but qualitatively normal, there was significant fibrosis in 82%. On the other hand, all walls that were quantitatively normal but qualitatively abnormal were free of significant fibrosis. In all of the cases together when there was disagreement, the quantitative technique correctly predicted the presence or absence of fibrosis in 86%.

These observer variability studies and comparisons of qualitative and quantitative analyses with postmortem findings clearly indicate the need to study resting and intervention ventriculography by quantitative methods. Although initial attempts were extremely time consuming and laborious, the widespread use of computer systems in data reduction has made such studies much easier to perform.

QUANTITATION OF VENTRICULAR ASYNERGY

All of the objective methods used to quantitate ventricular wall motion are based upon an empirical geometric reference figure. Each method has its own inherent assumptions and problems. The diastolic silhouette of the ventricle is generally used as the fixed reference from which the endocardial surface moves during contraction. Implicit in any mathematical model is the assumption that a given point on the endocardial surface in diastole can be represented by a specific point on the endocardium during systolic contraction. This is obviously impossible without the use of endocardial markers. The systolic silhouette is usually realigned along the long axis of the heart, which connects the middle of the aortic valve plane and apex. Two commonly used methods involve super-imposing the midpoint of this long axis for the systolic and diastolic images [52, 66] or superimposing the midpoints of the aortic valve [39, 44, 67]. Both methods assume that the long axis remains unchanged during ventricular con-traction, and that all points on the endocardial surface in diastole move sym-metrically toward this center axis in the first method and toward the base of the heart for the second method. Neither technique corrects for movement of the patient on the X-ray table, movement of the diaphragm, or a change in the long axis of the heart. In order to correct for these factors, Chaitman et al. [66] have used two fixed external reference points and the patient's diaphragm as an internal reference point. These investigators demonstrated better cor-relation of the external reference method with the electrocardiographic findings of infarct than either of the other two methods in a direct comparison of the same patients. Others have attempted to use a coronary sinus catheter as an internal reference point [68]. Unfortunately, a coronary sinus catheter also reflects cardiac motion and, since it fixes the position of the mitral valve, it will exaggerate apical to base shortening.

Having chosen the type of alignment, a variety of chord models have been used to express regional wall motion. Some authors have divided the long axis from the aortic valve to the apex of the heart into four equidistant segments, creating either three chords [68] or six hemiaxes [44], or alternately into five equidistant segments and a resultant eight hemiaxes for analysis [43]. In ad-dition to the chord method, Herman et al. have also utilized a radial technique whereby the center points of the long axes of the diastolic and systolic silhouet-tes are superimposed and four radii are constructed at 45° intervals [44]. All of these methods express the degree of hemiaxis or chord shortening during systole as a percent of the initial or diastolic length, i.e., thereby normalized for the initial length. Chaitman and co-workers [64] have also approached the problem by studying regional changes of the heart during systole. With this technique, the long axis in the right anterior oblique separates the heart into anterior and inferior zones while a perpendicular axis placed one-fourth the distance from the apex creates an apical region. Regional function was ex-pressed as a percent change in regional area and did not require superimposing the diastolic and systolic silhouettes. Gelberg et al. [69] have recently reported their findings of a direct comparison between the area, chord, and radial methods in 17 patients with a normal ventricle and 17 patients with one or more zones of severe asynergy. After statistically normalizing their data to represent the number of standard deviations that the abnormal value differed from the normal mean, the null hypothesis was tested using a 2×3 contingency table which demonstrated a difference among the three methods. Further testing showed that the difference was due to the area method which was found to have the lowest failure rate and the greatest ability to differentiate normal areas from abnormal areas.

Our laboratory uses an automated system for calculating both ventricular volume and regional wall motion data. Because of its automation, we are able to collect the data as a routine part of the procedure in over 90% of the patients undergoing study [7]. The biplane film pairs of the left ventricle at end-diastole and end-systole are traced onto clear plastic with a wax pencil on a rear projection screen. These images are then digitized by means of a sonic digitizer interfaced to a PDP 11/45 computer that stores the data as x, y coordinates on a data disk. This digitized information is then used to calculate biplane ventricular volume data using the area–length method of Dodge et al. [16] as modified in our laboratory [6], as well as for the quantitation of wall motion [43]. Three methods are currently being used to assess regional ventricular function in our laboratory, as shown in Figure 5A–C and in Tables 1–3. In the hemiaxial method, a longitudinal axis is contructed connecting the middle of the aortic valve plane and apex of the heart for both the end-diastolic and end-systolic silhouettes. This axis is then divided into five segments of equal length and hemiaxes perpendicular to the longitudinal axis are constructed to the borders of the silhouette as shown in Figure 5A. This results in nine hemiaxes for both the shallow right anterior oblique and steep left anterior oblique image. The percent shortening of each hemiaxis is calculated according to the formula: percent shortening = (diastolic length − systolic length/diastolic length) x 100. In the radial method, radii are constructed from the midpoint of the longitudinal axis to the edge of the ventricular silhouette at $15°$ intervals where hemiaxis 12 represents the apical segment for both the right anterior and left anterior oblique views (Figure 5b). In the area method, the longitudinal axis in the right anterior oblique view is divided into thirds and chords are constructed from these points to the edge of the left ventricular image (Figure 5c). The apical region is treated as a single area combining both anterior and inferior subdivisions. In the left anterior oblique view the longitudinal axis is divided in half with a single perpendicular line dividing the posterolateral left ventricle into two areas in addition to a single septal area. All three methods treat end-diastole and end-systole independently, thereby correcting for cardiac motion except for any rotation that may occur during ventricular contraction.

The normal values shown in Tables 1–3 were derived from 58 patients with normal coronary arteriograms and left ventriculograms, who had undergone

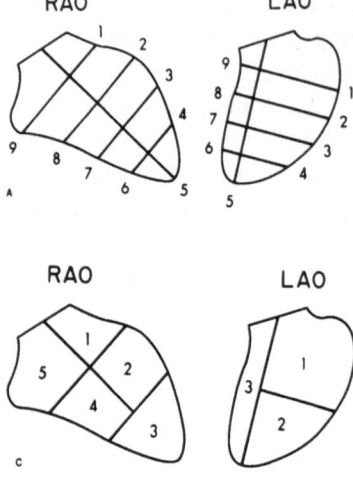

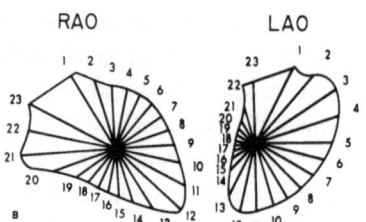

Figure 5A–C. (*A*) Hemiaxial method of determining regional abnormalities of wall motion in right anterior oblique (RAO) and left anterior oblique projections (LAO). Hemiaxes 1 and 9 in the RAO view and 1 in the LAO may overlie the mitral ring and therefore may not reflect left ventricular wall motion. (*B*) Radial method of determining regional abnormalities of wall motion in RAO and LAO views. As noted in the text, radial axes 1–3 in RAO and LAO views may be superimposed on the mitral ring as well as axes 21–23 in the RAO view. In addition, radial axis 23 in the LAO view may be superimposed on the aortic valve. In any of these situations, the involved axes are disregarded. (*C*) Area method for determining regional abnormalities of wall motion in RAO and LAO views.

cardiac catheterization because of atypical chest pain. Asynergy is defined quantitatively for each axis or area as decreased systolic hemiaxis shortening or area change greater than 2 standard deviations from the mean. In the right anterior oblique view, hemiaxes 1 and 9 and radial axes 1–3 and 21–23 frequently overlie the mitral annulus and in those situations should not be used. This may also be true of hemiaxis 1 and radial axes 1–3 in the left anterior oblique view.

Although biplane ventriculography would be expected to aid in the identification of more asynergic zones than single-plane ventriculography, this has not proven to be the case. Studies by Ideker et al. [43] as well as by Cohn et al. [25] have shown that asynergy was never seen exclusively in the left anterior oblique view indicating that all asynergic zones may be identified by single-plane right anterior oblique ventriculography. One might speculate, however, that biplane filming would provide the angiographer with a better estimate of the total extent of the asynergy.

Table 1. Hemiaxial system of analysis in 58 normal patients

Angiographic view		Hemiaxis	Systolic shortening Mean	(SD)	Lower limit of normal (based on 2 SD)
RAO	Anterior wall	1	47	10	27
		2	34	9	16
		3	30	7	16
		4	32	8	16
	Apex	5	17	3	11
	Inferior wall	6	40	11	18
		7	33	8	17
		8	29	6	17
		9	12	12	−12
LAO	Posterolateral wall	1	12	9	−6
		2	15	7	1
		3	18	8	2
		4	24	14	−4
	Apex	5	21	4	13
	Septum	6	44	19	6
		7	49	20	9
		8	50	27	−4
		9	−11	33	−77

CONCLUSIONS

In conclusion, contrast ventriculography has proven to be a useful clinical tool to characterize both global and regional ventricular function. Quantitative measures of global ventricular function have been shown to be important descriptors for survival in both medically [7, 8] as well as surgically treated patients [9]. And, finally, although the subjective interpretation of wall motion has proved useful in identifying ischemic regional myocardial dysfunction, the problems of observer variability and reproducibility have led many investigators to resort to automated, quantitative methods. Because of the ability of intervention ventriculography to unmask reversible asynergy, it is hoped that these automated methods of analysis can be of helf in the clinician's understanding of the pathophysiology of coronary artery disease and that they will aid in the better selection of patients for medical and surgical therapy.

Table 2. Radial system of analysis in 58 normal patients

Angiographic view		Radial axis	Systolic shortening Mean	(SD)	Lower limit of normal (based on 2 SD)
RAO	Anterior wall	1	17	6	5
		2	35	8	19
		3	36	7	22
		4	34	8	18
		5	32	8	16
		6	30	7	16
		7	29	7	15
		8	28	6	16
		9	27	6	15
		10	25	5	15
		11	22	4	14
	Apex	12	17	3	11
	Inferior wall	13	26	6	14
		14	31	7	17
		15	32	7	18
		16	31	7	17
		17	31	8	15
		18	31	7	17
		19	30	7	16
		20	27	7	13
		21	14	10	−6
		22	15	6	3
		23	13	3	7
LAO	Posterolateral wall	1	17	3	11
		2	21	6	9
		3	17	7	3
		4	13	8	−3
		5	14	7	0
		6	16	7	2
		7	19	7	5
		8	22	7	8
		9	23	7	9
		10	24	7	10
		11	23	6	11
	Apex	12	21	4	13
	Septum	13	33	13	7
		14	45	19	7
		15	49	21	7
		16	51	21	9
		17	51	21	9
		18	51	22	7
		19	50	22	6
		20	48	23	2
		21	41	32	−23
		22	26	42	−58
		23	11	45	−79

Table 3. Area system of analysis in 58 normal patients

Angiographic view		Area	Systolic area change Mean (SD)		Lower limit of normal (based on 2 SD)
RAO	Anterior	1	52	7	38
		2	40	6	28
	Apex	3	48	6	36
	Inferior	4	43	6	31
		5	28	9	10
LAO	High posterolateral	1	26	9	8
	Low posterolateral	2	38	8	22
	Septum	3	54	15	24

REFERENCES

1. Arvidsson H: Angiocardiographic observations in mitral disease. Acta Radiol [Suppl] 158:11, 1958.
2. Dodge HT, Hay RE, Sandler H: Pressure-volume of the diastolic left ventricle of man with heart disease. Am Heart J 64:503, 1962.
3. Chapman CB, Baker O, Reynolds J, Bonte FJ: Use of biplane cinefluorography for measurement of ventricular volume. Circulation 18:1105, 1958.
4. Bunnell IL, Grant C, Greene DG: Left ventricular function derived from the pressure-volume diagram. Am J Med 39:881, 1965.
5. Miller GAH, Kirklin JW, Swan HJC: Myocardial function and left ventricular volumes in acquired valvular insufficiency. Circulation 31:374, 1965.
6. Rackley CE, Behar VS, Whalen RE, McIntosh HD: Biplane cineangiographic determinations of left ventricular function: pressure-volume relationships. Am Heart J 74:766, 1967.
7. Harris PJ, Behar VS, Conley MJ, Rosati RA: Ventricular function and outcome in medically treated coronary artery disease. Circulation 60 [Suppl [2]:233, 1979.
8. Nelson GR, Cohn PF, Gorlin R: Prognosis in medically treated coronary artery disease. Influence of ejection fraction compared to other parameters. Circulation 52:408, 1975.
9. Oldham HN Jr, Kong Y, Bartel AG, Morris JJ Jr, Behar VS, Peter RH, Rosati RA, Young WG Jr, Sabiston DC Jr: Risk factors in coronary artery bypass surgery. Arch Surg 105:918, 1972.
10. Friesinger GC, Schaefer J, Criley JM, Gaertner RA, Ross RS: Hemodynamic consequences of the injection of radiopaque material. Circulation 31:730, 1965.
11. Brown R, Rahimtoola SH, Davis GD, Swan HJC: The effect of angiocardiographic contrast medium on circulatory dynamics in man. Cardiac output during angiocardiography. Circulation 31:234, 1965.
12. Behar VS, Waxman MB, Morris JJ Jr: The effects of a contrast medium (sodium iothalamate, 80%) on left ventricular function. Am J Med Sci 60:202, 1970.

13. Vine DL, Hegg TD, Dodge HT, Stewart DK, Frimer M: Immediate effect of contrast medium injection on left ventricular volumes and ejection fraction. A study using metallic epicardial markers. Circulation 56:379, 1977.
14. Wynne J, Green LH, Mann T, Levin D, Grossman W: Estimation of left ventricular volumes in man from biplane cineangiograms filmed in oblique projections. Am J Cardiol 41:726, 1978.
15. Rogers WJ, Smith LR, Hood WP Jr, Mantle JA, Rackley CE, Russell RO Jr: Effect of filming projection and interobserver variability on angiographic biplane left ventricular volume determination. Circulation 59:96, 1979.
16. Dodge HT, Sandler H, Ballew DW, Lord JD Jr: The use of biplane angiocardiography for the measurement of left ventricular volume in man. Am Heart J 60:762, 1960.
17. Greene DG, Carlisle R, Grant C, Bunnell IL: Estimation of left ventricular volume by one-plane cineangiography. Circulation 35:61, 1967.
18. Sandler H, Dodge HT: The use of single plane angiocardiograms for the calculation of left ventricular volume in man. Am Heart J 75:325, 1968.
19. Kasser IS, Kennedy JW: Measurement of left ventricular volumes in man by single-plane cineangiocardiography. Invest Radiol 4:83, 1969.
20. Kennedy JW, Trenholme SE, Kasser I: Left ventricular volume and mass from single-plane cineangiocardiogram. A comparison of anteroposterior and right anterior oblique methods. Am Heart J 80:343, 1970.
21. Fraker TD Jr, Wise NK, Harrell FE Jr, Behar VS: Comparison of biplane and single plane left ventricular volumes in atrial spetal defect. Cathet Cardiovasc Diagn 6:39, 1980.
22. Vogel JHK, Cornish D, McFadden RB: Underestimation of ejection fraction with singleplane angiography in coronary artery disease: role of biplane angiography. Chest 64:217, 1973.
23. Walsh W, Falicov RE, Pai AL: Comparison of single and biplane ejection fractions in patients with ischaemic heart disease. Br Heart J 38:388, 1976.
24. Gentzler RD II, Gault JH, Hunter AS, Liedtke AJ, Leaman DM: Asymmetric left ventricular contraction in patients with previous myocardial infarction. Comparison of volume and dimensional characteristics derived from frontal and lateral cineangiograms. Circulation 48:352, 1973.
25. Cohn PF, Gorlin R, Adams DF, Chahine RA, Vokonas PS, Herman MV: Comparison of biplane and single plane left ventriculograms in patients with coronary artery disease. Am J Cardiol 33:1, 1974.
26. Wégria R, Frank CW, Misrahy GA, Wang HH, Miller R, Case RB: Immediate hemodynamic effects of acute coronary occlusion. Am J Physiol 177:123, 1954.
27. Rushmer RF, Watson N, Harding D, Baker D: Effects of acute coronary occlusion on performance of right and left ventricles in intact unanesthetized dogs. Am Heart J 66:522, 1963.
28. Wong M, Escobar EE, Martinez G, Rapaport E: Effect of coronary artery embolization on ventricular volumes. Circ Res 16:518, 1965.
29. Harley A, Behar VS, McIntosh HD: Immediate hemodynamic effects of acute coronary occlusion and their modification by anesthesia. Am J Cardiol 22:559, 1968.
30. Simpson L, Behar VS, Ebert PA: Cardiac function after restoration of flow in acute coronary occlusion. Surg Forum 21:162, 1970.

31. Feild BJ, Russell RO Jr, Dowling JT, Rackley CE: Regional left ventricular performance in the year following myocardial infarction. Circulation 46: 679, 1972.
32. Feild BJ, Russell RO Jr, Moraski RE, Soto B, Hood WP Jr, Burdeshaw JA, Smith M, Maurer BJ, Rackley CE: Left ventricular size and function and heart size in the year following myocardial infarction. Circulation 50: 331, 1974.
33. Williams RA, Cohn PF, Vokonas PS, Young E, Herman MV, Gorlin R: Electrocardiographic, arteriographic and ventriculographic correlations in transmural myocardial infarction. Am J Cardiol 31:596, 1973.
34. Miller RR, Amsterdam EA, Bogren HG, Massumi RA, Zelis R, Mason DT: Electrocardiographic and cineangiographic correlations in the assessment of the location, nature and extent of abnormal left ventricular segmental contraction in coronary artery disease. Circulation 49:445, 1974.
35. Bodenheimer MM, Banka VS, Helfant RH: Q waves and ventricular asynergy: predictive value and hemodynamic significance of anatomic localization. Am J Cardiol 35:615, 1975.
36. Awan NA, Miller RR, Vera Z, Janzen DA, Amsterdam EA, Mason DT: Noninvasive assessment of cardiac function and ventricular dyssynergy by precordial Q wave mapping in anterior myocardial infarction. Circulation 55:833, 1977.
37. Maroko PR, Kjekshus JK, Sobel BE, Watanabe T, Covell JW, Ross J Jr, Braunwald E: Factors influencing infarct size following experimental coronary artery occlusion. Circulation 43:67, 1971.
38. Hillis LD, Askenazi J, Braunwald E, Radvany P, Muller JE, Fishbein MC, Maroko PR: Use of changes in the epicardial QRS complex to assess interventions which modify the extent of myocardial necrosis following coronary artery occlusion. Circulation 54:591, 1976.
39. Klein MD, Herman MV, Gorlin R: A hemodynamic study of left ventricular aneurysm. Circulation 35:614, 1967.
40. Rogers WJ, McDaniel HG, Smith LR, Mantle JA, Russell RO Jr, Rackley CE: Correlation of angiographic estimates of myocardial infarct size and accumulated release of creatine kinase MB isoenzyme in man. Circulation 56:199, 1977.
41. Rigaud M, Rocha P, Boschat J, Farcot JC, Bardet J, Bourdarias JP: Regional left ventricular function assessed by contrast angiography in acute myocardial infarction. Circulation 60:130, 1979.
42. Swan HJC, Forrester JS, Diamond G, Chatterjee K, Parmley WW: Hemodynamic spectrum of myocardial infarction and cardiogenic shock: a conceptual model. Circulation 45:1097, 1972.
43. Ideker RE, Behar VS, Wagner GS, Starr JW, Starmer CF, Lee KL, Hackel DB: Evaluation of asynergy as an indicator of myocardial fibrosis. Circulation 57:715, 1978.
44. Herman MV, Heinle RA, Klein MD, Gorlin R: Localized disorders in myocardial contraction. Asynergy and its role in congestive heart failure. N Engl J Med 277:222, 1967.
45. Herman MV, Gorlin R: Implications of left ventricular asynergy. Am J Cardiol 23:538, 1969.
46. Pasternac A, Gorlin R, Sonnenblick EH, Haft JI, Kemp HG: Abnormalities of ventricular motion induced by atrial pacing in coronary artery disease. Circulation 45:1195, 1972.

47. Wyatt HL, Forrester JS, Tyberg JV, Goldner S, Logan SE, Parmley WW, Swan HJC: Effect of graded reductions in regional coronary perfusion on regional and total cardiac function. Am J Cardiol 36:185, 1975.
48. Forrester JS, Wyatt HL, Da Luz PL, Tyberg JV, Diamond GA, Swan HJC: Functional significance of regional ischemic contraction abnormalities. Circulation 54:64, 1976.
49. Waters DD, Da Luz P, Wyatt HL, Swan HJC, Forrester JS: Early changes in regional and global left ventricular function induced by graded reductions in regional coronary perfusion. Am J Cardiol 39:537, 1977.
50. Tzivoni D, Diamond G, Pichler M, Staukus K, Vas R, Forrester J: Analysis or regional ischemic left ventricular dysfunction by quantitative cineangiography. Circulation 60:1278, 1979.
51. Chatterjee K, Swan HJC, Parmley WW, Sustaita H, Marcus H, Matloff J: Depression of left ventricular function due to acute myocardial ischemia and its reversal after aortocoronary saphenous-vein bypass. N Eng J Med 286:1117, 1972.
52. Chatterjee K, Swan HJC, Parmley WW, Sustaita H, Marcus HS, Matloff JM: Influence of direct myocardial revascularization on left ventricular asynergy and function in patients with coronary heart disease: with and without previous myocardial infarction. Circulation 47:276, 1973.
53. Banka VS, Bodenheimer MM, Helfant RH: Determinants of reversible asynergy. Effect of pathologic Q waves, coronary collaterals, and anatomic location. Circulation 50:714, 1974.
54. Banka VS, Bodenheimer MM, Helfant RH: Determinants of reversible asynergy: the native coronary circulation. Circulation 52:810, 1975.
55. Hamby RI, Aintablian A, Wisoff BG, Hartstein ML: Response of the left ventricle in coronary artery disease to postextrasystolic potentiation. Circulation 51:428, 1975.
56. Popio KA, Gorlin R, Bechtel D, Levine JA: Postextrasystolic potentiation as a predictor of potential myocardial viability: preoperative analyses compared with studies after coronary bypass surgery. Am J Cardiol 39:944, 1977.
57. Helfant RH, Pine R, Meister SG, Feldman MS, Trout RG, Banka VS: Nitroglycerin to unmask reversible asynergy: correlation with post coronary bypass ventriculography. Circulation 50:108, 1974.
58. Sniderman AD, Herscovitch P, Marpole D, Fallen EL: Restoration of regional wall motion by nitroglycerin therapy in patients with left ventricular asynergy. Chest 66:545, 1974.
59. McAnulty JH, Hattenhauer MT, Rösch J, Kloster FE, Rahimtoola SH: Improvement in left ventricular wall motion following nitroglycerin. Circulation 51:140, 1975.
60. Banka VS, Bodenheimer MM, Shah R, Helfant RH: Intervention ventriculography. Comparative value of nitroglycerin, post-extrasystolic potentiation and nitroglycerin plus post-extrasystolic potentiation. Circulation 53:632, 1976.
61. Klausner SC, Ratshin RA, Tyberg JV, Lappin HA, Chatterjee K, Parmley WW: The similarity of changes in segmental contraction patterns induced by postextrasystolic potentiation and nitroglycerin. Circulation 54:615, 1976.

62. Bodenheimer MM, Banka VS, Hermann GA, Trout RG, Pasdar H, Helfant RH: Reversible asynergy. Histopathologic and electrographic correlations in patients with coronary artery disease. Circulation 53:792, 1976.

63. Bodenheimer MM, Banka VS, Trout RG, Hermann GA, Pasdar H, Helfant RH: Local characteristics of the normal and asynergic left ventricle in man. Am J Med 61:650, 1976.

64. Chaitman BR, DeMots H, Bristow JD, Rösch J, Rahimtoola SH: Objective and subjective analysis of left ventricular angiograms. Circulation 52:420, 1975.

65. Zir LM, Miller SW, Dinsmore RE, Gilbert JP, Harthorne JW: Interobserver variability in coronary angiography. Circulation 53:627, 1976.

66. Chaitman BR, Bristow JD, Rahimtoola SH: Left ventricular wall motion assessed by using fixed external reference systems. Circulation 43:1043, 1973.

67. Ueda H, Ueda K, Morooka S, Nakanishi A, Ito I, Yasuda H, Takabatake Y, Sugishita Y, Uchida Y, Ozeki K: A cineangiographic study of the regional contraction sequence of the normal and diseased left ventricle in man. Jpn Heart J 10:95, 1969.

68. Sniderman AD, Marpole D, Fallen EL: Regional contraction patterns in the normal and ischemic left ventricle in man. Am J Cardiol 31:484, 1973.

69. Gelberg HJ, Brundage BH, Glantz S, Parmley WW: Quantitative left ventricular wall motion analysis: a comparison of area, chord and radial methods. Circulation 59:991, 1979.

8. RADIONUCLIDE VENTRICULOGRAPHY

FRANS J. TH. WACKERS, HARVEY J. BERGER, and BARRY L. ZARET

The morbidity and prognosis after a myocardial infarct have been shown to be related closely to the extent of myocardial necrosis and the degree of left ventricular dysfunction [1–6]. In patients with a first acute myocardial infarct, a direct correlation has been demonstrated between the magnitude of cardiac enzyme release in the blood and left ventricular hemodynamics [2], in particular, ejection fraction [4, 6] (see Roberts, p. 129). Thus, although assessment of ventricular performance does not provide a direct measure of infarct size, it is related to other estimates of this parameter. It also provides clinically relevant pathophysiologic insights. Data collected by the Seattle Heart Watch [7] and others [8] indicate that resting left ventricular ejection fraction is the single most valuable predictor of survival in patients with coronary heart disease.

Radionuclide techniques have been developed and validated for noninvasive assessment of left and right ventricular ejection fraction and regional left ventricular wall motion. Newly developed mobile gamma-camera/minicomputer systems and portable probe systems now make it possible to perform these studies in the coronary care unit at the patient's bedside, facilitating serial evaluation of cardiac performance in critically ill patients. Potentially important prognostic information also can be obtained in this way.

Cardiac performance can be evaluated by radionuclide techniques in several ways. First-pass radionuclide angiocardiography [9] and multiple-gated equilibrium cardiac blood imaging [10] are employed widely. For these techniques, analysis is based upon time-activity curves generated from cardiac images by using scintillation cameras interfaced to computer systems. Nonimaging probe devices also have been developed recently for assessing left ventricular performance [11].

This chapter will review these radionuclide techniques for studying cardiac performance, as well as the clinical data that have been obtained when the techniques have been applied to the patient with an acute myocardial infarct.

FIRST-PASS RADIONUCLIDE ANGIOCARDIOGRAPHY

For this method, the radionuclide (15–20 mCi of technetium-99m pertechnetate or other ^{99m}Tc compounds) is injected rapidly as a compact bolus into an

Wagner GS (ed): Myocardial Infarction: Measurement and Intervention, pp 199–233.
© 1982 Martinus Nijhoff Publishers, The Hague/Boston/London.

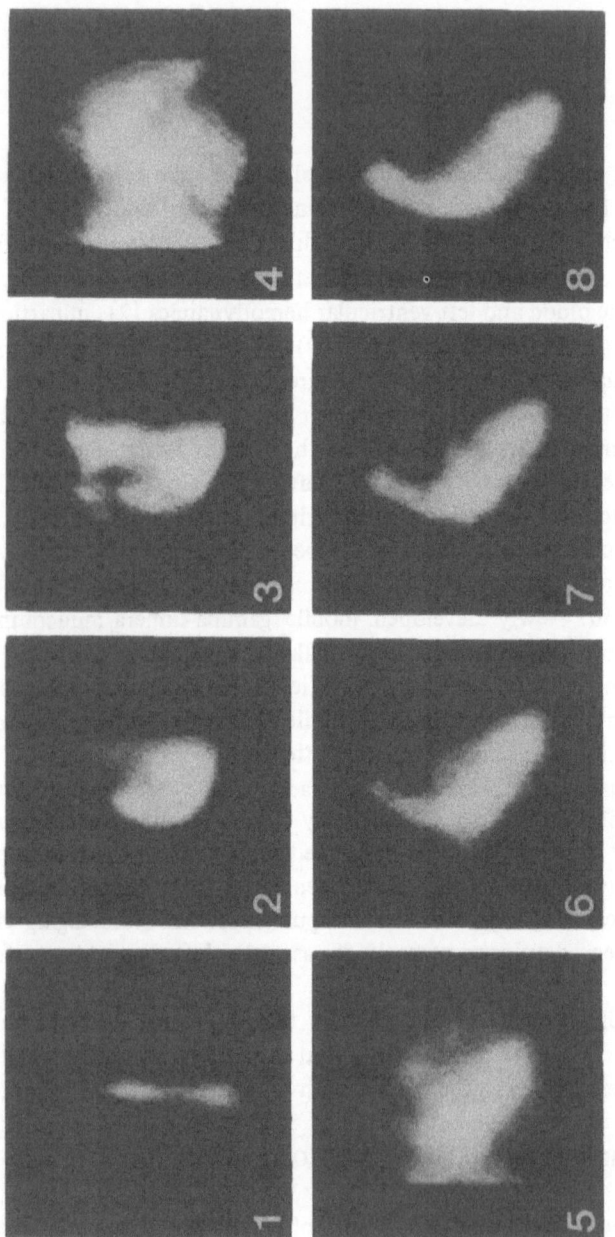

Figure 1. Sequential 1-s images obtained during the first pass of the radionuclide bolus through the central circulation. The normal temporal and anatomic separation of right (frame 3) and left ventricle (frame 7) is present. Reproduced with permission [9].

antecubital vein. Quantitative analysis of the transit of this bolus through the central circulation is based upon the principles of indicator dilution theory. It is assumed that homogeneous mixing of the radioactive tracer with blood has occurred by the time the bolus enters the ventricles. Thus, changes in externally detected counts are proportional to changes in chamber volumes during the cardiac cycle. The efficacy and reliability of the first-pass method depends upon obtaining sufficiently high count rates to assure statistical reliability. Conventional single-crystal scintillation cameras are limited in terms of maximal count rate efficiency. Since the count rate response is linear only up to 50–60,000 counts/s, further increase of the injected dose will not resolve this problem satisfactorily. Reasonable count rates can be obtained during the passage of the bolus through the right ventricle, but during the levo-phase, count rates generally

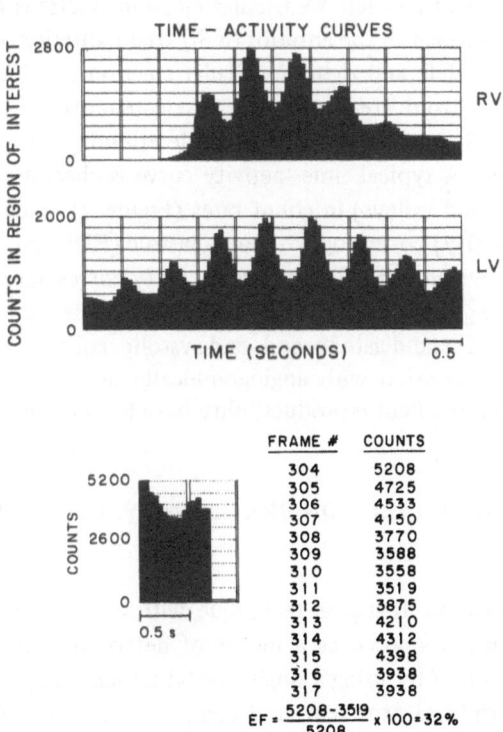

$$EF = \frac{5208 - 3519}{5208} \times 100 = 32\%$$

Figures 2 (top) and 3 (bottom). (*2*) Right ventricular (RV) and left ventricular (LV) time–activity curves obtained in 20 frames/s with the computerized multicrystal scintillation camera. Peaks and valleys in count rate correspond to end-diastole and end-systole, respectively. Reproduced with permission [9]. (*3*) Representative cardiac cycle (background corrected) used to calculate left ventricular ejection fraction (EF). The counts for each summed 0.05-s frame of the representative cycle (the equivalent of a volume curve) are shown along with the EF calculation. On this study, end-diastolic counts were 5208, end-systolic counts 3519, and calculated EF 32%.

are suboptimal. To overcome the statistical uncertainty of low count rate data, several mathematical manipulations have been proposed for determining left ventricular ejection fraction by the first-pass technique using a conventional single-crystal gamma camera [12]. In contrast, a multicrystal camera (with a mosaic of 294 individual sodium iodide crystals) is suited ideally for the performance of first-pass radionuclide angiocardiography, since it possesses a high count rate capability of up to 450,000 counts/s without significant data distortion [13]. An important practical limitation of the latter instrument is that it is not portable.

First-pass radionuclide angiocardiographic data are collected for approximately 20–30 s after bolus injection and are stored generally in computer memory as high-frequency data frames of 20- to 50-ms intervals. The anatomic and temporal separation of radioactivity within individual chambers enables calculation of both right and left ventricular ejection fractions (Figure 1). This study usually is performed in the anterior or 30° right anterior oblique position. For determination of left and right ventricular ejection fractions, time-activity curves are generated from areas of interest selected over the left and right ventricles [12–17]. Standardized methods for determining the region of interest have been developed. A typical time–activity curve is characterized by cyclical fluctuations (peaks and valleys) in count rates (Figure 2). Each peak (maximal ventricular radioactivity) corresponds to end-diastole (ED), and minimal activity corresponds to end-systole (ES). These time–activity curves have to be corrected for noncardiac background activity. Ejection fraction is calculated from the background-corrected end-diastolic and end-systolic count rates: ED–ES/ED (Figure 3). Good correlation with angiographically determined left ventricular ejection fraction and excellent reproducibility have been reported [12–18].

RIGHT VENTRICULAR EJECTION FRACTION BY GATED FIRST-PASS TECHNIQUE

Recently, a combination first-pass technique with electrocardiographic gating (see below) has been proposed as a means of determining reliably right ventricular ejection fraction by using a single-crystal camera [19]. The radionuclide is injected in a peripheral arm vein as a compact bolus. The data of the first transit through the right heart are accumulated in the 30° right anterior oblique position. Data collection is started as soon as the radioactive bolus enters the superior vena cava and is terminated at the beginning of the pulmonary phase. Electrocardiographic gating assures summation of scintillation data from different cardiac cycles. For this technique, data from 5 to 15 heartbeats usually are accumulated. Relatively high count rates can be obtained with this approach. No background correction is necessary when the study is performed in the 30°

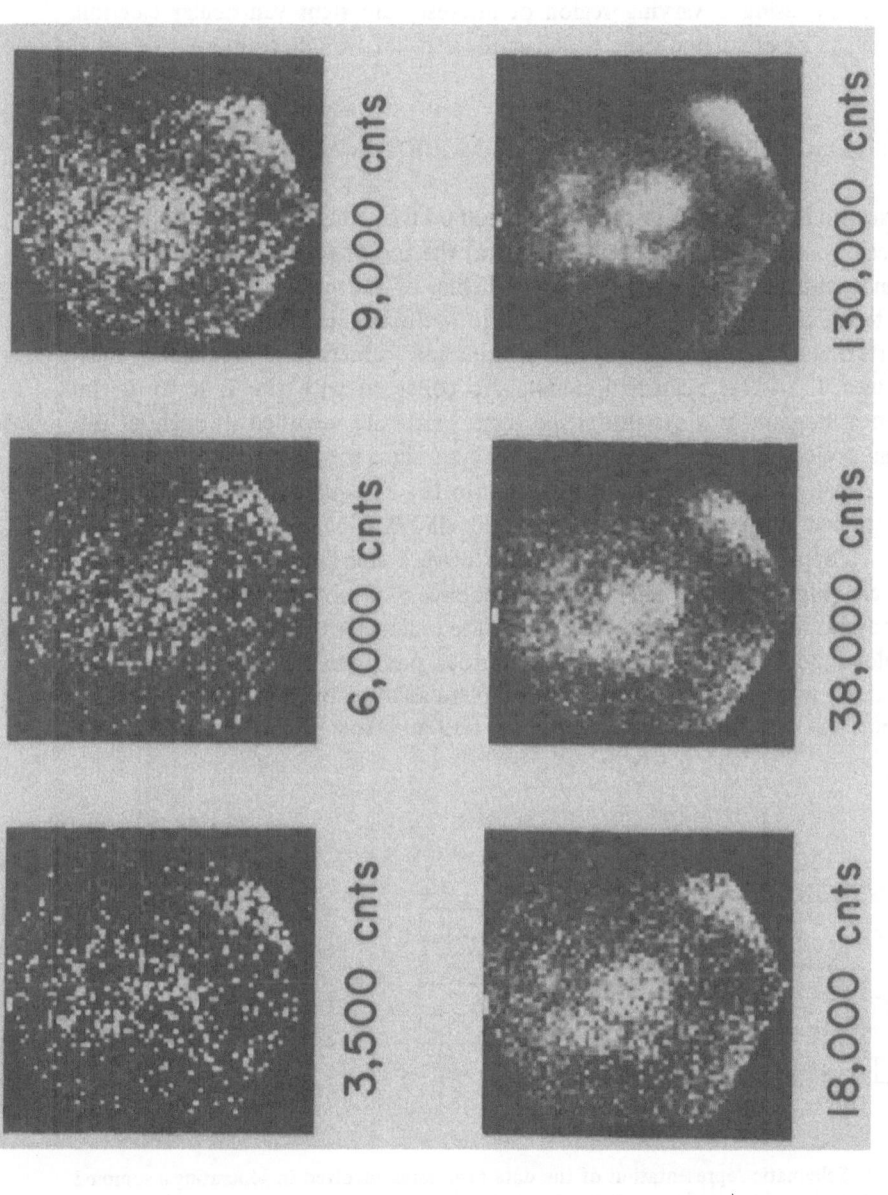

Figure 4. Effect of increasing count density per frame on the image quality of a multigated blood pool study. End-diastolic frames of six multigated studies, with count densities ranging from 3,500 to 130,000 counts per field of view are shown. The first study (3,500 counts) was collected from approximately ten cardiac cycles, whereas the last study (130,000 counts) represents data collected over approximately 350

204

right anterior oblique position, since there is virtually no overlap of the right atrium and right ventricle, and data collection is terminated before the radioactivity enters the lungs. A time—activity curve is generated over the right ventricle by using a varying region of interest, and right ventricular ejection fraction can be calculated from end-diastolic and end-systolic counts.

MULTIPLE-GATED EQUILIBRIUM BLOOD POOL IMAGING

The cardiac blood pool is imaged after blood pool labeling with technetium-99m. This can be achieved by two methods: (a) the use of technetium-99m-labeled human serum albumin, or (b) in vivo labeling of the patient's red blood cells with technetium-99m pertechnetate [20]. Multiple-gated blood pool imaging is performed with a single-crystal scintillation camera and dedicated mini-computer [21—23]. Scintillation data are collected with the R wave of the electrocardiogram as a synchronizing signal. Data are recorded throughout the cardiac cycle and stored separately, depending upon the relationship to each R wave. Usually the RR interval is divided into 16—28 equal time frames. Imaging is continued until acquisition of 150,000—250,000 counts per whole image frame or approximately 175—200 counts/picture element (pixel) over the left ventricle (Figures 4—6). This generally requires 5—8 min and accumulates data over several hundred cardiac cycles. Since the radioactivity has equilibrated with the blood pool, sequential imaging in various positions is possible. Usually, at least three positions are chosen for complete analysis of all cardiac chambers: anterior, 45° left anterior oblique (or the obliquity that gives best separation of

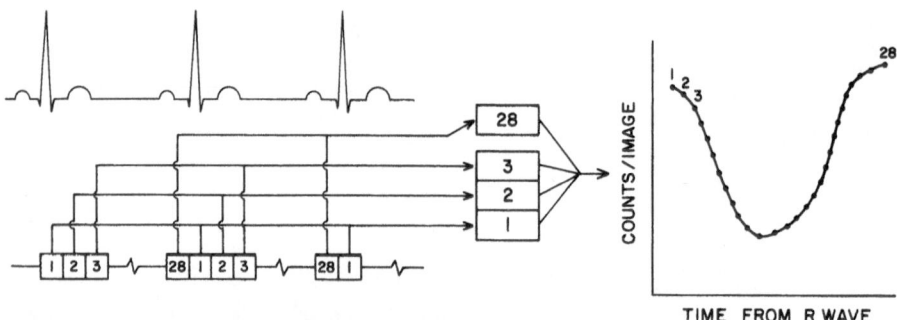

Figure 5. Schematic representation of the data processing involved in generating a summed left ventricular time—activity curve by using the multigated equilibrium blood pool technique. In this example, the cardiac cycle has been divided into 28 segments. Data occurring during the specific time intervals shown below are stored in computer memory for several hundred individual cardiac cycles. Following background correction, these individual data points are displayed as a relative volume curve as indicated on the right.

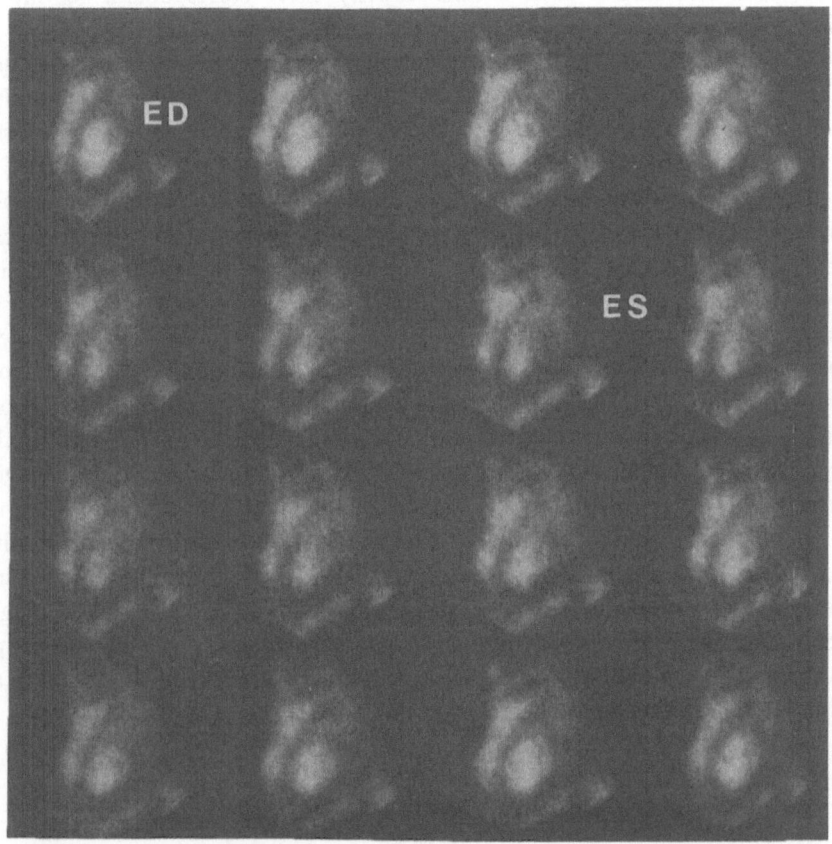

Figure 6. Serial images obtained from a multigated equilibrium blood pool study using 16 frames in a single cardiac cycle. All images were obtained in the left anterior oblique position. End-diastole (ED) is shown in the upper left-hand corner. The temporal sequence is read from left to right. The seventh image is end-systole (ES). In this study, normal uniform ventricular contraction can be appreciated throughout the cardiac cycle.

the two ventricles), and left lateral (with the patient lying on his right side). By displaying the data either as static images or as an endless loop movie, each chamber can be analyzed in terms of relative position, size, and contraction pattern.

Left ventricular ejection fraction can be determined from only the left anterior oblique position, because it is only in this view that radioactivity from the right and left ventricle is separated adequately. In individual patients, the angle of obliquity may be different, e.g., in patients with marked cardiac enlargement, only a steep left anterior oblique or even left lateral position may separate the two ventricles. Only the views with the best ventricular separation should be used for calculation of left ventricular ejection fraction. From the ECG-gated scintillation data, a time–activity curve corresponding to volume changes in the left ventricle is generated from a region of interest chosen to correspond anatomically to the left ventricle. Since background activity in equilibrium blood pool studies is considerably higher than in first-pass studies, definition of the left ventricular outline or edge is of crucial importance. Computer programs for detecting the edge, based upon either a second derivative or a defined count threshold, have been developed and are currently available. In individual instances, manually determined outlines also can be used. A *varying* region of interest that follows the ventricular outline throughout the cardiac cycle is preferable to a fixed region [24]. The time–activity curve has to be corrected for background activity, usually determined from an area immediately lateral to the left ventricle. Left ventricular ejection fraction is calculated from the conventional equation as with the first-pass technique. Good correlations have been reported between left ventricular ejection fraction determined by the multiple-gated equilibrium technique and that determined by contrast angiography [23–26] or the first-pass radionuclide technique [26] (Figure 7).

We believe that right ventricular ejection fraction is difficult to determine accurately from equilibrium studies because of the overlap with the right atrium. However, recent studies that used the equilibrium technique to measure right ventricular ejection fraction have had encouraging results [27–29]. Further evaluation of this method appears to be warranted, especially in patients with an enlarged right atrium and/or right ventricle.

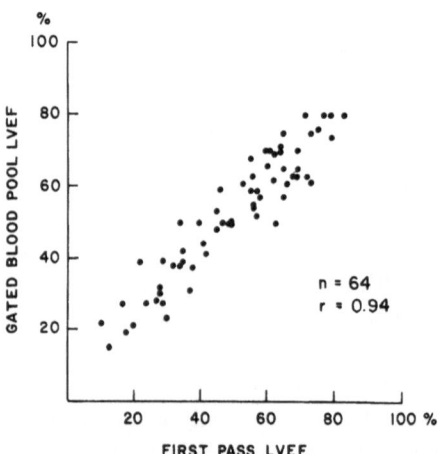

Figure 7. Correlation between left ventricular ejection fraction (LVEF) assessed with multigated blood pool imaging and first-pass radionuclide angiocardiography in 64 patients. Reproduced with permission [26].

REGISTONAL WALL MOTION

Segmental wall motion preferably should be analyzed qualitatively from an endless-loop movie display. The analysis of single end-diastolic and end-systolic frames generally is difficult and important details recognizable on movie display are lost.

Using the first-pass technique and superimposition of end-diastolic and end-systolic frames, Marshall et al. [13, 18] reported good accuracy (89%) and reproducibility to detect regional wall motion abnormalities when compared with contrast left ventriculography (Figure 8). This has been confirmed subsequently by several studies [14, 15].

On radionuclide multigated blood pool studies, the relative size and contraction of both atria and ventricles can be appreciated. Unfortunately, the interpretation of the images is highly subjective and observer experience is of decisive importance. Okada et al. [30] analyzed the variance among observers who interpreted multigated blood pool imaging. Intra- and interobserver variability was comparable to that reported for contrast ventriculography, except for the interventricular septum, which had a higher interobserver variance on multigated images. The same investigators also evaluated the accuracy of the detection of wall motion abnormalities compared with contrast angiography [31]. The agreement ranged from 88% for the anterolateral segment to 82% for the apex of the left ventricle.

In our experience, accuracy in detecting regional wall motion abnormalities is improved by adding a left lateral image to the traditional anterior and left anterior oblique views. The addition of this third view improved considerably the detection of inferoposterior wall motion abnormalities and, in particular, of posterobasilar aneurysms, without loss of specificity [32] (Figure 9). In addition, although the recognition of anterior wall motion abnormalities was not affected by the additional information of the left lateral view, the segmental nature of anteroapical aneurysms was appreciated better from the left lateral view (Figures 10, 11).

This geometric approach is qualitative and has limitations since only those segments of the ventricular wall tangential to the imaging device can be analyzed. To overcome this problem, ejection fraction functional images [33–35] can be created by displaying the ejection fraction per pixel. These images display the relative contribution of each pixel to global left ventricular ejection fraction, allowing better appreciation of three-dimensional volume changes. Further regional quantitative measurements may be obtained by assessing regional ejection fraction [33] or by measuring hemiaxes or radials [36]. These latter methods are as yet experimental. Maddox et al. [33] reported 90% agreement between analysis of regional wall motion by ejection fraction images and by contrast angiography. In our experience, ejection fraction images

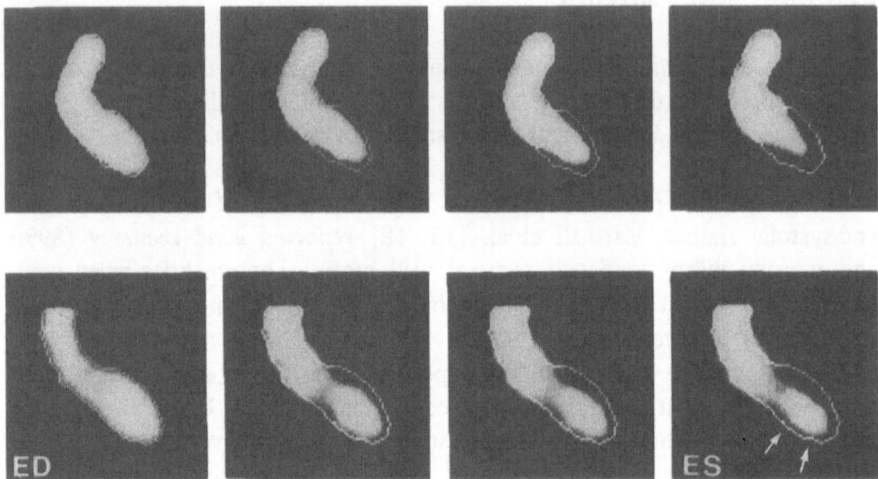

Figure 8. Analysis of left ventricular wall motion by first-pass radionuclide angiocardiography in the anterior position. The contracting left ventricle is shown superimposed over the end-diastolic perimeters generated by computer technique. End-diastole (ED) and end-

are particularly helpful for serial evaluation of patients with markedly impaired left ventricular function. Although global left ventricular performance may not change significantly during exercise [37] or after sublingual nitroglycerin, ejection fraction images may display significant regional changes.

VENTRICULAR VOLUME

Left ventricular ejection fraction is an extremely useful index of cardiac performance. However, ejection fraction depends on preload and afterload. A change in ejection fraction may be due to a change in the loading conditions of the ventricle, as well as its contractility. Therefore, additional physiologic parameters, such as pressure—volume relationships [38] are necessary in order to characterize cardiac performance completely.

Using first-pass radionuclide angiocardiography Rerych et al. [39] determined left ventricular end-diastolic volume by applying planimetry to scintigraphic images. They obtained good correlation with volumes calculated from catheterization data ($r = 0.89$). Recently, several nongeometric count based methods have been suggested to determine left ventricular volumes from multigated equilibrium cardiac blood pool studies [40, 41]. Counts in end-diastolic frames are converted to volume units by using the radioactivity measured from a small sample of the patient's blood as a reference. Regression equations

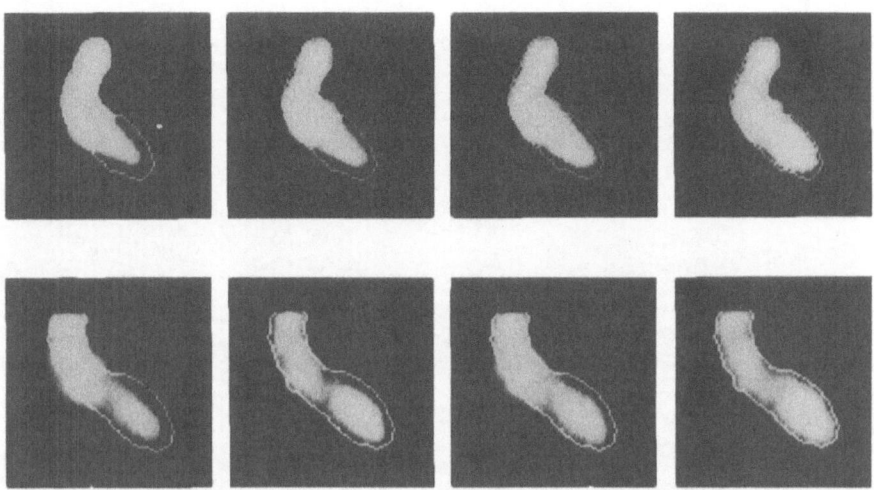

systole (ES) are indicated. The upper row of images shows normal left ventricular wall
motion, whereas the lower row demonstrates inferoapical hypokinesis (arrow).

are necessary to convert count rates to true ventricular volumes. A major theoretical and technical problem yet to be resolved is accurate correction for
radiation attenuation and for the depth of the left ventricle, especially in patients
with enlarged and/or aneurysmal ventricles. Once end-diastolic volume is determined accurately, stroke volume and end-systolic volume also can be derived
readily $[(1 - EF) EDV = ESV]$. Relative volume changes (end-diastolic volume,
end-systolic volume, stroke volume, and cardiac output) can now be obtained
when serial studies are performed for a limited period of time without moving
the gamma camera away from the patient. By simple correction for physical
decay of the radioisotope and correction for changes in heart rate and frame
length, it is possible to analyze relative volume changes.

NONIMAGING DEVICES

A recent modification of the gated blood pool imaging technique involves the
use of a specially collimated nuclear probe and dedicated microprocessor [11,
42]. This nonimaging approach provides various parameters of global left
ventricular function, but does not give insights into regional ventricular function
or right ventricular performance. By virtue of its true portability and decreased
size, this instrument is well suited for the study of critically ill patients with
acute infarction. Using equilibrium data, left ventricular ejection fraction,

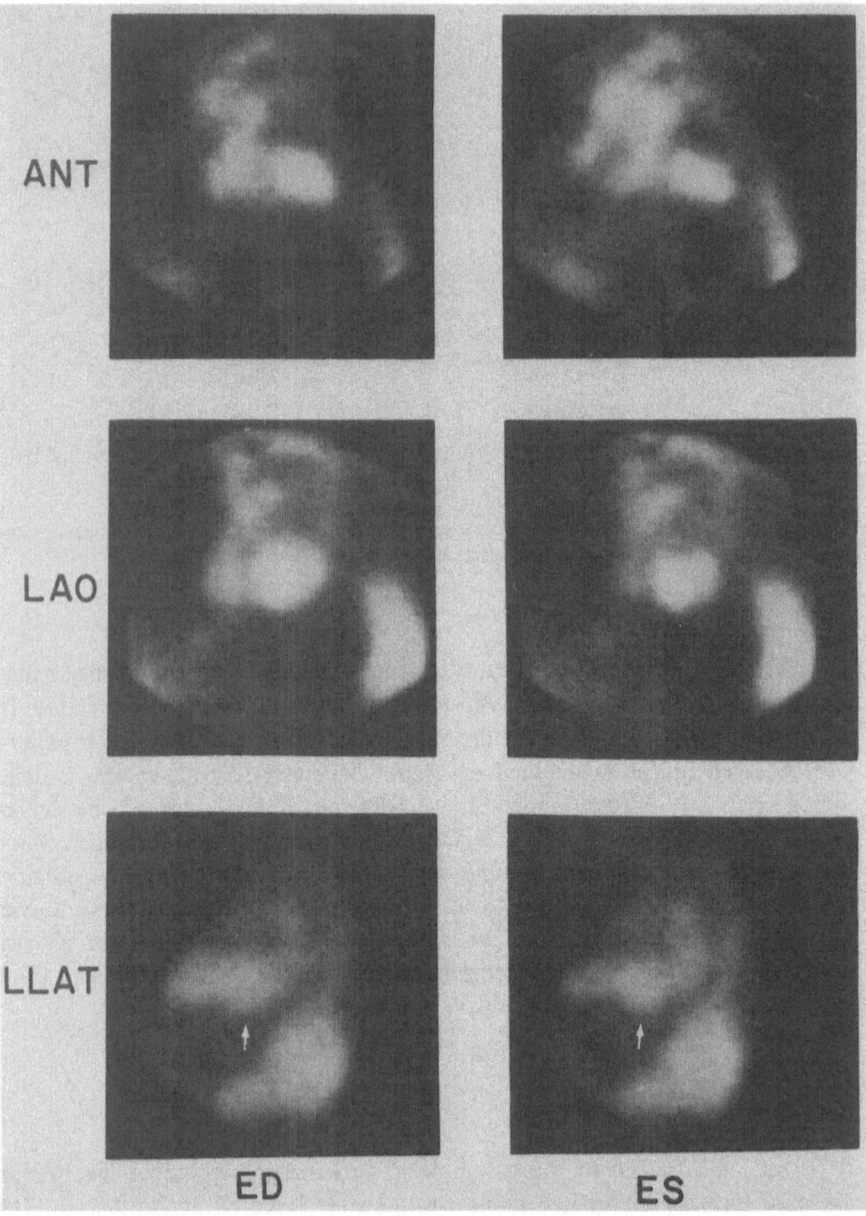

Figure 9. Multigated equilibrium blood pool images in a patient with a posterobasal aneurysm (arrow). Images are shown in the anterior (ANT), left anterior oblique (LAO), and left lateral (LLAT) position and at end-diastole (ED) and end-systole (ES). The aneurysm is best appreciated in the LLAT position. This study clearly indicates the need to obtain multigated studies in multiple positions in order to define aneurysm or significant regional wall motion abnormalities. Reproduced with permission [32].

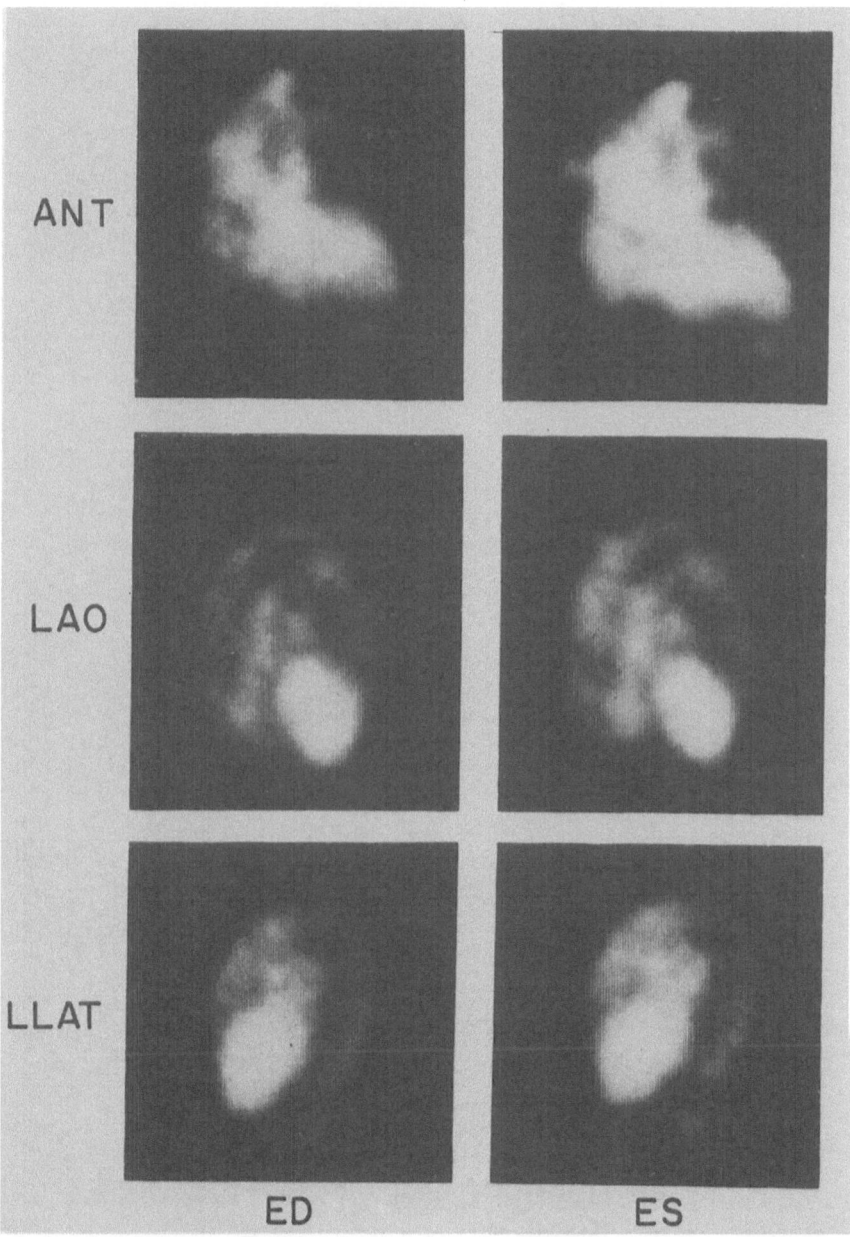

Figure 10. Multigated equilibrium cardiac blood pool images in a patient with diffuse hypokinesis. The format is the same as in Figure 9. Note the left ventricular enlargement, the normal right ventricular size, and the absence of a distinct regional wall motion abnormality.

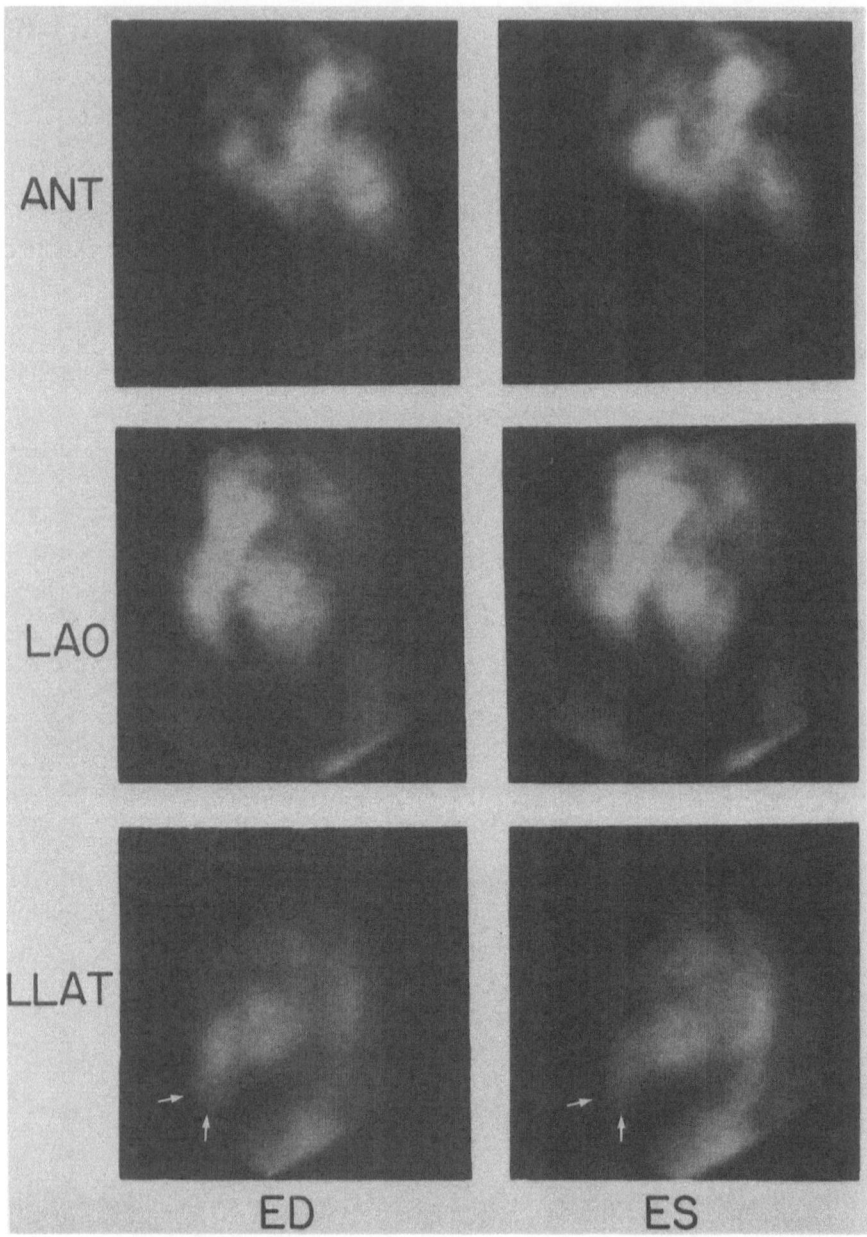

Figure 11. Multigated equilibrium cardiac blood pool images in a patient with an antero-apical aneurysm (arrow). The format is the same as in Figure 9. Although the aneurysm can be detected in the ANT and LAO position, it is best appreciated in the LLAT position. Reproduced with permission [32].

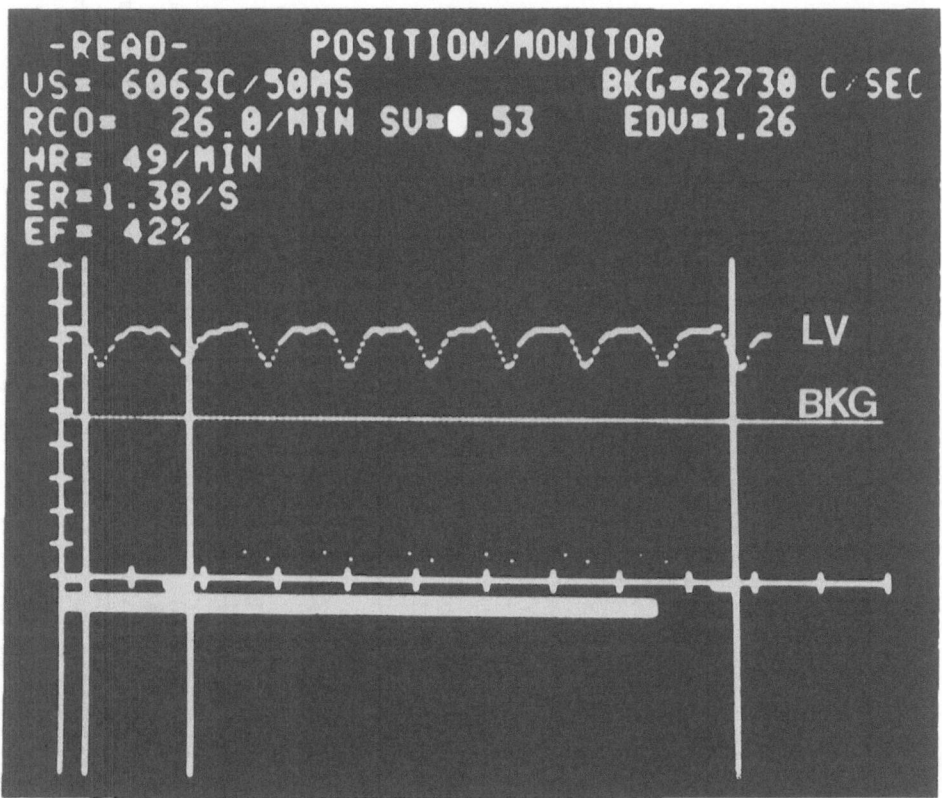

Figure 12. Actual real-time display of the count-rate data photographed directly from the cathode ray tube of the computerized nuclear probe. The real-time beat-to-beat left ventricular volume curve (LV) is displayed above the average background (BKG) level. The average left ventricular ejection fraction (EF) calculated by the microprocessor for the individual beats shown between the two vertical cursors is 42%.

ejection rate, and relative cardiac output and volumes can be obtained in the conventional electrocardiographically gated mode. Because of the increased sensitivity of the detector system, statistically reliable results can be generated in 15–30 s (Figure 12).

Radionuclide data also can be acquired and analyzed directly on a beat-to-beat basis without the need for gating [43–45]. The left ventricular volume curve can be displayed simultaneously with the electrocardiogram and arterial pressure. Analysis of these data enables evaluation of specific pathophysiologic questions that cannot be answered using conventional scintillation camera techniques. Particularly in the setting of acute coronary artery disease, the instantaneous effects of cardiac arrhythmias, cardiovascular reflexes, and acute pharmacologic interventions can be investigated (Figure 13).

214

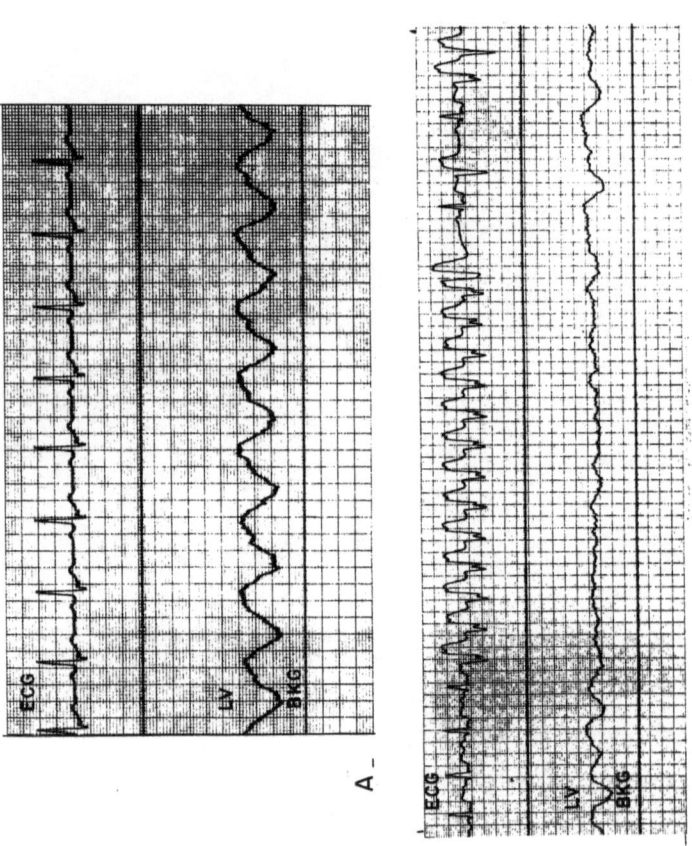

Figure 13. Strip-chart recordings of beat-to-beat display of background (BKG) activity level, left ventricular (LV) volume curve, and electrocardiogram (ECG) from a patient in sinus rhythm (*A*) and a patient with a short run of ventricular tachycardia (*B*). Note the constancy and uniform periodicity of the curves in *A*, in which left ventricular ejection fraction is 59%. In *B*, left ventricular ejection fraction during sinus rhythm is 46%. The onset of ventricular tachycardia is associated with a dramatic change in periodicity of left ventricular volume curve and fall of ejection fraction. After cessation of the tachycardia, each sinus beat generates a volume change, whereas the ventricular premature beats are ineffective. *A* is reproduced with permission [44].

Left ventricular ejection fraction obtained with the probe either on a beat-to-beat basis or with the gated mode correlates well with that measured by conventional camera techniques or contrast angiography [45]. In addition, the inter- and intraobserver variations and intrinsic single-beat variability are sufficiently low to enable statistically and clinically meaningful applications.

Recently, a miniaturized semiconductor nuclear probe has been developed [46]. This prototype system uses a cadmium telluride detector and lightweight collimator, which weigh less than 200 g. After further development, this technology may enable continuous noninvasive monitoring of left ventricular function over 24 h in critically ill patients in a manner similar to right-heart catheterization and assessment of left ventricular filling pressures. Preliminary results with the prototype system demonstrate the feasibility of this approach.

RESULTS OF PATIENT STUDIES IN ACUTE MYOCARDIAL INFARCT

When a patient is admitted to the coronary care unit after an acute episode of chest pain, several questions are clinically relevant. Did the patient sustain an acute myocardial infarct? If so, what is the site and extent of myocardial damage? To what extent is ventricular performance impaired? Most importantly, what is the immediate and long term prognosis?

For the *diagnosis* of acute myocardial infarct, radionuclide angiocardiography is of limited value. Many patients with an acute myocardial infarct may have only minimal wall motion abnormalities. In addition, global cardiac performance in many patients may be within the range of normal. In other patients, ventricular performance may be depressed as a result of a prior myocardial infarct or concomitant valvular disease. Thallium-201 myocardial perfusion scintigraphy (see Okada, p. 295) and technetium-99m–Sn-pyrophosphate myocardial scintigraphy (see Marcus, p. 325) are more appropriate radionuclide techniques for the diagnosis of acute infarct. Kostuk et al. [4] and Rigo et al. [5] were the first to apply radionuclide angiocardiography in patients with acute myocardial infarcts. In these early studies, left ventricular volumes and ejection fraction were derived by planimetry of the scintigraphic images. These results encouraged further development of count-based techniques.

CARDIAC PERFORMANCE AND LOCATION OF INFARCT

In patients with acute myocardial infarcts, the degree of impairment of left and right ventricular performance is dependent upon infarct site [47, 48]. Using first-pass radionuclide angiocardiography, Reduto et al. [49] evaluated

216

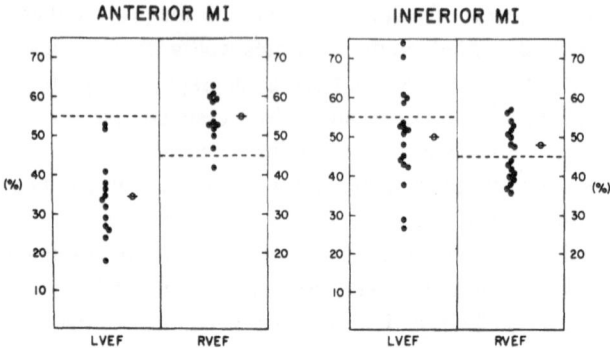

Figure 14. Left ventricular (LV) and right ventricular (RV) ejection fraction (EF) in patients with acute anterior and inferior myocardial infarct (MI). Individual patients are represented by closed circles and means by open circles. The lower limits of normal for LVRF and RVEF are shown by dashed horizontal lines. Although all patients with anterior infarcts had abnormal LVEF, only one had abnormal RVEF. Note that of 18 patients with inferior infarcts, five had normal LVEF, whereas nine of 18 had abnormal RVEF. Reproduced with permission [49].

31 patients with uncomplicated acute transmural myocardial infarct. Anterior wall infarcts resulted in a greater reduction in left ventricular ejection fraction than inferior wall infarcts (mean ± SEM: 34% ± 3% vs 50% ± 3%, $p < 0.01$) (Figure 14). In a recent study, Shah et al. [50], studying 56 patients with acute myocardial infarcts, reported a similar difference for mean left ventricular ejection fraction between patients with anterior and inferior wall infarcts. In addition, they identified a subgroup of patients with inferior wall infarct and precordial ST segment depression who had significantly lower left ventricular ejection fraction than the remaining patients with acute inferior wall infarct. They assumed that these patients had additional anterior wall myocardial ischemia. True posterior wall infarct may be an alternative explanation for this observation.

For right ventricular performance, Reduto et al. [49], Tobinick et al. [17] as well as others [51–54], noted that 35%–50% of patients with inferior wall myocardial infarcts have abnormal right ventricular ejection fraction, whereas this occurred in only approximately 5% of patients with anterior wall infarcts (Figure 14). This is consistent with findings by Wackers et al. [55] and others [53] that right ventricular necrosis, as assessed by myocardial imaging with ^{99m}Tc pyrophosphate, occurs frequently (37%) only in patients with acute inferior wall infarcts. The majority of these patients do not have clinical evidence of right ventricular failure. In patients who demonstrate the classic clinical picture of right ventricular infarction in association with an acute inferior infarct [56, 57], the gated equilibrium cardiac blood pool studies are characteristic [52, 53]. These studies show a normal or nearly normal-sized left ventricle with often preserved normal left ventricular ejection fraction, and a markedly enlarged, diffusely hypokinetic right ventricle (Figure 15). After the acute phase, right ventricular performance may return toward normal in some of these patients [54, 56].

Schelbert et al. [58] studied 50 patients with acute myocardial infarct during the first five days after the acute event. Among various hemodynamic measures (cardiac output, stroke work index), left ventricular ejection fraction, assessed by first-pass technique, best reflected the patient's clinical status when determined by Killip's classification. Left ventricular ejection fraction also was inversely related to pulmonary arterial wedge pressure ($r = -0.72$). These results are consistent with the early work by Kostuk et al. [4], who reported an inverse relationship between infarct size estimated by analysis of serial changes in CK activity and planimetric calculation of left ventricular ejection

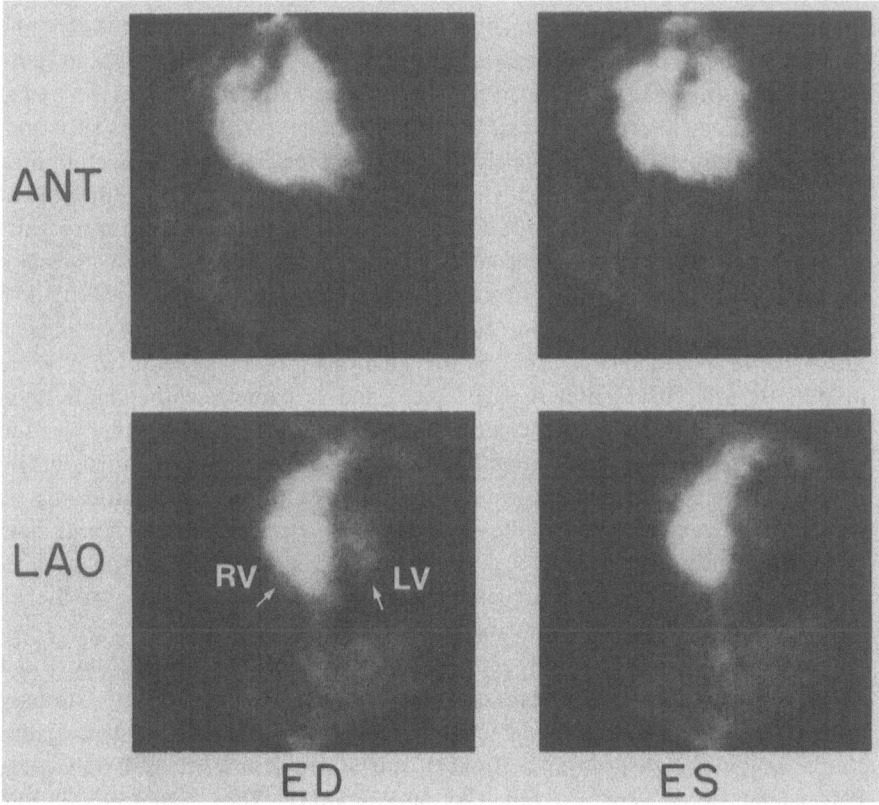

Figure 15. Multigated equilibrium blood pool images in a patient with acute inferior wall infarct and massive right ventricular infarct. Note the dilated, poorly contracting right ventricle (RV) and the excellent contraction of the left ventricle (LV).

fraction from radionuclide angiocardiography ($r = -0.71$). More recently, Morrison et al. [6] reported similar results. Ohsuzu et al. [59] recently reported preliminary findings in 127 patients with acute myocardial infarct in whom they correlated parameters of global left ventricular function (ejection fraction, systolic blood pressure, end-diastolic and end-systolic volume, and systolic pressure—end-systolic volume ratio) with infarct size estimated by semiquantitative assessment of segmental wall motion abnormalities. Again, left ventricular ejection fraction appeared to be the single most valuable indicator of the extent of myocardial damage in the early phase of myocardial infarct.

REGIONAL WALL MOTION ABNORMALITIES

Segmental wall motion abnormalities may be seen after infarct, but in some patients left ventricular wall motion may be almost normal. Especially in acute inferior wall myocardial infarct, segmental contractility may appear to be entirely normal on the anterior and left anterior oblique views. In this situation, a left lateral projection is extremely helpful to appreciate contraction abnormalities of the inferoposterior wall. Occasionally, however, dramatic improvement and almost complete reversal of an area of akinesis can be observed in patients with subendocardial or nontransmural infarcts. In general, patients with major segmental wall motion abnormalities have larger infarcts and lower global ejection fractions. Ramanatham et al. [36] studied the effects of sublingual nitroglycerin on segmental contraction abnormalities in patients with acute infarcts (6–24 h after onset of chest pain) and in patients with remote myocardial infarcts. No significant change occurred in *global* left ventricular ejection fraction in either group of patients after nitroglycerin. However, nitroglycerin improved the contractile performance in the area of infarct significantly in patients with acute infarcts, while no such change occurred in the infarct zone of patients with remote infarcts. Whether these changes reflect improved function of reversibly damaged myocardium or changes in compliance of the involved myocardial segment by nitroglycerin remains unclear.

Friedman and Cantor [60] reported that 61 (96%) of 64 left ventricular aneurysms demonstrated by contrast angiography in 138 patients with coronary artery disease were accurately detected by gated studies. The three false negative studies involved two posterobasal aneurysms and one anterior wall aneurysm. Left lateral views were not obtained in this study. Thus, gated equilibrium blood pool imaging in multiple views provides a reliable means to monitor noninvasively the development of a ventricular aneurysm following an infarct. Nichols et al. [61] also found good agreement between the pattern of left ventricular dysfunction revealed by multigated studies and findings at contrast left ventriculography. Dymond et al. [62] and Stephens et al. [63] further demonstrated the feasibility and accuracy of detecting left ventricular aneurysm by radionuclide techniques. True aneurysms characteristically display a wide-necked, poorly contracting, saccular protuberance throughout the cardiac cycle, clearly delineated from the remaining contractile myocardium. The wall of a true aneurysm is composed of fibrous scar tissue. Aneurysms commonly cause left ventricular failure and may be the source of emboli or arrhythmias, but they rarely rupture. False or pseudoaneurysms are caused by a small contained rupture of a recent infarct. Contained only by pericardium, false aneurysms have the tendency to rupture late after the infarct. Thus, identification of patients with this condition may be of criticla clinical significance. Botvinick et al. [64] and others [65] reported the typical appearance of a pseudoaneu-rysm: a third large chamber attached to the left ventricle by a narrow neck, displaying an hourglass configuration.

Regional ejection fraction functional images may be helpful in detecting *non-tangential* regional wall dysfunction by displaying the relative contribution of myocardial segments to global left ventricular ejection fraction.

Holman et al. [66] analyzed count-based regional left ventricular asynchrony by a computer-assisted method from multigated blood pool studies. Their results indicate that the earliest effects of myocardial ischemia involve left ventricular performance during early systole. This phenomenon is typically regional and occurs in regions with the most significant coronary stenosis. Areas of myocardial infarct are associated with severe abnormalities of asynchronous regional left ventricular wall motion, even when global ejection fraction appears to be normal. This approach [67] provides an index of relative ventricular contractility and increases the sensitivity for localization of regional contraction abnormalities.

SERIAL MEASUREMENT OF LEFT VENTRICULAR FUNCTION IN ACUTE MYOCARDIAL INFARCTS

Early observations by Shillingford and Thomas [68] and others [69, 70] using continuous hemodynamic monitoring of cardiac output, arterial pressure, stroke volume, peripheral resistance, and heart rate in patients with acute infarct suggested that significant improvement in hemodynamic function occurred during the first three days of infarct. Radionuclide techniques now can be used to obtain sequential measurements of right and left ventricular function at the bedside. Schelbert et al. [58] serially determined left ventricular ejection fraction by the first-pass technique in 63 patients with acute infarct. They reported that during the early post-infarct period (first five days), left ventricular ejection fraction improved in 54% of 50 patients, deteriorated in 26%, and remained unchanged in 20%. The changes occurred within an average time of 1.9 days. It was not clear how early after onset of infarct the first measurements were made. For the entire patient group, these individual changes did not result in a significant change in ejection fraction. These data are consistent with earlier studies by Kostuk et al. [4] and Rigo et al. [5] using planimetric analysis of radionuclide angiocardiograms. Reduto et al. [49] followed left and right ventricular ejection fraction sequentially in 31 patients with uncomplicated acute transmural myocardial infarcts from a mean of 16 h after admission until discharge (Figure 16). Relatively minimal mean changes occurred during the two weeks following acute myocardial infarct, although changes in individual patients did occur. Left ventricular ejection fraction improved in 13%, deteriorated in 22% and remained unchanged in 64%. These results, and also the late follow-up data reported by Schelbert et al. [58], suggest that significant changes in left ventricular ejection fraction do not occur once the patient has entered the subacute stage of infarct.

In a recent study from our laboratory, serial multigated blood pool imaging was performed during the initial 24 h of myocardial infarct in 34 patients with their first transmural myocardial infarcts [71]. Studies were begun at admission < 12 h after onset of chest pain (in 70% of the patients < 6 h). Preliminary results indicate that no significant trend in left ventricular ejection fraction occurs during this time period by analysis of variance. However, individual patients showed marked changes in ejection fraction that exceeded the intrinsic variability of this technique (± 5%) and ranged from + 30% to − 10% (Figure 17). In 22 patients (65%), left ventricular ejection fraction changed by more than 5%: in 12 patients there was an increase, and in ten a decrease of ejection fraction. These changes occurred independent of the time interval of the first study after chest pain, initial ejection fraction, site of infarct, or subsequent course, and occurred without major changes in rate−pressure product. Thus, although left ventricular ejection fraction appears to remain relatively stable during the subacute phase, marked changes occur during the first 24 h after infarct. These findings may be relevant to evaluations of therapeutic interventions during the early hours of a myocardial infarct.

Recently, Morrison et al. [72] studied the effect of digitalis on left ventricular ejection fraction by serial multigated blood pool imaging in 14 patients with acute myocardial infarct. In a control group of nine patients, they reported no change in mean left ventricular ejection fraction, comparing data obtained within the first 6 h of chest pain and at follow-up 4−5 days later. However, in the group of 14 patients who were treated with digitalis, a significant 4% increase was found. Based upon data on spontaneous changes in left ventricular ejection fraction in patients with acute infarct described above [71], we believe that these results should be interpreted with extreme caution. For statistical reasons, it appears that the effects of therapeutic interventions on left ventricular

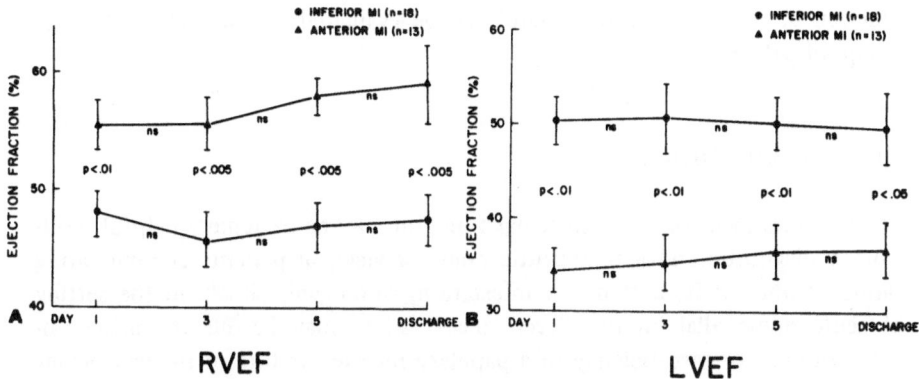

Figure 16. Sequential measurement of left ventricular (LV) and right ventricular (RV) ejection fractions (EF) in patients with inferior and anterior wall myocardial infarct (MI). RVEF and LVEF are significantly different at any time after infarct in patients with anterior and inferior MI. No significant sequential change occurs in either group from day 1 until discharge for LVEF or RVEF. Reproduced with permission [49].

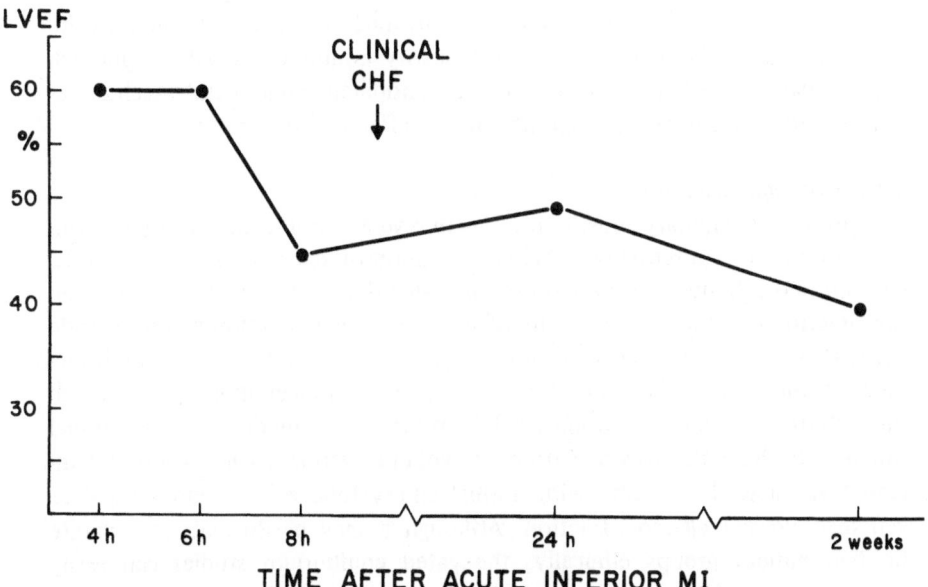

Figure 17. Sequential measurement of left ventricular ejection fraction (LVEF) in a patient with an acute inferior wall infarct. At 4 and 6 h after infarct, LVEF is 60%. At 8 h after infarct, LVEF has decreased to 44%, without apparent change in clinical condition. Only 4 h later, the patient developed clinical signs of congestive heart failure. LVEF remained at this level and was 42% at discharge.

function in acute myocardial infarct can be evaluated in only relatively large groups of patients.

CARDIOGENIC SHOCK

Bedside assessment of left ventricular function may be extremely helpful, both from a diagnostic and a therapeutic point of view, in patients demonstrating cardiac failure or its extreme manifestation, cardiogenic shock, in the setting of acute myocardial infarct. Severe heart failure may be due to massive infarct, rupture or insufficiency of a papillary muscle, rupture of the ventricular septum, or right ventricular infarct.

Massive myocardial infarct

Multigated equilibrium cardiac blood pool studies confirm the clinical impression and usually display marked enlargement of the left ventricle with markedly depressed contractility. Overall, left ventricular ejection fraction usually is 10%–20%. The poor overall cardiac function is not necessarily due to irreversible myocardial damage; severe myocardial ischemia may depress cardiac contractility to a similar extent. Cardiac function may improve spontaneously or by vasodilator therapy in individual patients. The objective information from radionuclide studies will justify a more conservative approach in these patients. When interventions are considered, radionuclide techniques provide a noninvasive means of monitoring the effects of treatment.

Rupture of papillary muscle

Rupture of a papillary muscle resulting in severe mitral regurgitation is a relatively uncommon, potentially lethal complication of acute myocardial infarcts. It occurs most frequently with posterior wall infarcts. Since cardiac function may deteriorate rapidly, assessment of left ventricular function at the bedside is crucial for further management of these patients and can be done by multiple-gated equilibrium cardiac blood pool imaging. Although most patients will demonstrate severely compromised left ventricular function, an occasional patient will show the classic pattern of volume-overloaded left ventricle: increased end-diastolic volume with normal end-systolic volume and normal or even high normal ejection fraction. Although it may be difficult to separate the two patient groups clinically, the gated equilibrium studies can easily separate them and may be extremely helpful to direct further surgical management.

Rupture of the ventricular septum

Rupture of the ventricular septum is another serious complication that usually occurs in the lower septum associated with either anteroseptal or posteroseptal infarcts. Although right-heart catheterization with sampling of oxygen saturation at various levels in the right heart is still the diagnostic procedure of choice to assess and quantitate the left-to-right shunt, radionuclide methods may provide useful qualitative and visual confirmation. Injection of a bolus of technetium-99m pertechnetate may demonstrate the transit of radioactivity through the lungs, left atrium and left ventricle and the subsequent shunt to the right ventricle to visually establish the diagnosis. Quantitation of the left-to-right shunt by first-pass radionuclide angiocardiography and computer analysis of the pulmonary flow components using a gamma variate function probably will be invalid, because these patients may have low cardiac output and consequently a prolonged pulmonary transit.

Right ventricular infarct

Right ventricular involvement in acute myocardial infarct is an important clinical entity to recognize. The clinical syndrome of right ventricular infarct as described by Cohn et al. [56] in 1974 is characterized by marked systemic hypotension and frank shock manifesting disproportionately elevated right ventricular pressures. These patients respond with an increase of cardiac output, and often survival, to volume loading. Right ventricular infarct occurs almost exclusively as a complication of inferoposterior and septal left ventricular infarct. The multigated cardiac blood pool studies in these patients may be quite characteristic [52, 53] (Figure 15). The right ventricle is markedly enlarged and hypokinetic, whereas left ventricular function often is preserved. Although the right ventricle may be enlarged because of preexistent pulmonary disease, in our experience multi-gated blood pool imaging has been extremely helpful to rule out right ventricular involvement in patients with acute inferior wall infarcts and hypotension.

LEFT VENTRICULAR EJECTION FRACTION AND PROGNOSIS

The overall size of a myocardial infarct will be reflected by the degree of left ventricular dysfunction. Schelbert et al. [58] noted an inverse relationship between the patient's functional class and left ventricular ejection fraction. Because of the wide range of normal ejection fractions (55%–80%), however, it is impossible to determine the precise amount of involved myocardium. Nevertheless, the left ventricular ejection fraction has prognostic significance after acute myocardial infarct and may be helpful in predicting early morbidity and mortality. Shah et al. [50] reported that all patients with a normal left ventricular ejection fraction survived the initial hospital course. Mean left ventricular ejection fraction was significantly lower in the nonsurvivors (17% vs 46%). These investigators concluded that an ejection fraction of 30% or less was a poor prognostic sign, and death related to pump failure occurred in 55% of such patients, whereas it did not occur in patients with ejection fractions exceeding 30%. In addition, all patients who developed congestive heart failure had initially depressed ejection fraction. Individual patients may have severely depressed left ventricular ejection fraction in the absence of clinical manifestations of heart failure, confirming the relative lack of sensitivity of clinical findings alone in detecting depressed ventricular function in the early stage of infarct (Figure 18). On the other hand, radionuclide assessment of right and left ventricular function may be extremely helpful in differentiating between cardiogenic shock due to massive left ventricular infarct or right ventricular infarct.

Similar observations have been reported by Lyons and Olson [73]. These investigators observed that during the acute phase of myocardial infarct, normal left ventricular ejection fraction ($\geqslant$ 50%) predicted a low (1.5%) risk of cardiac death during six months of follow-up, and none of these patients developed congestive heart failure. In contrast, patients with depressed left ventricular ejection fraction had a high risk of both cardiac death (22.1%) and developing congestive heart failure (33.7%).

Schulze et al. [74] assessed the relative role of depressed left ventricular ejection fraction and ventricular arrhythmias as indicators of poor prognosis following an acute myocardial infarct. Eighty-one patients were followed for one year after acute infarct. Sudden death occurred in eight patients, all with ejection fractions less than 40% and complicated ventricular arrhythmias. Approximately 90% of the patients with complicated ventricular premature contractions in the late hospital phase of their acute infarct had a left ventricular ejection fraction less than 40%, suggesting larger infarcts. Although mortality was higher in patients with depressed ejection fraction, the presence of complicated ventricular arrhythmias in the late hospital phase selected a subgroup of patients with even greater risk for (sudden) death.

Borer et al. [75] recently reported results in 45 patients who had 6–14 months of follow-up after acute infarct. Their results are slightly at variance with those of Schulze et al. Resting ejection fraction at discharge correlated with the complexity of ventricular arrhythmias. Of patients with an ejection fraction less than 35%, 93% manifested complex arrhythmias, whereas in patients with an ejection fraction of more than 35%, arrhythmias were much more difficult to predict. All five patients who died had ejection fractions less than 35% and four had complex arrhythmics. Although the data are still limited to a relatively small number of patients, these findings suggest that arrhythmias may not represent a risk factor independent of that imposed by left ventricular mechanical dysfunction.

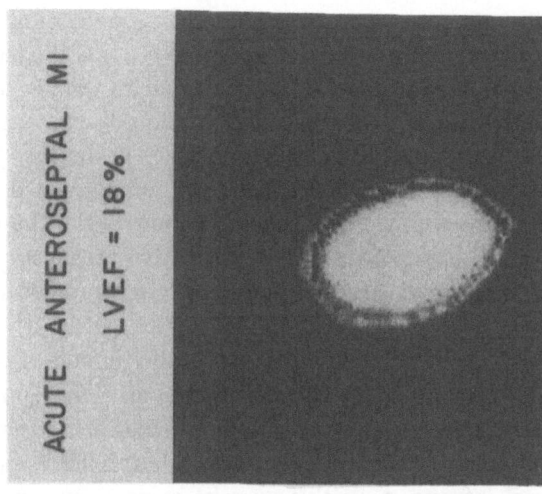

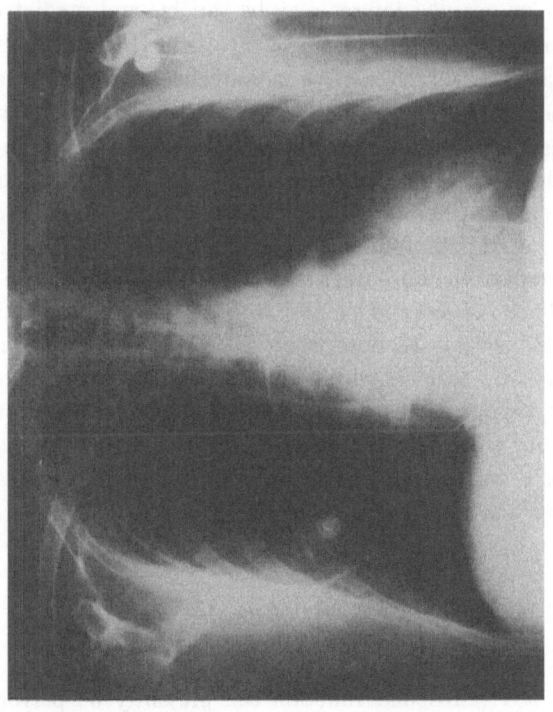

Figure 18. Disparity between findings at physical exam, chest X-ray, and radionuclide angiocardiography in a patient with acute anteroseptal myocardial infarct (MI). No signs of heart failure were present at physical exam; the chest X-ray reveals a normal cardiac size with possible left ventricular prominence. No signs of pulmonary venous hypertension are present. The pulmonary capillary wedge pressure was minimally elevated. First-pass radionuclide angiocardiography in the left anterior oblique position shows diffuse hypokinesis and septal akinesis. The computer-generated left ventricular end-diastolic perimeter is shown superimposed over the end-systolic image. Left ventricular ejection fraction (LVEF) is 18%.

LEFT VENTRICULAR FUNCTION DURING EXERCISE AFTER ACUTE
MYOCARDIAL INFARCT

Patients with an uncomplicated acute myocardial infarct have been shown to
be capable of performing submaximal exercise safely before hospital discharge;
important prognostic information can be obtained from exercise tests in these
patients [75–82]. Electrocardiographic ST segment depression during exercise
has been shown to be highly predictive of increased mortality in the first year
after an infarct [76, 79]. Similarly, angina during the stress test correlated well
with recurrence of stable angina during the follow-up period [79]. The presence of exercise-induced arrhythmias does not seem to have prognostic significance in patients without clinical heart failure soon after a myocardial
infarct [75, 80, 81].

The functional ventricular response after acute myocardial infarct appears
to differ depending on the location of the infarct. Pulido et al. [78] reported
that all patients with a recent anterior myocardial infarct manifested a significant reduction in left ventricular ejection fraction with submaximal exercise.
In inferior or nontransmural infarcts, a variable exercise response was noted.
In 26% of their patients, a normal response to exercise (increase of $\geqslant 5\%$)
occurred. Reduto et al. [82] also demonstrated that the exercise response in
patients who sustained a myocardial infarct may be variable and predicted by
neither the predischarge resting values nor the site of infarct (Figure 19). Borer
et al. [75] studied 45 patients by rest/exercise radionuclide angiocardiography
at hospital discharge and again 6–14 months later. During the early study,
mean left ventricular ejection fraction was abnormal (average 39% ± 5) and
showed little change during submaximal exercise. Only eight of the 45 patients
manifested a significant change (increase or decrease) in ejection fraction compared with values at rest. At late follow-up, the ejection fraction in seven
patients who had an exercise ejection fraction greater than 40% at the predischarge study improved both at rest and exercise. For the remaining 23 patients
at follow-up, no change in ejection fraction occurred both at rest and exercise.
These studies demonstrate that patients with a myocardial infarct may manifest
a normal left ventricular response to exercise (normal exercise reserve) in spite
of severely depressed resting function. It is likely that these patients will have a
better long-term prognosis, but this remains to be proven. The exercise response, including wall motion analysis, may enable identification of patients
with significant coronary stenoses outside the region of infarct [83].

CONCLUSION

Assessment of right and left ventricular function can presently be performed
noninvasively and reliably at the patient's bedside in the coronary care unit

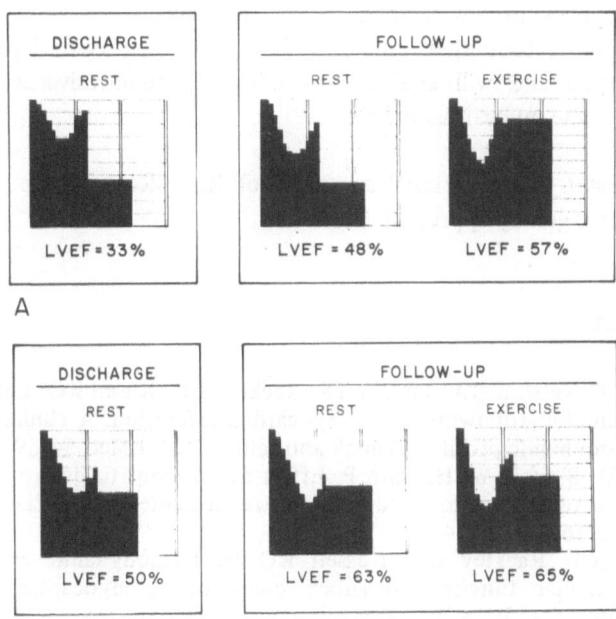

Figure 19. Normal (*A*) and abnormal (*B*) exercise left ventricular (LV) reserves in patients with recent myocardial infarct assessed by first-pass radionuclide angiocardiography. The patient in *A* had a decreased LV ejection fraction (EF) of 33% at hospital discharge. At follow-up this had improved to 48%, and further increased during exercise to 57%, a normal response. The patient in *B* also showed improvement of resting LVEF at follow-up (from 50% to 63%). However, at exercise, this patient was not able to increase LVEF more than 5%, which is an abnormal response.

using validated radionuclide techniques. Although providing only indirect evidence of the degree of myocardial damage and infarct size, these techniques provide a key functional assessment of the infarcted ventricle. It can be expected that data obtained by these methods will have a major impact on clinical decision making. Readily available information concerning right and left ventricular function in patients with complicated acute infarcts may be of crucial importance for patient management. Patients at increased risk may be recognized earlier, even before conventional clinical parameters become apparent. The data confirm that left ventricular ejection fraction is the most important predictor of the patient's prognosis after an acute myocardial infarct. Patients with significantly depressed ejection fraction (30%–35%) have a poorer outlook than those whose residual global left ventricular function remained preserved. Therefore, we believe that ventricular performance should be assessed prior to hospital discharge in most patients with an acute myocardial infarct. The role of exercise function tests after infarct remains to be defined, but it has the

228

potential to further identify patients at increased or decreased risk. In the near future, development of new radiopharmaceuticals, specialized cardiac detectors, and new computer techniques especially for determining regional performance can be expected and will enable more complete noninvasive evaluation of patients with acute myocardial infarct.

Acknowledgment. The secretarial assistance of Ruth Rosen in the preparation of this chapter is greatly appreciated.

REFERENCES

1. Weber KT, Ratshin RA, Janicki TS, Rackley CE, Rusell RO: Left ventricular dysfunction following acute myocardial infarction. A clinicopathologic and hemodynamic profile of shock and failure. Am J Med 54:697, 1973.
2. Mathey D, Bleifeld W, Hanrath P, Effert S: Attempt to quantitate relation between cardiac function and infarct size in acute myocardial infarction. Br Heart J 36:271, 1974.
3. Ratshin RA, Rackley CE, Russell RO Jr: Hemodynamic evaluation of left ventricular function in shock complicating myocardial infarction. Circulation 45:127, 1972.
4. Kostuk WJ, Ehsani A, Karliner JS, Ashburn WL, Peterson KL, Ross J Jr, Sobel BE: Left ventricular performance after myocardial infarction assessed by radioisotope angiocardiography. Circulation 47:242, 1973.
5. Rigo P, Murray M, Strauss HW, Taylor DR, Kelly DT, Weisfeldt ML, Pitt B: Left ventricular function in acute myocardial infarction evaluated by gated scintiphotography. Circulation 50:678, 1974.
6. Morrison J, Coromilas J, Munsey D, Robbins M, Zema M, Chiaramida S, Reiser P, Scherr L: Correlation of radionuclide estimates of myocardial infarction size and release of creatine kinase-MB in man. Circulation 62, 277, 1980.
7. Hammermeister KE, DeRouen TA, Dodge HT: Variables predictive of survival in patients with coronary disease. Selection by univariate and multivariate analyses from the clinical, electrocardiographic, exercise, arteriographic, and quantitative angiographic evaluations. Circulation 59:421, 1979.
8. Nelson GR, Cohn PF, Gorlin R: Prognosis in medically treated coronary artery disease: influence of ejection fraction compared to other parameters. Circulation 52:408, 1975.
9. Berger HJ, Matthay RA, Pytlik LM, Gottschalk A, Zaret BL: First-pass radionuclide assessment of right and left ventricular performance in patients with cardiac and pulmonary disease. Semin Nucl Med 9:275, 1979.
10. Strauss HW, McKusick KA, Boucher CA, Bingham JB, Pohost GM: Of linens and laces – the eighth anniversary of the gated blood pool scan. Semin Nucl Med 9:296, 1979.
11. Wagner HN Jr, Wake R, Nickoloff E, Natarajan TK: The nuclear stethoscope: a simple device for generation of left ventricular volume curves. Am J Cardiol 38:747, 1976.

12. Schelbert HR, Verba JW, Johnson AD, Brock GW, Alazraki NP, Rose FJ, Ashburn WL: Nontraumatic determination of left ventricular ejection fraction by radionuclide angiocardiography. Circulation 51:902, 1975.

13. Marshall RC, Berger HJ, Costin JC, Freedman GS, Wolberg J, Cohen LS, Gottschalk A, Zaret BL: Assessment of cardiac performance with quantitative radionuclide angiocardiography: sequential left ventricular ejection fraction, normalized left ventricular ejection rate, and regional wall motion. Circulation 56:820, 1977.

14. Jengo JA, Mena I, Blaufuss A, Criley JM: Evaluation of left ventricular function (ejection fraction and segmental wall motion) by single pass radioisotope angiography. Circulation 57:326, 1978.

15. Hecht HS, Mirell SG, Rolett EL, Blahd WH: Left-ventricular ejection fraction and segmental wall motion by peripheral first-pass radionuclide angiography. J Nucl Med 19:17, 1978.

16. Berger HJ, Matthay RA, Loke J, Marshall RC, Gottschalk A, Zaret BL: Assessment of cardiac performance with quantitative radionuclide angiocardiography: right ventricular ejection fraction with reference to findings in chronic obstructive pulmonary disease. Am J Cardiol 41:897, 1978.

17. Tobinick E, Schelbert HR, Henning H, LeWinter M, Taylor A, Ashburn WL, Karliner JS: Right ventricular ejection fraction in patients with acute anterior and inferior myocardial infarction assessed by radionuclide angiography. Circulation 57:1078, 1978.

18. Marshall RC, Berger HJ, Reduto LA, Gottschalk A, Zaret BL: Variability in sequential measures of left ventricular performance assessed with radionuclide angiocardiography. Am J Cardiol 41:531, 1978.

19. Winzelberg GG, Boucher CA, Pohost GM, McKusick KA, Bingham JB, Okada RD, Strauss HW: Right ventricular function in aortic and mitral valve disease: Relation of gated first pass radionuclide angiography to clinical and hemodynamic findings. Chest 79:520, 1981.

20. Pavel DG, Zimmer AM, Patterson VN: In vivo labeling of red blood cells with ^{99m}Tc: a new approach to blood pool visualization. J Nucl Med 18: 305, 1977.

21. Green MV, Ostrow HG, Douglas MA, Myers RW, Scott RN, Bailey JJ, Johnston GS: High temporal resolution ECG-gated scintigraphic angiocardiography. J Nucl Med 16:95, 1975.

22. Bacharach SL, Green MV, Borer JS, Douglas MA, Ostrow HG, Johnston GS: A real-time system for multi-image gated cardiac studies. J Nucl Med 18:79, 1977.

23. Burow RD, Strauss HW, Singleton R, Pond M, Rehn T, Bailey IK, Griffith LC, Nickoloff E, Pitt B: Analysis of left ventricular function from multiple gated acquisition cardiac blood pool imaging. Comparison to contrast angiography. Circulation 56:1024, 1977.

24. Sorensen SG, Hamilton GW, Williams DL, Ritchie JL: R-wave synchronized blood-pool imaging: A comparison of the accuracy and reproducibility of fixed and computer-automated varying regions-of-interest for determining the left ventricular ejection fraction. Radiology 131:473, 1979.

25. Green MV, Brody WR, Douglas MA, Borer JS, Ostrow HG, Line BR, Bacharach SL, Johnston GS: Ejection fraction by count rate from gated images. J Nucl Med 19:880, 1978.

26. Wackers FJ, Berger HJ, Johnstone DE, Goldman L, Reduto LA, Langou

RA, Gottschalk A, Zaret BL: Multiple gated cardiac blood pool imaging for left ventricular ejection fraction: validation of the technique and assessment of variability. Am J Cardiol 43:1159, 1979.

27. Maddahi J, Berman DS, Matsuoka DT, Waxman AD, Stankus KE, Forrester JS, Swan HJ: A new technique for assessing right ventricular ejection fraction using rapid multiple-gated equilibrium cardiac blood pool scintigraphy. Description, validation and findings in chronic coronary artery disease. Circulation 60:581, 1979.

28. Slutsky R, Hooper W, Gerber K, Battler A, Froelicher V, Ashburn W, Karliner J: Assessment of right ventricular function at rest and during exercise in patients with coronary heart disease: a new approach using equilibrium radionuclide angiography. Am J Cardiol 45:63, 1980.

29. Maddahi J, Berman DS, Matsuoka DT, Waxman AD, Forrester JS, Swan HJ: Right ventricular ejection fraction during exercise in normal subjects and in coronary artery disease patients: assessment by multiple-gated equilibrium scintigraphy. Circulation 62:133, 1980.

30. Okada RD, Kirschenbaum HD, Kushner FG, Strauss HW, Dinsmore RE, Newell JB, Boucher CA, Block PC, Pohost GM: Observer variance in the qualitative evaluation of left ventricular wall motion and the quantitation of left ventricular ejection fraction using rest and exercise multi-gated blood pool imaging. Circulation 61:128, 1980.

31. Okada RD, Pohost GM, Nichols AB, McKusick KA, Strauss HW, Boucher CA, Block PC, Rosenthal SV, Dinsmore RE: Left ventricular regional wall motion assessment by multigated and end-diastolic, end-systolic gated radionuclide left ventriculography. Am J Cardiol 45:1211, 1980.

32. Kelly MJ, Giles RW, Simon TR, Berger HJ, Zaret BL, Wackers FJ: Multigated equilibrium radionuclide angiocardiography: improved detection of left ventricular wall motion abnormalities and aneurysms with the addition of the left lateral view. Radiology 139:167, 1981.

33. Maddox DE, Holman BL, Wynne J, Idoine J, Parker JA, Uren R, Neill JM, Cohn PF: Ejection fraction image: a noninvasive index of regional left ventricular wall motion. Am J Cardiol 41:1230, 1978.

34. Bodenheimer MM, Banka VS, Fooshee CM, Gillespie JA, Helfant RH: Detection of coronary heart disease using radionuclide determined regional ejection fraction at rest and during handgrip exercise: correlation with coronary arteriography. Circulation 58:640, 1978.

35. Maddox DE, Wynne J, Uren R, Parker JA, Idoine J, Siegel LC, Neill JM, Cohn PF, Holman BL: Regional ejection fraction: a quantitative radionuclide index of regional left ventricular performance. Circulation 59:1001, 1979.

36. Ramanathan KB, Bodenheimer MM, Banka VS, Helfant RH: Severity of contraction abnormalities after acute myocardial infarction in man: response to nitroglycerin. Circulation 60:1230, 1979.

37. Williams B, Berger H, Wackers F, Brendel A, Lewis S, Gottschalk A, Zaret B: Left ventricular ejection fraction functional images at rest and bicycle exercise: Definition of normal and abnormal regional responses in coronary artery disease [abstr]. J Nucl Med 21:P65, 1980.

38. Levine HJ, Gaasch WH: Diastolic compliance of the left ventricle. I: causes of a noncompliant ventricular chamber. Mod Concepts Cardiovasc Dis 47:95, 1978.

39. Rerych SK, Scholz PM, Newman GE, Sabiston DC Jr, Jones RH: Cardiac function at rest and during exercise in normals and in patients with coronary heart disease: evaluation by radionuclide angiocardiography. Ann Surg 187:449, 1978.

40. Slutsky R, Karliner J, Ricci D, Kaiser R, Pfisterer M, Gordon D, Peterson K, Ashburn W: Left ventricular volumes by gated equilibrium radionuclide angiography: a new method. Circulation 60:556, 1979.

41. Dehmer GJ, Lewis SE, Hillis LD, Twieg D, Falkoff M, Parkey RW, Willerson JT: Nongeometric determination of left ventricular volumes from equilibrium blood pool scans. Am J Cardiol 45:293, 1980.

42. Bacharach SL, Green MV, Borer JS, Ostrow HG, Redwood DR, Johnston GS: ECG-gated scintillation probe measurement of left ventricular function. J Nucl Med 18:1176, 1977.

43. Camargo EE, Harrison KS, Wagner NH, Bourguignon MH, Reid PR, Alderson PO, Baxter RH: Noninvasive beat-to-beat monitoring of left ventricular function by a nonimaging nuclear detector during premature ventricular contractions. Am J Cardiol 45:1219, 1980.

44. Berger HJ, Davies RA, Batsford WP, Hoffer PB, Gottschalk A, Zaret BL: Beat-to-beat left ventricular performance assessed from the equilibrium cardiac blood pool using a computerized nuclear probe. Circulation 63: 133, 1981.

45. Berger H, Davies R, Batsford W, Hoffer P, Gottschalk A, Zaret B: Beat-to-beat assessment of left ventricular performance using a portable computerized nuclear probe: validation, analysis of variability, and initial study of ectopy [abstr]. J Nucl Med 21:P7, 1980.

46. Hoffer P, Berger H, Steidley J, Brendel A, Gottschalk A, Zaret B: Miniature cadmium telluride detector module for continuous monitoring left ventricular function. Radiology 138:477, 1981.

47. Rackley CE, Russell RO Jr: Left ventricular function in acute myocardial infarction and its clinical significance. Circulation 45:231, 1972.

48. Hamby RI, Hoffman I, Hilsenrath J, Aintablian A, Shanies S, Padmanabhan VS: Clinical, hemodynamic and angiographic aspects of inferior and anterior myocardial infarctions in patients with angina pectoris. Am J Cardiol 34: 513, 1974.

49. Reduto LA, Berger HJ, Cohen LS, Gottschalk A, Zaret BL: Sequential radionuclide assessment of left and right ventricular performance after acute transmural myocardial infarction. Ann Intern Med 89:441, 1978.

50. Shah PK, Pichler M, Berman DS, Singh BN, Swan HJ: Left ventricular ejection fraction determined by radionuclide ventriculography in early stages of first transmural myocardial infarction: relation to short-term prognosis. Am J Cardiol 45:542, 1980.

51. Rotman M, Ratliff NB, Hawley J: Right ventricular infarction: a haemodynamic diagnosis. Br Heart J 36:941, 1974.

52. Rigo P, Murray M, Taylor DR, Weisfeldt ML, Kelly DT, Strauss HW, Pitt B: Right ventricular dysfunction detected by gated scintiphotography in patients with acute inferior myocardial infarction. Circulation 52:268, 1975.

53. Sharpe DN, Botvinick EH, Shames DM, Schiller NB, Massie BM, Chatterjee K, Parmley WW: The noninvasive diagnosis of right ventricular infarction. Circulation 57:483, 1978.

54. Steele P, Kirch D, Ellis J, Vogel R, Battock D: Prompt return to normal of depressed right ventricular ejection fraction in acute inferior infarction. Br Heart J 39:1319, 1977.
55. Wackers FJ, Lie KI, Sokole EB, Res J, Van der Schoot JB, Durrer D: Prevalence of right ventricular involvement in inferior wall infarction assessed with myocardial imaging with thallium-201 and technetium-99m pyrophosphate. Am J Cardiol 42:358, 1978.
56. Cohn JN, Guiha NK, Broder MI, Limas CJ: Right ventricular infarction. Clinical and hemodynamic features. Am J Cardiol 33:209, 1974.
57. Cohn JN: Right ventricular infarction revisited. Am J Cardiol 43:666, 1979.
58. Schelbert HR, Henning H, Ashburn WL, Verba JW, Karliner JS, O'Rourke RA: Serial measurements of left ventricular ejection fraction by radio-nuclide angiography early and late after myocardial infarction. Am J Cardiol 38:407, 1976.
59. Ohsuzu F, Boucher CA, Osbakken MD, Bingham JB, Newell JB, Gold HK, Leinbach RC, Pohost GM, Strauss HW: Evaluation of left ventricular function in acute myocardial infarction using radionuclide ventriculo-graphy: relation of regional wall motion to the parameters of global left ventricular function [abstr]. J Nucl Med 21:P74, 1980.
60. Friedman ML, Cantor RE: Reliability of gated heart scintigrams for de-detection of left-ventricular aneurysm: concise communication. J Nucl Med 20:720, 1979.
61. Nichols AB, McKusick KA, Strauss HW, Dinsmore RE, Block PC, Pohost GM: Clinical utility of gated cardiac blood pool imaging in congestive left heart failure. Am J Med 65:785, 1978.
62. Dymond DS, Jarritt PH, Britton KE, Spurrell RA: Detection of post-infarction left ventricular aneurysms by first pass radionuclide ventriculo-graphy using a multicrystal gamma camera. Br Heart J 41:68, 1979.
63. Stephens JD, Dymond DS, Spurrell RA: Radionuclide and hemodynamic assessment of left ventricular functional reserve in patients with left ventri-cular aneurysm and congestive cardiac failure. Response to exercise stress and isosorbide dinitrate. Circulation 61:536, 1980.
64. Botvinick EH, Shames D, Hutchinson JC, Roe BB, Fitzpatrick M: Non-invasive diagnosis of a false left ventricular aneurysm with radioisotope gated cardiac blood pool imaging. Differentiation from true aneurysm. Am J Cardiol 37:1089, 1976.
65. Katz RJ, Simpson A, DiBianco R, Fletcher RD, Bates HR, Sauerbrunn BJ: Noninvasive diagnosis of left ventricular pseudoaneurysm: role of two dimensional echocardiography and radionuclide gated pool imaging. Am J Cardiol 44:372, 1979.
66. Holman BL, Wynne J, Idoine J, Neill J: Disruption in the temporal se-quence of regional ventricular contraction. I. Characteristics and Incidence in Coronary Artery Disease. Circulation 61:1075, 1980.
67. Slutsky R, Karliner JS, Battler A, Peterson K, Ross J Jr: Comparison of early systolic and holosystolic ejection phase indexes by contrast ventri-culography in patients with coronary artery disease. Circulation 61:1083, 1980.
68. Shillingford J, Thomas M: Hemodynamic effects of acute myocardial in-farction in man. Progr Cardiovasc Dis 9:571, 1967.

69. Kupper W, Bleifeld W, Hanrath P, Mathey D, Effert S: Left ventricular hemodynamics and function in acute myocardial infarction: studies during the acute phase, convalescence and late recovery. Am J Cardiol 40:900, 1977.

70. Rahimtoola SH, DiGilio MM, Ehsani A, Loeb HS, Rosen KM, Gunnar RM: Changes in left ventricular performance from early after acute myocardial infarction to the convalescent phase. Circulation 46:770, 1972.

71. Wackers F, Berger M, Zaret B: Spontaneous changes of global and regional left ventricular function during the first 24 hours of acute myocardial infarction: implications for evaluating thrombolytic therapy [abstr]. Circulation [Suppl 2]:IV-196, 1981.

72. Morrison J, Coromilas J, Robbins M, Ong L, Eisenberg S, Stechel R, Zema M, Reiser P, Scherr L: Digitalis and myocardial infarction in man. Circulation 62:8, 1980.

73. Lyons KP, Olson HG: Correlation between radionuclide left ventricular ejection fraction during acute myocardial infarction and cardiac death or CHF. J Nucl Med 21:P6, 1980.

74. Schulze RA Jr, Strauss HW, Pitt B: Sudden death in the year following myocardial infarction: relation to ventricular premature contractions in the late hospitals phase and left ventricular ejection fraction. Am J Med 62:192, 1977.

75. Borer JS, Rosing DR, Miller RH, Stark RM, Kent KM, Bacharach SL, Green MV, Lake CR, Cohen H, Holmes D, Donohue D, Baker W, Epstein S: Natural history of left ventricular function during 1 year after acute myocardial infarction: comparison with clinical, electrocardiographic and biochemical determinations. Am J Cardiol 46: 1980.

76. Markiewicz W, Houston N, DeBusk RF: Exercise testing soon after myocardial infarction. Circulation 56:26, 1977.

77. Wohl AJ, Lewis HR, Campbell W, Karlsson E, Willerson JT, Mullins CB, Blomqvist CG: Cardiovascular function during early recovery from acute myocardial infarction. Circulation 56:931, 1977.

78. Pulido JI, Doss J, Twieg D, Blomqvist GC, Faulkner D, Horn V, DeBates D, Tobey M, Parkey RW, Willerson JT: Submaximal exercise testing after acute myocardial infarction: myocardial scintigraphic and electrocardiographic observations. Am J Cardiol 42:19, 1978.

79. Théroux P, Waters DD, Halphen C, Debaisieux JC, Mizgala HF: Prognostic value of exercise testing soon after myocardial infarction. N Engl J Med 301:341, 1979.

80. DeBusk RF, DAvidson DM, Houston N, Fitzgerald J: Serial ambulatory electrocardiography and treadmill exercise testing after uncomplicated myocardial infarction. Am J Cardiol 45:547, 1980.

81. DeBusk RF, Haskell W: Symptom-limited vs heart-rate-limited exercise testing soon after myocardial infarction. Circulation 61:738, 1980.

82. Reduto LA, Johnstone DE, Berger HJ, Gottschalk A, Zaret BL: Radionuclide left ventricular performance and reserve following acute myocardial infarction: relationship to resting performance in the acute infarct period. Circulation [Suppl] 58:II, II-27, 1978.

83. DePuey EG, Sonnemaker RE, Garcia E, Burdine JA: Exercise radionuclide ventriculography in patients with prior myocardial infarction. J Nucl Med 21:P5, 1980.

9. ULTRASOUND

RICHARD S. STACK and JOSEPH KISSLO

Although echocardiography has been found to be very useful for evaluating valvular and congenital heart disease, its use for quantitating the amount of ischemic myocardium has not been as well documented. Echocardiography has been limited for this purpose because of two major factors. First, until recently ultrasonic examination of the heart was limited to the M-mode approach where a single beam provided limited information concerning movement of only the septum and posterior walls. Second, image quality is frequently impaired in patients with ischemic heart disease due to age, chest wall configuration, accompanying lung disease, and other ill-defined factors.

Two-dimensional echocardiography overcomes the limited access to the heart found in M-mode by providing spatial integration of the anatomic information in a tomographic or cross-sectional format. This wide field of view enables detection and intelligible interpretation of virtually every wall of the heart when image quality is satisfactory. When image quality is impaired, the spatial characteristics of the cross-sectional approach still frequently renders useful information despite poorly visualized targets. Thus, the two-dimensional approach shows greater promise for evaluating ventricular size, shape, and wall motion characteristics in patients with ischemic heart disease when compared with M-mode [1–6].

The fact that two-dimensional echocardiography provides dynamic information regarding both *chamber size and wall thickness* constitutes its most unique characteristic when compared with other imaging methods used to apply quantitative descriptors to ischemic myocardium. Cardiac images based on static (chest X-ray) or dynamic (flouroscopic, cineventriculographic, or radioisotope angiographic) approaches represent the heart and its chambers as silhouettes and are thus quite different from echocardiography in informational content. Silhouette methods usually provide an integrated image of overall ventricular size and movement and are therefore well suited for assessing ventricular chamber shape and volume. Although echocardiographic methods may be used with some difficulty for similar purposes, they are better suited for assessing regional abnormalities of chamber size or wall thickness.

This chapter describes the practical methods for examining the left ventricle by two-dimensional echocardiography and summarizes the recent literature

Wagner GS (ed): Myocardial Infarction: Measurement and Intervention, pp 235–260.
© 1982 Martinus Nijhoff Publishers, The Hague/Boston/London.

in the use of this technique for evaluating patients who have left ventricular myocardial ischemia.

ECHOCARDIOGRAPHIC TECHNIQUES

The simplest approach to understanding the multiple views utilized by two-dimensional echocardiography is to imagine two basic cardiac axis orientations: the long axis (Figure 1) and the short axis (Figure 2) Examination of the left ventricle is usually begun in the long axis (Figure 1, panel I) by placing the

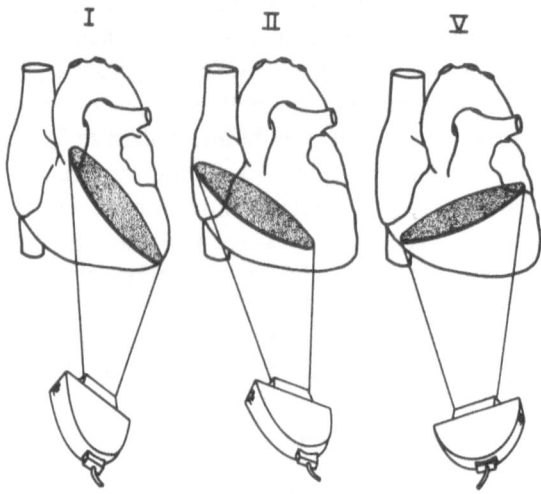

Figure 1. Transducer orientations for evaluation of the long axis of the left ventricle. For details, see text.

transducer on the chest wall in the second, third, or fourth left intercostal space and angling the scan plane parallel to an imaginary plane from the patient's right shoulder to the left subcostal margin. This plane intercepts the long axis of the left ventricle from the aortic root to the apex. The interventricular septum and the posterior ventricular wall can generally be evaluated in this view.

Another long-axis view, termed the apical long-axis or the apical four-chamber view is obtained by placing the transducer over the ventricular apex, rotating approximately 90° clockwise, and then angling cephalad through the ventricle [7]. This plane of view intercepts the apical, septal, and anterolateral walls of the left ventricle.

Serial short axes of the heart may be obtained by rotating the transducer

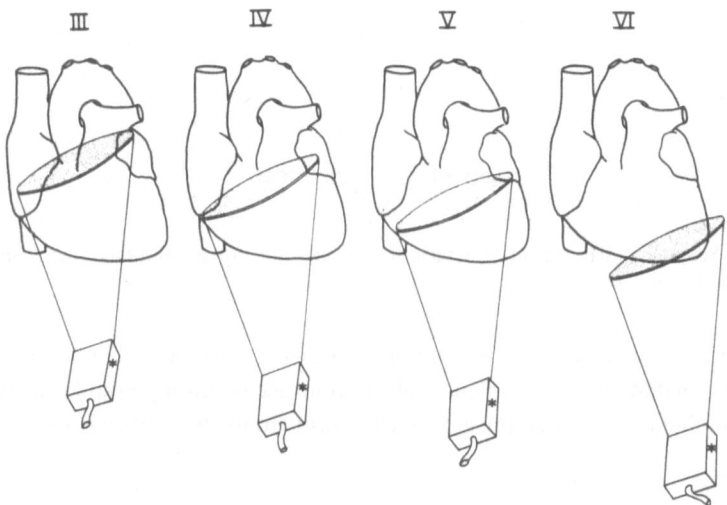

Figure 2. Transducer orientations for evaluation of the serial short axes of the left ventricle. For details, see text.

90° in the original left parasternal long axis and then sequentially angling the interrogating plane at the level of the aortic root (Figure 2, panel III), mitral valve orifice (panel IV), papillary muscles (panel V), and apex (panel VI). Evaluation of the left ventricular chamber in short axis is generally accomplished using the latter three views. They enable imaging of the posterolateral, antero-lateral, septal, and inferior walls from the base to the apex.

TRANSDUCER ANGULATION

Particular care must be taken during the examination procedure to angle the interrogating plane properly through the true long or short axis of the ventricle. Improper angulation of the scan plane tangentially through the ventricle will distort the appearance of the ventricular lond axis. The characteristic normal elliptical configuration will appear circular, or cut off, near the apex and origins of the papillary muscles. In the short axis, the problem is recognized when the normal circular appearance of the cavity in this axis appears elliptical or oval (Figure 3). In addition, the papillary muscles appear midway around the ven-tricular circumference rather than posteriorly, and there may be reciprocal thickening and thinning of the chamber walls on opposite sides of the ventricle. The presence of regional wall motion abnormalities secondary to ischemic heart disease will also produce distortion of the normal circular shape of the short-axis

238

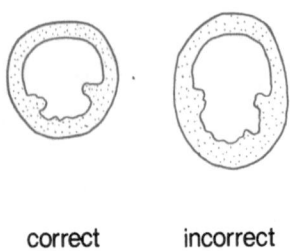

correct   incorrect

Figure 3. Schematic diagram showing images resulting from correct and incorrect transducer angulation. For details, see text.

view. This can generally be recognized, however, by the fact that the majority of the distortion due to ischemic wall motion occurs during systole, while the distortion due to tangential imaging is seen throughout the cardiac cycle.

ECHOCARDIOGRAPHIC IMAGING SYSTEM

Multiple ultrasonic systems have been devised for viewing the left ventricle in the cross-sectional format [8]. Each specific system has its own operational characteristics rendering differences in resolution, sector area size, or gray-scale presentation.

Illustrations in this chapter were obtained using a previously described [9, 10] real-time, phased-array imaging system. This device utilizes a handheld, 25-element transducer array that measures 14 x 24 mm at the site of skin contact and relies upon phased-array principles to electronically steer and focus the sound beam through the structures under investigation. Real-time, cross-sectional images of cardiac structures are presented in a circular sector format, 50°, 60°, or 90° in azimuth at a frame rate of 30/s. Images are permanently recorded on videotape for later playback and analysis.

Much detail is lost in the illustrations of the single-frame two-dimensional scan images which were made from videotape recordings by means of 35 mm photography of the sector arc in the stop-frame mode. As such, there is a loss of visual integration of motion that normally accompanies real-time playback. Moreover, there is a severe degradation of image quality caused by photographing a single video field from the videotape recording because of the fact that an individual field represents the scan information collected in 1/60th of a second. When operating in the 90°, 160-line format, therefore, each single video field shows only one-half (80 lines) of the information provided in the real-time scan.

ESTIMATION OF LEFT VENTRICULAR VOLUME

In order to reliably quantitate the amount of ischemic myocardium, the accuracy of echocardiographic dimension measurements utilized for the calculation of ventricular volumes and myocardial mass must first be explored. Several studies have shown a significant correlation between M-mode echocardiographic and angiographic estimates of left ventricular volumes and ejection fraction. However, when ventricles become grossly enlarged [1, 11], or contain significant regional wall abnormalities [2, 3, 12], the correlation with angiographic estimates of ventricular volume rapidly deteriorates. Most of the problems in estimating volumes with the M-mode technique are related to the small sampling area afforded by the beam from a single stationary ultrasonic crystal. Two-dimensional echocardiography, by providing more target information, could theoretically improve volume estimates. In vitro studies have shown a remarkable potential for accurate volume determinations by the cross-sectional technique. Initial clinical studies in vivo, however, have shown a greater variability in the relation between two-dimensional and other established measures of left ventricular volumes.

A recent study by Eaton et al. [13] has examined the accuracy of two-dimensional echocardiography to measure the volumes of latex balloons and formalin-fixed canine hearts in vitro by using Simpson's rule. Simpson's rule states that volume can be calculated by dividing a three-dimensional object into slices of known thickness and surface area. The volume of the object is equal to the sum of the volumes of each slice: Volume $(V) = \Sigma AH$, where A is the planimetered surface area and H is the height of each slice. By using this technique, the calculated volumes of the latex balloons and the formalin-fixed hearts correlated extremely well with direct volume measurements having correlation coefficients of 0.99 and 0.99 respectively. To approximate in vivo measurements, Eaton then used Simpson's rule to measure the volumes of isolated, cross-perfused, ejecting canine hearts compared with direct measurements using a volumetric displacement chamber. The correlation was again very close $(r = 0.97)$.

Several clinical studies have been performed to estimate left ventricular volumes in vivo in humans. Folland et al. [4] studied various geometric models to estimate volume by using two-dimensional echocardiographic images and compared them with angiographic and radionuclide volume estimates. Using a modified Simpson's rule approach with one long-axis and three short-axis images gave the closest correlation with angiographic volume estimates. Estimations of end-systolic volume (ESV) showed the closest agreement with single-plane angiographic estimates having a correlation coefficient of 0.86. Estimates of end-diastolic volume (EDV) and ejection fraction (EF) showed less consistent relationships to the angiographic measures. Combining all EDV and ESV data points improved the correlation ($r = 0.84$) but a large SEE (43 cc) remained. Comparison of echocardiographic and first-pass radionuclide angiographic estimates of ejection fraction gave a correlation coefficient that was similar to the comparison of the echocardiographic and cineangiographic estimates ($r = 0.75$). It should be noted that the study group consisted of 35 patients, 20 of whom showed regional contraction abnormalities by cineangiography, and eight of whom had ventricular volumes greater than 200 cc. Thus, although the relation between two-dimensional echocardiographic and cineangiographic estimates of ejection fraction were relatively weak, they showed a much closer agreement than did simultaneous M-mode echocardiographic estimates.

A similar study recently published by Schiller et al. [5] compared biplane angiographic and two-dimensional echocardiographic estimates of EDV, ESV, and EF among 30 patients. A closer relationship between the two techniques was shown in this study even though the percentage of patients with regional wall motion abnormalities due to coronary artery disease was slightly higher than the previously mentioned study group. The advantage of the integrated target information provided by the two-dimensional approach was again demonstrated when simultaneous M-mode volume estimates were compared with angiographic estimates in 23 of the patients. The intraobserver variation for cross-sectional echocardiographic volume estimates in Schiller's study was only ± 4%. Interobserver variation was tested by a regression analysis of the echocardiographic volume data that was calculated by two different observers and yielded correlation coefficients of 0.82, 0.95, and 0.95 for EDV, ESV, and EF, respectively.

Carr et al. [14] also studied the realtionship between two-dimensional echocardiographic and biplane angiographic volume determinations yielding a correlation of .93 for both the ejection fraction and the end-diastolic volume. While the data for the ejection fraction were close to the line of identity, the end-diastolic volume determinations by two-dimensional echocardiography were significantly less than the angiographic determinations.

Silverman and co-workers [15] compared angiographic and two-dimensional echocardiographic volume determinations in children and found an excellent correlation for end-diastolic ($r = 0.94$) and end-systolic ($r = 0.91$) volumes by using a Simpson's rule algorithm. M-mode volume calculations using a corrected cube method showed a somewhat less consistent relationship to angiography with correlations of 0.84, 0.85, 0.77 for EDV, ESV, and stroke volume (SV), respectively.

Despite these findings, certain factors limit the practical utility of two-dimensional echocardiography for the estimation of left ventricular volumes. Variations between in vitro and the range of in vivo correlations suggest that the difficulties imposed by viewing the heart through the intact chest wall are significant. Target acquisition and overall image quality tend to vary widely among patients. This represents the greatest limitation to the use of two-dimensional echocardiography for routine clinical volume determinations. This is particularly true among older patients who are studied for evaluation of coronary artery disease. In a recent study [16] comparing two-dimensional echocardiography with quantitative angiography for the detection of wall motion abnormalities, clinically useful information with clear visualization of isolated ventricular segments could be obtained in 89% of the patients. However, visualization of the entire left ventricle could be obtained in only 60% of the patients.

This problem is further complicated when exercise protocols are employed as part of the echocardiographic procedure. Increased respiratory rate and tidal volume make echocardiography very difficult during exercise or in the immediate postexercise period.

Using these approaches for the echocardiographic assessment of ventricular volume is also relatively laborious and time consuming. Thus, two-dimensional echocardiography may be generally less practical than other currently available techniques in applying global quantitative descriptors of left ventricular chamber size, particularly when target acquisition and image quality are suboptimal. To date, no large series utilizing two-dimensional echocardiography for this purpose in a wide variety of disease states has been published.

ESTIMATION OF LEFT VENTRICULAR MASS

Perhaps the most unique feature of two-dimensional echocardiography as compared with other descriptors of the left ventricle is its ability to image the myocardium noninvasively in realtime. Usually, gross inspection alone is adequate to determine whether the myocardium shows abnormal thickening or thinning. In Figure 4, three hearts with variable wall thicknesses are shown. Panel A shown a short-axis view of a normal left ventricle. In Panel B, there is increased wall thickness with a normal chamber circumference in a patient with symmetric ventricular hypertrophy. Panel C shows a combination of left ventricular hypertrophy and dilation.

Several experimental studies have been performed to attempt to quantitate the mass of the myocardium more precisely with two-dimensional echocardiography. Because of the lack of an adequate standard of measurement in vivo, most of these studies have involved the comparison of cross-sectional in vivo estimates with direct measures of left ventricular mass at autopsy in dogs. Wyatt et al. [17] recently published a study that analyzed seven different mathematical models for quantifying left ventricular mass from in vivo echocardiographic measurements in 21 dogs. Using a modified Simpson's rule model, they found an extremely close relationship between ultrasonic and postmortem

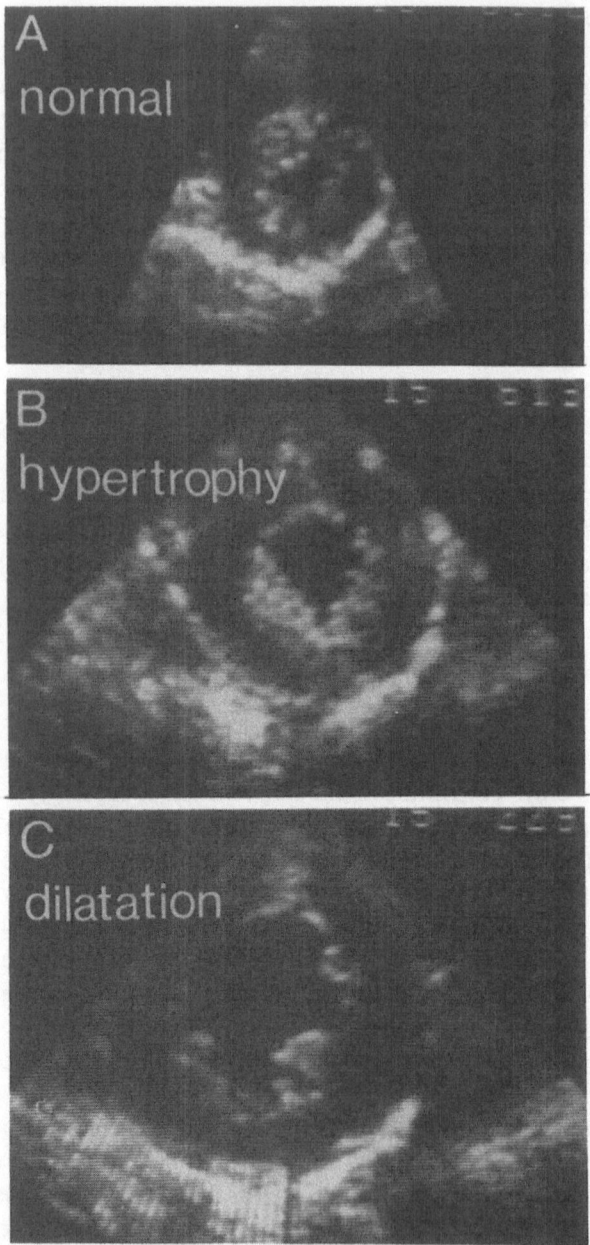

Figure 4. Systolic short-axis images from patients with normal ventricular contraction (*A*), left ventricular hypertrophy (*B*), and dilatation and hypertrophy (*C*). Chamber size and wall thickness are easily visualized.

measurements ($r = 0.95$). He also found a similar relationship using an area—length model with the left ventricle represented as an ellipsoid toward the apex and a cylinder near the base ($V = 5/6AL$). The correlation coefficient was 0.94 with an SEE of 11 g. Both methods enabled the data points to cluster closely about the line of identity and resulted in a percent error of only 6% ± 1%. These results have recently been confirmed by other investigators. Salcedo and co-workers [18] reported an r value of 0.97 when comparing two-dimensional estimates with anatomic left ventricular mass measurements in 19 dogs. Schiller et al. [19] showed similar results, reporting a correlation of 0.96 with postmortem measurements using paired long- and short-axis views in the dog model.

DIRECT IMAGING OF THE CORONARY ARTERIES

The proximal portions of both the right and left main coronary arteries can often be visualized by using two-dimensional echocardiography in patients with adequate target definition in the region of the aortic root (Figure 5). Slight degrees of angulation from the standard parasternal short-axis view of the aortic root often enables delineation of the proximal right coronary artery (Figure 5A) and the left main coronary artery to its bifurcation (Figure 5C). Weyman et al. [20] first confirmed the identity of such targets when they visualized the left main coronary artery lumen by using a mechanical sector scanner during the injection of indocyanine green dye directly into the lumen at catheterization. By further angling of the transducer, other more distal portions of the left anterior descending coronary to its midpoint may be identified (Figure 6). Multiple echocardiographic views are utilized for identification of other portions of the coronary tree, such as the short axis of the left ventricle for identifying portions of the posterior descending artery.

Preliminary data from a recent study [21] indicate that two-dimensional echocardiographic techniques can identify many portions of the proximal and distal coronary circulation. Cross-sectional echocardiograms were performed in 142 consecutive patients undergoing coronary arteriography. Coronary vasculature detected by cross-sectional echocardiography was validated by comparative and complex measurements of the lengths of major coronary arteries and branches from the aortic root visualized by angiography. The vessels detected included the left main coronary artery in 72% of the patients, and the distal portions of the circumflex coronary artery in the posterior atrio-ventricular groove in 27% of the patients. The left anterior descending coronary artery could be detected to its midportion in 26% of the patients. The first major anterolateral branch from the left anterior descending artery could be visualized in 12% of the patients, and the first major marginal branch from the

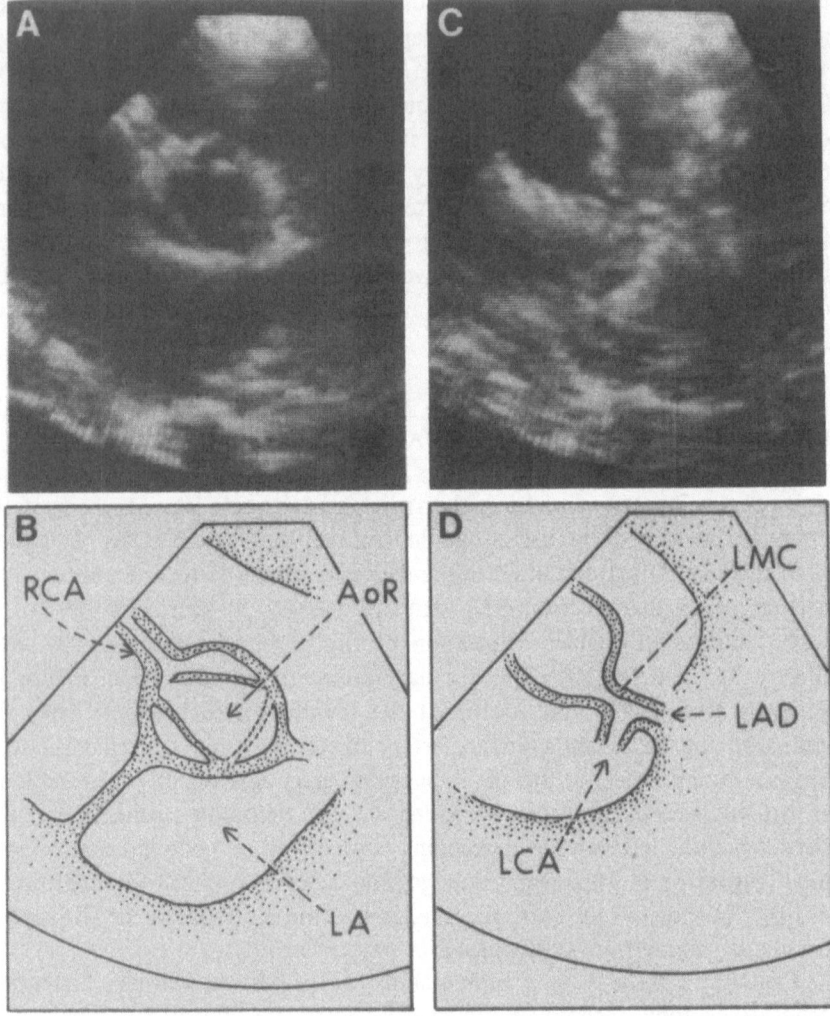

Figure 5. These stop-frame images of the short axis of the aortic root (AoR) delineate the proximal, right coronary artery (RC) (*A* and *B*) and the left main coronary (LMC) artery to its bifurcation into the left circumflex artery (LCA) and the left anterior descending (LAD) artery (*C* and *D*).

circumflex coronary artery was delineated in 10%. The proximal right coronary artery was visualized in 68% of the patients, and its midportion before the acute marginal could be seen in 12%. The posterior descending artery was visualized in 41% of the patients.

245

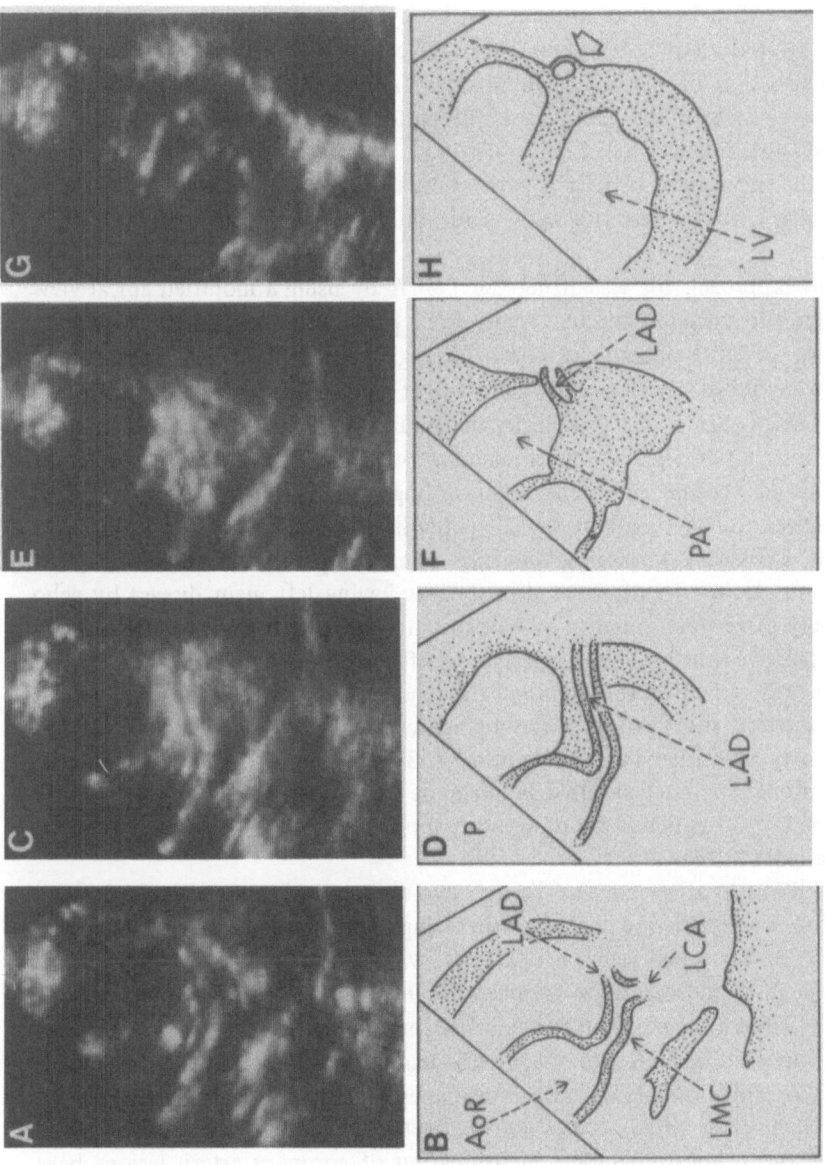

Figure 6. Sequential stop-frame images and paired schematic diagrams show the technique for following the course of the left anterior descending (LAD) coronary artery from the aortic root. (A) The left main as it bifurcates. The angulations of the transducer in C shows the course of the LAD to its midpoint. (E and G) The LAD in cross section as it dips over the brim of the left ventricle (LV); PA, pulmonary artery.

The clinical utility of two-dimension echocardiography for detecting atheromatous lesions within the coronary vessels, however, remains indeterminant at present. Weyman et al. [20] first described the echocardiographic appearance of normal and diseased left main coronary segments in a group of young normal volunteers and a group of patients with CAD who had undergone coronary cineangiography. The latter group consisted of three patients with greater than 75% obstruction of the left main coronary artery (LMCA), one patient with a large aneurysm of the LMCA, and 15 patients with coronary artery disease that did not involve the LMCA. Aronow and co-workers [22] have described the assessment of LMCA patency in a prospective study of 93 patients undergoing coronary arteriography with only one false positive for LMCA disease.

A new approach for visualizing the LMCA by using a modified apical view has recently been published by Ogawa et al. [23]. They studied three separate groups of patients undergoing coronary angiography. Of the 35 patients, 27 (77%) were judged to have adequate target definition to enable description of the LMCA. Six of the technically inadequate studies were ascribed to chest wall abnormalities while in the remaining two patients the LMCA could not be visualized because of intense echocardiographic reflections from calcified aortic valves. In 26 (96%) of the 27 patients, the patency of the LMCA was correctly assessed echocardiographically when compared with the subsequent angiograms. Four patients were described as having left main disease by echo while only three were found to have obstruction of the left main by angiography (a false positive echo). The final group consisted of 30 patients who were studied prior to catheterization to determine the relative usefulness of the apical versus the parasternal short-axis echocardiographic approach. Use of the short-axis view clearly identified the LMCA in 16 (53%) of the 30 patients. The apical cross-sectional approach resulted in adequate identification of the LMCA in 21 (70%) of the 30 patients. By using both approaches, the LMCA was visualized in 28 patients (93%).

In addition to atheromatous disease, two-dimensional echocardiography may be useful in certain rare disorders involving the coronary arteries, including coronary artery aneurysms in patients with mucocutaneous lymph node syndrome [24] and vegetative endocarditis involving the coronary arteries [21] Figure 7 shows a large bacterial vegetation entering the left main and circumflex coronary arteries in a 16-year-old girl who had anginal chest pain and fever. This echocardiographic finding was cause for immediate surgical intervention.

Although these initial studies are intriguing, the actual specificty and sensitivity of the echocardiographic identification of coronary artery lesions have not been adequately determined at the present time. The potential for false positive and false negative results due to incorrect or inadequate target recognition is significant. The system utilized for the illustrations in this chapter has

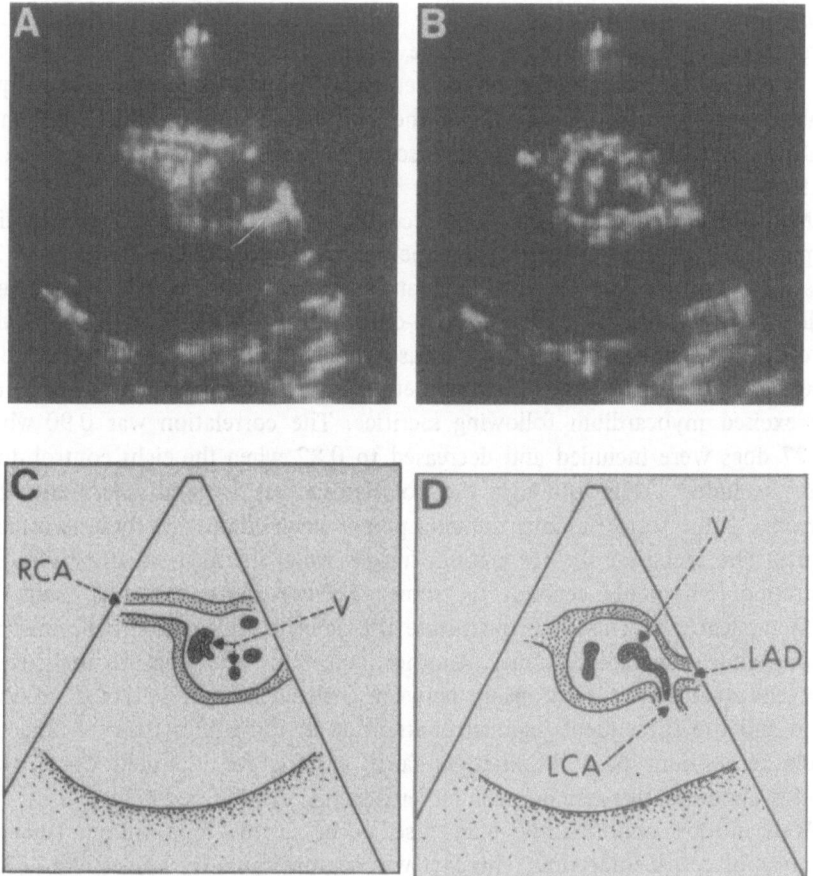

Figure 7. Stop-frame images show the right (*A* and *C*) and left (*B* and *D*) coronary arteries in a young girl with vegetative endocarditis. A vegetative lesion (V) is seen to enter the left main and circumflex coronary arteries.

an azimuthal resolution of 1.5° and a range resolution of 1.5 mm [9]. However, the resolution characteristics of commercially available two-dimensional systems may vary considerably. In addition, it has been our experience that noncalcified atheromatous plaques may not be detected ultrasonically in some patients. The use of direct visualization of the coronary arteries must await further large-scale prospective studies before its clinical utility can be adequately defined.

REGIONAL WALL MOTION ABNORMALITIES

Two-dimensional echocardiography is unique among the currently available imaging techniques for its ability to actually image reflections of the ventricular myocardium and its dynamic motion in real time. Previous studies using M-mode techniques for detecting regional wall motion abnormalities in patients with coronary artery disease met with some success [25–29], but were limited by the inability to scan all areas of the ventricle. The two-dimensional technique enables greater spatial integration of the available target information and thus enables better recognition and comparison of normal and abnormal contraction patterns of the ventricular myocardium.

Meltzer and co-workers [30] have recently used two-dimensional echocardiography to attempt to quantitate experimental myocardial infarction in 27 closed-chest dogs. They compared quantitative estimates of percent regional wall motion abnormality by using two-dimensional echocardiography with the percent of myocardium showing increased technetium pyrophosphate activity imaged 6 h after infarction. The technetium scans were performed directly on the excised myocardium following sacrifice. The correlation was 0.90 when all 27 dogs were included and decreased to 0.82 when the eight control dogs were excluded. Thus although the correlation was a good one there still remained some scatter among the data points when comparing these two techniques. The fact that the technetium images were obtained so soon after the infarction (6 h) could account for some of these discrepancies as could the mathematical model used to quantitate the percent wall motion abnormalities in the echocardiographic studies. Another important factor may be the lack of a precise quantitative relationship between a given mass of infarcted myocardium and the subsequent regional contraction abnormalities that are induced. While technetium pyrophosphate is fairly specific for infarcted tissue, wall motion abnormalities may occur in either ischemic or infarcted tissue.

Wall motion abnormalities may also occur in the myocardium adjacent to areas of actual infarction. This fact was demonstrated by Ideker et al. [31] in a pathologic study in humans comparing the percentage of fibrosis in areas of myocardium that had shown regional wall motion abnormalities by quantitative angiographic studies during life. They found that walls showing normal motion had a mean percentage of fibrosis of 0.4% while those showing hypokinesis contained only 6.3% fibrosis. The more severe wall motion abnormalities showing complete akinesis had 14.3% fibrosis, while walls having frank dyskinesis showed only 30.1% (see chapter 8). These findings are important in considering the hemodynamic response to a given mass of infarcted tissue. It has been shown in recent years that most hospitalized patients who die of myocardial infarction succumb to pump failure rather than dysrhythmia [32]. Thus while the actual mass of a myocardial infarction is important, the resultant decrease in functional myocardial contraction may be the more pertinent clinical concern.

The ability to alter the percentage of wall motion abnormality by pharmacologic intervention designed to alter infarct size in dogs was echocardiographically explored by Meltzer et al. [30], who found that infusions of nitroglycerin significantly decreased while phenylephrine significantly increased the percent abnormal wall motion over a period from 20 min to 5½ h following coronary occlusion. Control dogs, which were given saline alone, showed no significant change in percent wall motion abnormality after the initial 20 min following occlusion.

The relationship between two-dimensional echocardiography and quantitative biplane cineangiography in localizing asynergy in man has recently been defined [16]. Movement in five wall segments were compared in 105 consecutively catheterized patients (525 total segments). On double-blind analysis, 95 segments were not adequately visualized echocardiographically (Figure 8, left panel).

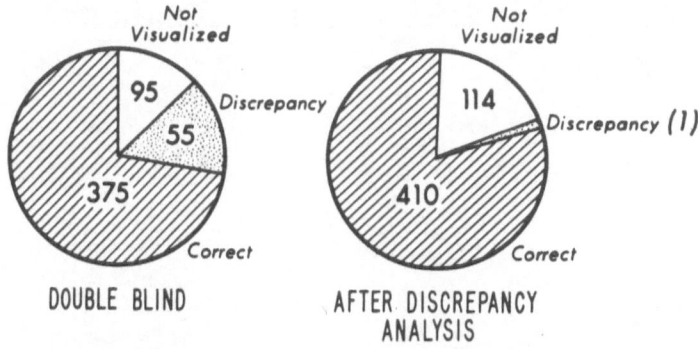

Figure 8. Results of double-blind analysis (*left*) and after descrepance analysis (*right*) in comparison of two-dimensional echocardiography and cineangiography in the detection of asynergy. For details, see text.

Among the remaining 430 segments, echocardiography and cineangiography agreed in 375 (87%) while discrepancies occurred in 55 segments (13%). A restrospective review of these discrepancies showed easily recognizable reasons for the differences in 54 segments (Figure 8, right panel): 34 discrepancies were attributed to echocardiography, 15 to angiography, and six were termed indeterminate. Of the 35 discrepancies attributable to echocardiography, ten resulted from observer error and 19 from inadequately visualized echo targets that were previously judged adequate. Despite the care taken to position the transducer properly on the chest wall, four errors were caused by tangential angulation of the transducer.

Most of the 15 discrepancies from angiography resulted from the superimposition of abnormally contracting wall regions over the normally contracting portions of the ventricle (Figures 9 and 10). For example when severe anterior wall asynergy was present, the abnormally contracting anterior wall was superimposed over the interventricular septum in the LAO angiographic view, thus

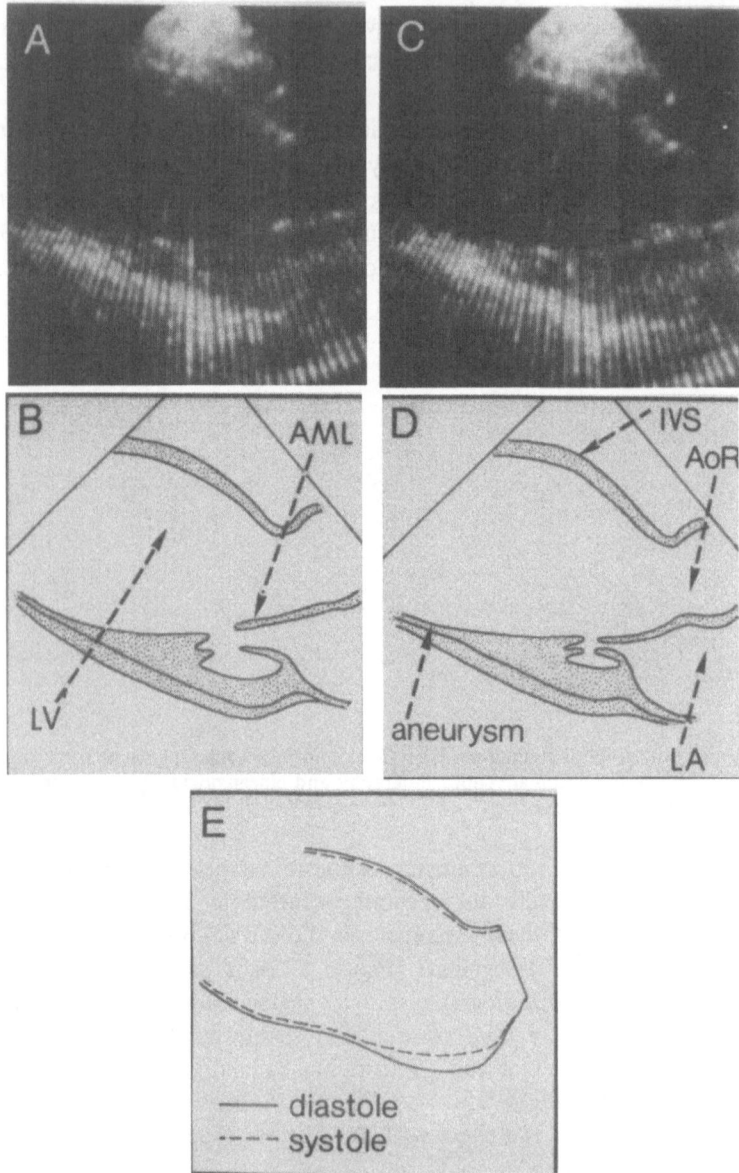

Figure 9. Sequential diastolic (*A*) and systolic (*C*) stop-frame scan images in the 90° sector arc through the long axis of the left ventricle of a patient with coronary artery disease and a huge left ventricular aneurysm. The corresponding schematic diagrams (*B* and *D*) have been added to help locate structures since these images are typical of the somewhat degraded images seen in patients with ventricular asynergy. (*E*) Diffuse asynergy with relative preservation of motion along the posterior wall region at the base of the heart; LV, left ventricular cavity; IVS, interventricular septum; AoR, aortic root; LA, left atrium; AML, anterior mitral valve leaflet.

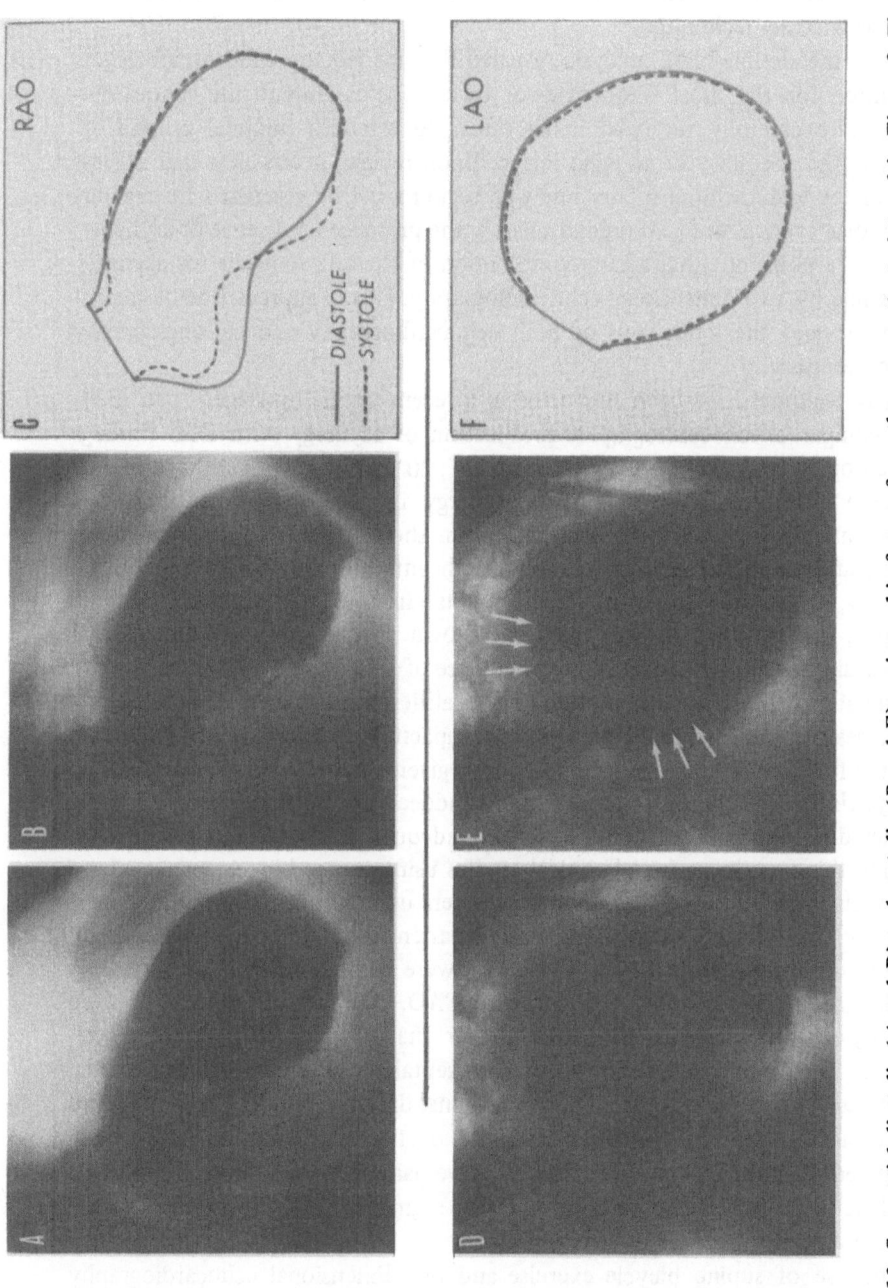

Figure 10. Sequential diastolic (*A* and *D*) and systolic (*B* and *E*) angiographic frames from the same patient pictured in Figure 8. The RAO view is pictured on the top row while the LAO view is on the bottom. Note the large ventricular aneurysm and contracting base in *C*. The arrows in *E* point to the contracting base that is poorly visualized through the silhouette of the aneurysm in the LAO view (*F*). These findings were similar to those predicted by two-dimensional echocardiography.

obscuring true septal wall motion. The six discrepancies that were termed indeterminate were so classified because they could not readily be attributed to either imaging technique.

Since the double-blind analysis revealed that inadequate endocardial targets accounted for the most frequent error by echocardiography, the echocardiograms were carefully reviewed in an effort to establish minimal criteria for assessing the adequacy of an echo image. Upon review, it was clear that at least 50% of the endocardium in any one wall region must be visualized throughout the cardiac cycle in order to predict reliably the presence or absence of asynergy. These data point out that accurate evaluation of the left ventricle for asynergy is possible by two-dimensional echocardiography. Proper appreciation of correct technique and the limitations of both echocardiography and cineangiography is also necessary.

These findings have been supported in a recent article by Heger et al. [33], who compared echocardiographic localization of asynergy with ECG findings and autopsy evidence of necrosis. Out of 20 patients with ECG evidence of acute inferior infarction, 19 had asynergy in posterior segments, 14 out of 14 patients with acute anterior infarction showed asynergy in anterior segments, and three out of three patients with anteroinferior infarction showed asynergy in anterior and posterior segments. In four patients who went to autopsy, 21 of 22 segments that had shown asynergy by two-dimensional echocardiography also had pathologic evidence of infarction.

The ability to detect wall motion abnormalities at rest, however, does not enable assessment of impaired cardiac reserve capacity and thus may underestimate the true functional impairment imposed by a given anatomic lesion in a coronary artery. Unfortunately, movement artifacts induced by dynamic exercise impose further difficulties in acquiring technically adequate echocardiographic images. Despite this fact, some initial clinical studies using supine bicycle exercise have met with some success. Mason and co-workers used M-mode echocardiography to study wall motion abnormalities in 13 patients with angiographically documented coronary artery disease [34], and were able to study 25 echocardiographic segments in the 13 patients with CAD. Of these segments, 22 were supplied by coronary arteries with greater than 70% stenosis. During peak exercise, there was a significant decrease in septal and posterior wall thickening, a decrease in septal and posterior wall maximal diastolic thinning velocities, and a decrease in percent systolic shortening of the minor-axis diameter when compared with the resting state. Each of these parameters was shown to increase significantly, however, in 22 corresponding segments in 11 normal volunteers without evidence of coronary artery disease.

The use of supine bicycle exercise and two-dimensional echocardiography has recently been studied by Wann et al. [35] in 28 patients undergoing cardiac catheterization for evaluation of angina pectoris. Technically adequate exercise echocardiograms were obtained in 20 patients (71%). Ten of these patients showed reversible asynergy in regions supplied by coronary arteries with significant obstruction. Among these, six patients underwent exercise thallium-201 perfusion scanning. All six patients showed reversible perfusion defects in the areas of reversible wall motion abnormality demonstrated echocardiographically. Among the ten patients without wall motion abnormality by echo, there was one patient with significant stenosis of the midportion of the LAD who had a positive exercise thallium study. On subsequent analysis of the echocardiogram, abnormalities in the motion of the anterior wall were confirmed, and this single false negative test result was ascribed to observer error.

Quantitative analysis of wall motion abnormalities has been shown to be superior to qualitative visual inspection in the detection of asynergy by cineangiography [36]. In a recent abstract, quantitative analysis of regional wall motion abnormalities was applied to two-dimensional echocardiography in the short-axis views. [37]; 28 patients who had undergone diagnostic cardiac catheterization were divided into two groups based on the presence of normal coronary arteries or of proximal single-vessel coronary artery disease associated with asynergy on the angiogram. Mean and standard deviation normal values for absolute and relative end-diastolic and end-systolic wall thickness and hemiaxial shortening were determined from patients in the normal group. These measurements were obtained from 24 radii adjusted for rotation about the short axis and determined from the centroid of the left ventricle. Compared with the normals, the patients with coronary artery disease showed abnormal (greater than 2 standard deviation) reduction in percent wall thickening (15 out of 15), diminished hemiaxial shortening (14 out of 15), and increased end-diastolic radius to wall thickness ratio (13 out of 15) along the radii affected by the distribution of the coronary involvement.

This propensity for ischemic myocardium to thin during systole is shown in the following samples. Figure 11 shows sequential diastolic and systolic frames from the short axis of the left ventricle in a resting patient with minor coronary obstructive disease. Systolic chamber circumference and radial shortening are normal. Wall thickening is uniform. In contrast, the sequence of postexercise systolic wall thinning shown in Figure 12 occurred in a patient who manifested normal thickening at rest. Subsequent catheterization revealed severe obstructive disease in a dominant circumflex coronary artery supplying the area of noted wall thinning. Despite the striking differences in these patients, practical clinical experience in the assessment of wall motion abnormalities by this approach is limited at the present time.

In addition to the detection of asynergy, two-dimensional echocardiography has now been used to actually observe sequential changes in the myocardium following acute infarction [38]. Eight dogs were followed sequentially for six days after ligation of the midportion of the left anterior descending coronary

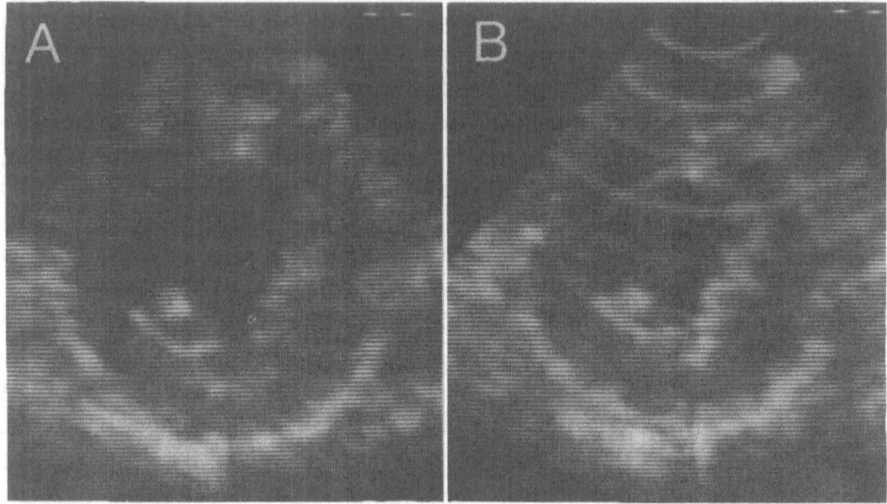

Figure 11. Sequential diastolic (*A*) and systolic (*B*) stop-frames at the level of the papillary muscles in the short axis from a patient with minor coronary artery disease. Ventricular wall thickening is uniform.

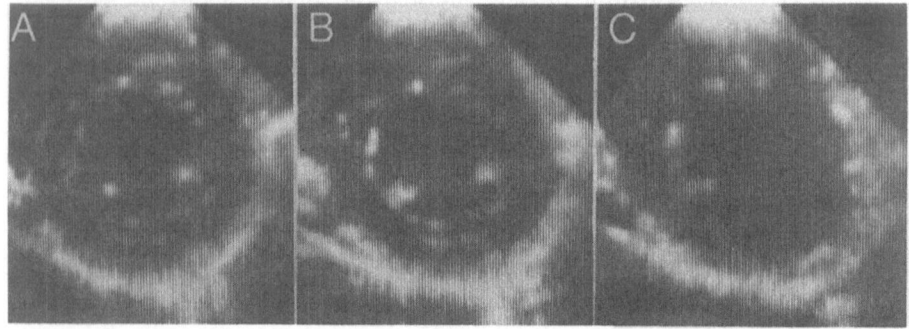

Figure 12. Sequential diastolic (*A*), midsystolic (*B*), and end-systolic (*C*) stop-frames at the level of the papillary muscles. Echo was obtained postexercise in a patient with severe coronary occlusive disease and shows posterolateral and inferior wall systolic thinning.

artery distal to the first septal perforator. Alterations in systolic radial shortening and wall thickening along 24 equidistant radii about the ventricular short axis were analyzed and compared with baseline measurements. Initial diffuse lengthening of radii during systole and absence of wall thickening were noted involving a segment from the anterior interventricular groove to the anterior papillary muscle. Serially, there was a progressive return of radial shortening, preceded by increased wall thickening along the margins of the involved segment. Ultimately, a well-demarcated area characterized by the absence of both systolic radial shortening and wall thickening remained where increased ultrasonic speckle and shadowing corresponded to early scar formation on postmortem examination.

This ability to detect changes in regional wall configuration following acute myocardial infarction has recently been applied in humans. Postmortem studies [39] have shown that among patients who die within 30 days of acute infarction as many as 72% will show histologic evidence of regional thinning and dilatation of the infarcted area beginning within one week of acute infarction. This process generally occurs without histologic evidence of infarct extension after the acute event and has been termed 'infarct expansion.' Pathologic evidence suggests that it results from intramyocardial rupture of necrotic muscle fibers and it appears to be of much greater hemodynamic and prognostic importance than actual infarct extension [40].

Eaton and co-workers [41] have recently used two-dimensional echocardiography in an attempt to detect significant infarct expansion in the first two weeks after acute infarction in 28 patients. Eight of these patients showed gross infarct expansion by echo beginning within three days of the infarction. These patients could not be separated from the patients without significant expansion by the usual clinical indicators of an extended infarction. One important difference soon became evident: the eight-week mortality in the patients with infarct expansion was 50% while there were no deaths in patients who did not show infarct expansion by serial two-dimensional echocardiographic examinations. All the surviving patients who had been shown to have infarct expansion by echo remained in congestive heart failure following discharge from the hospital.

ASSESSMENT OF COMPLICATIONS

Echocardiography finds its most practical clinical use in the assessment of complications of ischemic heart disease. In addition to the detection of acute infarct expansion, two-dimensional echocardiography has been shown to be useful in the diagnosis of ventricular aneurysm [42] and pseudoaneurysm [43].

Acute systolic murmurs with hemodynamic compromise in the setting of acute infarction may occur secondary to acute mitral regurgitation or ventricular septal rupture. Clinically, the differential diagnosis may frequently be difficult or impossible without cardiac catheterization [44]. Two-dimensional echocardiography, especially when combined with saline contrast techniques, has now been shown to be useful in identifying ventricular septal defect [45, 46]. The rupture of a papillary muscle in the setting of acute infarction, on the other hand, gives an echocardiographic appearance similar to that described for a flail mitral leaflet [47]. The spectrum of two-dimensional echocardiographic findings in papillary muscle dysfunction has recently been reviewed by Ogawa et al. [48].

Echocardiography is also useful for detecting mural thrombi following myocardial infarction [49] DeMaria et al. [50] recently compared two-dimensional echocardiography and angiography in 25 patients with anterior myocardial infarction. Five of the patients had clinical evidence of systemic embolization while the remaining 20 served as control patients. Two-dimensional echocardiography showed a distinct irregular apical mass in all five patients in the embolus group, but in none of the patients without evidence of embolus. These findings were confirmed in all patients by subsequent cineangiographic evaluation or during surgery for resection of ventricular aneurysm.

USE OF TWO-DIMENSIONAL ECHOCARDIOGRAPHY

These studies indicate that two-dimensional echocardiography can be a useful tool for the noninvasive evaluation of the left ventricle in patients with ischemic heart disease when image quality is adequate. The spatial integration of target information into tomographic sections of the heart provides important information regarding dynamic changes in chamber size, wall thickness, and motion characteristics in real time.

Although experiments designed to test in vitro two-dimensional echocardiographic measurements as well as in vivo studies in dogs have demonstrated a remarkable potential for accurate analysis of chamber size and global ventricular performance, in vivo studies in humans have been unable to reproduce as high a degree of precision and are cumbersome in clinical practice. The major limitation to in vivo measurements has been inadequate target acquisition and insufficient signal to noise ratio in some patients, which may prohibit adequate definition of myocardial targets. This may cause major areas of drop-out in any given tomographic plane, precluding accurate global ventricular analysis.

On the other hand, the unique capabilities of two-dimensional echocardiography to simultaneously study regional dynamic changes in chamber circumference, wall thickness, and motion characteristics may be more practical. It is likely that some combination of quantitative descriptors based on regional ventricular alterations will become useful. Two-dimensional echocardiography appears to demonstrate hitherto unknown sequential changes in wall thickness and motion in selected patients with infarct expansion following myocardial infarction. The ability to noninvasively detect infarct expansion may also have very important prognostic and possibly therapeutic implications. Two-dimensional echocardiography also appears useful in the diagnosis of several complications of myocardial infarction.

The ultimate role of two-dimensional echocardiography in the assessment of ischemic myocardium will likely depend on its ability to detect alterations in regional chamber size and wall thickness. Echocardiographic changes following infarction are related to alterations in wall motion, and thickness, and acoustic changes within the myocardium. The exact relation between these changes and the extent of histologic infarction has not been adequately delineated. Continued improvement in system performance and target acquisition should enable more precise definition of myocardial boundaries and, hence, the acquisition of more reliable descriptors of wall movement and thickness changes.

Acknowledgments. Supported by the Multidisiciplinary Cardiovascular Research Training National Research Service Award grant HL 07101, National Heart, Lung and Blood Institute Research grant HL 17670, and the Henry J. Kaiser Family Foundation.

REFERENCES

1. Popp RL, Alderman EL, Brown OR, Harrison DC: Sources of error in calculation of left ventricular volumes by echocardiography [abstr]. Am J Cardiol 31:152, 1973.
2. Ratshin RA, Boyd CN, Rackley CE, Moraski RE, Russell R: Quantitative echocardiography: correlation with ventricular volume by angiocardiography in patients with coronary artery disease with and without wall motion abnormalities [abstr]. Circulation [Suppl 4] 48:48, 1973.
3. Teichholz LE, Kreulen T, Herman MV, Gorlin R: Problems in echocardiographic volume determinations: echocardiographic—angiographic correlations in the presence or absence of asynergy. Am J Cardiol 37:7–11, 1976.
4. Folland ED, Parisi AF, Moynihan PF, Jones DR, Feldman CL, Tow DE: Assessment of left ventricular ejection fraction and volumes by real-time, two-dimensional echocardiography. A comparison of cineangiographic and radionuclide techniques. Circulation 60:760–766, 1979.
5. Schiller NB, Acquatella H, Ports TA, et al: Left ventricular volume from paired biplane two-dimensional echocardiography. Circulation 60:547–555, 1979.
6. Kisslo JA: Comparison of M-mode and two-dimensional echocardiography. Circulation 60:734–736, 1979.
7. Silverman NH, Schiller NB: Apex cardiography: a two-dimensional technique for evaluation congenital heart disease. Circulation 57:503–511, 1978.
8. Feigenbaum H: Echocardiography, 2nd edn. Philadelphia: Lea and Febiger, 1976, pp. 30–50.
9. Von Ramm OT, Thurstone FL: Cardiac imaging using a phased-array ultrasound system. I: System design. Circulation 53:258–262, 1976.

10. Kisslo JA, von Ramm OT, Thurstone FL: Cardiac imaging using a phased array ultrasound system. II: Clinical technique and application. Circulation 53:262–267, 1976.
11. Ratshin RA, Rackley CE, Russel RC: Quantitative echocardiography: accuracy of ventricular volume analysis by area length, linear regression and quadratic regression formulae [abstr]. Am J Cardiol 35:165, 1975.
12. Ludbrook P, et al: Comparison of ultrasound and cineangiographic measurements of left ventricular performance in patients with and without wall motion abnormalities. Br Heart J 35:1026–1032, 1973.
13. Eaton LW, Maughan WL, Shoukas AA, Weiss JL: Accurate volume determination in the isolated ejecting canine left ventricle by two-dimensional echocardiography. Circulation 60:320–326, 1979.
14. Carr K, Engler R, Forsythe J, Johnson A, Gosink B: Measurement of left ventricular ejection fraction by mechanical cross-sectional echocardiography and comparison with angiography [abstr]. Circulation [Suppl 2] 58:40, 1978.
15. Silverman NH, Schiller NB, Yarger RL, Ports TA: Left ventricular volume analysis by two-dimensional echocardiography in children [abstr]. Circulation [Suppl 2] 58:202, 1978.
16. Kisslo JA, Robertson D, Gilbert BW, von Ramm OT, Behar VS: A comparison of real-time, two-dimensional echocardiography and cineangiography in detecting left ventricular asynergy. Circulation 55:134–141, 1977.
17. Wyatt HL, Heng MK, Meerbaum S, et al: Cross-sectional echocardiography. I: Analysis of mathematical models for quantifying mass of the left ventricle in dogs. Circulation 60:1104–1113, 1979.
18. Salcedo E, Gockowski K, Tarazi R: Experimental study of left ventricular mass by two-dimensional echocardiography [abstr]. Circulation [Suppl 2] 60:137, 1979.
19. Schiller N, Skioldebrand C, Schiller E, et al: In vivo assessment of left ventricular mass by two-dimensional echocardiography [abstr]. Circulation [Suppl 2] 60:137, 1979.
20. Weyman AE, Feingenbaum H, Dillon JC, Johnston KW, Eggleton RC: Noninvasive visualization of the left main coronary artery by cross-sectional echocardiography. Circulation 54:169–173, 1976.
21. Kisslo J: Two-dimensional echocardiography. Radiol Clin North Am 18:105, 1980.
22. Aronow WS, Chandraratna PAN, Murdock K, Milholland H: Left main coronary artery patency assessed by cross-sectional echocardiography and coronary arteriography. Circulation [Suppl 2] 60:145, 1979.
23. Ogawa S, et al: New approach to visualize the left main coronary artery using apical cross-sectional echocardiography. Am J Cardiol 45:301–304, 1980.
24. Yoshikawa J, et al: Cross-sectional echocardiographic diagnosis of coronary artery aneurysms in patients with the mucocutaneous lymph node syndrome. Circulation 59:133–139, 1979.
25. Jacobs JJ, Feingenbaum H, Corya BC, Phillips JF: Detection of left ventricular asynergy by echocardiography. Circulation 48:263–271, 1973.
26. Corya BC, Rasmussen S, Knoebel SB, Feingenbaum H: Echocardiography in acute myocardial infarction. Am J Cardiol 37:1–10, 1975.

27. Feigenbaum H, et al: Role of echocardiography in patients with coronary artery disease. Am J Cardiol 37:775–786, 1976.
28. Dortimer AC, et al: Distribution of coronary artery disease. Circulation 54:724–729, 1976.
29. Kolibash AJ, et al: The relationship between abnormal echocardiographic septal motion and myocardial perfusion in patients with significant obstruction of the left anterior descending artery. Circulation 56:780–785, 1977.
30. Meltzer RS, Woythaler JN, Buda AJ, et al: Two-dimensional echocardiographic quantification of infarct size alteration by pharmacologic agents. Am J Cardiol 44:257–269, 1979.
31. Ideker RS, Behar VS, Wagner GS, et al: Evaluation of asynergy as an indicator of myocardial fibrosis. Circulation 57:715–725, 1978.
32. Weil MH, Shubin H: Shock following acute myocardial infarction. Prog Cardiovasc Dis 11:1–17, 1968.
33. Heger JJ, Weyman AE, Wann LS, Dillon JC, Feigenbaum H: Cross-sectional echocardiography in acute myocardial infarction: detection and localization of regional left ventricular asynergy. Circulation 60:531–538, 1979.
34. Mason SJ, et al: Exercise echocardiography: detection of wall motion abnormalities during ischemia. Circulation 59:50–59, 1979.
35. Wann LS, et al: Exercise cross-sectional echocardiography in ischemic heart disease. Circulation 60:1300–1308, 1979.
36. Leighton RF, Wilt SM, Lewis RP: Detection of hypokinesis by a quantitative analysis of left ventricular cineangiograms. Circulation 50:121–127, 1974.
37. Kisslo, JA, von Ramm OT, Behar VS: Echocardiographic evaluation of ischemia: descriptors of the ventricular short axis [abstr]. Circulation [Suppl 2] 58:40, 1978.
38. Kisslo JA, Ideker R, Harrison L, Scallion R, von Ramm OT, Pilkington T: Serial wall changes after acute myocardial infarction by two-dimensional echo [abstr]. Circulation [Suppl 2] 60:151, 1979.
39. Hutchins GM, Bulkley BH: Infarct expansion versus extension: two different complications of acute myocardial infarction. Am J Cardiol 41:1127–1132, 1978.
40. Willerson JT: Echocardiography after acute myocardial infarction. N Engl J Med 300:87–88, 1979.
41. Eaton LW, Weiss JL, Bulkley BH, Garrison JB, Weisfeldt ML: Regional cardiac dilatation after acute myocardial infarction. N Engl J Med 300:57–62, 1979.
42. Weyman AE, et al: Detection of left ventricular aneurysms by cross-sectional echocardiography. Circulation 54:936–944, 1976.
43. Sears TD, Ong YS, Starke H, Forker AD: Left ventricular pseudoaneurysm identified by cross-sectional echocardiography. Ann Int Med 90:935–936, 1979.
44. Dugall JC, Pryor R, Blount SG: Systolic murmur following myocardial infarction. Am Heart J 87:577–583, 1974.
45. Farcot JC, et al: Two-dimensional echocardiographic visualization of ventricular septal rupture after acute anterior myocardial infarction. Am J Cardiol 45:370–377, 1980.

46. Scanlan JG, Seward JB, Tajik AJ: Visualization of ventricular septal rupture utilizing wide angle two-dimensional echocardiography. Mayo Clin Proc 54:381–384, 1979.
47. Ahmad S, Kleiger RE, Connors J, Krone R: The echocardiographic diagnosis of rupture of a papillary muscle. Chest 73:232–234, 1978.
48. Ogawa S, Hubbard FE, Mardelli TJ, Dreifus LS: Cross-sectional echocardiographic spectrum of papillary muscle dysfunction. Am Heart J 97:312–321, 1979.
49. Van den Bos AA, Vletter WB, Hagemeijer F: Progressive development of a left ventricular thrombus. Chest 74:307–309, 1978.
50. DeMaria AH, et al: Left ventricular thrombi identified by cross-sectional echocardiography. Ann Int Med 90:14–18, 1979.

10.   COMPUTERIZED TOMOGRAPHY

J. WILLIAM WHITAKER and ERIK L. RITMAN

Computerized tomography (CT) is a powerful tool for quantifying regional roentgen density of various tissues. When coronary blood flow is interrupted, a number of changes occur in the ischemic myocardium. These changes result in regional differences in tissue roentgen attenuation. Roentgen attenuation of a material is usually expressed as the change in X-ray beam intensity after passing through one centimeter of the material. It is often called roentgen density or CT number of the tissue.

Early studies employed commercially available CT scanners to estimate the regional roentgen density of the myocardium in canine hearts excised following coronary artery ligation [1–4]. In hearts excised at least 2 h after coronary ligation, the myocardium distal to the coronary occlusion was less roentgen opaque than the normally perfused myocardium. Once an area of decreased roentgen attenuation became apparent, the average value of roentgen attenuation for the area did not change appreciably from the second to the 48th hour following coronary ligation, although the border between normal and infarcted tissue became more distinct as the time after occlusion increased.

Wittenberg et al. measured wet–dry weight ratios in areas of normal myocardium and in areas with decreased roentgen attenuation [5]. Their data clearly showed that the decrease in roentgen attenuation was due to localized edema since the regions with decreased CT numbers had an increased wet–dry ratio compared with the normal myocardium. Such edema has prognostic significance since correlation between the extent of eventual myocardial necrosis and the degree of intracellular edema has been demonstrated [6]. Reperfusion, thought to accelerate the process of localized cellular and extracellular edema, results in earlier detection of areas with decreased roentgen attenuation. Such areas become apparent after 1 h occlusion followed by 40 min reperfusion [5].

Iodinated contrast agents have been employed to aid in the evaluation of myocardial ischemia and infarct by computerized tomography. During the first minutes after the injection of a bolus of contrast into a peripheral vein, there is a rise in roentgen attenuation in the normally perfused myocardium. Investigators have noted, however, that in areas of myocardium distal to occluded vessels, there is little change in regional roentgen attenuation with the passage of a contrast agent [7, 8]. Doherty et al. have observed an increase in regional

Wagner GS (ed): Myocardial Infarction: Measurement and Intervention, pp 261–276.
© *1982 Martinus Nijhoff Publishers, The Hague/Boston/London.*

attenuation in reperfused areas with the passage of contrast, which they attributed to reactive hyperemia [8].

In addition to the preferential lack of appearance of contrast medium in hypoperfused areas of the myocardium in the first minutes following a bolus injection, there is also a preferential uptake of contrast medium in infarcted tissue at later times. Higgins et al. [4] have scanned excised canine hearts at 2, 8, and 48 h following coronary ligation. Several minutes before the hearts were excised, iodinated contrast was injected. At 8 and 48 h after occlusion, they noted an infarct avidity for the iodinated contrast agent in that the damaged myocardium had an increased roentgen attenuation compared with the normal myocardium. An increased tissue concentration of iodine has been detected in these areas by a fluorescent excitation method in amounts that account for the increased attenuation, but the exact anatomic or biochemical basis for the sequestration is uncertain [9].

The anatomic extent of infarcted tissue as estimated from the extent of decreased CT regional roentgen attenuation of the myocardium has been correlated with histochemical estimations of infarct extent by Siemers et al. [10]. The correlation between the volume of infarcted tissue as estimated using the CT scan and the area of histochemical staining was excellent with the smallest infarct studied being 1.1 cm^3. The CT technique had a 100% sensitivity as compared with histochemical staining and accurately localized the infarcted tissue. The results of these early experiments clearly indicate the potential of computerized tomography for quantitative evaluation of the location, extent, and duration of myocardial ischemia and infarct. These studies, however, were performed under highly artificial experimental conditions that are of a limited relevance to the clinical setting.

The applicability of conventional systems of computerized tomography in studies of the cardiovascular system is severely limited because these systems require more than one second to complete a scan for one cross section. This results in motion artifacts in the images of the moving heart and requires multiple scans to ensure that the suspected region of infarct or ischemia is incorporated in the image. To overcome these constraints, a system that can obtain synchronous reconstructions over the entire axial range of the heart within a very short time period has been constructed and is currently undergoing evaluation. This system enables stop-action imaging of the entire volume of the heart at a rapid sampling rate throughout the cardiac cycle.

THEORETICAL BASIS FOR CT OF THE HEART

The mathematical and physical basis of computerized tomography is described in detail elsewhere [11, 12]. A brief outline of the general principles is provided here.

Conventional radiographs are two-dimensional representations of three-dimensional anatomy and, as such, record the intensity of transmitted X-rays after attenuation by superimposed anatomic structures. The roentgen attenuation coefficients of individual tissues included in a conventional roentgenogram and their actual three-dimensional locations cannot be accurately determined, however, due to the superimposition of other structures. A computerized tomographic image provides more accurate information regarding tissue density and location than the conventional roentgenogram since it is a two-dimensional representation of a two-dimensional slice through the body.

In computerized tomography, X-rays from multiple angles of view are transmitted through a slice, producing a projection image of the slice from each angle of view. These transmitted X-ray profiles contain information concerning the cross-sectional distribution of X-ray density across the volume of study (see Figure 1). The mathematical techniques required to reconstruct three-dimensional anatomy from the two-dimensional projection roentgen opacity profiles have been known for over a half-century. Their application has only been practical in recent years, however, with the advent of modern computer systems. Several mathematical techniques have been employed in reconstruction algorithms, but all require roentgen-intensity measurements from a number of different angles. Spatial and density resolution of the CT images can be improved by increasing the number of sampling angles, but even with the minimum number of angles required for suitable reconstructions, the equivalent of thousands of equations must be solved to obtain an approximate roentgen density value for each picture element (pixel) of reconstruction. By graphically displaying the roentgen density of these pixels, computerized tomography provides an accurate anatomic representation. Such a display enables a quantitative look *into* an organ rather than *through* an organ, which is the case with conventional two-dimensional projection images.

For studies of the cardiopulmonary system, it is necessary to synchronously image a volume containing the entire heart if accurate measurements are to be made of three-dimensional cardiac structures. To achieve the necessary axial range for synchronous volume reconstructions of the entire heart, a scanning system was developed that employs a cone-beam X-ray source. The temporal resolution necessary for stop-action imaging of the beating heart can be achieved by rapid sequential pulsing of multiple X-ray sources and imaging systems. By rotating the multiple X-ray sources and imaging chains on a gantry to which they are attached, the number of angles of view per scan can be increased in order to obtain images with increased spatial and density resolution at the cost of increased scan time. Such a system, the Dynamic Spatial Reconstructor (DSR), was installed at our institution in the fall of 1979 and is portrayed in Figure 2 [13, 14]. The DSR system presently employs 14 X-ray sources and 14 video-camera chains mounted on a circular gantry that can be rotated at

264

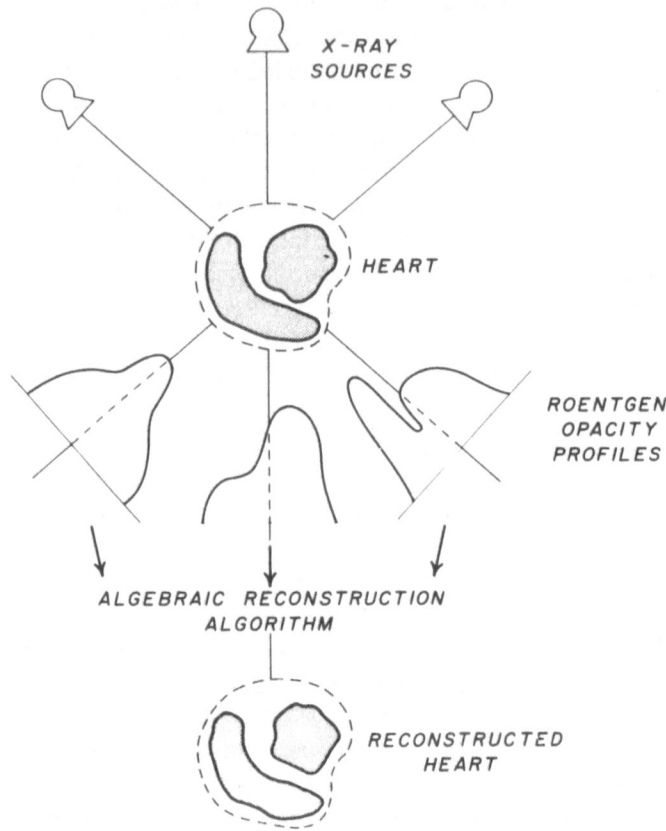

Figure 1. Intuitive representation of the reconstruction process. Each individual roentgen opacity profile contains information about the cross-sectional distribution of roentgen density. By employing several roentgen opacity profiles from different angles of view, the three-dimensional roentgen-density distribution in an organ can be estimated and displayed by computer techniques. In addition to the algebraic reconstruction algorithm, many other principles such as filtered back-projection can be used. Reproduced with permission from Robb et al., *Proceedings of the Society of Photo-Optical Instrumentation Engineers* 40:11, 1973.

15 rpm, but is designed to ultimately employ 28 X-ray video-camera chains. X-rays from each source, after passing through the body, are converted to light by a fluoroscopic screen and the resulting television image is recorded on video disc for subsequent computer processing.

A cylindrical volume, 25 cm in height and up to 37 cm in diameter, can be reconstructed with this system. All 28 X-ray sources and video chains can be activated in rapid sequence within 0.011 s and this scanning sequence can be repeated

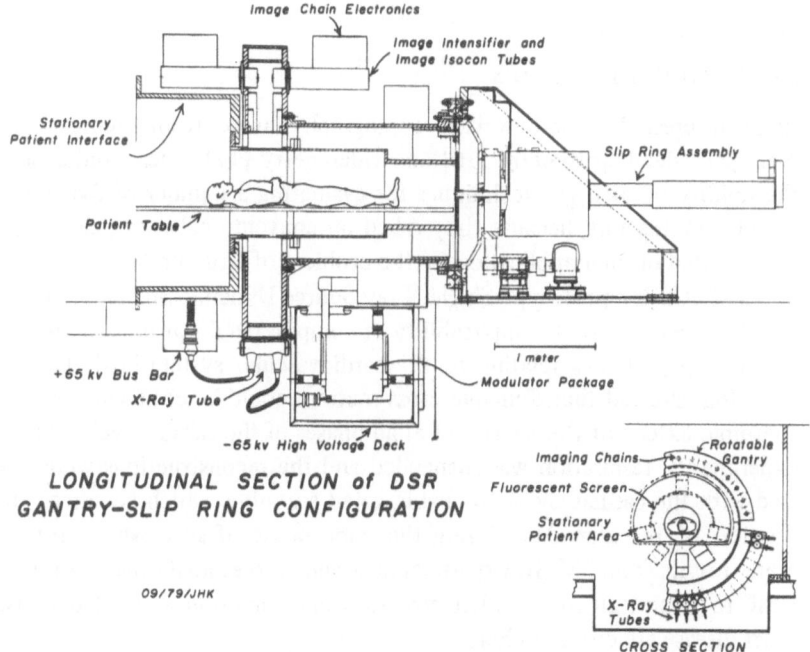

Image Chain Electronics

Image Intensifier and
Image Isocon Tubes

Stationary
Patient Interface

Slip Ring Assembly

Patient Table

+65 kv Bus Bar

X-Ray Tube

1 meter

Modulator Package

-65 kv High Voltage Deck

**LONGITUDINAL SECTION of DSR
GANTRY–SLIP RING CONFIGURATION**

09/79/JHK

Imaging Chains

Fluorescent Screen

Stationary
Patient Area

Rotatable
Gantry

X-Ray
Tubes

CROSS SECTION

Figure 2. Schematic representation of the DSR system. From 14 to 28 X-ray sources are mounted along a semicircle below the patient so that the corresponding projection images are formed on a 12-inch-wide semicircular fluorescent screen suspended above the patient. Video-camera chains are positioned behind the fluorescent screens. The X-ray sources, fluorescent screens, and video cameras are attached to a gantry that can be rotated at 15 rpm. Reproduced with permission from Kinsey et al., The DSR – a high temporal resolution volumetric roentgenographic CT scanner, *Herz* 5 (3):177–188, 1980.

60 times/s. Since the endocardium moves at approximately 100mm/s during systole, its movement should be less than 1 mm over the 0.01 s when image data are obtained from each scan.

The spatial, density, and temporal resolutions of reconstructed images are interdependent. Maximum spatial and density resolution is achieved by increasing the number of angles of view, which results, however, in compromise of temporal resolution. Increased density resolution can be achieved by increasing the number of X-rays passing through each reconstructed volume. The DSR, with its modular design of multiple X-ray video-camera chains, can be flexibly programmed so as to emphasize spatial, density, or temporal resolution, depending on the information desired. However, most of the 'trade-off' of spatial, density, and temporal resolution can be selected after the scan has been completed. The importance of this flexibility to control the number of angles of view used in a reconstruction was shown in computer simulations [15]. Such

266

a capability is an important feature necessary to broaden the applicability of the DSR as a research device.

EXPERIMENTAL STUDIES

Early interest in computerized tomography arose from studies employing roentgen videodensitometry [16] and videometry [17]. These studies supported the validity of roentgen techniques for evaluating a number of dynamic cardiovascular events but, because they relied on conventional roentgen images, they were limited in their application by the problem of structural superimposition.

The SSDSR, a prototype Single X-ray Source Dynamic Spatial Reconstructor, was designed to test the applicability of computerized transmission tomography for solving problems relating to the cardiovascular system [18]. Early studies with dogs showed that dynamic cross sections could be obtained over the entire anatomic extent of the heart and at all phases of the cardiac cycle. During these experiments, respiration was suspended and the reconstructions were synchronized with the cardiac cycle to enable gated scanning, which acquires a different fraction of the scan data during the same phase of successive cardiac cycles. Some results from SSDSR experiments designed to evaluate the capability of the DSR to quantitate myocardial structure and function as related to ischemic heart disease are discussed here.

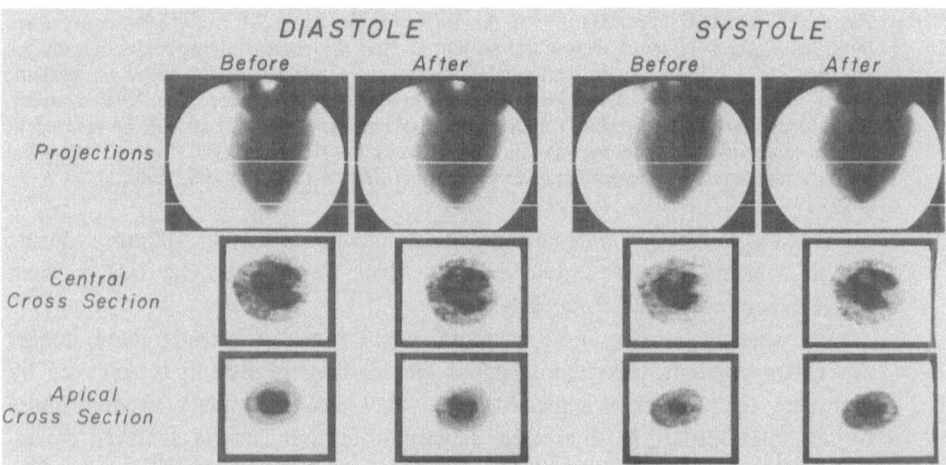

Figure 3. (Top) X-ray video projection images of a working metabolically supported isolated canine left ventricle recorded during diastole and systole before and after ligation of the circumflex coronary artery. *(Bottom)* Reconstructed cross sections of the ventricle, at the two levels indicated by brightened lines in top panel, determined for diastole and systole before and after ligation of the circumflex coronary artery. Reproduced with permission from Robb et al., *Proceedings of the Society of Photo-Optical Instrumentation Engineers* 89:69, 1976.

Figure 3 shows the results of an experiment designed to study the left ventricle before and after coronary ligation in systole and diastole. Reconstructions at the level of the horizontal white lines show evidence of regional systolic dysfunction in the distribution of the left circumflex artery. This information is not apparent in the projection data unless the affected wall is silhouetted appropriately. This clearly demonstrates the value of the three-dimensional reconstruction process for obtaining information lost in the conventional two-dimensional projection image. The reconstructed images provide a much more precise localization of structures in space than do conventional roentgenograms and, as has been demonstrated by others using commercially available scanners, more accurate estimates of myocardial muscle mass, left ventricular volume, and regional wall dynamics can be made [20]. Of particular value is the demonstration with the SSDSR that alterations in regional rates of wall thickening can be evaluated. The rate of wall thickening appears to be a good indicator of regional ischemia and infarct [21, 22]. The rapid repetition imaging capability of the DSR could enable accurate evaluation of this index of regional myocardial function.

The spatial resolution of the DSR approach has been tested by sewing Tygon tubes, as simulated coronary arteries of various diameters, to the epicardium of beating canine hearts [23]. The reconstructed vessels filled with different amounts of contrast were identified and their transverse cross-sectional area was measured from the CT images. The brightness x area product was calculated for each vessel. This value consists of the sum of the CT X-ray density values, i.e., (tube CT number) — (heart wall CT number), for all voxels within the image of each lumen. Voxel is a three-dimensional, that is volume, picture element. The relationship between true lumen cross-sectional area and the brightness x area product enables quantitation of much smaller stenoses than would be expected from the actual spatial resolution capabilities of the DSR imaging system. The rationale for this index is that the total number of X-ray photons absorbed by the cross section of a tube filled with contrast agent determines the total brightness of its reconstructed image even though this image may be spread out (blurred) to a size that is determined by the limits of spatial resolution of the system. By employing such an analysis, the percent stenosis of vessels as small as 0.6 mm in diameter can be detected (Figure 4).

The regional roentgen attenuation of an area of myocardium following the injection of a contrast agent should vary in proportion to the regional blood volume. Experiments employing a constant infusion of iodinated contrast and sampling roentgen attenuation in the subepicardium, midwall, and subendocardium every 1/30th of a second have shown phasic changes in regional roentgen attenuation consistent with known data concerning phasic regional myocardial blood content [23, 24]. Contrast infusions can also be employed to assess regional perfusion in areas distal to coronary obstructions. Figure 5 shows two levels from a reconstruction obtained after an injection of contrast in a dog with

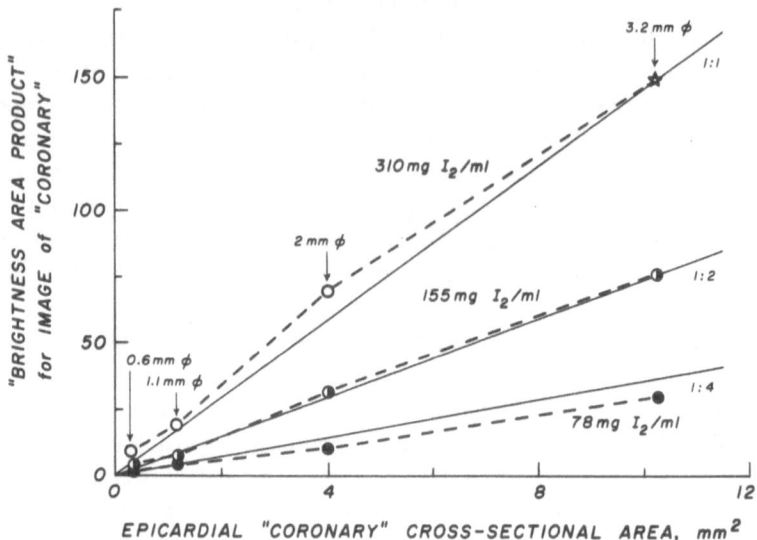

Figure 4. Brightness X area product from reconstructions of simulated coronary arteries filled with three concentrations of contrast (100%, 50%, and 25%) correlates well with relative cross-sectional area of the vessel with diameters ranging from 0.6 mm to 3.2 mm. Reproduced with permission from Scanlan et al. [23].

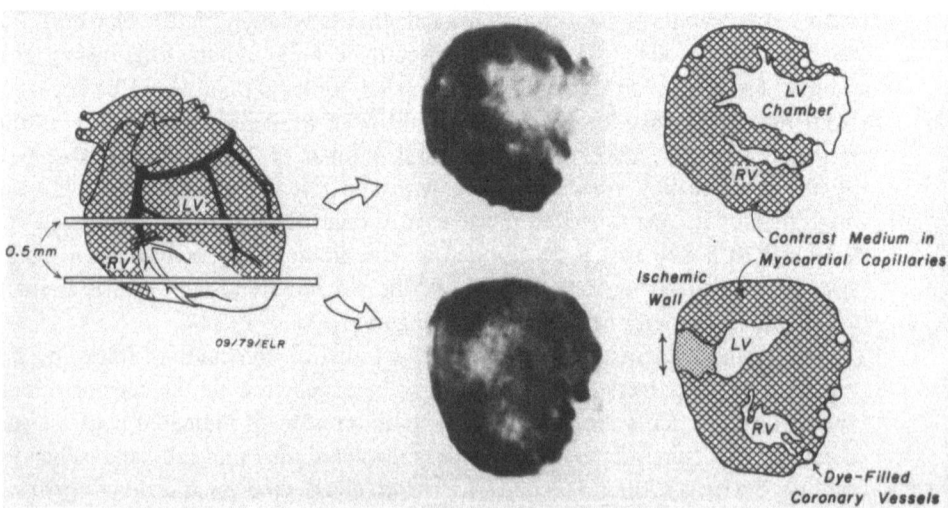

Figure 5. Transverse section images of an in situ canine heart (at locations indicated in *left* panel) indicate transmural distribution of contrast agent. The region distal to a ligated branch of the left anterior descending coronary artery contains less contrast agent and is less roentgen opaque. Reproduced with permission from Scanlan et al. [23].

a ligated left anterior descending coronary artery. The myocardium distal to the ligated vessel is clearly less roentgen opaque than the normally perfused myocardium [23]. These preliminary experimental studies demonstrate the potential of a system of computerized tomography to obtain quantitative information about regional coronary anatomy, myocardial perfusion, and function.

Ischemic heart disease has a broad range of clinical manifestations depending upon the extent and magnitude of obstructive atherosclerotic lesions, collateral blood flow, and the degree to which regional myocardial reserve and overall cardiac function are compromised. Multiple independent tests are commonly employed to provide independent measures of structure and function that might be affected by the disease process. These tests are generally performed at different times and under different physiologic conditions so that the relative importance of the interacting manifestations of ischemic heart disease is often not apparent. One objective in the design of the DSR was to provide a system to make simultaneous evaluations of the multiple manifestations of ischemic heart disease. Figure 6 summarizes the parameters relating to ischemic heart disease that might be assessed with a DSR scan following a single injection of a roentgen opaque contrast agent to improve density differential between blood and surrounding tissue. Preliminary experimental results from early DSR scans demonstrate the feasibility of the approach.

Figure 7 is an image of a sagittal section through the left ventricle from a reconstruction obtained after the injection of contrast agent into the right atrium. This stop-action image comes from the first study of a living, anaesthetized dog by employing the DSR. The cross-sectional display may be oriented

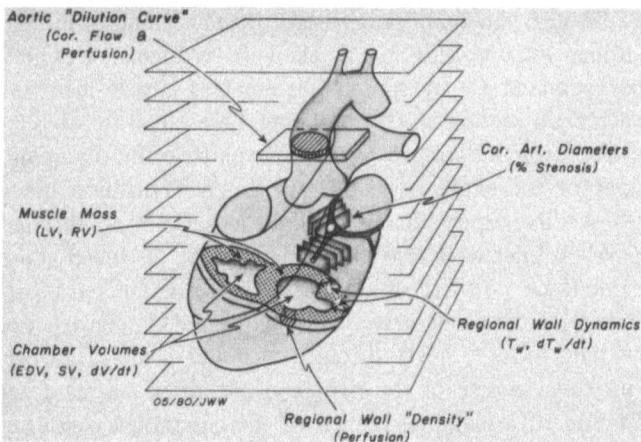

Figure 6. Schematic representation of the aspects of cardiac structure and function that might be evaluated simultaneously with DSR scans employing a single injection of roentgen opaque contrast agent into a cardiac chamber. This evaluation involves retrospective generation of multiple oblique section images.

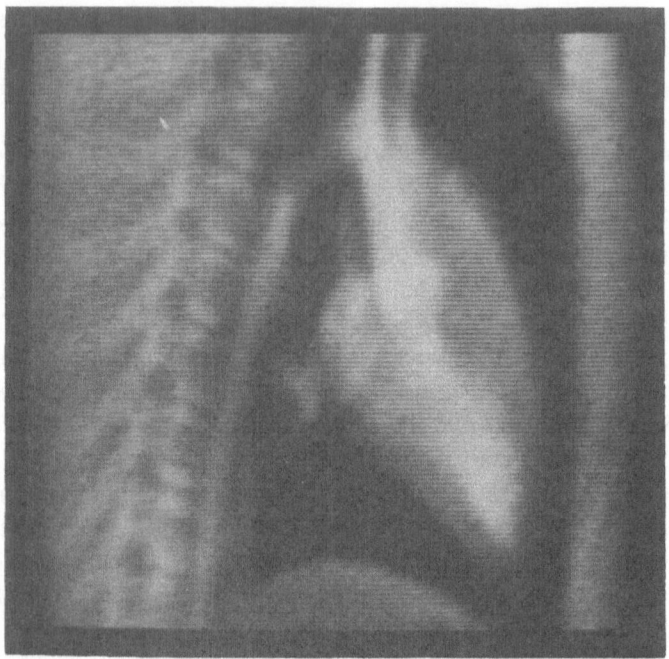

Figure 7. A computer-generated sagittal section image obtained with the DSR through the left ventricle and aortic root of a beating, in situ, canine heart following the injection of iodinated contrast agent into the right atrium.

in any plane through the cylindrical reconstructed volume to better appreciate selected anatomic relationships and detail. Left ventricular volume and muscle mass can be estimated by measuring (planimetry) muscle mass and chamber volume in each cross section and by summing these values for each cross section through the reconstructed volume of the left ventricle. By obtaining sequential reconstructions of the entire heart 60 times/s, the dynamics of regional wall motion and three-dimensional chamber volume can also be appreciated.

The coronary arteries were also imaged in the dog discussed above. Figure 8 shows a 12-mm-thick postmorten section of the reconstructed heart through a plane at the level of the aortic valve, and a 2-mm-thick reconstruction obtained from the beating, in situ, heart through a similar plane. The reconstruction shows the proximal course of the right and cirumflex coronary arteries with good visualization of a marginal branch of the circumflex measuring less than 1 mm in diameter.

Figure 9 shows a sagittal reconstruction through the aortic arch and left ventricle after the injection of contrast into the aortic root. A single injection of contrast provides all the information necessary to draw conclusions about

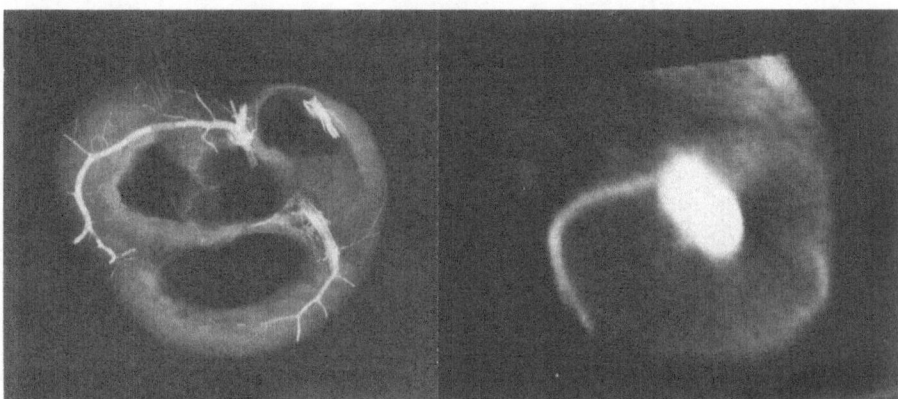

Figure 8. Contact X-ray image of 12-mm postmorten section of a dog heart through a plane at the level of the atrioventricular groove and a 2-mm-thick oblique cross section reconstruction obtained through a similar plane in the beating, in situ, heart. The proximal course of the circumflex coronary artery with a maginal branch less than 1 mm in diameter and the proximal right coronary artery were demonstrated. (Courtesy of Dr. L.D. Harris.)

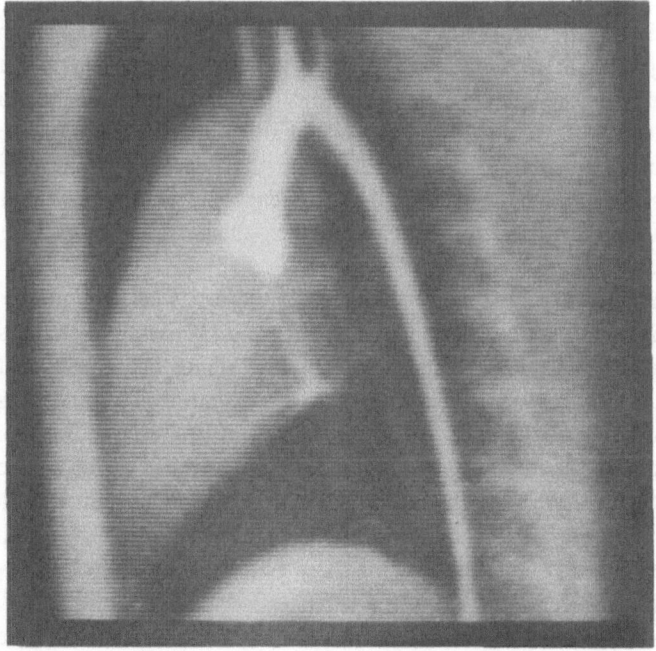

Figure 9. Sagittal section image obtained with the DSR through the aorta and left ventricle of a beating, in situ, canine heart following the injection of iodinated contrast agent into the aortic root.

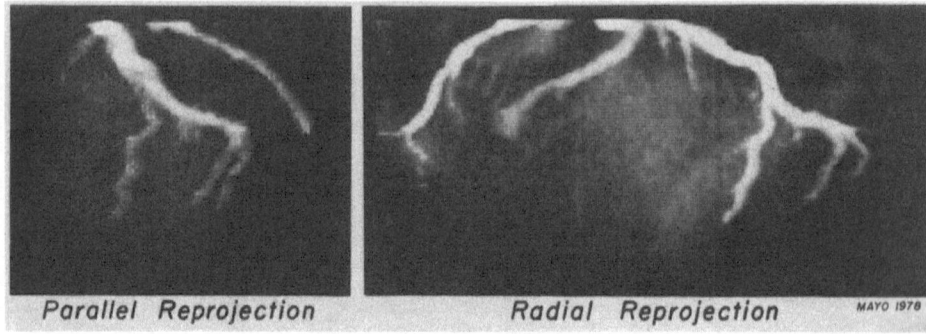

Parallel Reprojection   Radial Reprojection   MAYO 1978

Figure 10. Parallel reprojection and radial reprojection of the reconstructed images of a canine coronary tree following the ligation of the left anterior descending coronary artery. The radial reprojection facilitates recognition of the occluded LAD. Reproduced with permission from Harris et al., *Journal of Computer Assisted Tomography* 3:439, 1979.

coronary anatomy since the reconstructed volume of the coronary tree can be displayed in a number of ways. One display technique is demonstrated in Figure 10. In this figure, the reconstructed cross sections are mathematically reprojected in a radial manner that facilitates detection and localization of coronary artery stenoses and occlusions. Details of this and the related technique of selective tissue dissolution are essential for identification of a lesion's location and orientation in order to determine the degree of stenosis. Plans exist for an oscillating mirror system that will enable a true three-dimensional display of the reconstructed image to further facilitate structural recognition and analysis [25].

The reconstructed aorta and coronary arteries can be employed to estimate coronary blood flow as depicted in Figure 6. If dynamic changes in density are recorded from reconstructions in sampling planes orthogonal to the aorta and a selected coronary artery after a roentgen opaque contrast agent is injected, then a densogram of the mass of the contrast agent in the sampling plane is generated. Previous work with roentgen videodensitometry has shown a strong correlation between the inverse of the integrated area of the densogram and blood flow [26]. By comparing the area under densograms generated from the aorta and a coronary artery, relative flow in these two vessels can be estimated (Figure 11). By knowing cardiac output and relative flow between the aorta and a coronary artery, absolute flow in the coronary artery can then be estimated. By observing the relationship between areas under the densograms generated with the passage of a suitable roentgen opaque contrast agent through equal-sized sampling volumes at selected myocardial sites, a similar analysis can be employed to estimate relative myocardial perfusion.

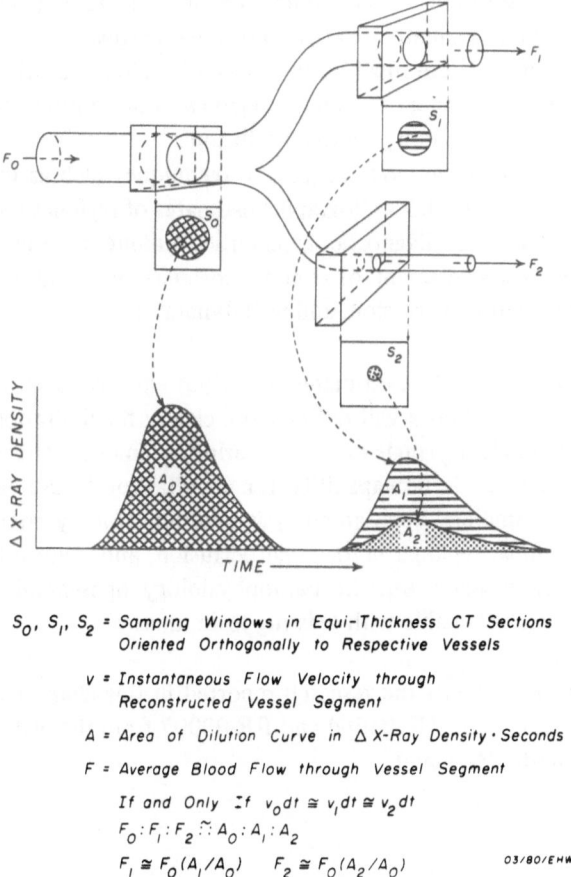

$S_0,\ S_1,\ S_2$ = Sampling Windows in Equi-Thickness CT Sections
Oriented Orthogonally to Respective Vessels

v = Instantaneous Flow Velocity through
Reconstructed Vessel Segment

A = Area of Dilution Curve in Δ X-Ray Density · Seconds

F = Average Blood Flow through Vessel Segment

If and Only If $\int v_0 dt \cong v_1 dt \cong v_2 dt$

$F_0 : F_1 : F_2 \therefore A_0 : A_1 : A_2$

$F_1 \cong F_0 (A_1/A_0) \qquad F_2 \cong F_0 (A_2/A_0)$

03/80/EHW

Figure 11. Schematic representation of the DSR capability for estimating relative blood flow. If the velocity profile is the same for densograms generated through equal-thickness sampling planes orthogonal to the aorta and a selected coronary artery during the passage of a roentgen opaque contrast agent, then the ratio of the areas under the densograms is a measure of a relative flow in the two vessels. (Courtesy of Dr. E.H. Wood.)

FUTURE

The DSR is undergoing preliminary evaluation at this time, so that the impact of it and similar techniques is not known at this time. However, future cardio-vascular applications of the DSR are expected to fall into four areas.

(1) Clarification of pathophysiologic mechanisms, such as the mechanism(s) controlling transmural perfusion. The relative importance of aortic

pressure, coronary artery stenosis, transmural compression, and transmural distribution of metabolic demand due to regional myocardial tension can be evaluated relative to regional perfusion.

(2) Identification of the most useful index of regional location and severity of myocardial ischemia such as regional wall motion, coronary morphology, or regional myocardial perfusion.

(3) Evaluation of single-mode diagnostic techniques such as the accuracy of two-dimensional echocardiographic estimates of regional wall motion.

(4) Identification of diagnostic capabilities unique to the DSR such as simultaneous assessment of regional coronary anatomy, coronary blood glow, myocardial perfusion, and wall dynamics.

At present, quantitative DSR estimates of various cardiovascular parameters are being assessed. These studies will define more clearly the limitations of the DSR as compared with existing single-mode measuring techniques. The unique feature of the DSR, however, is its capability for simultaneously evaluating multiple cardiovascular parameters. Such an analysis relating coronary artery anatomy to coronary blood flow, regional myocardial perfusion, and myocardial mechanics may provide new insights into the pathophysiology of ischemic heart disease that have not been obtainable with existing techniques.

Acknowledgment. Some of the research reported in this chapter was supported in part by research grants HL-04664 and RR-00007 from the National Institutes of Health, Bethesda, Maryland.

REFERENCES

1. Adams DF, Hessel SJ, Judy PF, Stein JA, Abrams HL: Differing attenuation coefficients of normal and infarcted myocardium. Science 192:467, 1976.
2. Ter-Pogossian MM, Weiss ES, Coleman RE, Sobel BE: Computed tomography of the heart. Am J Roentgenol 127:79, 1976.
3. Powell WJ, Wittenberg J, Maturi RA, Dinsmore RE, Miller SW: Detection of edema associated with myocardial ischemia by computerized tomography in isolated, arrested canine hearts. Circulation 55:99, 1977.
4. Higgins CB, Siemers PT, Schmidt W, Newell JD: Evaluation of myocardial ischemic damage of various ages by computerized transmission tomography. Time-dependent effects of contrast material. Circulation 60:284, 1979.
5. Wittenberg J, Powell W Jr, Dinsmore RE, Miller SW, Maturi RA: Computerized tomography of ischemic myocardium: quantitation of extent and severity of edema in an in vitro canine model. Invest Radiol 12:215, 1977.
6. Powell WJ Jr, Dibona DR, Flores J, Leaf A: The protective effect of hyperosmotic mannitol in myocardial ischemia and necrosis. Circulation 54:603, 1976.

275

7. Carlsson E, Lipton MJ, Berninger WH, Doherty P, Redington RW: Selective left coronary myocardiography by computed tomography in living dogs. Invest Radiol 12:559, 1977.
8. Doherty P, Lipton MJ, Skioldebrand C, Berninger WH, Redington RW, Carlsson E: The detection of coronary stenosis and reactive hyperaemia by computed tomography [abstr]. Circulation [Suppl 2] 58:II–5, 1978.
9. Newell JC, Higgins W Schmidt, Kelly M: Computerized tomographic image of evolved myocardial infarctions [abstr]. Circulation [Suppl 2] 60:II–27, 1979.
10. Siemers PT, Higgins CB, Schmidt W, Ashburn W, Hagan P: Detection, quantitation, and contrast enhancement of myocardial infarction utilizing computerized axial tomography: comparison with histochemical staining and ^{99m}Tc-pyrophosphate imaging. Invest Radiol 13:103, 1978.
11. Ledley RS, Di Chiro G, Luessenhop AJ, Twigg HL: Computerized transaxial X-ray tomography of the human body. Science 186:207, 1974.
12. Brooks RA, Di Chiro G: Theory of image reconstuction in computed tomography. Radiology 117:561, 1975.
13. Ritman EL, Robb RA, Johnson SA, Chevalier PA, Gilbert BK, Greenleaf JF, Sturm RE, Wood EH: Quantitative imaging of the structure and function of the heart, lungs, and circulation. Mayo Clin Proc 53:3, 1978.
14. Ritman EL, Kinsey JH, Robb RA, Harris LD, Gilbert BK: Physics and technical considerations in the design of the DSR: a high temporal resolution volume scanner. Am J Radiol 134:369, 1980.
15. Ruegsegger PE, Harris LD, Rowland SW, Ritman EL: Predictions of the performance of a dynamic spatial reconstruction system based on mathematical simulations. In: Heintzen PH, Bürsch JH (eds) Roentgen-video-techniques for dynamic studies of structure and function of the heart and circulation. Stuttgart: Thieme; Littleton MA: PSG, 1978, pp. 313–317.
16. Smith HC, Sturm RE, Wood EH: Videodensitometric system for measurement of vessel blood flow, particularly in the coronary arteries, in man. Am J Cardiol 32:144, 1973.
17. Ritman EL, Sturm RE, Wood EH: Biplane roentgen videometric system for dynamic (60-sec) studies of the shape and size of circulatory structures, particularly the left ventricle. Am J Cardiol 32:180, 1973.
18. Sturm RE, Ritman EL, Johnson SA, Wondrow MA, Erdman DI, Wood EH: Prototype of a single X-ray video imaging chain designed for high temporal resolution computerized tomography by means of an electronic scanning dynamic spatial reconstruction system. Proc San Diego Biomed Symp 15:181, 1976.
19. Robb RA, Harris LD, Chevalier PA, Ritman EL: Quantitative dynamic three-dimensional imaging of the heart and lungs by computerized synchronous cylindrical scanning reconstruction tomography. In: Heintzen PH, Bürsch JH (eds) Roentgen-video-techniques for dynamic studies of structure and function of the heart and circulation. Stuttgart: Thieme; Littleton MA: PSG, 1978, pp. 285–299.
20. Lipton MJ, Hayashi TT, Boyd D, Carlsson E: Measurement of left ventricular cast volume by computed tomography. Radiology 127:419, 1978.
21. Dumesnil JG, Ritman EL, Frye RL, Gau GT, Rutherford BD, Davis GD: Quantitative determination of regional left ventricular wall dynamics by roentgen videometry. Circulation 50:700, 1974.

22. Franklin D, Sasayama S, McKown D, Kemper S, Ross J Jr: Regional ventricular wall dynamics during acute coronary artery occlusion and reperfusion in conscious dogs [abstr]. Physiologist 18:218, 1975.
23. Scanlan JG, Gustafson DE, Chevalier PA, Robb RA, Ritman EL: Evaluation of ischemic heart disease with a prototype volume imaging "CAT" scanner. Am J Cardiol 46:1263–1268, 1980.
24. Griggs DM Jr: Blood flow and metabolism in different layers of the left ventricle. Physiologist 22:36, 1979.
25. Harris LD, Robb RA, Yuen TS, Ritman EL: Display and visualization of three-dimensional reconstructed anatomic morphology: experience with the thorax, heart, and coronary vascular of dogs. J Comput Assist Tomogr 3:439, 1979.
26. Lantz B: Relative flow measured by roentgen videodensitometry in hydrodynamic model. Acta Radiol [Diagn] (Stockh) 16:503, 1975.

11. REGIONAL MYOCARDIAL BLOOD FLOW: A MODEL FOR ASSESSING INTERVENTION THERAPY IN THE CONSCIOUS ANIMAL

FREDERICK R. COBB, ROBERT H. MURDOCK, JR., and KENNETH G. MORRIS

The extent of myocardial infarct that results from acute occlusion of a major coronary artery in experimental animals is highly variable [1, 2]. The concept that myocardial ischemia results in alterable as well as variable irreversible injury is well supported in the literature [3–5]. The variable response to coronary artery occlusion, however, complicates the evaluation of intervention designed to alter ischemic injury especially when the basis for analysis is mean infarct size in a treated versus an untreated group. Considerable effort has thus been directed toward the development of techniques that provide indices that predict the extent of eventual necrosis early in the course of ischemic injury [1–8]. An optimum model for assessing the effects of an intervention on the course of an infarct should provide quantitative measurements or indices of the extent of ischemia before the onset of irreversible injury; these measurements should relate closely to the extent of final myocardial necrosis.

Quantitation of the relationship between regional myocardial blood flow after acute coronary artery occlusion and the subsequent extent of histologic myocardial infarction has been a major area of investigation in our laboratory [1, 8–13]. The objective of these efforts has been to test the hypothesis that regional myocardial blood flow to an ischemic region is the major determinant of the size of a myocardial infarct. We reasoned that if the relationship proved to be sufficiently close, it would provide a model that could be used to assess the effects of interventions that may influence the course of ischemic injury. Several observations provide the rationale for this model. Under basal conditions the myocardium extracts near maximum amounts of oxygen from the arterial blood [14]. Because the metabolism of the myocardium is predominantly aerobic and the capacity for anerobic metabolism is limited during ischemia [15, 16], the integrity of myocardial metabolism is critically dependent on blood flow. The myocardium would be expected to be extremely vulnerable to disease processes or experimental conditions that reduce myocardial blood flow. It follows that blood flow to the ischemic region should be a major determinant of the extent of an infarct. The relationship between regional myocardial blood flow after acute coronary occlusion and subsequent infarct should improve if variables introduced by anesthesia, acute thoracotomy, and the perioperative period could be avoided. Our studies were carried out in chronically

Wagner GS (ed): Myocardial Infarction: Measurement and Intervention, pp 277–294.
© 1982 Martinus Nijhoff Publishers, The Hague/Boston/London.

instrumented animals by using techniques that provided quantitative measurements of regional blood flow and tissue necrosis but enabled conduction of the experiments under conditions that approximated those of clinical infarction.

ANIMAL PREPARATION

Healthy mongrel dogs, 18–23 kg in weight, were selected for study on the basis of temperament and absence of anemia (hematocrit greater than 38%) and infection. A left thoracotomy was performed and a polythylene snare-type occluder was positioned on the left circumflex coronary artery proximal to the first marginal branch. The base of the snare was sutured to the fibrous tissue adjacent to the coronary artery. A number-four silk thread was tied to the base of the stabilized snare and looped loosely around the coronary artery. The silk was then threaded through a small-diameter polyethylene tubing that was then threaded through the larger arm of the snare. A loose loop of silk was left around the coronary artery. The coronary artery can be completely occluded by restricting the inner polyethylene tubing. This type of snare has the advantage of reliably producing a controlled complete permanent occlusion without producing premature closure; it is not suitable for studies that require repeated release of the occlusion. Heparin-filled catheters were placed in the aortic arch via the internal thoracic artery and in the left antrium via the atrial appendage. The catheters and snares were tunneled to subcutaneous pouches so that they could be exteriorized prior to study by small subcutaneous incisions.

During the recovery period, the animals were trained to lie quietly on a laboratory table and were checked frequently to assure that they were free of infection or anemia. Studies were carried out 7–10 days after surgery, while the dogs lay loosely restrained and resting quietly on a laboratory table. The laboratory was dimly illuminated and kept free of noise or other environmental conditions that might have disturbed the dogs. A standard limb lead electrocardiogram and aortic and left atrial pressures were recorded continuously. Acute infarction was induced by complete coronary artery occlusion. Since occlusion of a large coronary artery frequently results in discomfort as manifest by restlessness, morphine sulfate, total dose 0.5 mg/kg, was infused slowly before the occlusion. Lidocaine 2 mg/kg was given as a bolus injection 5 min before the coronary occlusion to minimize ventricular arrhythmias. The administration of antiarrhythmic agents and analgesics was the same in each animal and was limited to the period of acute occlusion. Using this protocol, the incidence of ventricular fibrillation was approximately 20%. Animals that developed ventricular fibrillation were excluded from further study.

Regional blood flow was determined by injecting 9 ± 1-μ microspheres labeled with gamma-emitting nuclides, ^{46}Sc, ^{85}Sr, ^{141}Ce, ^{51}Cr, ^{125}I, and ^{95}Nb.

Each blood flow measurement was made by injecting 1 ml of the microsphere suspension containing 3 million microspheres via the left atrial catheter. Serial injections of this quantity of microspheres produced no effects on systemic or coronary hemodynamics. Regional blood flow measurements were obtained before coronary occlusion and 45 s, 2, 6, and 24 h after complete coronary occlusion.

Five days after the acute myocardial infarction, the heart was removed and placed in 10% buffered formalin for 4–5 days to facilitate sectioning and fix the tissue for later histologic sectioning. The left ventricle was then sectioned from base to apex into four transverse rings of equal thickness as

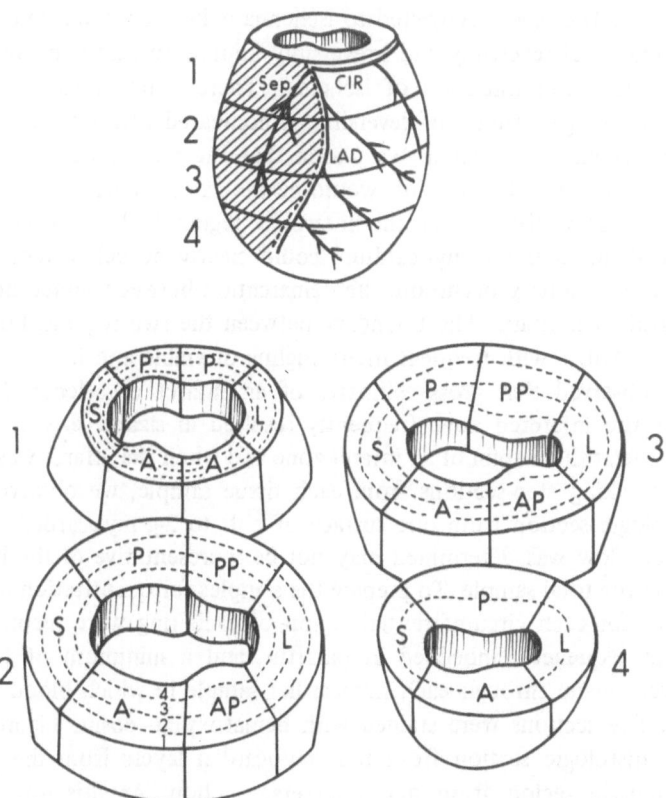

Figure 1. This schematic diagram illustrates the technique for sectioning the left ventricle. The atrial tissue and right ventricle were removed as indicated by the stippled and lined area. The left ventricle was sectioned into circumferential regions, i.e., anterior (A), septal (S), posterior (P), posterior papillary (PP), lateral (L), and anterior papillary (AP). Each circumferential region in rings 1, 2, and 3 was divided into four equal transmural layers. Regions in ring 4 were divided into equal epicardial and endocardial layers. Reprinted by permission of the American Heart Association Inc. [1].

illustrated in Figure 1. Each transverse ring was sectioned into circumferential regions. Each circumferential region was subsectioned into four transmural layers, sample size 1–2 g. Blood flow was then determined by measuring the radioactivity in each myocardial sample by using standard procedures [1, 17, 18], and the following formula:

$$Q_m = Q_r \times (C_m/C_r)$$

where Q_m = myocardial blood flow (ml/min), Q_r = reference blood flow (ml/min), C_m = counts per minute in myocardium, and C_r = counts per minute in reference blood flow.

An essential element of a model used to assess interventions that may protect ischemic myocardium includes the careful quantitation of the extent of final tissue necrosis. The region subjected to ischemia is heterogeneous and contains varying amounts of reversibly and irreversibly injured myocardium for variable periods of time after initiation of ischemia. There is no uniform agreement concerning histologic criteria of reversible as compared with irreversible injury early after ischemia is initiated. We reason that the most precise method for measuring the extent of infarction would be the careful quantitation of histologic necrosis at a time when the infarcted region had stabilized and the infarcted and noninfarcted myocardium could clearly be delineated. Three to four days after coronary occlusion, the demarcation between intact and infarcted myocardium is sharp. The boundary between the two regions, however, is often very irregular with frequent intermingling of viable and infarcted muscle fibers. We observed that gross estimates of an infarct or selected histologic sections of the infarcted zone frequently resulted in sizable errors. This was especially true at the margin of an infarct zone and when the infarct was small or patchy. By taking step-sections from each tissue sample, we observed that a single histologic section from one surface of a 1- to 2-g myocardial sample in which blood flow was determined may not be representative of the histologic infarction in the total sample. To prepare the samples for quantitation of infarct, the samples for each circumferential region of each ring were recombined in their precut sequence, embedded in paraffin, and a minimum of four step-sections were made through each myocardial sample in which blood flow was calculated. The sections were stained with hematoxylin–eosin. Figure 2 illustrates one histologic section from four myocardial layers from the posterior papillary muscle region from one transverse section. At this interval there was sharp delineation between infarcted and intact myocardium. The extent of histologic infarct was quantitated using a projection microscope to produce sketches of the infarcted and noninfarcted tissue that were then planimetered with a graphpen ultrasonic digitizer and computer interface. These procedures enable detailed measurement of regional myocardial blood flow and the extent of infarction in each sample from the ischemic zone.

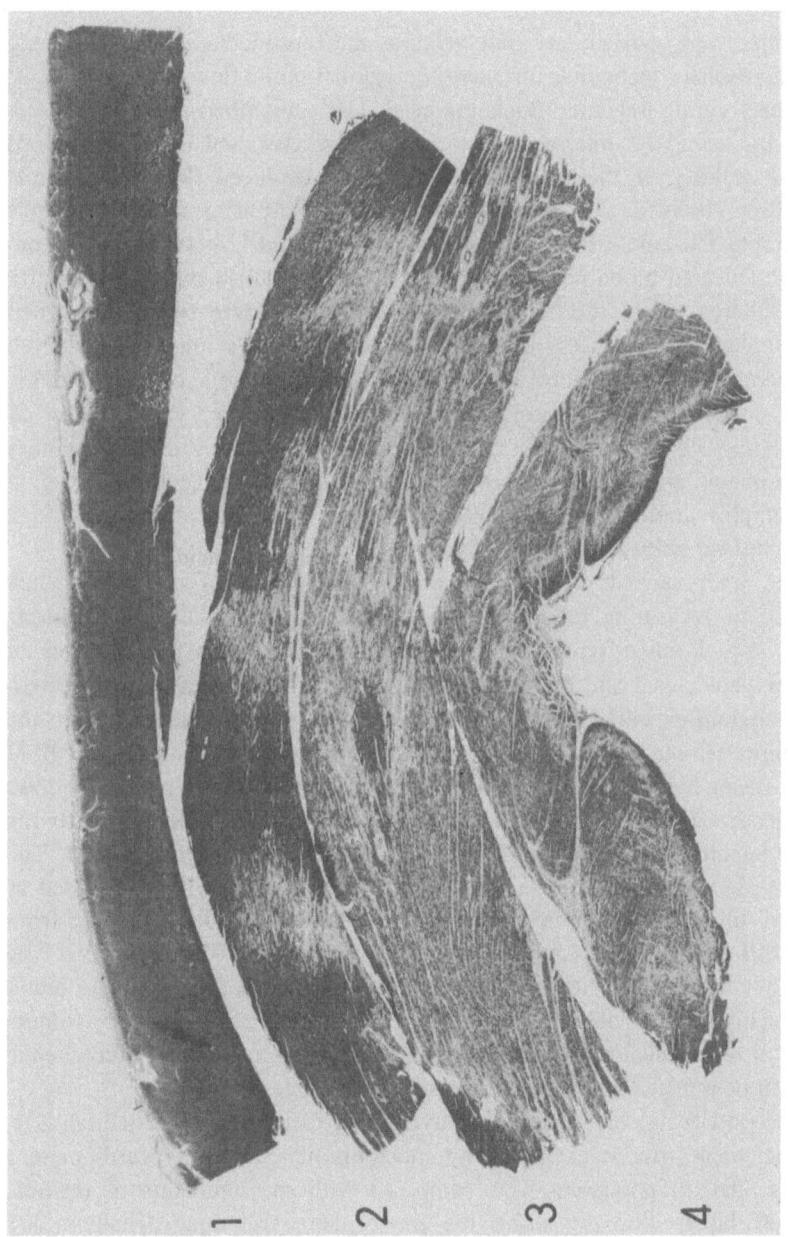

Figure 2. Histologic section of myocardial samples from the posterior papillary muscle region of one ring: 1 is the outer epicardial and 4 the inner endocardial layer. The extent of infarction was 2%, 30%, 91%, and 100% in sections 1, 2, 3, and 4, respectively.

VALIDATIONS OF THE MICROSPHERE TECHNIQUE FOR MEASURING
BLOOD FLOW TO SMALL MYOCARDIAL REGIONS

Two studies were carried out that validate the reproducibility and accuracy
of the microsphere technique for assessing regional blood flow in small myocardial samples during ischemia. Buckberg et al. [19], described potential sources
of error by using the microsphere technique, which raised certain questions
about the validity of the technique for assessing reduced flow rates. These
investigators observed that as the number of microspheres in the reference
blood sample fell below 500, the measurement variability between two simultaneously collected blood samples increased. They concluded that the variability
in microspheres would reflect a similar variability in organ blood flow when
tissue samples contained less than 500 microspheres. We inject 3–4 million
microspheres to deliver approximately 1000 microspheres/g of myocardium,
assuming a heart size of approximately 150 g and a coronary blood flow of
approximately 5% of the cardiac output. We reasoned that even if the number
of microspheres per injection were increased, during ischemia the number in
certain samples would drop below 500 and possibly result in prohibitively high
measurement variability.

Studies were carried out to determine the accuracy of the microsphere
technique for measuring blood flow in 1- to 2-g myocardial samples during
ischemia [1]. Four different isotopes containing 3 million microspheres of
each label were mixed and injected simultaneously after occlusion of the proximal left circumflex coronary artery in a group of six dogs. Blood flow to the
nonischemic sample varied from 1.36 ± 0.10 to 1.66 ± 0.11 ml/g/min $\pm$ SEM
with the mean blood flow difference between simultaneously measured flows
ranging from 0.09 ± 0.02 to 0.12 ± 0.03 ml/g/min $\pm$ SEM. Blood flow to the
ischemic region varied from 0.02 ± 0.01 to 0.56 ± 0.12 ml/g/min $\pm$ SEM. The
differences between simultaneously measured blood flow when expressed as
volume of blood flow were very small in the ischemic regions, ranging from
0.01 ± 0.001 ml/g/min at lowest flow rates to 0.06 ± 0.02 ml/g/min at the
higher flow rates. These data indicate that the assessment of ischemic blood
flow is highly reproducible so that very small changes in the absolute volume
of blood flow in small myocardial segments in both ischemic and nonischemic
regions can be assessed with the microsphere technique.

In a second group of studies, the myocardial distribution of thallium-201,
a tracer element that is extracted by metabolically active myocardium in a
fashion similar to potassium, was compared with measurements of regional
myocardial blood flow by using the microsphere technique. Thallium-201
and radioisotope-labeled microspheres were injected simultaneously during
treadmill exercise and acute coronary occlusion. This protocol resulted in
regions of severe ischemia (blood flow less than 0.1 ml/g/min) and regions

with marked increases in blood flow (3.3- to 7.2-fold increases) in each animal. It was thus possible to compare two dissimilar techniques for assessing myocardial perfusion in small myocardial samples over a wide range of blood flow values [20]. There was a close linear relationship between the two dissimilar techniques; linear regression analyses demonstrated correlation coefficients equal to or greater than 0.98 in each animal. These studies indicate that the radioisotope-labeled microsphere technique provides highly reproducible and accurate measurements of regional perfusion in small regions of the myocardium over a wide range of reduced and increased blood flow.

MICROSPHERE LOSS FROM INFARCTED MYOCARDIUM AS A POTENTIAL SOURCE OF ERROR IN EVALUATING ISCHEMIC BLOOD FLOW

The use of the microsphere technique for assessing regional blood flow is based on the observation that the microspheres are permanently trapped in the coronary microvasculature during the initial passage [19, 21]. Certain reports have indicated that infarcted myocardium may effect loss of microspheres, which may prohibit assessment of collateral blood flow [22, 23]. Interpretation of microsphere loss is based on the observation that in the absence of myocardial infarct, regional myocardial blood flow is relatively homogeneous in the left ventricle; i.e., the ratio of blood flow in circumflex to anterior descending coronary regions equals 1 [14], but after infarct the ratio of preocclusion regional blood flow in infarcted/noninfarcted regions decreases [22, 23]. The percent reduction in the ratio reflects the percent of apparent microsphere loss due to infarction. Some investigators have concluded that the reduction in the ratio can be explained by tissue swelling resulting from increased fluid content and/or inflammatory cell infiltration after acute infarct [24], whereas others have concluded that a combination of true loss and tissue swelling occurs [23].

We carried out studies to determine the effects of apparent microsphere loss on the ischemic blood flow measurements and to what extent these effects altered interpretation of serial measurements of collateral blood flow [10]. We reasoned that the infarcting process should affect the microspheres present in a myocardial sample in a random fashion. Thus, the microspheres injected before and after ischemia would be affected in a similar fashion and the apparent loss of all microspheres present in the sample prior to infarct would be comparable. The effects of infarcted myocardium on ischemic blood flow were assessed by calculating a correction factor for individual samples based on the ratio of preocclusion blood flow in ischemic/nonischemic samples. The correction factor was used to determine the effects of apparent microsphere loss on

Table 1. Relationship of apparent microsphere loss and blood flow correction to the degree of ischemia

| | | Blood flow ranges (ml/min/g) | | | | | |
		0–0.10	0.11–0.20	0.21–0.35	0.36–0.50	0.51–0.75	0.76–1.00
Epicardial	% Loss	19.4 ± 5.4*	10.3 ± 4.4*	10.8 ± 4.2*	3.1 ± 4.7	3.5 ± 2.8	− 3.3 ± 7.4
	Flow corr	0.018 ± 0.005*	0.024 ± 0.009*	0.048 ± 0.018*	0.031 ± 0.027	0.030 ± 0.017	− 0.020 ± 0.058
		7/28	12/43	12/36	11/25	13/40	5/7
Endocardial	% Loss	15.5 ± 3.9*	17.6 ± 4.7*	11.1 ± 6.9	14.3 ± 4.0*	4.4 ± 4.9	7.4 ± 4.1
	Flow corr	0.010 ± 0.003*	0.047 ± 0.019*	0.052 ± 0.025*	0.077 ± 0.022*	0.033 ± 0.031	0.077 ± 0.034*
		12/113	8/23	9/17	8/16	6/11	3/4

Apparent microsphere loss in % ± SEM and blood flow correction in ml/min/g in samples grouped according to the degree of ischemia 15 min after coronary artery occlusion: negative values indicate apparent microsphere gain. * = $p < 0.05$. Ratios = number of dogs contributing to each particular value/total number of myocardial samples. The values were obtained by first calculating an average % loss and flow correction for each dog and then obtaining the averages of both values for the group. The animals were sacrificed three days after acute infarction. Reprinted by permission of the American Heart Association, Inc. [10].

the ischemic blood flow measurements. The apparent microsphere loss (% ± SEM) and blood flow correction (ml/min/g) as a function of ischemic blood flow ranges are presented in Table 1 for a group of animals subjected to permanent circumflex coronary artery occlusion and then sacrificed three days later [10]. Significant microsphere loss occurred in samples with less than 0.35 ml/min/g in the epicardial layers and less than 0.5 ml/min/g in the endocardium; maximum loss was 19.4%, which is comparable to the degree of microsphere loss observed by Jugdutt et al [23]. The significant apparent microsphere loss resulted in statistically significant but very small absolute changes in ischemic blood flow. The corrections for ischemic blood flow ranged from 0.05 to 0.02 ml/min/g in the epicardial regions and from 0.08 to 0.01 ml/min/g in the endocardial regions.

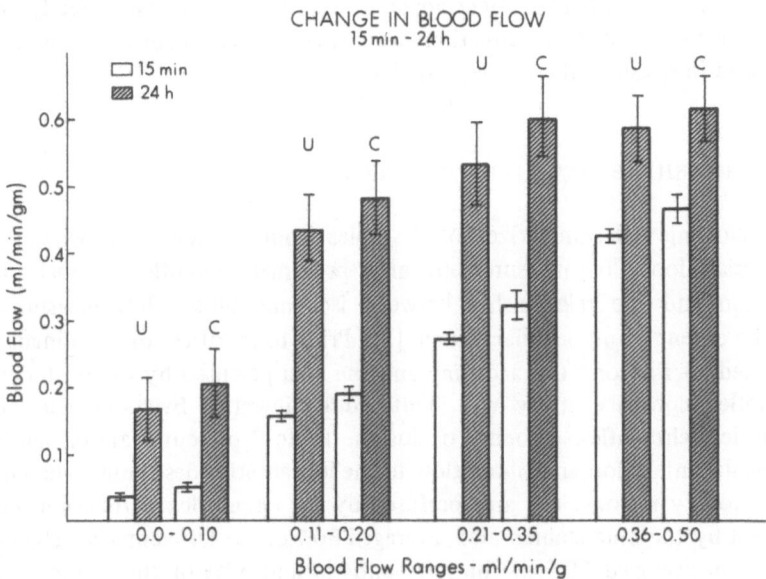

Figure 3. Mean blood flow ± SEM at 15 min and 24 h after occlusion in dogs killed at three days. Samples have been grouped according to ischemic blood flow ranges; mean value represents uncorrected (u) and corrected (c) measurements. Reprinted by permission of the American Heart Association, Inc. [10].

Figure 3 illustrates the change in regional blood flow between 15 min and 24 h post occlusion before and after correction for apparent microsphere loss. Both corrected and uncorrected measurements of collateral blood flow increased significantly in each ischemic blood flow range below 0.5 ml/min/g. The relative change in blood flow between 15 min and 24 h were comparable before and after correction. Because the effects of correction were small relative to the large change in collateral blood flow, correction had minimal effects on the interpretation of changes in collateral blood flow. Thus, although significant apparent microsphere loss is effected by infarcted myocardium, the effects on regional blood flow to an ischemic region are so small that one may question whether they are of biological significance. Studies in our laboratory and others [10, 22, 23], demonstrated that the tissue changes that effect apparent microsphere loss are present between 6 and 24 h after occlusion; there is minimal loss prior to or after these intervals. It is appropriate to apply a correction factor to blood flow measurements obtained prior to the onset of microsphere loss, i.e., less than 6 h after occlusion [24], but once apparent microsphere loss begins or is complete, a correction will overcorrect ischemic blood flow values. In the previous study, correction of the 24-h blood flow measurements may have been excessive since events that effect apparent microsphere loss had already begun. In any event, blood flow corrections were small so that uncorrected and corrected blood flow values at 24 h were similar.

RELATIONSHIP BETWEEN BLOOD FLOW AND INFARCT

The following will summarize initial studies from our laboratory which examined serial blood flow measurements after proximal circumflex coronary artery occlusion and the relationship between ischemic blood flow measurements and the extent of myocardial infarct [1]. Prior to sacrifice, these animals were subjected to a second thoracotomy and the area perfused by the occluded left circumflex coronary artery was identified by injecting Evans blue dye distal to the left circumflex coronary occlusion. Table 2 presents data on mean left ventricular infarction and blood flow to the left anterior descending and circumflex coronary regions. The area perfused by the circumflex coronary artery, as outlined by the blue stained area, averaged 36% of the left ventricle. The infarcted region averaged 19% of the left ventrical and 52% of the region supplied by the occluded circumflex coronary artery. Collateral flow to the ischemic region afforded protection for a considerable but highly variable amount of ischemic myocardium, i.e., 12%–84% of the ischemic region was infarcted. Mean flow to the ischemic region increased from 0.25 ± 0.03 following occlusion to 0.53 ± 0.07 at 24 h. In more recent studies, we have used postmortem injections of the coronary vasculature with barium sulfate gel as described by Jugdutt et al. [25, 26] to define the occluded bed regions. This technique enables identification of the epicardial and transmural distribution of the occluded vessel from radiographs of the left ventricle before and after sectioning into transverse rings. We feel these techniques are easier than injecting the coronary vasculature in vivo with dyes and also may reduce potential error from staining

Table 2. Left ventricular infarct and blood flow to left anterior descending and left circumflex coronary artery regions

Dog no.	LV wt (g)	% LV cir.	% LV inf.	% cir. inf.	LAD blood flow (ml/min/g)				LCCA blood flow (ml/min/g)			
					45 s	2 h	6 h	24 h	42 s	2 h	6 h	24 h
1	117	37	23	63	0.76	0.90	1.04	1.69	0.18	0.22	0.26	0.63
2	94	33	20	60	1.37	1.42	1.24		0.12	0.25	0.28	
3	134	34	13	38	1.32	1.90	1.56	2.07	0.18	0.41	0.46	0.84
4	124	36	23	64	1.66	1.42	1.13	1.01	0.24	0.35	0.34	0.36
5	128	40	23	58	1.14	1.00	1.01	0.88	0.27	0.33	0.30	0.44
6	117	35	20	57	1.49	1.74	1.27	1.05	0.27	0.39	0.35	0.45
7	114	39	33	84	1.22	1.14	0.90	1.23	0.13	0.14	0.11	0.21
8	91	43	27	62	0.99	1.02	1.42	1.06	0.25	0.39	0.39	0.38
9	89	28	4	12	0.65	0.98	0.62	0.51	0.30	0.58	0.57	0.50
10	130	36	16	46	1.54	1.46	1.39	1.60	0.29	0.56	0.51	0.63
11	60	29	8	26	0.87	1.45	1.19	0.86	0.52	0.63	0.76	0.86
Mean	109	36	19	52	1.18	1.31	1.16	1.20	0.25	0.39	0.39	0.53
SEM	± 7	± 1	± 3	± 6	± 0.10	± 0.10	± 0.08	± 0.15	± 0.03	± 0.05	± 0.05	± 0.07
p						NS	NS	NS	< 0.01	< 0.05	< 0.05	0.02

Tabulation of the left ventricular weight (LV wt, in grams), percent of left ventricle perfused by the left circumflex coronary artery (% LV cir.), percent of left ventricle infarcted (% LV inf.), percent circumflex region infarcted (% cir. inf.), and mean blood flow measurements (ml/min/g) in the areas perfused by the left anterior descending coronary artery (LAD) and the left circumflex coronary artery (LCCA) 45 s, and 2, 6, and 24 h post occlusion. p values compare the blood flow values at each interval with the preceding value; $p > 0.05 =$ NS (not significant). Reprinted by permission of American Heart Association, Inc. [1].

regions outside the original occluded region as a result of newly developed collateral vessels between occluded and nonoccluded vessels.

Table 3 presents the mean percentage of infarction and blood flow values in each transmural layer. There was an inverse relationship between transmural infarct and blood flow. Transmural blood flow was not evenly distributed; blood flow to endocardial layer 4 was approximately one-half that to epicardial layer 1. Blood flow increased in each layer between 45 s and 24 h.

Table 3. Mean myocardial infarct and blood flow in transmural layer from the LCCA region

Transmural layer	Infarcted myocardium (%)	LCCA region blood flow (ml/min/g)			
		45 s	2 h	6 h	24 h
1	19 ± 6	0.36 ± 0.05	0.58 ± 0.07	0.58 ± 0.07	0.78 ± 0.10
2	46 ± 9	0.22 ± 0.04	0.35 ± 0.05	0.38 ± 0.06	0.56 ± 0.09
3	70 ± 8	0.15 ± 0.02	0.25 ± 0.04	0.26 ± 0.04	0.41 ± 0.08
4	76 ± 6	0.16 ± 0.02	0.23 ± 0.03	0.23 ± 0.04	0.34 ± 0.06

Mean percent infarcted myocardium and sequential measurements of myocardial blood flow (ml/min/g) in samples from transmural layers 1–4 of the region perfused by the left circumflex coronary artery (LCCA). Reprinted by permission of American Heart Association, Inc. [1].

The relationship between blood flow at 45 s and 2, 6, and 24 h after occlusion, and the percent of myocardial infarction in samples from the four transmural layers in the ischemic area are illustrated in Table 4. The data are grouped in flow ranges of 0–0.10, 0.11–0.20, 0.21–0.35, 0.36–0.50, 0.51– 0.75, and 0.76–1.00 ml/min/g. In each transmural layer, the percent myocardial infarct was inversely related to blood flow. For a given range of blood flow, the percent of infarcted myocardium in endocardial samples exceeded the percent of infarct in epicardial samples, indicating that the relationship between blood flow and the extent of myocardial infarct varied in different transmural layers of the myocardium. The relationship between blood flow 45 s and 2 h after occlusion and the extent of infarct is illustrated graphically in Figures 4 and 5. The infarct values in layers 3 and 4 are combined in the graphs because, with the exception of values in the blood flow range of 0.36–0.50 at 2 h, the percent of infarct was not significantly different in these layers.

There are at least two possible explanations for the disproportionately greater infarct in endocardial regions. As blood flow increased to the ischemic region, the number of samples in the low blood flow ranges decreased and the number in the high blood flow ranges increased. There was a greater tendency for samples in the epicardial layers, as compared with samples in the endocardial layers, to shift to higher blood flow ranges, indicating that the increments in blood flow to the ischemic region were preferentially delivered to the epicardial

Table 4. Relationship between blood flow and percent infarct in transmural myocardial layers

| | Myocardial blood flow ranges (ml/min/g) | | | | | |
	0.00–0.10	0.11–0.20	0.21–0.35	0.36–0.50	0.51–0.75	0.76–1.00
	% Infarct					
45 s after occlusion						
Layer 1	35 ± 12	28 ± 9	17 ± 5	10 ± 3	7 ± 2	7 ± 3
	(5/11)	(8/14)	(8/19)	(8/16)	(9/12)	(3/5)
Layer 2	73 ± 7	46 ± 10	34 ± 10	26 ± 4	14 ± 4	1
	(8/24)	(8/18)	(8/12)	(2/3)	(6/6)	(1/1)
Layer 3	79 ± 8	73 ± 8	56 ± 10	62 ± 20	15 ± 7	
	(10/39)	(6/12)	(6/8)	(3/3)	(4/4)	
Layer 4	91 ± 4	84 ± 6	63 ± 15	40 ± 15	19 ± 6	12 ± 11
	(11/43)	(7/13)	(6/10)	(4/4)	(2/3)	(2/2)
2 h after occlusion						
Layer 1	89	37 ± 11	27 ± 9	19 ± 5	10 ± 3	6 ± 1
	(1/4)	(4/7)	(5/10)	(7/16)	(10/20)	(6/18)
Layer 2	90 ± 5	82 ± 6	48 ± 8	32 ± 7	20 ± 4	9 ± 6
	(4/14)	(5/7)	(9/19)	(7/11)	(8/12)	(2/2)
Layer 3	96 ± 1	84 ± 4	72 ± 8	45 ± 10	30 ± 9	15 ± 7
	(6/21)	(7/13)	(9/19)	(6/6)	(3/4)	(4/4)
Layer 4	96 ± 1	90 ± 5	68 ± 8	80 ± 9	34 ± 13	24 ± 11
	(10/33)	(9/16)	(6/11)	(4/4)	(6/8)	(2/3)
6 h after occlusion						
Layer 1	89	44 ± 12	31 ± 14	21 ± 5	10 ± 3	6 ± 2
	(1/4)	(3/5)	(3/7)	(7/14)	(10/29)	(9/15)
Layer 2	93 ± 3	76 ± 4	56 ± 6	29 ± 5	21 ± 3	9 ± 4
	(5/14)	(5/16)	(7/16)	(8/12)	(8/14)	(4/4)
Layer 3	95 ± 2	83 ± 4	73 ± 8	50 ± 11	33 ± 6	3 ± 1
	(7/21)	(8/14)	(9/14)	(6/8)	(6/7)	(2/2)
Layer 4	96 ± 1	90 ± 5	68 ± 6	70 ± 15	22 ± 4	21 ± 5
	(10/34)	(9/17)	(6/9)	(5/5)	(6/6)	(4/4)
24 h after occlusion						
Layer 1	88	100	57 ± 14	39 ± 14	13 ± 4	10 ± 3
	(1/2)	(1/1)	(4/5)	(3/7)	(7/21)	(6/18)
Layer 2	100	95 ± 3	85 ± 2	49 ± 4	32 ± 9	14 ± 4
	(1/4)	(4/6)	(5/11)	(5/13)	(6/14)	(5/8)
Layer 3	96 ± 2	89 ± 8	85 ± 5	73 ± 6	45 ± 9	33 ± 15
	(7/16)	(4/7)	(7/13)	(4/5)	(7/13)	(3/4)
Layer 4	98 ± 1	94 ± 3	88 ± 5	66 ± 10	63 ± 14	23 ± 4
	(8/21)	(7/12)	(8/13)	(5/7)	(6/9)	(5/8)

Relationship between ischemic blood flow and percent of subsequent myocardial infarct in samples from transmural layers 1–4, 45 s, and 2, 6, 24 h after complete occlusion of the left circumflex coronary artery in 11 dogs. Samples in each transmural layer are grouped according to blood flow ranges, and the percent of myocardial infarct ± SEM in each range and layer are tabulated. Ratios (in parentheses) = number of dogs contributing to each particular value/total number of myocardial samples. The infarct values were obtained by first calculating an average infarct value for each dog and then obtaining the average of the percent infarct for the group. Reprinted by permission of American Heart Association, Inc. [1].

290

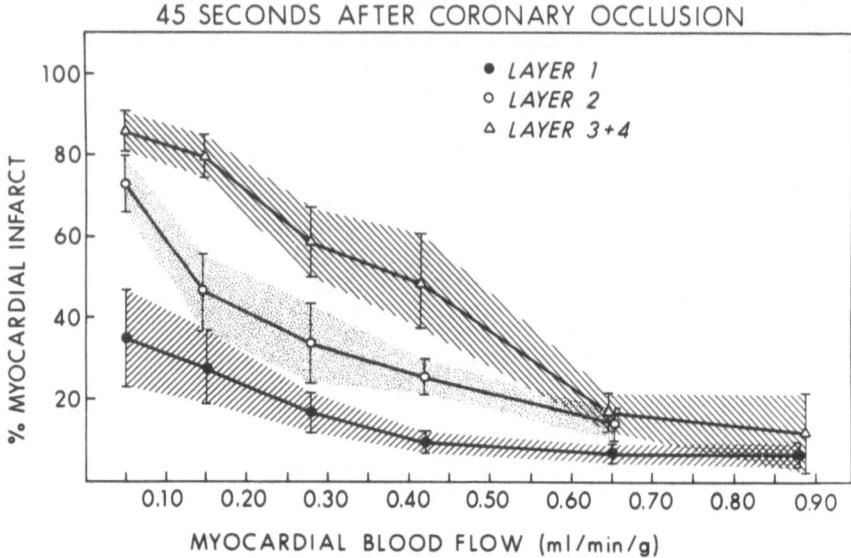

Figure 4. The percent myocardial infarct ± SEM in myocardial samples from transmural layers 1, 2, and 3 plus 4 are plotted as a function of myocardial blood flow 45 s after coronary occlusion. Reprinted by permission of the American Heart Association, Inc. [1].

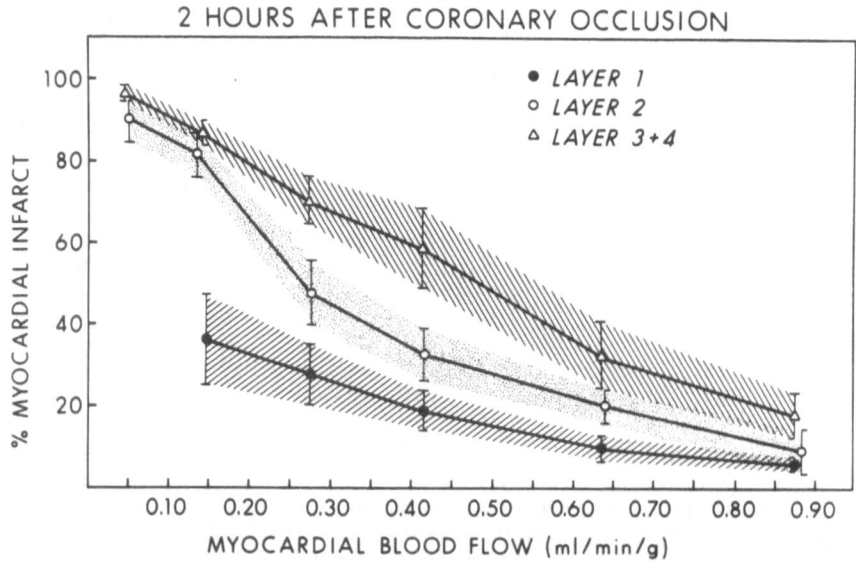

Figure 5. The percent myocardial infarct ± SEM in myocardial samples from transmural layers 1, 2, and 3 plus 4 are plotted as a function of myocardial blood flow 2 h after coronary occlusion. Reprinted by permission of the American Heart Association, Inc. [1].

layers. For example, 45 s after occlusion, there were 44 samples in layer 1 and 66 samples in layer 4 in the flow ranges of 0–0.35 ml/min/g, whereas 24 h after occlusion, 8 samples in layer 1 and 46 samples in layer 4 remained in these flow ranges. Although disproportionate endocardial infarct was still apparent when samples were grouped 24 h after occlusion, the differences between endocardial and epicardial infarction for comparable blood flow ranges was less striking.

Alternatively, it is possible that factors operating independently of blood flow may have contributed to the disproportionate endocardial infarct. Griggs et al. [27] observed that coronary artery occlusion resulted in significant transmural metabolic gradients. They considered the possibility that the transmural metabolic gradients may have resulted from transmural gradients in wall stress as well as blood flow. Although the factors that contribute to the apparent disproportionate endocardial infarct have not been clearly delineated, these data indicate that the transmural location of the myocardial samples is an important determinant of the relationship between blood flow after acute coronary occlusion and the extent of the subsequent infarct.

The relationship between measurements of blood flow early after acute coronary artery occlusion and the extent of subsequent myocardial infarct in samples grouped according to blood flow ranges and transmural layers provides reference data that can be used to evaluate interventions that alter the extent of infarct. The mean percent infarct ± 2 SEM should predict with 95% confidence limits a similar amount of infarct in a different group of dogs sub-jected to the same experimental conditions. The standard error of each percent infarct value in a given flow range is a measure of the variability of the relation-ship between blood flow and subsequent infarct. The standard error of each infarct value thus determines the minimum change in infarct size that can be detected in a given flow range and layer.

In studies designed to evaluate the effects of a given intervention on infarct size, the same protocol will be followed. Blood flow will be measured at 15 min, and 2, 6, and 24 h after occlusion. We have elected to make the first measure-ment after occlusion 15 min rather than 45 s to allow systemic hemodynamics to be at a more steady state. The intervention to be evaluated will be initiated after the 15-min, 2-h or 6-h blood flow measurement. The effects of intervention therapy on the extent of infarct is determined by using the ischemic blood flow measurements before initiation of therapy to predict the expected infarct based on infarct measurements for a comparable degree of ischemia in a nontreatment or control group. The blood flow measurements obtained after initiation of the intervention will be compared with serial blood flow measurements in a non-treated group. Thus, any alteration in the extent of infarct will be related to changes in blood flow.

Studies by Jennings and Reimer [28, 29] using anesthetized animals indicate that infarct begins first in the papillary muscle areas of the endocardium. As the duration of the occlusion was increased, the initial infarct area progressively increased and involved varying amounts of the epicardium. β-Adrenergic blockade with propranolol reduced infarct at the periphery rather than in the endocardial region [5]. If these data prove to apply to the conscious dog model, then certain interventions may reduce infarct first in epicardial layer 1 and less ischemic regions in layers 2, 3, and 4. Thus, certain interventions that result in relatively small changes in total infarct size may prevent or greatly enhance infarct in these border areas and thus be detected by this technique. Alternatively, if transmural wall tension is an important determinant of the distribution of infarct, interventions that influence the generation of wall tension, such as increases and decreases in aortic pressure, may be expected to alter ischemic injury to a greater extent in the endocardium. It is possible that certain interventions will alter the extent of infarct independently of changes in blood flow whereas other interventions will alter infarct coincidentally with increases or decreases in blood flow to the ischemic region.

By permitting blood flow to be measured at intervals after acute coronary occlusion and the relationship between blood flow and the extent of infarct to be determined in separate transmural layers rather than in the total region of ischemia, this model should provide (a) a sensitive technique for evaluating interventions that reduce or extend infarct (b) data about the mechanism whereby an intervention alters an infarct i.e., alteration in infarct in the epicardial or endocardial region, or both, and (c) reference data that can be used to determine whether alterations in the relationship between blood flow and infarct occurred coincidentally with alterations in blood flow. By using an awake dog, this model avoids the variables introduced by general anesthesia and acute surgery.

Acknowledgments. The following persons have been collaborating investigators on the studies: Dr. F. Rivas, Dr. R.J. Bache, Dr. P.A. McHale, Dr. J.C. Rembert, Dr.A.P. Nielsen, and Dr. J.C. Greenfield. This work is supported in part by the research grant HL 18537 from the National Heart, Lung and Blood Institute and the Medical Research Service of the Veterans Administration Medical Center. Dr. Frederick R. Cobb received support from the American Heart Association as an Established Investigator.

REFERENCES

1. Rivas F, Cobb FR, Bache RJ, Greenfield JC Jr: Relationship between blood flow to ischemic regions and extent of myocardial infarction: serial measurement of blood flow to ischemic regions in dogs. Circ Res 38:439–447, 1976.

2. Roe CR, Cobb FR, Starmer CF: The relationship between enzymatic and histologic estimates of the extent of myocardial infarction in conscious dogs with permanent coronary occlusion. Circulation 55:438–449, 1977.

3. Maroko PR, Kjekshus JK, Sobel BE, Watanabe T, Covell JW, Ross J Jr, Braunwald E: Factors influencing infarct size following experimental coronary artery occlusion. Circulation 43:67–82, 1971.

4. Maroko PR, Libby P, Covell JW, Sobel BE, Ross J Jr, Braunwald E: Precordial S–T segment elevation mapping: an atraumatic method for assessing alterations in the extent of myocardial ischemic injury: the effects of pharmacologic and hemodynamic interventions. Am J Cardiol 29:223–230, 1972.

5. Rasmussen MM, Reimer KA, Kloner RA, Jennings RB: Infarct size reduction by propranolol before and after coronary ligation in dogs. Circulation 56:794–798, 1977.

6. Shell WL, Kjekshus JK, Sobel BE: Quantitative assessment of the extent of myocardial infarction in the conscious dog by means of analysis of serial changes in serum creatine phosphokinase activity. J Clin Invest 50:2614–2625, 1971.

7. Shell WE, Lavelle JF, Covell JW, Sobel BE: Early estimation of myocardial damage in conscious dogs and patients with evolving acute myocardial infarction. J Clin Invest 52:2579–2590, 1973.

8. Irvin, RG, Cobb FR: Relationship between epicardial ST-segment elevation, regional myocardial blood flow, and extent of myocardial infarction in awake dogs. Circulation 55:825–832, 1977.

9. Cobb FR, Murdock RH, McHale PA, Greenfield JC Jr: Relationship between regional blood flow and myocardial infarction: effects of apparent microsphere loss and/or tissue swelling [abstr]. Circulation [Suppl 2] 60:II–117, 1979.

10. Murdock RH Jr, Cobb FR: Effects of infarcted myocardium on regional blood flow measurements to ischemic regions in canine hearts. Circ Res 47:701–709, 1980.

11. Murdock R Jr, Morris J, Pryor W, Cobb FR: Time-course for salvaging ischemic myocardium [abstr]. Circulation [Suppl 3]: 62:III–144, 1980.

12. Cobb FR, Bache RJ, Rivas F, Greenfield JC Jr: Local effects of acute cellular injury on regional myocardial blood flow. J Clin Invest 57:1359–1368, 1976.

13. Cobb FR, McHale PA, Rembert JC: Effects of acute cellular injury on coronary vascular reactivity in awake dogs. Circulation 57:962–967, 1978.

14. Gregg DE, Fisher LC: Blood supply to the heart. In: Hamilton WF, Dow P (eds) Handbook of physiology, sect 2, vol 2: Circulation. Washington American Physiological Society, 1963, pp 1517–1584.

15. Braasch W, Gudbjarnason S, Puri PS, Ravens KG, Bing RJ: Early changes in energy metabolism in the myocardium following acute coronary artery occlusion in anesthetized dogs. Cir Res 23:429–438, 1968.

16. Kubler W, Spieckermann PG: Regulation of glycolysis in the ischemic and the anoxic myocardium. J Mol Cell Cardiol 1:351–377, 1970.

17. Domenech RJ, Hoffman JIE, Noble MIM, Saunders KB, Henson JR, Subijanto S: Total and regional coronary blood flow measured by radioactive microspheres in conscious and anesthetized dogs. Circ Res 25:581–587, 1969.

18. Cobb FR, Bache RJ, Greenfield JC Jr: Regional myocardial blood flow in awake dogs. J Clin Invest 53:1618–1625, 1974.
19. Buckberg GD, Luck JC, Payne DB, Hoffman JIE, Archie JP, Fixler DE: Some sources of error in measuring regional blood flow with radioactive microspheres. J Appl Physiol 31:598–604, 1971.
20. Nielsen AP, Morris KG, Murdock R, Bruno FP, Cobb FR: Linear relationship between the distribution of thallium-201 and blood flow in ischemic and nonischemic myocardium during exercise. Circulation 61:797–801, 1980.
21. Utley J, Carlson EL, Hoffman JIE, Martinez HM, Buckberg GD: Total and regional myocardial blood flow measurements with $25\,\mu$, $15\,\mu$, $9\,\mu$, and filtered $1-10\,\mu$ diameter microspheres and antipyrine in dogs and sheep. Circ Res 34:391–405, 1974.
22. Capurro NL, Goldstein RE, Aamodt R, Smith HJ, Epstein SE: Loss of microspheres from ischemic canine cardiac tissue: an important technical limitation. Circ Res 44:223–227, 1979.
23. Jugdutt BI, Hutchins GM, Bulkley BH, Becker LC: The loss of radioactive microspheres from canine necrotic myocardium. Circ Res 45:746–756, 1979.
24. Reimer KA, Jennings RB: The changing anatomic reference base of evolving myocardial infarction: underestimation of myocardial collateral blood flow and overestimation of experimental anatomic infarct size due to tissue edema, hemorrhage and acute inflammation. Circulation 60:866–876, 1979.
25. Jugdutt BI, Grover CB, Hutchins GM, Bulkley BH, Pitt B, Becker LC: Effect of indomethacin on collateral blood flow and infarct size in the conscious dog. Circulation 59:734–743, 1979.
26. Jugdutt BI, Hutchins GM, Bulkley BH, Becker LC: Salvage of ischemic myocardium by ibuprofen during infarction in the conscious dog. Am J Cardiol 46:74–82, 1980.
27. Griggs DM Jr, Tchokoev W, Chen CC; Transmural differences in ventricular tissue substrate levels due to coronary constriction. Am J Physiol 222:705–709, 1972.
28. Reimer KA, Jennings RB: The 'wavefront phenomenon' of myocardial ischemic cell death. II. Transmural progression of necrosis within the framework of ischemic bed size (myocardium at risk) and collateral flow. Lab Invest 40:633–644, 1979.
29. Jennings RB, Reimer KA: Salvage of ischemic myocardium. Mod Concepts Cardiovasc Dis 43:125–130, 1974.

12. RADIONUCLIDE PERFUSION TECHNIQUES

ROBERT D. OKADA, CHARLES A. BOUCHER, and GERALD M. POHOST

Radionuclide perfusion imaging to quantitate ischemic and infarcted myocardium employs four general groups of tracers (Tables 1 and 2). The first group of tracers are analogues of potassium that are taken up rapidly and maximally by normal myocardium and slower (depending on the degree of ischemia) by

Table 1. Perfusion techniques for quantitation of myocardial ischemia and infarct

Indicator type	Radionuclide	Administration route
Potassium analogues	^{43}K, ^{131}Cs, ^{129}Cs, ^{201}Tl, ^{81}Rb	Intravenous
Radioactive particles (albumin macroaggregates or microspheres)	^{99m}Tc, ^{133}In, ^{131}I	Intracoronary, aorta, or left heart
Diffusible tracers	^{133}Xe, ^{81m}Kr	Intracoronary, aorta, or left heart

ischemic zones. Infarcted myocardium accumulates very little, if any, tracer. The second group of tracers used for perfusion imaging employ biodegradable particles labeled with short-lived radionuclides. These particles are injected into the left atrium or directly into a coronary artery and are trapped in capillaries or precapillary beds in proportion to the amount of blood flow through the particular region of the myocardium. The third group of indicators are diffusible tracers such as the inert gas xenon-133, whose regional myocardial washout rate after an intracoronary infusion is proportional to regional myocardial blood flow. Metabolically active substrates such as ^{11}C-palmitate, ^{13}NH$_3$, and ^{18}F-2-deoxyglucose represent a fourth group of tracers (Table 2).

This chapter emphasizes the noninvasive approaches for quantitating ischemic and infarcted myocardium by using perfusion imaging. Perfusion imaging with a positron camera will be discussed at the end of this chapter.

Wagner GS (ed): Myocardial Infarction: Measurement and Intervention, pp 295–324.
© 1982 Martinus Nijhoff Publishers, The Hague/Boston/London.

Table 2. Important positron-emitting radionuclides for imaging ischemia

Radionuclide	$t\frac{1}{2}$ (min)	Production reaction	Production source	Radiopharmaceuticals
Carbon-11 (^{11}C)	20	^{10}B (d, n)	Cyclotron	^{11}C-palmitate
Nitrogen-13 (^{13}N)	10	^{12}C (d, n)	Cyclotron	^{13}NH$_3$, ^{13}N-amino acids
Oxygen-15 (^{15}O)	2	^{14}N (d, n)	Cyclotron	H$_2$ ^{15}O
Fluorine-18 (^{18}F)	110	^{20}Ne (d, α)	Cyclotron	^{18}F-fatty acids, ^{18}F-2-deoxyglucose
Gallium-68 (^{68}Ga)	68	^{68}Ge (E.C.)	Generator	^{68}Ga microspheres
Rubidium-82 (^{82}Rb)	1.3	^{82}Sr (E.C.)	Generator	^{82}RbCl

POTASSIUM ANALOGUES

Background and theoretical basis for technique

The most widely used noninvasive technique for detecting clinical coronary artery disease in patients is exercise electrocardiography. The test requires the development of an exercise-induced imbalance between myocardial supply and demand distal to a coronary artery stenosis. The resultant myocardial ischemia is detected by the appearance of electrocardiographic changes and angina pectoris. The sensitivity of the test for detecting coronary artery disease is limited, particularly in patients with poor conditioning, since only myocardial supply and demand imbalances severe enough to produce ischemia can be detected. Furthermore, although the ischemic electrocardiographic changes can be localized to a particular left ventricular segment, the extent and severity of ischemia are difficult or impossible to quantitate. Radionuclide myocardial perfusion imaging during stress has several theoretical advantages over exercise electrocardiography. First, the technique should detect imbalances in myocardial perfusion before ischemia is apparent on the electrocardiogram. Second, the visualization of the ischemic myocardium in comparison with the normally perfused myocardium makes possible a quantitative estimate of the under-perfused area.

Prior to 1973, several gamma-emitting radionuclides had been employed to qualitatively assess regional myocardial perfusion at rest in patients with suspected coronary artery disease. These agents included radioisotopes of potassium (^{42}K, ^{43}K) and its analogues (^{129}Cs, ^{131}Cs, ^{86}Ru, ^{84}Ru) [1, 2]. These agents, which were efficiently extracted from the blood by the sodium–potassium ATPase system, were useful for detecting infarct. It was not until 1973, however, that potassium-43 was used to detect exercise-induced ischemia [3]. Rubidium-81 was used for myocardial imaging [4], and was found to have increased diagnostic accuracy in detecting coronary artery disease during exercise imaging compared with electrocardiographic exercise testing alone [5].

Kawana and associates suggested the use of thallium as a perfusion imaging agent based on its biologic similarities to potassium [6]. Thallium is similar to potassium in terms of organ distribution [7]. The principal photopeaks of thallium-201 are at 135 and 167 keV. Imaging is generally performed using the abundance of mercury X-rays at 69–83 keV. Thallium-201 has the advantages of more optimal lower photon energies and greater myocardial extraction (1.7%–3.7% of the administered dose) compared with potassium-43, rubidium-81, and cesium-129 [8, 9]. Strauss and associates [8] and Nielson and co-workers [10] have shown that the initial myocardial distribution of thallium-201 has a close linear relationship to regional myocardial blood flow. The first-pass myocardial extraction fraction is 88% [11], and the uptake of thallium-201 by cultured myocardial cells is described by a single exponential [12]. Used to obtain myocardial scintiscans in the goat, thallium-201 demonstrated peak myocardial concentrations 10–25 min after injection [7]. In 1976, thallium-201 imaging was combined with exercise as a noninvasive test for exercise-induced ischemia due to coronary artery disease [13, 14].

In 1977, Pohost and associates reported the disappearance of thallium-201 myocardial defects on initial postexercise images over a 2-h period following transient ischemia [15]. Defects observed on early postexercise images which filled in on the delayed images (thallium-201 redistribution) were felt to represent ischemia, whereas those that persisted were felt to represent scar (Figure 1). Since that time, numerous reports have appeared comparing the diagnostic accuracies of the qualitatively interpreted thallium-201 stress test and the electrocardiographic stress test. In a recent review, data summarized from multiple centers demonstrated a sensitivity of 82% for thallium-201 imaging compared with 60% for electrocardiographic stress testing ($p < 0.0001$) [16]. The specificities for the thallium-201 and electrocardiographic stress tests were 91% and 81%, respectively ($p < 0.05$).

Rest thallium-201 imaging has been used to detect remote and acute myocardial infarct [17, 18]. Wackers and associates demonstrated a thallium-201 defect in all 44 patients imaged within 6 h of an acute myocardial infarct [18]. After 24 h, only 72% of patients with acute myocardial infarct had defects detectable by thallium-201 imaging.

Pathophysiologic correlates of thallium-201 myocardial uptake have been studied in experimental canine infarct. In a canine model, regional thallium-201 uptake correlated well with the magnitude of tissue creatine phosphokinase depletion and microsphere estimates of transmural blood flow [19]. Even slight reductions in thallium-201 uptake (86% of normal) were associated with histopathologic evidence of necrosis. Buja and associates demonstrated a progressive reduction in myocardial blood flow between normal myocardium and the centers of experimental infarcts that correlated well with progressive reduction in thallium-201 uptake [20].

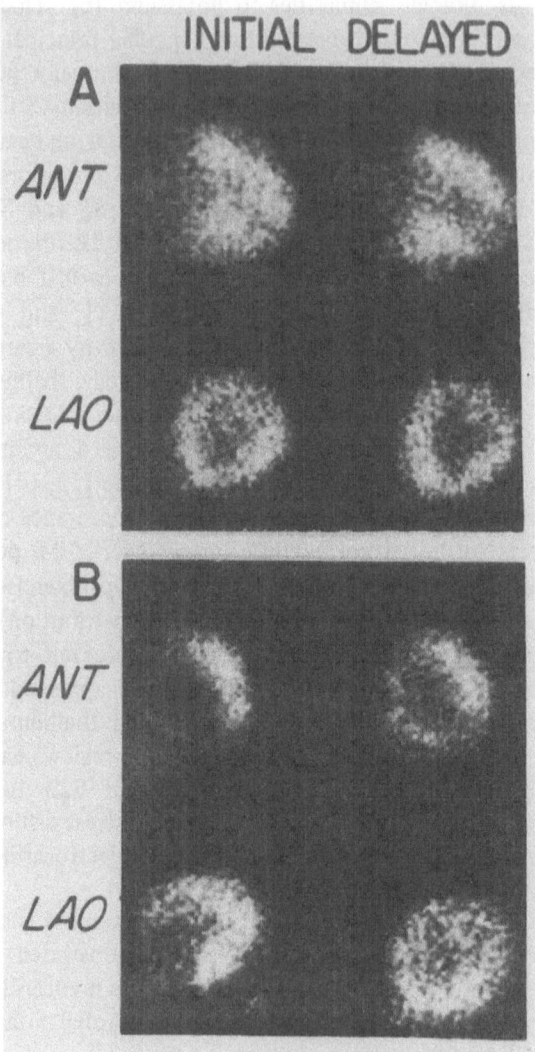

Figure 1. (*A*) Normal thallium-201 myocardial images immediately following exercise (initial) and 4 h later (delayed). Note the homogeneous distribution of tracer except for the apical and apical-inferior segments, where activity can normally be slightly lower. (*B*) Abnormal thallium-201 myocardial images. Note the inferior and apical defects on the initial anterior (ANT) view, and septal and apical-inferior defects on the initial left anterior oblique view (LAO). There is complete redistribution into the septal and apical-inferior segments (transient defect), partial redistribution into the inferior segment, and no redistribution into the apical segment (persistent defect).

Experimental studies

Although thallium-201 imaging is relatively sensitive for myocardial ischemia and infarct, there is considerable interobserver variance in the qualitative interpretation of thallium-201 defects [21]. Quantitative, semiautomated techniques might improve diagnostic accuracy. Such techniques might be useful for quantitating both the severity of ischemia and the extent of ischemic insult.

Thallium-201 defect size can be determined in a semiquantitative way and expressed as a percent of either the total left ventricular myocardial image or the left ventricular circumference [22]. Early attempts to measure the extent of ischemic insult (including ischemia and infarct) involved planimetry of the left ventricular outline and then the defect, expressing the defect as a percent of the total area or circumference (Figure 2). Using this type of approach,

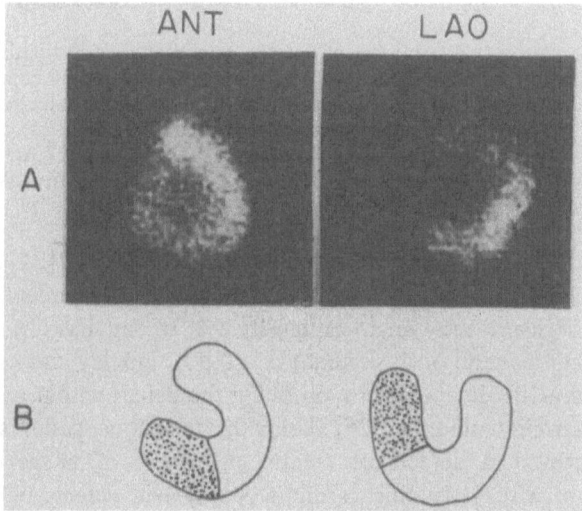

Figure 2. (*A*) Rest thallium-201 images with defects in a patient with an acute myocardial infarct. (*B*) Outlines of the left ventricular myocardium and the thallium-201 defect that were subsequently planimetered. The size of the infarct was the total area of the defect expressed as a percent of the total left ventricular area; ANT, anterior; LAO, left anterior oblique.

Wackers and associates found that thallium-201 defect size correlated with post-mortem infarct size in 23 patients who died from acute myocardial infarcts [23]. The size of infarct, as determined from schematic drawings of postmortem slices of heart, correlated well with the size determined from schematic drawings of the thallium-201 images ($r = 0.91$ for anterior infarct, $r = 0.97$ for inferior infarct, $r = 0.86$ for anterior-inferior infarct) (Figure 3). Niess and co-workers

300

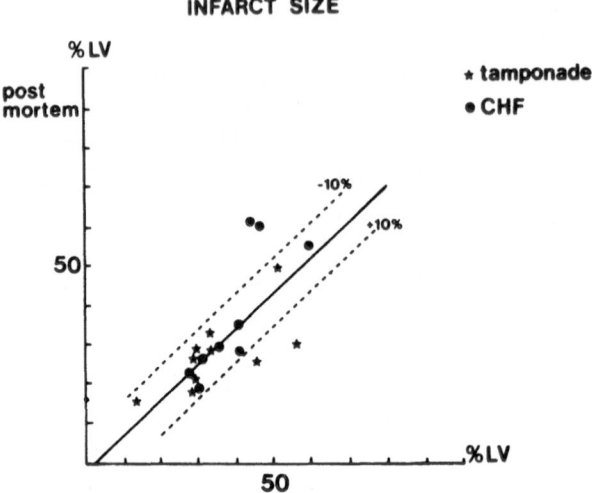

Figure 3. Relationship between size of infarct determined on the basis of postmortem findings and size of scintigraphically abnormal area as calculated by computer processing of schematic drawing of thallium-201 scintiscans. The dotted lines indicate a shift of the regression line by 10% of the total left ventricle; $n = 19$; $y = (0.88 \pm 0.21)x - (0.36 \pm 7.89)$; $r = 0.72$ for the whole group; $r = 0.91$ for anterior infarcts; $r = 0.97$ for inferior infarcts; $r = 0.86$ for anterior-inferior infarcts; CHF, congestive heart failure; LV, left ventricle. Reproduced from Wackers et al. [23] with permission of *Circulation.*

studied 32 patients an average of seven months after infarct [24]. Thallium-201 defect size (% circumference) correlated closely with the percent of abnormally contracting segment seen angiographically (% of end-diastolic circumference that was either akinetic or dyskinetic) ($r = 0.80$). Bulkley and associates determined thallium-201 defect size by outlining the defect within an outline of the left ventricular circumference [25]. Using this technique, patients with ischemic cardiomyopathy had defects of greater than 40% of image circumference, whereas those with idiopathic cardiomyopathy had defects of less than 20% of image circumference.

The application of computer approaches to planar thallium-201 image interpretation may provide a means for quantitating the severity as well as the extent of ischemia. The technique begins with an algorithm for subtracting the background for the thallium-201 image. The relative abnormal to normal myocardial concentration ratio of thallium-201 (and thus, perfusion) is then determined from the average of peak counts per picture element (pixel) in the abnormal and normal regions. Early use of this technique employed operator placed regions of interest over several segments of the left ventricular image. The average counts per pixel were then calculated by the computer for each region of interest. The region with the greatest number of counts per pixel was considered normally perfused. Regions with over 25% reduction in counts per pixel were considered abnormal. Using this technique, Verani et al. quantitated the extent of redistribution of thallium-201 on serial images after exercise in patients with coronary artery disease [26]. The quantitative technique was used to enhance objectivity in determining relative regional changes in activity over time. The authors were able to demonstrate that both infarcted and non-infarcted but jeopardized myocardium may display thallium-201 redistribution, especially when good-quality collaterals are present. Rubin and associates used this technique for interpreting stress thallium-201 images in patients with idiopathic hypertrophic subaortic stenosis and anginal symptoms [27]. No significant exercise-induced thallium-201 perfusion defect was found in nine of ten patients with idiopathic hypertrophic subaortic stenosis and normal coronary arteries. They concluded that this technique could assist in ruling out significant coronary artery disease in such patients.

Nelson and associates used a similar approach for determining infarct size in experimental canine myocardial infarction [28]. Thallium-201 images were obtained in the left lateral and left anterior oblique projections 48 h after ligation of the left anterior descending artery. Scintigraphic results were compared with tissue measurements of infarct volume calculated from thallium-201 autoradiograms and nitro-blue tetrazolium-stained tissue slices. After background subtraction and outline of the left ventricular perimeter, a region of interest selected to represent normal myocardial tissue was defined near the basal left ventricular border remote from the area of perfusion defect. Picture elements (representing an area of approximately 2 x 2 mm) that had count levels less than a given percent (threshold) of the average level for the normal region were considered to represent infarcted tissue. Scintigraphic infarct size was calculated as the total number of picture elements with subthreshold counts divided by the total number of picture elements in the left ventricular region. Scintigraphic infarct size in the left lateral and left anterior oblique projections correlated with tissue infarct size with $r = 0.88$, and 0.75, respectively, for thallium autoradiography, and $r = 0.71$ and 0.70, respectively, for tissue staining (Figure 4). These data suggest that thallium-201 imaging is a reasonably reliable approach for evaluating infarct size. However, initial thallium-201 distribution does not always depict infarcted zones only. Gewirtz and co-workers have demonstrated reduced distribution of thallium-201 to ischemic zones at rest in patients with severely stenotic but not occluded coronary arteries [29]. When zones of ischemia are depicted on the initial images, delayed images will generally demonstrate thallium-201 redistribution. Furthermore, Berger and colleagues have demonstrated, using dual radionuclide studies of experimental acute canine myocardial infarct, that infarcts on thallium-201 images are smaller than on technetium-99m images [30]. The smaller thallium-201 estimate of infarct size may be due to relatively normal perfused subepicardium overlying infarcted subendocardium at the infarct periphery.

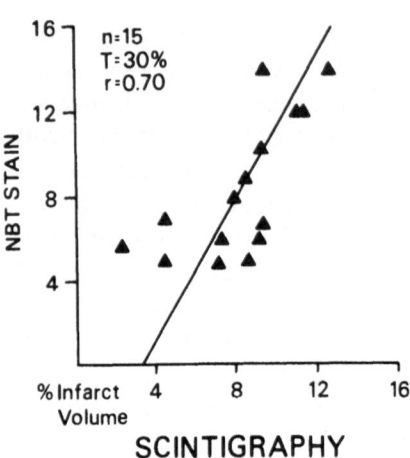
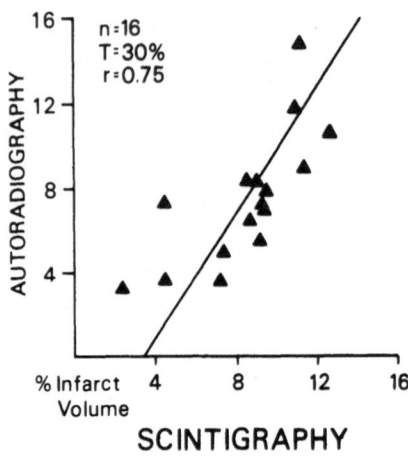

Figure 4. Relation of scintigraphic to tissue infarct size at 30% threshold level in the left anterior oblique projection. Solid line represents the regression relation; *n*, number of dogs studied; *r*, correlation coefficient; T, threshold level; NBT, nitro-blue tetrazolium. Reproduced from Nelson et al. [28] with permission of the *American Journal of Cardiology*.

More recently, planar thallium-201 images have been quantitated using a computer circumferential profile method [31]. After background subtraction, an operator-selected point is placed in the center of the ventricular cavity (Figure 5). Radii are then constructed from the image center to the periphery. The greatest count per pixel along each radius is plotted against angular position. The resultant plot is superimposed in an activity band representing the mean ± 2 standard deviations determined from normal volunteers. Activity falling below the 2 standard deviation limit is considered a defect. The percentage of radii with decreased peak activity represents defect size. Bulkley and associates have used this technique to correlate scintigraphic and postmortem infarct size in patients with fatal myocardial injury [32]. Using an operator-defined outer border of the left ventricle, this group determined the average thallium-201 activity per picture element along each radius from the center to the periphery of the ventricle. In 24 autopsied hearts those with large scintigraphic defects generally had large infarcts. However, the correlation between absolute thallium-201 defect score and the percent necrosis was poor ($r = 0.27$). Berger and colleagues have developed a similar technique for quantitating thallium-201 images [33]. These investigators determined relative myocardial activity by observing profiles crossing preselected regions on the myocardial image. Time—activity curves were then constructed from peak profile counts from various myocardial regions. Segments with greater than 25% reduction in activity relative to the area of most intense uptake were considered abnormal. Using this technique, these investigators have demonstrated thallium-201 redistribution at rest in patients with stable and unstable angina pectoris.

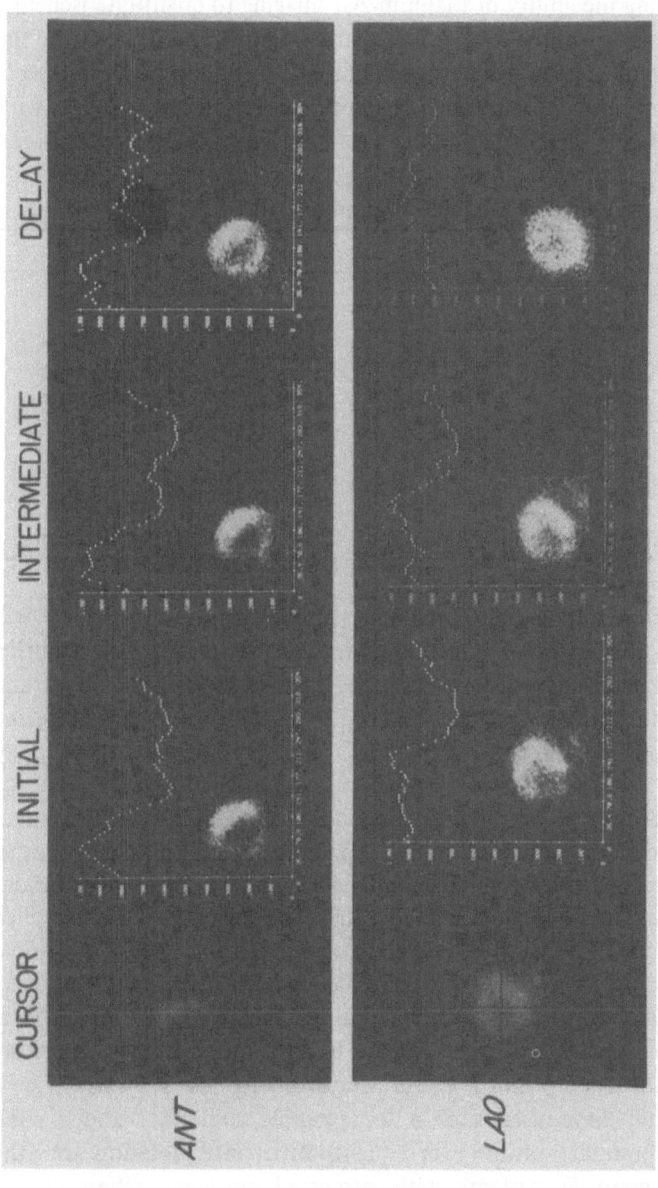

Figure 5. Quantitation of myocardial thallium-201 distribution using the circumferential profile method. The *left column* demonstrates the position of the cursors that have been set by the operator at the center of the ventricular cavity. Starting as 12 o'clock and proceeding *clockwise*, the program constructs radial lines from the center to the periphery and plots the maximal picture element counts on the *x*, *y* graph. This figure demonstrates quantitation of the transient and persistent defects observed in the same patient presented in Figure 2B.

Recent developments in collimators, computer programs, and cameras have made possible emission tomography using thallium-201. These techniques hold promise for improving the ability of thallium-201 imaging to quantitate ischemia and infarct. Subtraction of background activity is a major difficulty to the planar techniques that can be reduced or eliminated by the tomographic techniques. Furthermore, tomography enables depth resolution not possible with two-dimensional planar imaging. Table 3 lists some approaches to emission

Table 3. Emission tomography techniques using myocardial perfusion tracers

Technique	Camera type
Techniques using unmodified standard gamma camera	
a) 7-Pinhole	Standard gamma
b) Slanthole (rotating)	Standard gamma
c) Coded-aperture	Standard gamma
Techniques requiring special cameras	
a) Positron coincidence	Positron
b) Single-photon	Humongotron
c) Fresnel zone-plate	Zone-plate camera

tomography. Emission tomographic techniques using the positron camera will be discussed later. Single photon emission computerized tomography requiring modified gamma camera systems are described by Keyes [34], Dymond and associates [35], and Murphy and co-workers [36, 37]. The reader is referred to the article by Holman et al. for a discussion of Fresnel zone-plate tomography [38].

Tomographic techniques employing unmodified standard gamma cameras utilize special collimators containing multiple pinholes or multiple slant parallel holes that collect sets of data from different angles. The data from these various perspectives are used for tomographic reconstruction. The most widely applied such technique employs a stationary seven-pinhole collimator and a wide-field Anger scintillation camera. The seven pinholes acquire data simultaneously and project the data onto seven independent regions of the camera crystal (Figure 6). Multiple planes are reconstructed using a multiplicative algorithm and variation of the superposition relationships among the projected views. Vogel and associates have used such a tomographic collimator and a computerized circumferential profile for quantitative interpretation of the thallium-201 tomogram in patients with suspected coronary artery disease [31, 39]. In 42 patients, tomographic images and quantitative interpretation were more sensitive for coronary artery disease (95%) than standard planar imaging (74%). Unfortunately, the seven-pinhole tomographic technique has considerable depth distortion such that near resolution is approximately 0.5 cm

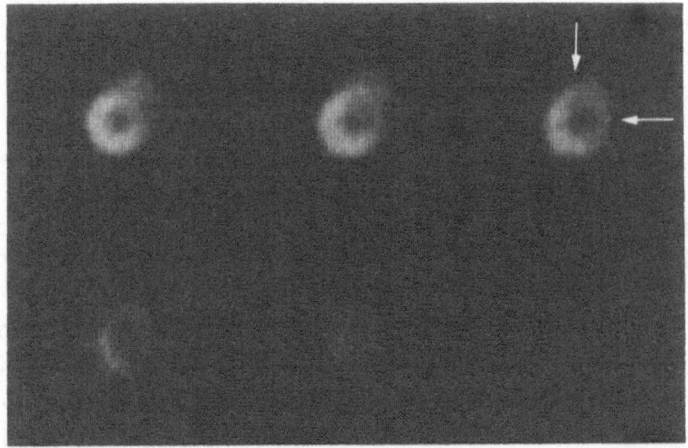

Figure 6. Tomographic reconstructions of seven-pinhole collimator 50° left anterior oblique image obtained 2 h after thallium-201 administration in a patient with occlusions of the left anterior descending and right coronary arteries. Tomographic planes start at apex (*top left image*) and proceed to base (*bottom right image*). Arrows indicate septal and apical-inferior defects.

while far resolution is approximately 2–3 cm. Thus, absolute quantitation is impossible. Francisco et al. used thallium-201, seven-pinhole tomography and quantitative circumferential profile analysis after maximal coronary vasodilation with dipyridamole [40]. These techniques in combination were highly sensitive (94%) and specific (100%) for coronary artery disease.

High-quality thallium-201 tomographic images have also been produced with a coded aperture collimator that opens and closes multiple pinholes in a predetermined sequence [41], and with a rotating collimator containing multiple slant holes [42]. Although each of these techniques hold promise for improved quantitation of myocardial perfusion images, the advantage of multipinhole imaging over planar imaging remains to be demonstrated.

RADIOACTIVE PARTICLES

Background and theoretical basis for technique

Ueda and associates first described canine regional myocardial blood flow measurement by ^{131}I-labeled macroaggregated albumin in 1965 [43]. When these small particles were injected into the coronary circulation, they were distributed in proportion to regional myocardial blood flow. The particles were trapped in precapillary and capillary beds, and their activity could be counted in a well counter. The relative density of deposition is generally higher in the endocardial region, and large particles are deposited preferentially in regions of high flow [44]. In 1966, myocardial imaging using radioactive particles was first done in canine models [45]. This technique demonstrated small vessel occlusions and flush coronary branch occlusions in experimental animals when the coronary angiograms appeared normal [46]. The injection of radioactive particles directly into the coronary arteries in man with subsequent myocardial imaging was reported by Endo and associates in 1970 [47]. The procedure has been shown to produce no adverse effects when particle size and numbers are not excessive [46, 48–50].

Human myocardial imaging with radioactive particles utilizes either macro-aggregates of albumin (MAA) or human albumin microspheres (HAM) labeled with ^{99m}Tc, ^{113m}In, ^{123}I, or ^{133}I. Particle sizes ranging from 10 to 50 microns are commercially available. Rest studies are performed by selectively injecting the right and left coronary arteries with MAA or HAM labeled with two different radioisotopes. Composite images are then produced by computer summation of the right and left coronary images. Rest studies can also be performed with one radioisotope by injecting one-third of the labeled MAA or HAM selectively into the right coronary artery and two-thirds into the left coronary artery. Unfortunately, this percentage of microspheres injected into each coronary artery must be an estimate of the actual distribution of coronary artery blood flow. Since the relative flows are unlikely to be precisely estimated, inhomogeneities on images between the right and left coronary artery distributions must be interpreted with caution. Furthermore, streaming can lead to selective accumulation of activity in either the left anterior descending or the left circumflex artery during the left main coronary artery injection and lead to apparent inhomogeneities.

A second radioisotope can be selectively injected into the left main coronary artery after contrast-agent-induced coronary hyperemia (Figure 7). This approach provides a physiologic basis for assessing the significance of a coronary artery stenosis [51]. Following catheterization, imaging is performed with a standard gamma camera in several projections. Images are collected for each isotope when multiple isotopes are employed.

Experimental studies and applications

Myocardial defects seen after injection of radioactive particles in the basal state have correlated with clinical evidence of a prior myocardial infarct and angiographic evidence of left ventricular contraction abnormalities [52–54]. Hamilton and associates demonstrated scar by direct inspection at the time of surgery in nine of 13 patients with scan defects at rest, and no evidence of scar

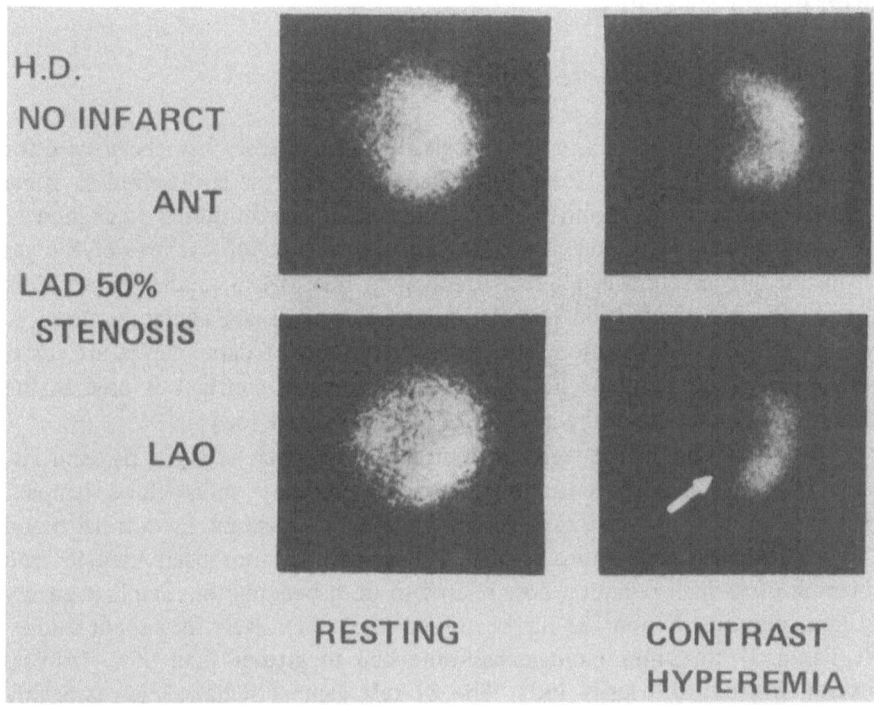

H.D.
NO INFARCT

ANT

LAD 50%
STENOSIS

LAO

RESTING

CONTRAST
HYPEREMIA

Figure 7. Radioactive microsphere anterior (ANT) and left anterior oblique (LAO) images at rest with one isotope (*left column*) and a second isotope 6 s after the induction of coronary hyperemia by radiographic contrast material (*right column*). The resting images are normal. Following hyperemia, there is a maldistribution of activity (arrow) away from the stenotic left anterior descending coronary artery bed. Reproduced from Ritchie et al. [53] with permission of *Radiology.*

in eight of eight patients with no scan defects at rest [55]. Stress-induced regional malperfusion can be assessed using injection of radioactive particles during contrast hyperemia [56]. Of 39 patients with coronary artery disease, 37 were found to have abnormal images at rest or during coronary hyperemia [57].

Methods for quantitating ischemic myocardium by using radioactive particle imaging have not been well studied in man. However, Gould et al. evaluated regional myocardial perfusion in dogs during coronary hyperemia in order to quantify stress-induced maldistribution of flow [56]. Left coronary artery flow was determined by using electromagnetic flowmeters on the anterior descending and circumflex coronary arteries and by double radionuclide studies. Coronary flows varied from basal to maximum hyperemia. Malperfusion due to coronary stenosis quantified with the gamma camera correlated closely with electromagnetic flowmeter results ($r = 0.96$).

DIFFUSIBLE TRACERS

Background and theoretical basis for technique

Several chemically inert and physiologically inactive gases have been used for determining myocardial blood flow. The radioactive gas is dissolved in saline and infused into the coronary artery. The initial distribution is a function of regional myocardial blood flow. The subsequent rate of washout of the gas from the myocardium is a direct function of myocardial capillary flow. Most frequently, the early (nonrecirculation) washout data are computer fitted to a monoexponential equation, although other forms of data analysis are sometimes used. The resultant myocardial clearance rate constant is used in the Kety formula that yields the myocardial blood flow rate [58].

Early nonradionuclide techniques utilized gases such as N_2O, H_2, and He, and measured gas concentrations in serial coronary sinus blood samples. Krypton-85 was the first radioactive gas used to measure myocardial blood flow in experimental animals [59]. Krypton-85 has not been used in man because of its high radiation dose related to both beta photons and high-energy gamma photons. Xenon-133 has been used most extensively for patient studies. It has a 1- to 2-min biologic half-time due to greater than 95% first-pass excretion from the lungs [60]. The 81-keV gamma radiation is reasonably good for external imaging. Single global myocardial washout curves were initially obtained using ^{133}Xe and a single-crystal gamma camera [61]. More recently, multiple regional myocardial washout curves have been obtained by using multicrystal gamma cameras or single-crystal gamma cameras and compartmental regional blood flow analysis [62, 63].

Krypton-81m is another radionuclide used for patient studies. The 190-keV gamma-ray energy is good for external myocardial imaging. The radiation hazard for imaging doses is negligible. The ultrashort half-line of 13 s enables sequential experiments repeated at brief intervals [64].

Experimental studies and applications

Xenon-133 myocardial perfusion studies demonstrate homogeneous myocardial distribution initially in patients with normal coronary arteries [65]. Left ventricular regional myocardial blood flow rates are slightly inhomogeneous in these patients (Figure 8). Patients with angina pectoris and normal coronary arteries have been found to have normal regional myocardial blood flow patterns [66]. Cannon and associates have determined mean left ventricular myocardial blood flows in patients with and without significant coronary artery disease [67]. Mean blood flows were not significantly different from normal in patients with single-vessel disease and subcritical disease. Mean left ventricular blood

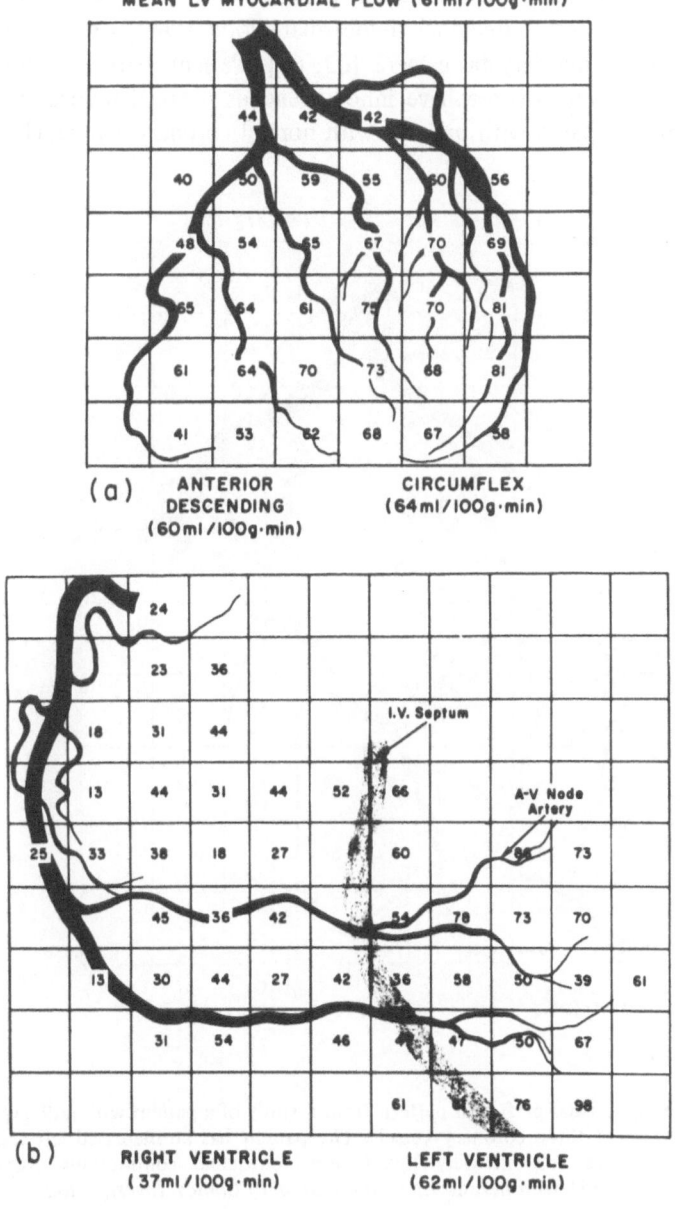

Figure 8. (*a*) The myocardial perfusion pattern from a study of a subject with a normal left coronary arteriogram. (*b*) The myocardial perfusion pattern from a study of a patient with an arteriographically normal dominant right coronary artery. Reproduced from Cannon et al. [67] with permission of the *Journal of Clinical Investigation*.

310

flows were significantly decreased in patients with two- and three-vessel coronary artery disease. Regional myocardial blood flow patterns have been examined using a multicrystal camera [63, 67]. Patients with two- and three-vessel coronary artery disease have inhomogeneous regional myocardial blood flow patterns compared with patients with normal coronary arteries (Figure 9).

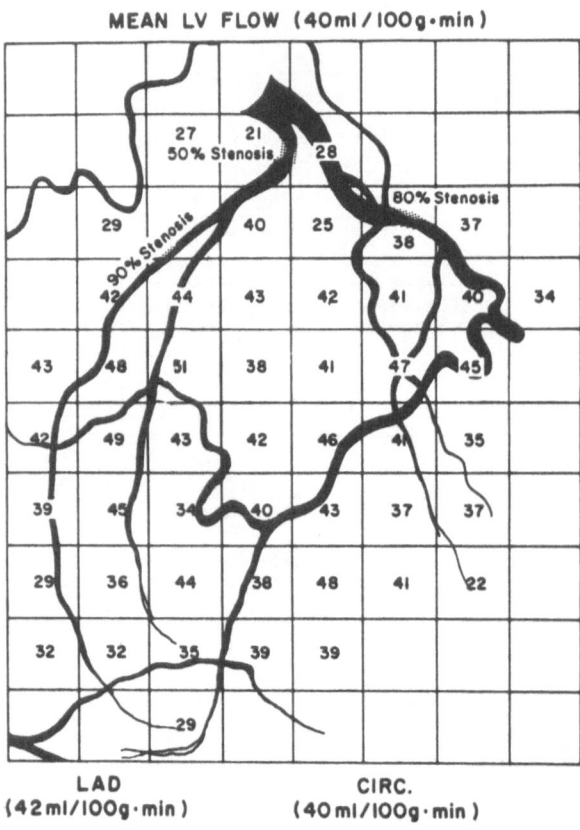

Figure 9. The myocardial perfusion pattern from a study of a patient with radiographically significant disease of three coronary vessels. The patient has an increased left ventricular end-diastolic pressure and diffusely hypokinetic ventricular contractions. Reproduced from Cannon et al. [67] with permission of the *Journal of Clinical Investigation*.

Patients with myocardial infarct have markedly decreased regional blood flow [68], and patients with myocardial aneurysm have almost no washout [69]. Patients with stable coronary artery disease may have normal regional myocardial flow patterns at rest, yet abnormal patterns after pacing [70] and after taking coronary vasodilators [71, 72].

Selwyn and co-workers have used the ultrashort half-line properties of ^{81m}Kr to obtain continuous gamma camera myocardial images during a constant infusion of ^{81m}Kr into the right and left aortic sinuses and before, during, and after atrial pacing [73]. Six patients with no significant coronary artery disease (less than 50% luminal stenosis) had uniform regional myocardial perfusion at rest and during stress. Seven patients with greater than 70% stenosis of one or more coronary arteries demonstrated reversible regional defects in myocardial perfusion during pacing stress.

Determination of regional myocardial blood flow patterns with ^{133}Xe and ^{81m}Kr requires cardiac catheterization and has several technical difficulties associated with myocardial fat uptake, tracer recirculation, cardiac motion, and the inability to distinguish endocardial from epicardial blood flow. Furthermore, images of tracer distribution relate not only to its myocardial concentration but also to the thickness of myocardium in a particular region. Thus, the appearance of reduced activity with pacing may be related in part to ventricular dilatation or changes in regional wall motion consequent to pacing-induced ischemia. Although this technique holds promise for quantitating regional myocardial blood flow patterns and thus the degree of ischemia, these factors may limit its ultimate clinical utility.

POSITRON IMAGING AND PERFUSION TECHNIQUES

Although positron camera imaging systems are not yet widely available, there is widespread interest in their use in quantifying myocardial perfusion. This is because this imaging method takes advantage of certain unique properties of positron-emitting radionuclides. In this section, the technical aspects and experience with positron imaging of ischemia will be reviewed.

Background and theoretical basis for technique

Radionuclides

The relevant positron-emitting radionuclides are listed in Table 2 [74, 75]. All have a relative excess of nuclear protons and emit positrons (positively charged particles of similar mass to electrons). Most have a relatively short half-life, which has two advantages. First, a greater quantity of activity can be given with a lower or equal dose of radiation and, second, multiple studies can be performed within a short time. On the other hand, the short radionuclide half-life has the disadvantage of requiring on-site radionuclide production, generally using a cyclotron close to the positron camera. Of the radionuclides listed, only ^{68}Ga and ^{82}Rb can be produced within a generator as the daughter of a much longer-lived parent radionuclide. Major industrial organizations, using the generator, can produce these radionuclides for a long period of time and then distribute them to institutions that do not have cyclotrons. All other radionuclides used with the positron camera require on-site cyclotron production, which necessitates a large investment of space and money, although recently developed, smaller tabletop cyclotrons may make such acquisitions more feasible.

Carbon, nitrogen, and oxygen are basic constituents of organic compounds and enable the potential labeling of a large variety of biologic compounds with positron-emitting radionuclides (^{11}C, ^{13}N, ^{15}O). Alternatively, these tracers can be administered as simple compounds, such as ^{11}CO, $C^{15}O_2$, ^{13}NH$_3$, or $H_2^{15}O$. Because these radionuclides may substitute for components of metabolic substrates, such as carbohydrates, fatty acids and amino acids, tracer uptake in the myocardium is related in part to myocardial metabolism of the particular substrate. Therefore, biochemical as well as structural data may be derived. Rubidium-82 can be used as a monovalent cation similar to thallium-201, as previously explained. Its uptake is slower in regions of ischemia since its supply to these regions is reduced. Gallium-68 is eluted from a generator and can be used to label albumin, microspheres, or phosphonates.

The mechanism by which these radionuclides emit photons is unique and offers special advantages for imaging. When a positron emitted from the nucleus interacts with an orbiting electron, these two particles annihilate. The mass of the particles is totally converted into energy in the form of two gamma rays that travel in opposite directions. Each has an energy of 511 keV. Opposing scintillation detectors within the positron camera are used to detect these two photons, as illustrated in Figure 10. Because these gamma photons have relatively high energy, they are less attenuated by the chest wall compared with lower-energy photons used in conventional gamma camera imaging. On the other hand, the beta particles produced by positron-emitting radionuclides have low energy and upon escape from the atom of origin are likely to deposit their kinetic energy in surrounding tissues. This results in a significantly higher radiation dose for a given quantity of radionuclide compared with conventional single gamma photon radiotracers.

Instrumentation

The ability to perform positron camera imaging is primarily limited by the availability of a medical cyclotron and the ability to develop radiopharmaceuticals [76]. The positron camera is characterized by a configuration of multiple detectors arranged in a multicrystal array opposite one another. There are two basic types. One type developed by Brownell and colleagues at Massachusetts General Hospital consists of two opposing multicrystal detector heads. These heads rotate around the patient in order to obtain tomographic information. The second configuration first developed by Ter-Pogossian et al.

POSITRON DECAY AND CONVERSION

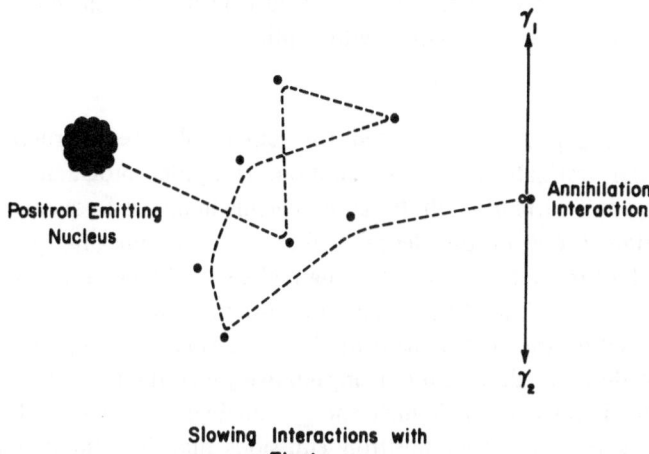

Figure 10. Illustration of the fate of a positron emission. The positron is emitted from the nucleus at high energy. It then loses kinetic energy as it interacts with nearby electrons. Eventually, the positron slows enough to combine with an electron and the two particles annihilate. This produces two back-to-back gamma emissions each having an energy of 511 keV (labeled γ_1 and γ_2).

at Washington University is a ring of paired opposing detectors that collects tomographic information by repositioning the patient within the ring. More recent versions employ multiple rings to collect several tomographic sections simultaneously. The ring configuration is more widely employed at the present time.

Only photons hitting opposing crystals simultaneously or within an extremely short time (i.e., 10s) are registered within the image. This process, called coincident detection, provides electronic collimation by not allowing scattered emissions, which would present as single events on only one of the two opposing crystals. However, not all coincident events are true. Random coincidences may occur as a result of random scatter simultaneously striking opposing detectors. These are often due to partially deflected photons and therefore are in part filtered by low-energy collimation. A built-in correction is necessary, however, because the number of random coincident events is substantial, increasing with the square of the activity to be detected. This is accomplished by sampling the events arriving at opposing detectors after adding a finite dead time to one of the two detectors. This provides a coincident kind of background correction to be subtracted from the total coincidence events. Because of the logarithmic increase in the occurrence of random coincident events with higher levels of activity, total activity that may be administered must be limited.

This approach has two advantages over gamma imaging. First, it is tomographic in nature. Second, because each coincident event is a result of two photons traveling a similar total distance, no matter how near or far the source is from the detector, there is no attenuation with depth.

Tomography

Positron imaging is ideally suited for tomographic reconstruction. Using rotational and translateral detector motion, computer programs can isolate the emissions at a certain depth. Because ischemia in man is frequently regional, its localization is one of the desirable features of an imaging system. Tomography enables separation of overlapping regions of the heart and in this way improves resolution. The development of positron emission tomography has been facilitated by the development of X-ray transmission-computerized tomography, providing a method of producing relatively high-resolution cross-sectional images [77]. Because of their high energy and high penetrance, the back-to-back photons resulting from positron emissions may be computer processed in a manner similar to X-ray tomography. At present, tomographic slices obtained using positron-emission tomography are 1–2 cm thick and the intrinsic resolution is 1–2 cm. The intrinsic resolution of X-ray transmission tomography is in the millimeter range.

Experimental studies and applications

Tracers with flow-related uptake

The potassium analogue, thallium-201, is being widely utilized clinically to evaluate regional blood flow and myocardial integrity. Rubidium-82 can also be used to obtain myocardial perfusion images [75, 78–80]. Because of the short half-life of this substance (75 s), only early distribution (perfusion) images can be obtained. The redistribution phenomenon cannot be assessed. However, this tracer is ideally suited for serial evaluation of regional blood flow using multiple injections. It also has the advantage of being generator produced, thereby obviating the need for a nearby medical cyclotron. However, since its half-life is so short, tomography is possible only after injection of a very large dose or during multiple or continuous infusions.

Rubidium-82 uptake is determined by myocardial blood flow to viable myocardial cells. Experimental studies using planar and transverse images have clearly demonstrated the feasibility of using this agent to detect regions of diminished flow. In a study of eight dogs, intravenous nitroglycerin (30–75 µg/min) was begun 20 min after occlusion of the left anterior descending coronary artery [79]. The sum of ST segment elevations in the 12 epicardial leads and [82]Rb images were obtained prior to occlusion, 15 min post occlusion and 15 min post nitroglycerin. Transmural myocardial blood flow was serially assessed by the left atrial injection of radiolabeled microspheres. Nitroglycerin resulted in a decrease in mean arterial pressure, a 50% decrease in the sum of ST segment elevations, and a 55% increase in ischemic blood flow. These changes correlated well ($p < 0.05$) with improvement in rubidium images as determined by comparing computer-derived regions of interest over ischemic and normal myocardium. A similar approach has been used to quantitate the hyperemic response occurring after transient coronary occlusion in dogs. Pilot studies have been performed in man, but are limited by the need to wait at least 60 s after the infusion is complete to clear blood activity, the loss of tracer activity due to the short (75 s) physical half-life, and the availability of a generator with insignificant breakthrough of the parent isotope, ^{82}Sr ($t_{1/2} = 27$ days).

Freely diffusible tracer

Preliminary work has been performed utilizing oxygen-15-labeled water as a freely diffusible tracer to quantitate myocardial blood flow after the intracoronary injection [75, 81, 82]. Perfusion rates were calculated using data processing analogous to studies of xenon washout. This work confirms that a positron imaging system can quantitate blood flow, although advantages over the conventional xenon method have not been demonstrated.

Metabolic substrates

The use of positron-emitting radionuclides to label metabolic substrates is a unique application of positron imaging. The most widely used substrate is ^{13}N-labeled ammonia [75, 83–86]. The radiopharmaceutical exists in two forms, ^{13}NH$_3$ and ^{13}NH$_4^+$, which are in equilibrium. At physiologic pH, the ionized form predominates. After intravenous injection, NH$_4^+$ is cleared rapidly from the blood with as much as 80%–90% being taken up in the first pass. Similar to other monovalent cations, extraction is related to myocardial blood flow and Na$^+$-K$^+$-ATPase membrane transport. However, extraction of ^{13}NH$_4^+$ is not entirely flow related. Extraction fraction is reduced with increased flow and increased with decreased flow. This may happen in part because the tracer, in the form of ^{13}NH$_3$, is also freely diffusible and is metabolized in the synthesis of glutamine and urea. Therefore, tracer extraction kinetics is complex [83, 85].

Nitrogen-13 ammonia defects demonstrated experimentally and clinically have corresponded to regions of ischemia and infarct, although the images have been limited by overlap due to lung and liver uptake. Quantitation of ^{13}NH$_3$ uptake in tomographic images has been reported by Gould et al. [84]. Stenoses of 43%–66% diameter narrowing were applied to the left circumflex artery of three chronically instrumented dogs and ^{13}NH$_3$ emission computed tomography was performed before and after infusing dipyridamole. Quantitation involved deriving absolute activity per mCi of the injected dose in multiple regions of interest. Absolute activity in corresponding regions of interest in neighboring planes was averaged. Activity in regions of reduced flow (circumflex artery territory) was compared with activity in the region of normal flow (left anterior descending artery territory). The data indicated that stenoses as low as 47% produced detectable reductions in $^{13}NH_3$ uptake on positron tomograms.

This technique was also applied clinically to 23 patients, five normal volunteers and 18 patients with coronary artery disease, having a total of 31 stenoses of 40%–100% diameter [86]. No perfusion defects were seen in the five normals. Of the 31 stenoses, 24 were detected. The seven stenoses not detected included the least severe stenosis in four of the five patients with triple-vessel coronary artery disease. Therefore, positron-emission tomography using $^{13}NH_3$ and dipyridamole-induced hyperemia can detect coronary stenoses, although the value of this approach compared with thallium-201 imaging in patients remains to be demonstrated.

Carbon-11-labeled palmitic acid is another substrate that has been studied, [75, 87, 88]. In normal dogs, regional ^{11}C-palmitate uptake has been shown to be homogeneous. When ^{11}C-palmitate time-activity data were derived from 1.5-cm^3 segments of the myocardium, both at rest and with augmentation of cardiac work by atropine or cardiac pacing, the average rate constant varied regionally by less than 11% [89]. During ischemia, there was diminished uptake of ^{11}C-palmitate as a result of reduced perfusion and reduced fatty acid oxidation.

This technique was recently applied to 28 patients with acute myocardial infarcts [88]. Infarct size was not assessed based on absolute uptake, but determined by a geometric reconstruction of the tomographic sections. Regions with 50% or less of maximal uptake were considered regions of acute infarct. These areas were planimetered and the areas of infarct within each slice were then summed to derive a volume that was then converted to a mass of myocardium infarcted. This value correlated closely with an enzymatic estimate of infarct size derived from creatine kinase curves ($r = 0.92$). Furthermore, in four patients, myocardial infarct size was determined by ^{11}C-palmitate imaging one month later and the method was found to be highly reproducible.

Although ^{11}C-palmitate emission tomography appears capable of assessing the size of an acute myocardial infarct (in the absence of a prior infarct), its use to quantitate fatty acid oxidation remains questionable. The kinetics of ^{11}C-palmitate are complex. Its distribution is related in part to regional perfusion and in part to metabolic factors. For example, an inverse relationship has been shown between the half-life of ^{11}C-palmitate and cardiac work. The tracer entering the cell may be included in the metabolic pathway of the fatty acid, or it may be incorporated into triglyceride stores. It is not presently possible to distinguish between uptake related to fatty acid oxidation and uptake due to storage by external imaging.

Because of the problem of sorting out the potential complex metabolic fate of both NH_3 and palmitate, the use of a tracer that participates in only one pathway would be preferred. One substrate that may satisfy this requirement is 2-deoxyglucose [75, 90–92]. This has been labeled with ^{18}F and has been used for studies of cerebral metabolism. Preliminary work in the heart suggests that it may be initially metabolized in a manner similar to glucose (via phosphorylation), but then is trapped in the cell as a hexose monophosphate, not entering any more of the metabolic pathways that glucose enters. Therefore, measurement of its presence reflects only glucose uptake. In five dogs, ischemia was produced by left anterior descending coronary artery stenosis and atrial pacing. Quantitation of $^{13}NH_3$ images in regions of ischemia in these dogs suggested a 47% decrease in flow and ^{18}F-deoxyglucose images indicated a 19% decrease in glucose uptake. Therefore, there was less reduction in tracer uptake than the decrease in regional blood flow. This suggests that ischemic myocardium extracts more glucose than normal myocardium.

Although the above substances have been the most widely used ones, others have been suggested, including ^{11}C-acetate, ^{13}N-glutamine, ^{13}N-asparagine, and ^{18}F-long-chain fatty acids. Few extensive quantitative imaging studies have been performed on these substances [75, 93, 94].

Radionuclide particles

Gallium-68 microspheres have been used to quantitate regional blood flow [75, 95]. The use of microspheres requires direct injection into the left heart or coronary arteries. Although the feasibility of this approach has been demonstrated, it has not been widely applied.

In summary, although positron emission tomography has great potential for studying cardiac metabolism and determining the extent of ischemic damage or infarct, its use is greatly compromised by the need for an on-site cyclotron. As with any tracer, the myocardial uptake of the substances after intravenous injection is largely determined by perfusion and it is difficult to separate metabolic from perfusion factors in tracer kinetics. The more widespread use of this modality awaits the development of radionuclide generators or smaller, less expensive cyclotrons. Furthermore, the clinical advantages of positron-emission tomography remain to be demonstrated.

RECOMMENDATIONS FOR CLINICAL USE

Although the use of positron imaging has been limited, the method has important potential applications. It can potentially analyze perfusion kinetics in a manner similar to gamma camera imaging, although this alone may not justify the expense of such studies. Its value lies in the fact that the techniques are ideally suited for quantitation and tomographic reconstruction because of the lack of attenuation with depth and coincident detection. Furthermore, the radionuclides enable imaging with physiologic as well as pharmacologic tracers, which provide noninvasive studies of both perfusion and metabolism. Further studies in developing radiopharmaceutical imaging techniques and quantitative programs are needed before its clinical value can be determined. At present, the high cost of a positron camera and cyclotron limit the clinical utility of the technique. Determination of regional myocardial flow patterns with ^{133}Xe requires cardiac catheterization and has several technical difficulties associated with myocardial fat uptake, ^{133}Xe recirculation, cardiac motion, and the inability to distinguish endocardial from epicardial blood flow. Myocardial imaging with radioactive particles also requires cardiac catheterization. Streaming and the necessity of separate right and left coronary artery injections are serious disadvantages. Myocardial perfusion imaging using potassium analogues is noninvasive and requires a standard gamma camera. The quantitation of ischemic and infarcted myocardium is limited by two-dimensional imaging with the possible superimposition of normal and abnormal myocardium. Tomographic techniques hold promise for improving the ability of thallium-201 imaging to quantitate ischemic and infarcted myocardium.

REFERENCES

1. Romhildt DW, Adolph RJ, Sodd VJ, Levenson NI, August LS, Nishiyama H, Berke RA: Cesium-129 myocardial scintigraphy to detect myocardial infarction. Circulation 48:1242, 1973.
2. Romhildt DW, Ashare AB, Adolph RJ, Levenson NI, Wee WG, Sodd VJ, August LS: Cesium-129 myocardial scintigraphy to quantify myocardial infarction in dogs. J Nucl Med 17:247, 1976.
3. Zaret BL, Strauss HW, Martin ND, Wells HP, McGowan RL, Flamm MD: Noninvasive regional myocardial perfusion with radioactive potassium. Study of patients at rest, with exercise and during angina pectoris. N Engl J Med 288:809, 1973.
4. Carr EA Jr, Beierwaltes WH, Wegst AV, Bartlett JD Jr: Myocardial scanning with rubidium-86. J Nucl Med 3:76, 1962.
5. Berman DS, Salel AF, DeNardo GL, Mason DT: Noninvasive detection of regional myocardial ischemia using rubidium-81 and the scintillation camera: comparison with stress electrocardiography in patients with arteriographically documented coronary stenosis. Circulation 52:619, 1975.
6. Kawana M, Krisek H, Porter J, Lathrop KA, Charleston D, Harper PV: Use of ^{199}Tl as a potassium analogue in scanning [abstr]. J Nucl Med 11:333, 1970.
7. Bradley-Moore PR, Lebowitz E, Greene MW, Atkins HL, Ansari AN: Thallium-201 for medical use. II. Biologic behavior. J Nucl Med 16:156, 1975.

8. Strauss HW, Harrison K, Langan JK, Lebowitz E, Pitt B: Thallium-201 for myocardial imaging: relation of thallium-201 to regional myocardial perfusion. Circulation 51:641, 1975.

9. Lebowitz E, Greene MW, Fairchild R, Bradley-Moore PR, Atkins HL, Ansari AN, Richards P, Belgrave E: Thallium-201 for medical use. I. J Nucl Med 16:151, 1975.

10. Nielson A, Morris KG, Murdock RH, Bruno FP, Cobb FR: Linear relationship between distribution of thallium-201 and blood flow in ischemic and nonischemic myocardium during exercise. Circulation [Suppl 2] 59 and 60:148, 1979.

11. Weich HF, Strauss HW, Pitt B: The extraction of thallium-201 by the myocardium. Circulation 56:188, 1977.

12. Zimmer L, McCall D, D'Addabbo L, Whitney K: Kinetics and characteristics of thallium exchange in cultured cells. Circulation [Suppl 2] 59 and 60:138, 1979.

13. Shames D, Taradash M, Botvinick E, Parmley W: Comparison of Tl-201 stress myocardial perfusion imaging to stress electrocardiography [abstr]. J Nucl Med 17:522, 1976.

14. Ritchie JL, Trobaugh GB, Williams DL, Hamilton GW: Myocardial imaging with thallium-201 at rest and exercise: correlation with coronary anatomy and exercise electrocardiography. Circulation [Suppl 2] 53 and 54:216, 1976.

15. Pohost GM, Zir LM, Moore RH, McKusick KA, Guiney TE, Beller GA: Differentiation of transiently ischemic from infarcted myocardium by serial imaging after a single dose of thallium-201. Circulation 55:294, 1977.

16. Okada RD, Boucher CA, Strauss HW, Pohost GM: Exercise radionuclide imaging approaches to coronary artery disease. Am J Cardiol 46:1188, 1980.

17. Hamilton GW, Trobaugh GB, Ritchie JL, Williams DL, Weaver WD, Gould KL: Myocardial imaging with intravenously injected thallium-201 in patients with suspected coronary artery disease: analysis of technique and correlation with electrocardiographic, coronary anatomic and ventriculographic findings. Am J Cardiol 39:347, 1977.

18. Wackers FJ, Sokole EB, Samson G, Van Der Schoot JB, Lie KI, Leim KL, Wellens HJJ: Value and limitations of thallium-201 scintigraphy in the acute phase of myocardial infarction. N Engl J Med 295:1–5, 1976.

19. DiCola VC, Downing SE, Donabedian RK, Zaret BL: Pathophysiological correlates of thallium-201 myocardial uptake in experimental infarction. Cardiovasc Res 11:141, 1977.

20. Buja LM, Parkey RW, Stokely EM, Bonte FJ, Willerson JT: Pathophysiology of technetium-99m stannous pyrophosphate and thallium-201 scintigraphy of acute anterior myocardial infarcts in dogs. J Clin Invest 57:1508, 1976.

21. Okada RD, Boucher CA, Kirshenbaum HD, Kushner FG, Strauss HW, Pohost GM: Thallium stress test: improved diagnostic accuracy for an individual observer using criteria derived from interobserver analysis of variance [abstr]. Clin Res 27:191A, 1979.

22. Henning H. Schelbert HR, Righetti A, Ashburn WL, O'Rourke RA: Dual myocardial imaging with technetium-99m pyrophosphate and thallium-201 for detecting, localizing and sizing acute myocardial infarction. Am J Cardiol 40:147, 1977.

23. Wackers FJ, Becker AE, Samson G, Sokole EB, Van Der Schoot JB, Vet AJT, Lie KI, Durrer D, Wellens H: Location and size of acute transmural myocardial infarction estimated from thallium-201 scintiscans. A clinico-pathological study. Circulation 56:72, 1977.

24. Niess GS, Logic JR, Russell RO Jr, Rackley CE, Rogers WJ: Usefulness and limitations of thallium-201 myocardial scintigraphy in delineating location and size of prior myocardial infarction. Circulation 59:1010, 1979.

25. Bulkley BH, Hutchins GM, Bailey I, Strauss HW, Pitt B: Thallium-201 imaging and gated cardiac blood pool scans in patients with ischemia and idiopathic congestive cardiomyopathy. A clinical and pathologic study. Circulation 55:753, 1977.

26. Verani MS, Jhingran S, Attar M, Rizk A, Quinones MA, Miller RR: Post-stress redistribution of thallium-201 in patients with coronary artery disease, with and without prior myocardial infarction. Am J Cardiol 43:1114, 1979.

27. Rubin KA, Morrison J, Padnick MB, Binder AJ, Chiaramida S, Margouleff D, Padamanabhan VT, Gulotta SJ: Idiopathic hypertrophic subaortic stenosis: evaluation of anginal symptoms with thallium-201 myocardial imaging. Am J Cardiol 44:1040, 1979.

28. Nelson AD, Khullar S, Leighton RF, Budd GC, Gohara A, Ross JN Jr, Andrews LT, Windham J: Quantification of thallium-201 scintigrams in acute myocardial infarction. Am J Cardiol 44:664, 1979.

29. Gewirtz H, Beller GA, Strauss HW, Dinsmore RE, Zir LM, McKusick KA, Pohost GM: Transient defects of resting thallium scans in patients with coronary artery disease. Circulation 59:707, 1979.

30. Berger HJ, Gottschalk A, Zaret BL: Dual radionuclide study of acute myocardial infarction: comparison of thallium-201 and technetium-99m stannous prophosphate imaging in man. Ann Intern Med 88:145, 1978.

31. Vogel RA, Kirch DL, LeFree MT, Rainwater JO, Jensen DP, Steele PP: Thallium-201 myocardial perfusion scintigraphy: results of standard and multi-pinhole tomographic techniques. Am J Cardiol 43:787, 1979.

32. Bulkley BH, Silverman K, Weisfeldt ML, Burow R, Pond M, Becker LC: Pathologic basis of thallium-201 scintigraphic defects in patients with fatal myocardial injury. Circulation 60:785, 1979.

33. Berger BC, Watson DD, Burwell LR, Crosby IK, Wellons HA, Teates CD, Beller GA: Redistribution of thallium at rest in patients with stable and unstable angina and the effect of coronary artery bypass surgery. Circulation 60:1114, 1979.

34. Keyes JW: Emission computerized tomography of the myocardium. In: Strauss HW, Pitt B (eds) Cardiovascular nuclear medicine, 2nd edn. St. Louis: CV Mosby, 1979.

35. Dymond DS, Stone DL, Elliott AT, Britton KE, Spurrell RAJ: Cardiac emission tomography in patients using 201 thallium. A new technique for perfusion scintigraphy. Clin Cardiol 2:192, 1979.

36. Murphy PH, Thompson WL, Moore ML, Burdine JA: Radionuclide computed tomography of the body using routine radiopharmaceuticals. I. System characteristics. J Nucl Med 20:102, 1979.

37. Burdine JA, Murphy PH, DePuey EG: Radionuclide computed tomography of the body using routine radiopharmaceuticals. II. Clinical applications. J Nucl Med 20:108, 1979.
38. Holman BL, Idoine JD, Sos TA, Tancrell R, DeMeester G: Tomographic scintigraphy of regional myocardial perfusion. J Nucl Med 18:764, 1977.
39. Vogel RA, Kirch D, LeFree M, Steele P: A new method of multiplanar emission tomography using a seven pinhole collimator and an Anger scintillation camera. J Nucl Med 19:648, 1978.
40. Francisco D, Go R, Van Kirk O, Ehrhardt J, Marcus M: Tomographic thallium-201 perfusion scintigraphy following maximal coronary vasodilatation with dipyridamole. Circulation [Suppl 2] 59 and 60:174, 1979.
41. Rogers WL, Koral KF, Mayans R, Leonard PF, Thrall JH, Brady TJ, Keyes JW Jr: Coded aperture imaging of the heart. J Nucl Med 21:371, 1980.
42. Parker JA, Uren RF, Jones AG, Maddox DE, Zimmerman RE, Neill JM, Holman L: Radionuclide left ventriculography with the slant hole collimator. J Nucl Med 18:848, 1977.
43. Ueda H, Kaihara S, Ueda K, Sugishita Y, Sasaki Y, Iio M: Regional myocardial blood flow measured by I-131 labelled macroaggregated albumin (I-131 MAA). Jpn Heart J 6:534, 1965.
44. Yipintsoi T, Dobbs, WA Jr, Scanlon PD, Knopp TJ, Bassingthwaighte JB: Regional distribution of diffusible tracers and carbonized microspheres in the left ventricle of isolated dog hearts. Circ Res 33:573, 1973.
45. Quinn JL III, Serratto M, Kezdi P: Coronary artery bed photoscanning using radioiodine albumin macroaggregates (RAMA). J Nucl Med 7:107, 1966.
46. Weller DA, Adolph RJ, Wellman HN, Carroll RG, Kim Q: Myocardial perfusion scintigraphy after intracoronary injection of ^{99m}Tc-labeled human albumin microspheres. Toxicity and efficacy for detecting myocardial infarction in dogs; preliminary results in man. Circulation 46:963, 1972.
47. Endo M, Yamazaki T, Konno S, Hiratsuka H, Akimoto T, Tanaka T, Sakakibara S: The direct diagnosis of human myocardial ischemia using ^{133}I-MAA via the selective coronary catheter. Preliminary report. Am Heart J 80:498, 1970.
48. Schelbert HR, Ashburn WL, Covell JW, Simon AL, Braunwald E, Ross, J Jr: Feasibility and hazards of the intracoronary injection of radioactive serum albumin macroaggregates for external myocardial perfusion imaging. Invest Radiol 6:379, 1971.
49. Pie ND: The effects of coronary arterial injection of radioalbumin macroaggregates on coronary hemodynamics and myocardial function. J Nucl Med 12:724, 1971.
50. Grames GM, Jansen C, Gander MP, Wieland HC, Judkins MP: Safety of the direct coronary injection of radiolabelled particles. J Nucl Med 15:2, 1974.
51. Gould KL, Lipscomb K, Hamilton GW: Physiologic basis for assessing critical coronary stenosis. Instantaneous flow response and regional distribution during coronary hyperemia as measures of coronary flow reserve. Am J Cardiol 33:87, 1974.
52. Ashburn WL, Braunwald E, Simon AL, Peterson KL, Gault JH: Myocardial perfusion imaging with radioactive-labeled particles injected directly into the coronary circulation of patients with coronary artery disease. Circulation 44:851, 1971.

53. Ritchie JL, Hamilton GW, Williams DL, Kennedy JW: Myocardial imaging with radionuclide-labelled particles. Analysis of the normal image, abnormal image, and technical consideration. Radiology 121:131, 1976.
54. Jansen C, Judkins MP, Grames GM, Gander M, Adams R: Myocardial perfusion color scintigraphy with MAA. Radiology 109:369, 1973.
55. Hamilton GW, Ritchie JL, Allen D, Lapin E, Murray JA: Myocardial perfusion imaging with 99m-Tc or 113m-In macroaggregated albumin: correlation of the perfusion image with clinical, angiographic, surgical, and histologic findings. Am Heart J 89:708, 1975.
56. Gould KL, Hamilton GW, Lipscomb K, Ritchie JL, Kennedy W: Method for assessing stress-induced regional malperfusion during coronary arteriography. Experimental validation and clinical application. Am J Cardiol 34:557, 1974.
57. Ritchie JL, Hamilton GW, Gould KL, Allen D, Kennedy JW, Hammermeister KE: Myocardial imaging with indium-113m- and technetium-99m-macroaggregated albumin. New procedure for identification of stress-induced regional ischemia. Am J Cardiol 35:380, 1975.
58. Kety SS: Theory of blood-tissue exchange and its application to measurement of blood flow. Methods Med Res 8:223, 1960.
59. Herd JA, Hollenberg M, Thorburn GD, Kopald HH, Barger AC: Myocardial blood flow determined with krypton 85 in unanesthetized dogs. Am J Physiol 203:122, 1962.
60. Chidsey CA III, Fritts HW Jr, Hardewig A, Richards DW, Courrand A: Fate of radioactive krypton (Kr-85) introduced intravenously in man. J Appl Physiol 14:63, 1959.
61. Ross RS, Ueda K, Lichtlen PR, Rees JR: Measurement of myocardial blood flow in animals and man by selective injection of radioactive inert gas into the coronary arteries. Circ Res 15:28, 1964.
62. Cannon PJ, Haft JI, Johnson PM: Visual assessment of regional myocardial perfusion utilizing radioactive Xenon and scintillation photography. Circulation 40:277, 1969.
63. Holman BL, Adams DF, Jewitt D, Eldh P, Idoine J, Cohn PF, Gorlin R, Adelstein, SJ: Measuring regional myocardial blood flow with [133] Xe and the Anger camera. Radiology 112:99, 1974.
64. Kaplan E, Mayron LW, Friedman AM, Gindler JE, Frazin L, Moran JM, Loeb H, Gunnar RM: Definition of myocardial perfusion by continuous infusion of krypton-81m. Am J Cardiol 37:878, 1976.
65. Cannon PJ, Dell RB, Dwyer EM Jr: Measurement of regional myocardial perfusion in man with 133 xenon and a scintillation camera. J Clin Invest 51:964, 1972.
66. Dwyer EM, Dell RB, Cannon PJ: Regional myocardial blood flow in patients with angina and normal coronary arteries. Circulation [Suppl 2] 46:6, 1973.
67. Cannon PJ, Schmidt DH, Weiss MB, Fowler DL, Sciacca RR, Ellis K, Casarella WJ: The relationship between regional myocardial perfusion at rest and arteriographic lesions in patients with coronary atherosclerosis. J Clin Invest 56:1442, 1975.
68. Dwyer EM Jr, Dell RB, Cannon PJ: Regional myocardial blood flow in patients with residual anterior and inferior transmural infarction. Circulation 48:924, 1973.

69. Cannon PJ, Sciacca RR, Fowler DL, Weiss MB, Schmidt DH, Casarella WJ: Measurement of regional myocardial blood flow in man: description and critique of the method using xenon-133 and a scintillation camera. Am J Cardiol 36:783, 1975.

70. Maseri A, L'Abbate A, Pesola A, Michelassi C, Marzilli M, De Nes M: Regional myocardial perfusion in patients with atherosclerotic coronary artery disease at rest and during angina pectoris induced by tachycardia. Circulation 55:423, 1977.

71. Scheibel RL, Moore R, Korbuly D, Ovitt TW, Payne JT, Tuna N, Amplatz K: Regional myocardial blood flow measurement in the evaluation of patients with coronary artery disease. Radiology 115:379, 1975.

72. Holman BL, Cohn PF, See JR, Idoine J, Adams DF: Measurement of regional myocardial blood flow with Xe-133 both at rest and after contrast hyperemia [abstr]. J Nucl Med 16:536, 1975.

73. Selwyn AP, Steiner R, Kivisaari A, Fox K, Forse G: Krypton-81m in the physiologic assessment of coronary arterial stenosis in man. Am J Cardiol 43:547, 1979.

74. Brownell GL, Burnham CA, Hoop B Jr, Kazemi H: Positron scintigraphy with short-lived cyclotron-produced radiopharmaceuticals and a multicrystal positron camera. In: Medical radioisotope scintigraphy, vol 1. International Atomic Energy Agency. (IAEA) New York: Unipub, 1972, pp 313–330.

75. Weiss ES, Siegel BA, Sobel BE, Welch MJ, Ter-Pogossian MM: Evaluation of myocardial metabolism and perfusion with positron-emitting radionuclides: Prog Cardiovasc Dis 20:191, 1977.

76. Brownell GL, Correia JA, Zamenhof RG: Positron instrumentation. In: Lawrence JH, Budinger TF (eds) Recent advances in nuclear medicine, vol 5. New York: Grune and Stratton, 1978, pp 1–49.

77. Phelps ME, Hoffman EJ, Huang SC, Kuhl DE: ECAT: a new computerized tomographic imaging system for positron-emitting radiopharmaceuticals. J Nucl Med 19:635, 1978.

78. Hoop B Jr, Beh RA, Beller GA, Brownell GL, Burnham CA, Hnatowich DJ, Moore RH, Parker JA, Roux-Lough PO, Smith TW: Myocardial positron scintigraphy with short-lived [82]Rb. IEEE. Transactions on Nuclear Science 23:584, 1976.

79. Beller GA, Alton WJ, Moore RH, Cochavi S: Detection of nitroglycerin-induced changes in regional myocardial perfusion during acute ischemia by serial imaging with [82]Rb$^+$ [abstr]. Circulation 54:II-216, 1976.

80. Budinger TF, Yano Y, Derenzo SE, Huesman RH, Cahoon JL, Atoyer BR, Greenberg WL, O'Brien HA Jr: Myocardial uptake of rubidium-82 using positron emission tomography [abstr]. J Nucl Med 20:603, 1979.

81. Parker JA, Beller GA, Hoop B. Holman BL, Smith TW: Assessment of regional myocardial blood flow and fractional oxygen extraction using ^{15}O-water and ^{15}O-hemoglobin [abstr]. Circulation 54:II-110, 1976.

82. Hack SN, Eichling JO, Bergmann SR, Sobel BE: External quantification of perfusion [abstr]. Circulation 60:II-269, 1979.

83. Walsh WF, Fill HR, Harper PV: Nitrogen-13-labeled ammonia for myocardial imaging. Semin Nucl Med 7:59, 1977.

84. Gould KL, Schelbert HR, Phelps ME, Hoffman EJ: Noninvasive assessment of coronary stenoses with myocardial perfusion imaging during pharmacologic coronary vasodilatation. V. Detection of 47 percent diameter coronary stenosis with intravenous nitrogen-13 ammonia and emission-computed tomography in intact dogs. Am J Cardiol 43:200, 1979.

85. Bergmann SR, Hack S, Tewson T, Welch MJ, Sobel BE: The dependence of accumulation of $^{13}NH_3$ by myocardium on metabolic factors and its implications for quantitative assessment of perfusion. Circulation 61:34, 1980.

86. Schelbert HR, Wisenberg G, Gould KL, Marshall R, Phelps M, Hoffman E, Gomes A, Kuhl D: Detection of coronary artery stenosis in man by positron emission computed tomography and N-13 ammonia [abstr]. Circulation 60:II-60, 1979.

87. Weiss ES, Ahmed SA, Welch MJ, Williamson JR, Ter-Pogossian MM, Sobel BE: Quantification of infarct in cross sections of canine myocardium in vivo with positron emission transaxial tomography and ^{11}C-palmitate. Circulation 55:66, 1977.

88. Ter-Pogossian MM, Klein MS, Markham J, Roberts R, Sobel BE: Regional assessment of myocardial metabolic integrity in vivo by positron-emission tomography with ^{11}C-labeled palmitate. Circulation 61:242, 1980.

89. Lerch R, Ter-Pogossian MM, Sobel BE: Tomographic quantification of regional myocardial metabolism in vivo [abstr]. Am J Cardiol 45:465, 1980.

90. Phelps ME, Hoffman EJ, Selin C, Huang SC, Robinson G, MacDonald N, Schelbert HR, Kuhl DE: Investigation of ^{18}F-2-fluoro-2-deoxyglucose for the measure of myocardial glucose metabolism [abstr]. Am J Cardiol 45:465, 1980.

91. Phelps M, Schelbert H, Huang SC, Hoffman E, Marshall R, Wisenberg G, Kuhl D: Validation of positron computed tomography (PCT) measure of local myocardial metabolic rate for glucose (LMMRGlu) [abstr]. Circulation 60:II-60, 1979.

92. Schelbert H, Phelps M, Selin C, Hoffman E, Kuhl D: Glucose metabolism of regional myocardial ischemia evaluated by ^{18}Fluoro-2-deoxyglucose and positron emission computed tomography [abstr]. Am J Cardiol 45:465, 1980.

93. Knust EJ, Kupfernagel C, Stöcklin G: Long-chain F-18 fatty acids for the study of regional metabolism in heart and liver; odd-even effects of metabolism in mice. J Nucl Med 20:1170, 1979.

94. Allan RM, Selwyn AP, MacArthur CCG: Labeled metabolic substrates for positive imaging in ischemia [abstr]. Am J Cardiol 45:465, 1980.

95. Wisenberg G, Schelbert H, Hoffman E, Huang H, Phelps M, Skorton D, Child J: Quantitation of regional myocardial blood flow by positron emission tomography [abstr]. Am J Cardiol 45:465, 1980.

13. INFARCT-AVID IMAGING TECHNIQUES

MELVIN L. MARCUS, RAYMUNDO T. GO, and JAMES C. EHRHARDT

During the past 20 years, an enormous amount of progress has been made in the development of infarct-avid techniques to image myocardial infarcts. Although currently available methods cannot accurately determine the size of an acute infarct, it is possible to ascertain the location of almost all acute myocardial infarcts by using infarct-avid radiopharmaceuticals. In some instances, the relative size of the infarct can be determined.

In 1958, Dreyfuss and his associates [1] were the first to show that an acute myocardial infarction in man could be detected by using iodine-133. Between 1958 and 1974, two infarct-avid imaging agents (^{97}Hg-fluorescein and ^{203}Hg-fluorescein) were evaluated, but the scintigrams produced were unsatisfactory [2, 3]. In 1974, progress in this area took a major step forward when Holman et al. [4, 5] demonstrated that excellent-quality infarct scintigrams could be obtained with ^{99m}Tc-(Sn)-tetracycline. In the same year, Bonte et al. [6] presented experimental data that demonstrated that ^{99m}Tc-pyrophosphate (^{99m}Tc-PYP) concentrated in acutely infarcted myocardium. Several months later, Willerson et al. [7, 8] demonstrated that superb infarct scintigrams could be obtained following i.v. ^{99m}Tc-PYP in a high percentage of patients with acute infarction.

In a very short time, ^{99m}Tc-PYP became the radiopharmaceutical of choice for infarct imaging. This occurred because two inherent problems with ^{99m}Tc-(Sn)-tetracycline were quickly recognized. First, ^{99m}Tc-(Sn)-tetracycline concentrated in the liver, interfering with the diagnosis of inferior wall myocardial infarct. Second, because ^{99m}Tc-(Sn)-tetracycline concentrated very slowly in areas of acute infarct, it was necessary to wait 24 h after injecting the radiopharmaceutical before imaging could commence. Since the calcium-chelating ^{99m}Tc complexes did not have these deficiencies, they became the agents of choice for infarct imaging. Today, the overwhelming majority of infarct scintigrams employ ^{99m}Tc-PYP. Although other related radiopharmaceuticals have been tested [9], most investigators have found that ^{99m}Tc-PYP is superior.

THEORETICAL BASIS

For any infarct-avid agent to be effective, it must bind to or form some type of complex with a substance that predominantly occurs in infarcted muscle. If

Wagner GS (ed): Myocardial Infarction: Measurement and Intervention, pp 325–346.
© 1982 Martinus Nijhoff Publishers, The Hague/Boston/London.

the infarct-avid agent is to discriminate between acute and chronic infarct, it must bind to a constituent of the infarct that is present for a finite time period. The concentration of the agent should not be influenced by other characteristic features of infarct, such as decreased blood flow or altered membrane permeability. Finally, the isotope should have ideal imaging characteristics.

^{99m}Tc-PYP probably forms a complex with various forms of tissue calcium stores that accumulate in areas of acute infarct [10–13]. Because the Ca^{++} is removed from most infarcts over a period of one to several weeks, ^{99m}Tc-PYP accumulation occurs mainly in areas of acute necrosis. ^{99m}Tc-PYP has very good imaging characteristics.

Polymorphonuclear leukocytes labeled with indium-111 (^{111}In) have also been used to identify areas of acute infarct [14]. This approach is of interest because the time course of polymorphonuclear infiltration and subsequent removal from areas of infarct is shorter (2–7 days) and less variable than that of various tissue calcium stores. Unfortunately, the imaging characteristics of ^{111}In are relatively poor.

Although other infarct-avid radiopharmaceuticals have been suggested, e.g., anticardiac myosin (Fab)$_2$ fragments [15], labeled polymorphonuclear cells [14], ^{99m}Tc-PYP is the only one that is widely used [7, 8].

EXPERIMENTAL STUDIES

Since 1975, many investigators have explored a host of important questions that relate to the ^{99m}Tc-PYP infarct scintigrams. These studies address several major questions.

Can ^{99m}Tc-PYP scintigrams discriminate between ischemic and infarcted myocardium?

Several studies have demonstrated beyond any reasonable doubt that ^{99m}Tc-PYP accumulation can discriminate between infarcted and ischemic myocardium. First, intense transient ischemia unassociated with infarction has been shown not to result in ^{99m}Tc-PYP accumulation [12, 16, 17]. Second, when excessive ^{99m}Tc-PYP accumulation does occur, studies in both experimental animals [17–20] and man [21] have almost invariably demonstrated histologic evidence of myocardial necrosis. In view of the impressive ability of ^{99m}Tc-PYP to detect acutely infarcted cardiac muscle, it is surprising that this radio-pharmaceutical is not commonly used as a research tool. It is easy to employ and far less expensive and time-consuming than histologic analysis. Unfortunately, although ^{99m}Tc-PYP correctly identifies myocardial segments that contain infarcted tissue, the extent of infarct cannot be predicted from the magnitude of the ^{99m}Tc-PYP accumulation.

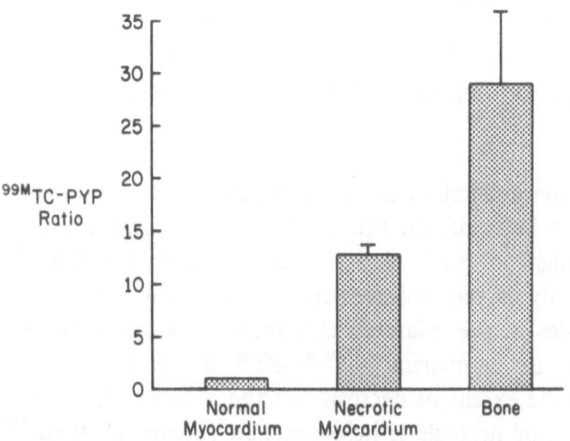

Accumulation of ^{99M}TC-PYP by
Normal Myocardium, Necrotic Myocardium and Bone

Figure 1. Concentration of ^{99m}Tc-PYP in normal myocardium, necrotic myocardium, and bone. These data were obtained in dogs sacrificed 48 h following permanent coronary occlusion. ^{99m}Tc-PYP was injected i.v. 2 h prior to sacrifice. The uptake of ^{99m}Tc-PYP in necrotic myocardium is less than that in bone but 13 times greater than that observed in normal myocardium [20].

What is the time course of ^{99m}Tc-PYP accumulation and disappearance following acute coronary ligation?

Infarcted myocardium accumulates a significant amount of ^{99m}Tc-PYP within 6 h following coronary occlusion [22]. However, images of diagnostic quality can seldom be obtained less than 12 h following coronary occlusion and accumulation may not be maximum for 72 h [7, 8, 12, 13]. Infrequently, accumulation is not maximal for 5–7 days [21, 23]. In experimental animals, average concentrations of ^{99m}Tc-PYP at 48 h after coronary occlusion are eleven times greater in the infarcted zone than in normal myocardium, and about one-half as great as the concentration in normal bone (Figure 1) [20].

The disappearance of ^{99m}Tc-PYP from acutely infarcted myocardium also follows a variable time course. In dogs subjected to permanent coronary occlusion, the scintigraphic abnormality fades substantially by seven days following occlusion [12]. In clinical studies, however, some patients have persistently positive scintigrams many months following an acute infarct in the absence of clinical evidence of a recurrent ischemic episode [21, 24, 25]. Although this may represent continuing low-grade myocardial necrosis in some instances [21], it is apparent that the time course of the accumulation and disappearance of

^{99m}Tc-PYP from areas of acute infarct is variable. The best results with ^{99m}Tc-PYP will be obtained in medical centers that perform serial examinations of their patients with suspected infarcts.

Does the concentration of ^{99m}Tc-PYP depend on the perfusion of the infarcted zone?

Several experimental studies [19, 20, 26] have shown that the concentration of ^{99m}Tc-PYP in an infarcted zone is flow dependent. If a coronary artery is occluded long enough to produce myocardial necrosis (> 20 min) and the occlusion subsequently is released to permit reflow, the rate at which the ^{99m}Tc-PYP accumulates in the infarcted area increases substantially [27]. If the coronary occlusion is permanent, ^{99m}Tc-PYP accumulation will depend on two factors — the extent of necrosis and the collateral flow to the involved zone. If the extent of necrosis is held constant (Figure 2), then ^{99m}Tc-PYP will vary directly with the extent of collateral flow [20]. If both the extent of necrosis and collateral flow are permitted to vary (which is the case clinically), the relationship between ^{99m}Tc-PYP accumulation and flow will be nonlinear [26]. This occurs because segments with extensive necrosis will tend to have very low flows, and involved segments with high flows will tend to have minimal amounts of necrosis. In both instances, the ^{99m}Tc-PYP accumulation will be less than that which occurs if both the extent of necrosis and the collateral flow in a given myocardial segment are in the moderate range [26].

The dependence of ^{99m}Tc-PYP accumulation in infarcted myocardium on collateral flow is a confounding variable. It contributes to the complex evolution of ^{99m}Tc-PYP scintigraphic abnormalities in a single patient because collateral flow is probably changing during the course of an infarct. Furthermore, at a single point in time, it prevents one from using the intensity of the scintigraphic abnormality as an indicator of infarct size.

How sensitive is the ^{99m}Tc-PYP scintigram for detecting infarcted myocardium?

In the experimental laboratory, the sensitivity of ^{99m}Tc-PYP for detecting areas of myocardial necrosis is exquisite. Autoradiographic studies [27] have shown that necrosis in individual cells can be detected with ^{99m}Tc-PYP. If a well-counter is employed to detect gamma emissions, 5% necrosis is a 1 g segment of myocardium will be readily detectable [20]. If the gamma emissions are detected with a scintillation camera imaging an in vivo heart, sensitivity will depend upon the characteristics of the imaging equipment and the location of the infarct. Several experimental studies [16, 18, 27, 28] and one clinical study [21] suggest

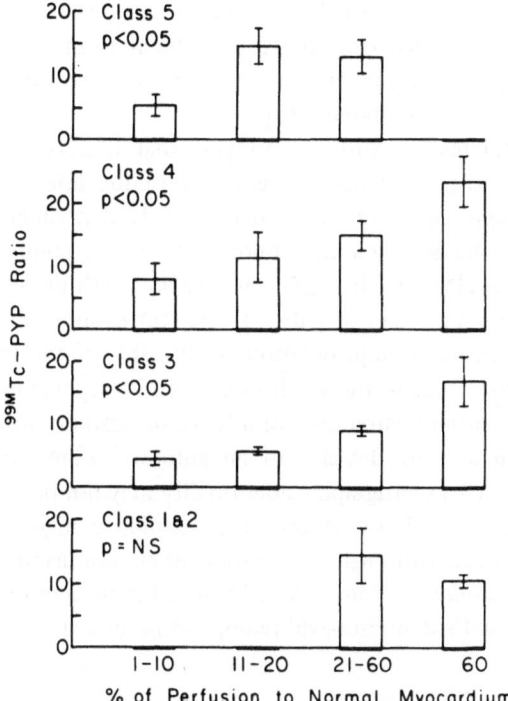

Figure 2. Effects of collateral flow and extent of necrosis on ^{99m}Tc-PYP accumulation. These data were obtained from dogs sacrificed 48 h following permanent coronary occlusion. ^{99m}Tc-PYP was injected i.v. 2 h prior to sacrifice. The left ventricle of each dog was divided into 96 segments, and in each segment we determined perfusion with microspheres, ^{99m}Tc-PYP concentration, and the extent of necrosis by histologic examination. The extent of necrosis by histologic examination. The extent of necrosis was divided into five classes, 1–5; these classes correspond to 1%–20%, 21%–40%, 41%–60%, 61%–80%, and greater than 81% necrosis in the segment examined. By examining the data at a given myocardial perfusion (21%–60% of control), it is obvious that the extent of necrosis (classes 1–5) is not a major determinant of ^{99m}Tc-PYP uptake. With the extent of necrosis held constant, ^{99m}Tc-PYP accumulation increases progressively with increases in myocardial perfusion (see class 3 and 4 panels) [20].

that infarcts that exceed 3–5 g are detectable. In general, the sensitivity of ^{99m}Tc-PYP is much greater than that which can be obtained with serial electrocardiograms and about equivalent to measurements of MB-CPK in plasma if the enzyme concentrations are monitored frequently in the proper time frame with a sensitive method [16, 28].

Can the size of a myocardial infarct be determined with a ^{99m}Tc-PYP scintigram?

If one employs conventional planar images, the size of a myocardial infarct usually cannot be accurately assessed with a ^{99m}Tc-PYP scintigram. Although experimental studies have shown that the size of an anterior transmural myocardial infarct can be estimated from the size of the abnormality of a ^{99m}Tc-PYP scintigram [18, 29], less favorable results were reported in a study that employed inferior and subendocardial infarcts [30].

There are several reasons why sizing myocardial infarcts with ^{99m}Tc-PYP is difficult. First, the three-dimensional geometry of the infarct is complex and without a tomographic imaging system it is unlikely that superb results will be obtained. Second, the scintigraphic abnormality has a complex evolutionary pattern, and it is not clear which stage correlates best with the size of the infarct. Third, in a significant number of patients, the scintigraphic abnormality is not localized [7]. In this subgroup, determining the size of the infarct would be particularly difficult. Fourth, the resolution of scintigraphic images deteriorates with distance, and thus measurements of inferior or posterior infarcts will be less accurate that estimates of the size of an anterior infarct. Finally, in some patients, the border of a scintigraphic abnormality may not be properly localized because a superimposed bony structure containing a high concentration of ^{99m}Tc-PYP obscures it. Although these problems are not insurmountable, major advances will be required before it will be possible to determine the size of a myocardial infarct with an infarct-avid radiopharmaceutical.

TECHNICAL ASPECTS OF THE PROCEDURE

To obtain ^{99m}Tc-PYP scintigrams of diagnostic quality, many technical aspects of the procedure must be rigorously controlled [31]. Two technical aspects are particularly critical.

The quality of commercially prepared ^{99m}Tc-PYP varies. Therefore, it is an absolute necessity that the binding of the ^{99m}Tc-PYP be independently assessed. If binding in a given batch of ^{99m}Tc-PYP does not exceed 95%, the radiopharmaceutical should not be used. ^{99m}Tc that is not bound to PYP will bind in vivo to the red blood cells, labeling the blood pool for the duration of the study. Under these conditions, the diffuse pattern is not a reliable indicator of infarct since it simply represents blood pool labeling. This problem can lead to a very high incidence of false positive studies. If one disregards the diffuse pattern, sensitivity will substantially decrease [32].

The technical point that requires emphasis relates to obtaining repeated ^{99m}Tc-PYP scintigrams. The first scintigram should be obtained 3 h following an intravenous injection of ^{99m}Tc-PYP. If the examination is negative or demonstrates a localized defect, additional views later in the day are not required. If it reveals a diffuse pattern, the examination should be repeated several hours later. If the diffuse abnormality persists, it almost always represents infarct if the binding of the ^{99m}Tc to PYP was excellent. Additional scintigrams at a later date should be obtained in almost all patients. If the initial scintigram is negative, a repeat procedure several days later may yield a positive result because the evolution of positive scintigraphic abnormalities in patients with acute infarcts is highly variable. If the initial infarct scintigram is positive, a repeat image one week later will yield additional information of diagnostic importance. If, at this point, the scintigraphic abnormality has faded significantly, the original scintigraphic abnormality was almost certainly due to an acute infarct. On the other hand, if the abnormality on the repeat scintigram is unchanged, it may be due to a previous infarct, left ventricular aneurysm, or continuing low-grade myocardial necrosis.

The superb results with ^{99m}Tc-PYP infarct scintigrams reported by the group at Southwestern [7, 8, 21] will be obtained only by groups that routinely employ serial application of this imaging technique.

CLINICAL STUDIES RELATED TO THE SENSITIVITY AND SPECIFICITY OF ^{99m}TC-PYP SCINTIGRAMS

Scintigraphic abnormalities are usually classified as localized or diffuse. In addition, the intensity of the abnormality is usually graded on a scale of 0 to 4 + as described by Willerson [7, 8] (see Table 1 and Figures 3–6). Earlier studies suggested that the localized pattern was characteristic of transmural myocardial infarct and the diffuse pattern was usually associated with subendocardial infarcts [7, 8]. Detailed pathologic studies have shown that the transmural extent of an infarct cannot be reliably predicted by the scintigraphic pattern [21] with one exception: the doughnut pattern that occurs in a small percentage of patients with myocardial infarct is almost invariably associated with massive transmural infarct [33].

Many clinical reports [8, 25, 33–40] suggest that 98% of patients with a transmural myocardial infarct will have a positive scintigraphic abnormality if the study is performed within the first six days of the infarct. The reported sensitivity of detecting subendocardial or smaller infarct varies in different series form 51% to 100% [25, 32–35, 37, 39]. The sensitivity in this patient subset is critically dependent on two factors: quality control of the ^{99m}Tc-PYP binding, which will tend to eliminate diffuse pattern abnormalities that represent blood pool labeling by free ^{99m}Tc, and serial imaging in equivocal cases. In hospital centers where the ^{99m}Tc-PYP is skillfully applied, about 90% of patients with a subendocardial infarct will have positive scintigrams [7]. Furthermore, in some patients, multifocal myocardial necrosis will be detectable [21].

If blood pool imaging is eliminated, false positive ^{99m}Tc-PYP scintigrams occur in less that 1%–2% of patients with normal hearts [8, 25, 33, 35–38]. Although many noncardiac causes of positive ^{99m}Tc-PYP scintigrams have been

Table 1. Grading scale for ^{99m}Tc-PYP infarct scintigrams

0	No activity and a negative myocardial scintigram
1 +	Questionable increased activity, but not absolutely definite, and also considered to be a negative scintigram (less intense than the ribs)
2 +	Definite but faint activity and a positive myocardial scintigram (equal to intensity of rib uptake)
3 +	Definite increased activity within the myocardial image (greater than intensity of rib uptake)
4 +	Definite increased activity within the myocardial image (equal to or greater than intensity of sternal uptake)

Table 2. Causes of localized uptake of ^{99m}Tc-PYP

Noncardiac causes
Persistent blood pool activity 37, 40
Rib fractures 41
Skeletal muscle damage usually related to cardioversion 42
Calcified costal cartilage 43
Breast conditions (tumors, inflammation, functional parenchyma in premenopausal females) 44
Skin lesions 45

Cardiac causes
Previous myocardial infarct (6 weeks to > 6 months old) 25
Left ventricular aneurysm 21, 46
Unstable angina 8, 21, 34, 39, 47
Multifocal myocardial necrosis 21
Myocardial contusion 48, 49
Valvular calcification 50
Cardiomyopathy 51

reported (see Table 2), with the exception of rib fractures they occur infrequently (Figure 7). Positive scintigrams in patients with heart disease who do not have an acute infarct are almost always due to myocardial necrosis [21]. In some instances (e.g., continuing low-grade myocardial necrosis associated with ventricular aneurysm, and multifocal myocardial necrosis, ^{99m}Tc-PYP scintigrams provide the only means short of pathologic examination of detecting this type of necrosis.

RECOMMENDATIONS CONCERNING THE CLINICAL USE OF ^{99m}TC-PYP SCINTIGRAMS

At present, ^{99m}Tc-PYP scintigrams are not of great value in patients who present with a typical myocardial infarct confirmed by characteristic abnormalities in MB-CK and localized by classic electrocardiographic criteria. In such patients, the scintigrams will usually not add sufficient information to justify the cost of the procedure.

20° LAO

LT. LAT.

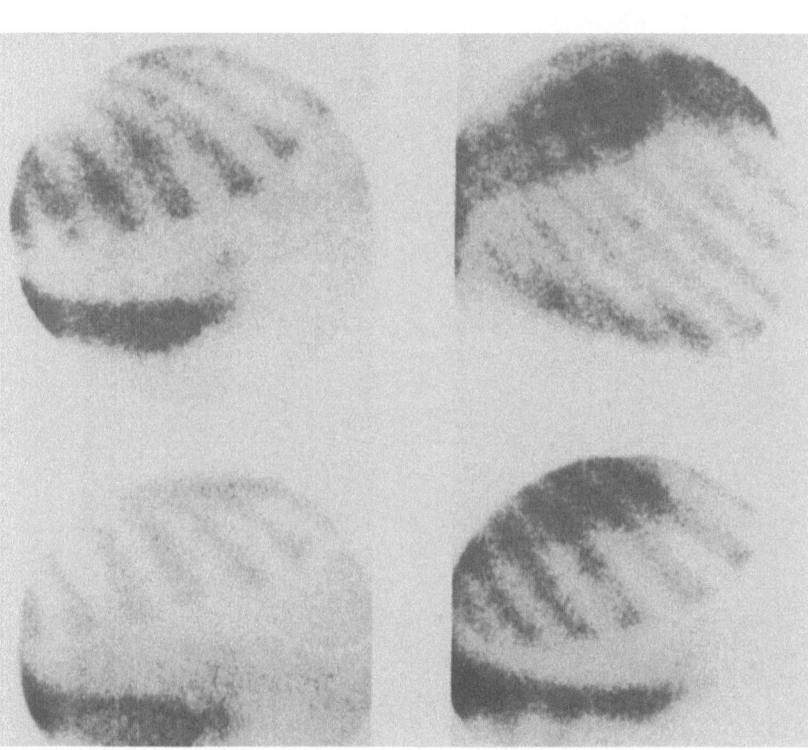

ANT.

45° LAO

Figure 3. In this figure and those to follow, ⁹⁹ᵐTc-PYP infarcts scintigrams were obtained in four views (ANT), anterior; 20° and 40° LAO, 20° and 40° left anterior oblique; LT. LAT., left lateral) 3 h following injection of ⁹⁹ᵐTc-PYP. This figure shows a normal ⁹⁹ᵐTc-PYP examination. Note that the sternum and ribs are clearly demarcated, and there is virtually no ⁹⁹ᵐTc-PYP accumulation in the area occupied by the heart.

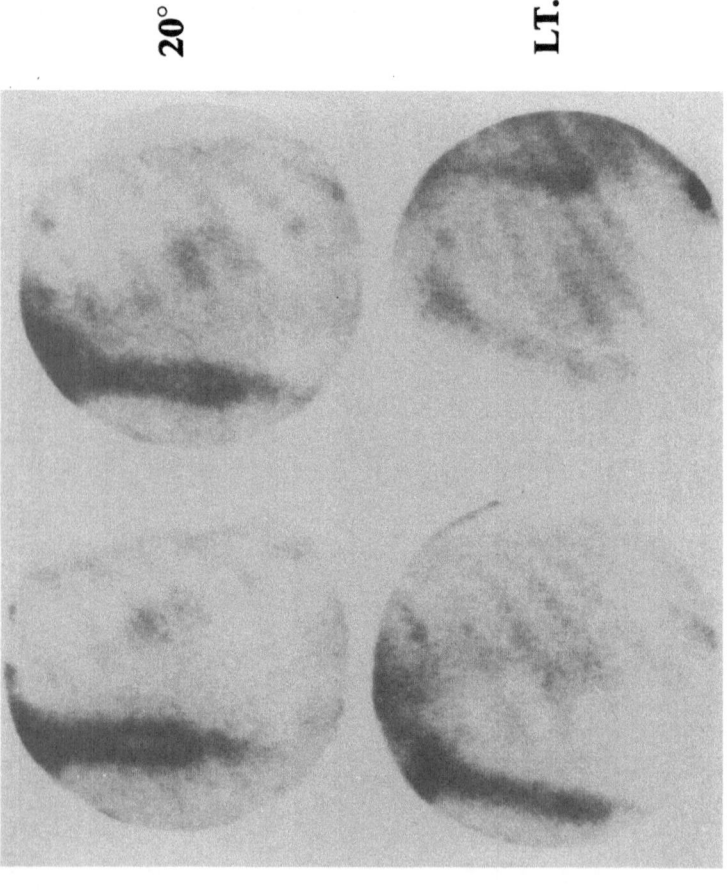

20° LAO

LT. LAT.

ANT.

45° LAO

Figure 4. Scintigram showing a localized accumulation of ^{99m}Tc-PYP in the lateral wall of the left ventricle. The abnormality is most apparent in the anterior and 20° LAO views. The intensity of the accumulation is about equal to that in the ribs and hence would be designated 2+.

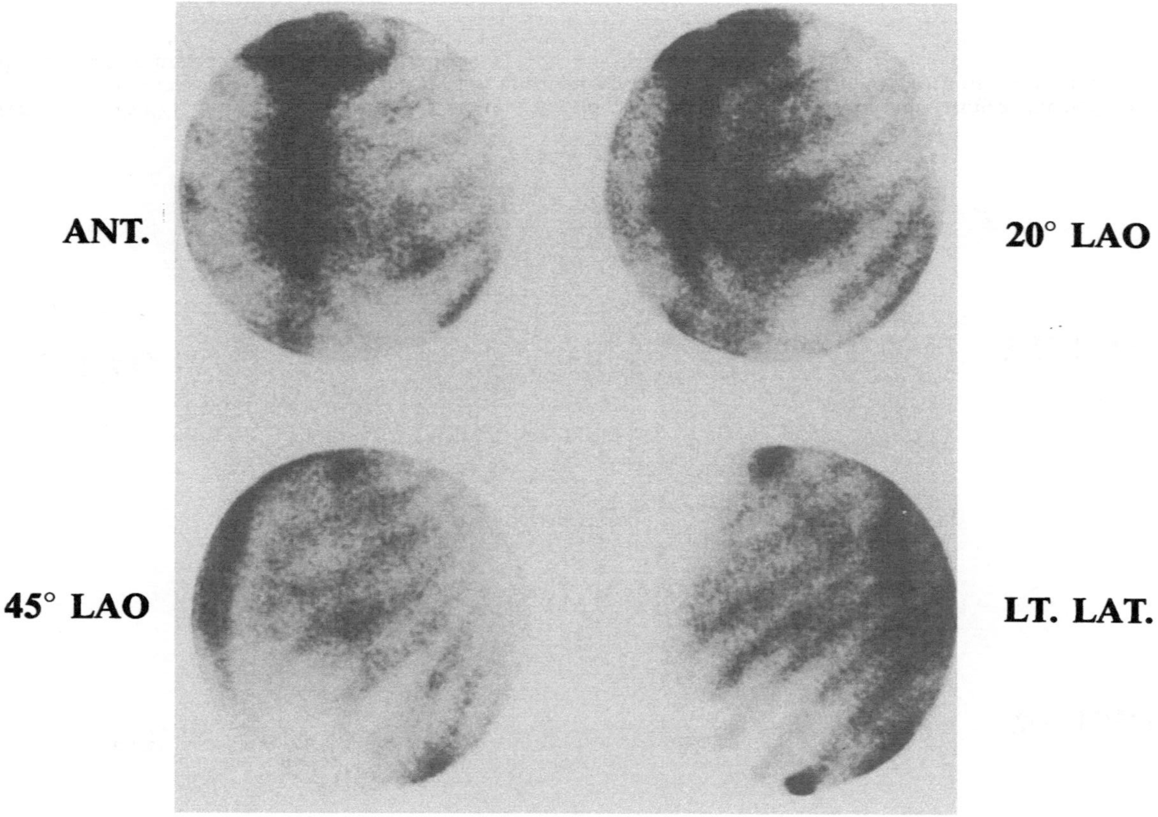

20° LAO

LT. LAT.

ANT.

45° LAO

Figure 5. Diffuse accumulation of ^{99m}Tc-PYP in the cardiac region. The intensity of the abnormality is greater than the ^{99m}Tc-PYP uptake in the ribs and less than the sternum. Hence, it would be graded 3 +. To help exclude a blood pool abnormality, the scintigrams should be repeated 2–3 h later. With time, blood pool activity will clear whereas ^{99m}Tc-PYP within necrotic myocardium will persist.

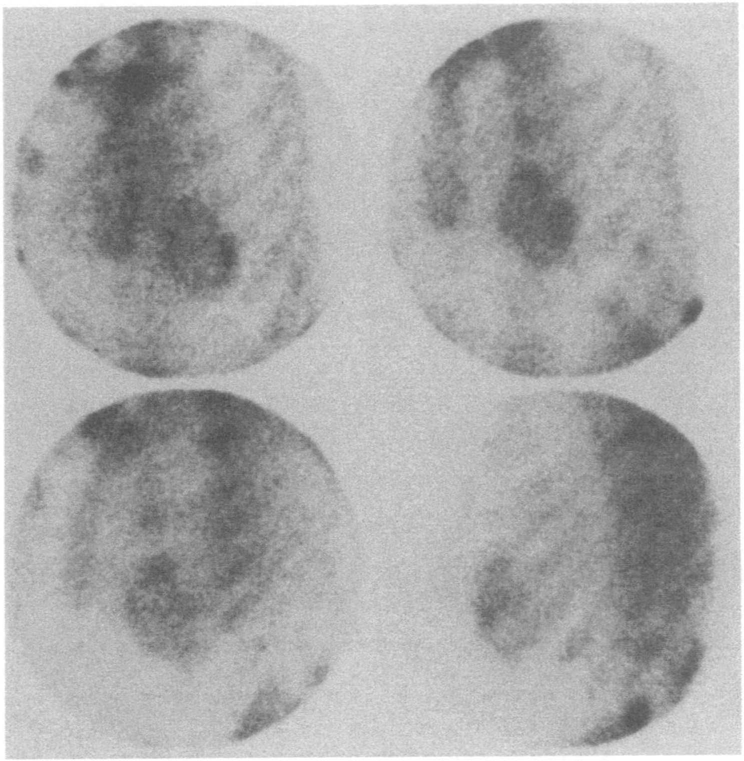

Figure 6. A typical ^{99m}Tc-PYP doughnut abnormality. Note that the intensity of the ^{99m}Tc-PYP accumulation at the periphery of the abnormality is greater than the intensity in the center. This is most apparent on the anterior view. The intensity of the abnormality is equal to or greater than that in the sternum, and hence would be graded **4** +.

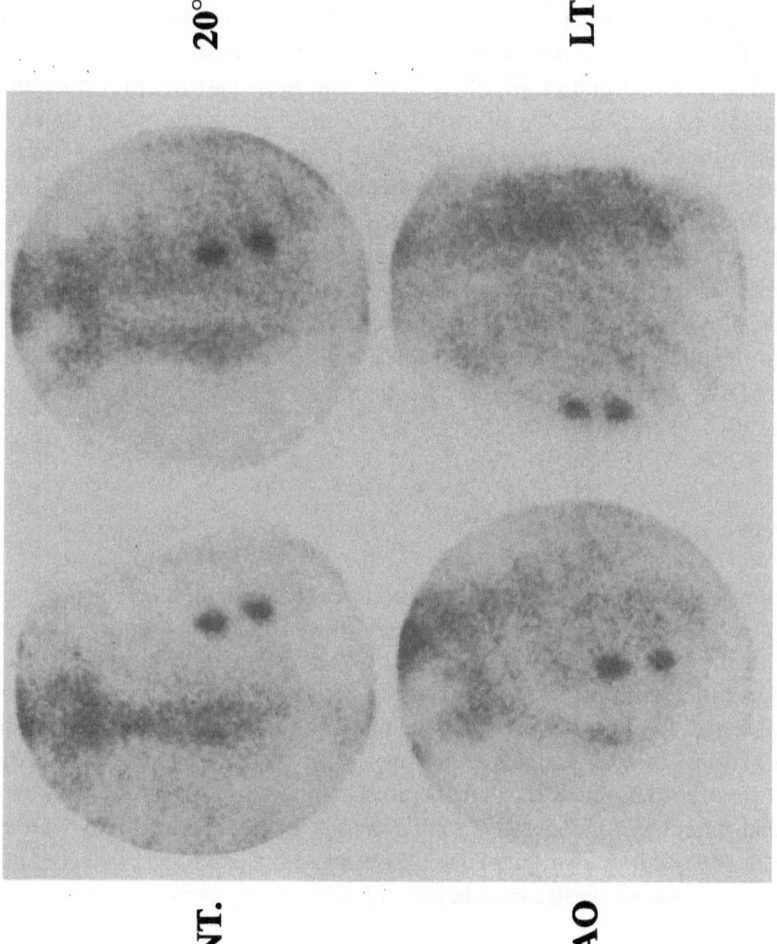

Figure 7. Scintigram depicting the most frequent noncardiac abnormality observed – multiple rib fractures.

In contrast, there are several patient subsets in whom the ^{99m}Tc-PYP scintigram does provide unique diagnostic information.

Infarcts 3–10 days old

Characteristic electrocardiographic and enzymatic abnormalities are most prominent during the first three days of an infarct. Thereafter, these tests may be completely normal or nondiagnostic. In contrast, almost all patients with transmural myocardial infarct [8, 25, 33–40] and most patients with subendo-cardial infarct [25, 32–35, 37, 39] will have positive scintigrams up to six days following an infarct. Furthermore, 10%–40% of patients with transmural myo-cardial infarct [21, 24, 25] will have scintigraphic abnormalities that persist for six months or longer. If a patient with a suspected infarct of 3–10 days' duration has a positive ^{99m}Tc-PYP scintigram, the test should be repeated in 1–2 weeks. If the second scintigram is normal or the abnormality is much less prominent, it is very likely that the patient sustained a recent myocardial infarct. If the scintigraphic abnormality on the second scrintigram is unchanged, the age of the infarct responsible for the scintigraphic abnormality is indetermi-nate [24, 25].

Perioperative myocardial infarct

Electrocardiographic and enzymatic methods of confirming the diagnosis of perioperative infarct are frequently nondiagnostic following major surgery because electrolyte and surgical trauma seriously interferes with these tests. This is a serious problem in patients who have had cardiac surgery because the minor cardiac damage associated with cardiopulmonary bypass may increase serum levels of MB-CK. In such patients, a positive ^{99m}Tc-PYP scintigram is diagnostic of acute myocardial infarct if a preoperative scintigram is diagnostic of acute myocardial infarct if a preoperative scintigram is diagnostic of acute myocardial infarct if a preoperative scintigram was negative and the operative procedure did not involve excision of cardiac muscle [36, 52, 53].

Suspected right ventricular infarct

The diagnosis of a right ventricular infarct is usually suspected when a patient with a transmural inferior wall infarct has venous hypertension in the absence of concomitant left ventricular failure. Unfortunately, other conditions that can complicate inferior infarcts such as pulmonary embolism, cardiac tamponade, or cor pulmonale secondary to chronic lung disease may yield a similar clinical picture [54, 55]. The diagnosis of right ventricular infarct can be accomplished with certainty in only two ways: a ^{99m}Tc-PYP scintigram in the left anterior projection that demonstrates accumulation of the radionuclide in the free wall of the right ventricle or pathologic examination. The ^{99m}Tc-PYP scintigram will detect evidence of right ventricular infarct in about one-third of patients with transmural inferior infarct [56]. In most cases, the right ventricular infarction is not associated with any clinical sequelae.

Localization of a myocardial infarct in patients with left bundle branch block

In most hospitals, the localization of an acute myocardial infarct depends upon classic electrocardiographic abnormalities. In patients with left bundle branch block or certain other interventricular conduction disturbances, the electrocardiogram is of little value in localizing the infarct. Furthermore, other cardiac imaging procedures such as gated blood pool ventriculograms (see Wackers, p. 215) or thallium-201 perfusion scintigrams (see Okada, p. 296) cannot discriminate between old and new areas of infarct. In this patient group, a ^{99m}Tc-PYP scintigram will usually enable localization of the infarct. If the scintigraphic abnormality present acutely is much less prominent on a second examination 1–2 weeks later, this establishes the diagnosis and location of the acute infarct with a high degree of certainty.

Coronary insufficiency syndrome

Patients with prolonged episodes (> 30 min) of severe precordial pain unassociated with conclusive enzymatic or electrocardiographic evidence of a myocardial infarct may have variable aspects of the spectrum of cardiac ischemia. These may include unstable angina, variant angina, subclinical localized subendocardial infarcts, low-grade continuing myocardial necrosis surrounding a previous area of infarct, and multifocal foci of myocardial necrosis. It may be possible to classify this heterogeneous group of phenomena into those with and without cardiac necrosis with the aid of a ^{99m}Tc-PYP scintigram. A recent detailed pathologic study [21] suggests that a positive ^{99m}Tc-PYP scintigram in such patients is almost always associated with pathologic evidence of recent myocardial necrosis. It is possible that when the coronary insufficiency syndrome is associated with evidence of recent myocardial necrosis, it follows a different course than when recent myocardial necrosis is not present. Obviously, many additional studies are needed in this area.

Myocardial contusion

Myocardial contusion occurs primarily in patients who have had major trauma involving the chest. The electrocardiographic findings are often nonspecific and the enzymatic abnormalities are difficult to dissociate from those that reflect concomitant skeletal muscle injury. Both experimental [48] and clinical studies [49] suggest that cardiac damage secondary to myocardial contusion can be detected with a ^{99m}Tc-PYP scintigram (Figure 8). Since the complications of myocardial contusion are similar to those associated with a myocardial infarct, the diagnosis will alert the patient's physician to possible life-threatening arrhythmias. In patients who have sustained chest trauma, a ^{99m}Tc-PYP scintigram should be performed if myocardial contusion is suspected.

Clinical applications of ^{99m}Tc-PYP scintigrams of less certain value

Two other clinical applications of the ^{99m}Tc-PYP scintigram may be of value. They are: diagnosis of infarct extension and predicting the patient's long-term prognosis. The diagnosis of infarct extension can occasionally be inferred from serial ^{99m}Tc-PYP scintigrams. If a second ^{99m}Tc-PYP scintigram shows a new area of involvement, this probably represents extension of the infarct. Also, if a series of infarct scintigrams reveals that the intensity of the abnormality in the involved area changed (e.g., 4 +, 2 +, 4 +) in a manner that differs from the typical evolution (e.g., 4 +, 2 +, 1 +), this is probably due to infarct extension.

There are several reasons why ^{99m}Tc−PYP scintigrams are usually not helpful in confirming the diagnosis of infarct extension. First, without tomographic images that are analyzed quantitatively, the resolution of the procedure is limited. Second, the evolutionary pattern of serial ^{99m}Tc-PYP scintigrams in patients with infarct varies. Finally, the accumulation of ^{99m}Tc-PYP in the involved zone depends on two variables that may be changing during the course of the infarct: the extent of necrosis and collateral flow.

Several recent studies (24, 25, 33) suggest that the ^{99m}Tc-PYP scintigram can help to identify patients with acute myocardial infarcts who are at high risk for developing late complications. If the initial ^{99m}Tc-PYP scintigram shows a doughnut pattern or if the scintigraphic abnormalities persist for 1−2 months following infarct, the likelihood of major late complications is increased. In general, patients with such scintigraphic findings have had a large transmural myocardial infarct. The role that the ^{99m}Tc-PYP infarct scintigram will play in identifying these patients is uncertain because it is possible that other diagnostic procedures (thallium perfusion scintigrams, gated blood flow scans, graded exercise tolerance tests) may be equally effective in identifying this same patient subgroup.

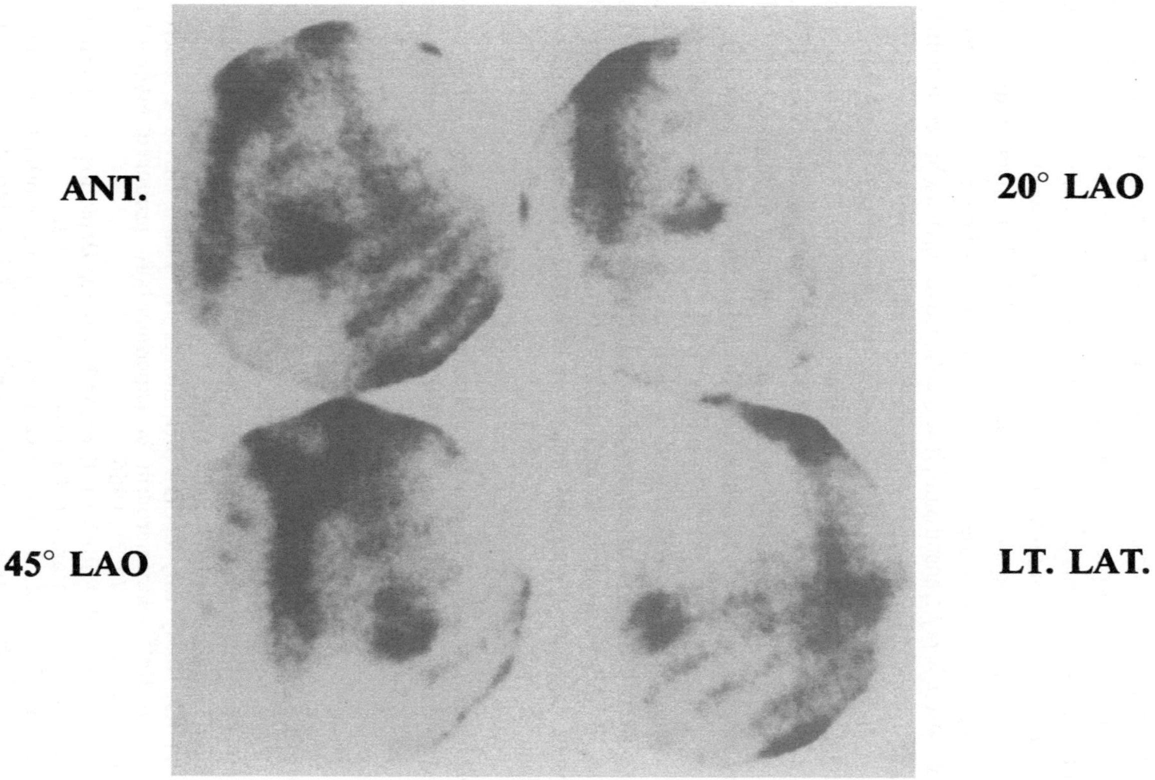

Figure 8. Scintigram showing a 4 + localized abnormality primarily involving the cardiac apex. This examination, in a 23-year-old man, was obtained 48h following severe chest trauma. Thus, the ^{99m}Tc-PYP accumulation is due to necrosis secondary to myocardial contusion.

Future developments

Advances in this area depend upon tomographic imaging techniques to the infarct scintigram and developing better radiopharmaceuticals. At present, at least 14 different systems designed to obtain tomographic images from gamma- or positron-emitting isotopes are being evaluated. In one study that employed tomographic images of ^{99m}Tc-PYP [57], it was possible to assess the size of an anterior wall myocardial infarct in dogs with considerable accuracy ($r = 0.98$). Perhaps the most exciting new application of ^{99m}Tc-PYP involves its use to enhance computed axial tomographic scans of myocardial infarct [58]. Because ^{99m}Tc-PYP alters X-ray transmission, it will enhance differences between acutely infarcted and normal muscle that can be detected with computed axial tomography (see Whitaker, p. 261). In one experimental study recently reported from the Mayo Clinic, it was possible to use this unique combination to determine the three-dimensional shape of acute myocardial infarct with astounding clarity [59].

Several new radiopharmaceuticals are being employed to identify areas of infarct by labeling white blood cells with ^{111}In [11], anticardiac myosin (Fab)$_2$ fragments [15], and ^{11}C-labeled palmitate [59]. The clinical usefulness of these radiopharmaceuticals will depend on their biologic characteristics and the resolving power of the system employed to image them. During the 1980s, it is likely that it will be possible to accurately determine the three-dimensional geometry of an acute myocardial infarct in man with one or more of these approaches.

Acknowledgment. Some of the original studies reported in this review were supported by Program Project Grant HL14388 and Research Career Development Award HL00328 to M.L.M.

REFERENCES

1. Dreyfuss F, Hochman A, Ben-Porath M, et al: Uptake of radioiodine by the infarcted heart. Isr Med J 17:219, 1958.
2. Gorten RJ, Hardy LB, McCraw BH, Stokes JR, Lumb GD: The selective uptake of Hg^{203}-chlormerodrin in experimentally produced myocardial infarcts. Am Heart J 72:71, 1966.
3. Málek P, Vavrejn B, Ratuský J, Kronrad L, Kolc J: Detection of myocardial infarction by in vivo scanning. Cardiologia 51:22, 1967.
4. Holman BL, Lesch M, Zweiman FG, Temte J, Lown B, Gorlin R: Detection and sizing of acute myocardial infarcts with ^{99m}Tc(Sn) tetracycline. N Engl J Med 291:159, 1974.
5. Holman BL, Idoine J, Fliegel CP, Dewanjee MK, Davis MA, Treves S, Eldh P: Detection and localization of experimental myocardial infarction with ^{99m}Tc-tetracycline. J Nucl Med 14:595, 1973.

6. Bonte FJ, Parkey RW, Graham KD, Moore J, Stokely EM: A new method for radionuclide imaging of myocardial infarcts. Radiology 110:473, 1974.

7. Willerson JT, Parkey RW, Bonte FJ, Meyer SL, Stokely EM: Acute subendocardial myocardial infarction in patients. Its detection by technetium 99-m stannous pyrophosphate myocardial scintigrams. Circulation 51:436, 1975.

8. Willerson JT, Parkey RW, Bonte FJ, Meyer SL, Atkins JM, Stokely EM: Technetium stannous pyrophosphate myocardial scintigrams in patients with chest pain of varying etiology. Circulation 51:1046, 1975.

9. Davis MA, Holman BL, Carmel AN: Evaluation of radiopharmaceuticals sequestered by acutely damaged myocardium. J Nucl Med 17:911, 1976.

10. Shen AC, Jennings RB: Myocardial calcium and magnesium in acute ischemic injury. Am J Pathol 67:417, 1972.

11. D'Agostino AN: An electron microscopic study of cardiac necrosis produced by 9 alpha-fluorocortisol and sodium phosphate. Am J Pathol 45:633, 1964.

12. Buja LM, Parkey RW, Dees JH, Stokely EM, Harris RA Jr, Bonte FJ, Willerson JT: Morphologic correlates of technetium-99m stannous pyrophosphate imaging of acute myocardial infarcts in dogs. Circulation 52:596, 1975.

13. Buja ML, Tofe AJ, Kulkarni PV, Mukherjee A, Parkey RW, Francis MD, Bonte FJ, Willerson JT: Sites and mechanisms of localization of technetium-99m phosphorus radiopharmaceuticals in acute myocardial infarcts and other tissues. J Clin Invest 60:724, 1977.

14. Thakur ML, Gottschalk A, Zaret BL: Imaging experimental myocardial infarction with indium-111-labeled autologous leukocytes: effects of infarct age and residual regional myocardial blood flow. Circulation (60): 297, 1979.

15. Khaw BA, Gold HK, Leinback RC, Fallon JT, Strauss W, Pohost GM, Haber E: Early imaging of experimental myocardial infarction by intracoronary administration of ^{131}I-labeled anticardiac myosin (Fab')$_2$ fragments. Circulation 58:1137, 1978.

16. Coleman RE, Klein MS, Ahmed SA, Weiss ES, Buchholz WM, Sobel BE: Mechanisms contributing to myocardial accumulation of technetium-99m stannous pyrophosphate after coronary arterial occlusion. Am J Cardiol 39:55, 1977.

17. Martonffy K, Reimer KA, Henkin RE, Jennings RB, Quinn JL: Technetium-99m pyrophosphate concentration in experimental myocardial infarcts [abstr]. J Nucl Med 16:548, 1975.

18. Botvinick EH, Shames D, Lappin H, Tyberg JV, Townsend R, Parmley WW: Noninvasive quantitation of myocardial infarction with technetium-99m pyrophosphate. Circulation 52:909, 1975.

19. Buja LM, Parkey RW, Stokely EM, Bronte FJ, Willerson JT: Pathophysiology of technetium-99m stannous pyrophosphate and thallium-201 scintigraphy of acute anterior myocardial infarcts in dogs. J Clin Invest 57:1508, 1976.

20. Marcus ML, Tomanek RJ, Ehrhardt JC, Kerber RE, Brown DD, Abboud FM: Relationships between myocardial perfusion, myocardial necrosis, and technetium-99m pyrophosphate uptake in dogs subjected to sudden coronary occlusion. Circulation 54:647, 1976.

21. Poliner LR, Buja LM, Parkey RW, Bonte FJ, Willerson JT: Clinicopathologic findings in 52 patients studied by technetium-99m stannous pyrosphosphate myocardial scintigraphy. Circulation 59:257, 1979.

22. Doherty PW, McLaughlin PR, Billingham M, Kernoff R, Goris ML, Harrison DC: Cardiac damage produced by direct current countershock applied to the heart. Am J Cardiol 43:225, 1979.

23. Falkoff M, Parkey RW, Bonte FJ, Lewis S, Buja LM, Dehmer G, Willerson JT: Technetium-99m stannous pyrophosphate myocardial scintigraphy: serial imaging to detect myocardial infarcts in patients. Clin Cardiol 1:163, 1978.

24. Buja LM, Poliner LR, Parkey RW, Pulido JI, Hutcheson D, Platt MR, Mills LJ, Bonte FJ, Willerson JT: Clinicopathologic study of persistently positive technetium-99m stannous pyrophosphate myocardial scintigrams and myocytolytic degeneration after myocardial infarction. Circulation 56:1016, 1977.

25. Olson HG, Lyons KP, Aronow WS, Brown WT, Greenfield RS: Follow-up technetium-99m stannous pyrophosphate myocardial scintigrams after acute myocardial infarction. Circulation 56:181, 1977.

26. Zaret B, DiCola VC, Donabedian RK, Puri S, Wolfson S, Freedman GS, Cohen LS: Dual radionuclide study of myocardial infarcton. Relationships between myocardial uptake of potassium-43, technetium-99m stannous pyrophosphate, regional myocardial blood flow and creatine phosphokinase depletion. Circulation 53:422, 1976.

27. Budd GC, Gohara A, White P, Schott DR, Kopel JA, Ross JN Jr, Leighton RF: Application of a serial frozen sectioning technique to the analysis of myocardial infarct size. Lab Invest 38:533, 1978.

28. Poliner LR, Buja LM, Parkey RW, Stokely EM, Stone MJ, Harris R, Templeton GH, Bonte FJ, Willerson JT: Comparison different noninvasive methods of infarct sizing during experimental myocardial infarction. J Nucl Med 18:517, 1977.

29. Stokely EM, Buja LM, Lewis SE, Parkey RW, Bonte FJ, Harris RA, Willerson JT: Measurement of acute myocardial infarcts in dogs with ^{99m}Tc-stannous pyrophosphate scrintigrams. J Nucl Med 17:1, 1976.

30. Willerson JT, Parkey RW, Harris RA, Bonte FJ, Stokely EM, Buja LM: Sizing actute myocardial infarction utilizing technetium stannous pyrophosphate myocardial scintigrams in dogs and man [abstr]. Clin Res 23:214A, 1975.

31. Marcus ML, Kerber RE: Present status of the [99m]technetium pyrophosphate infarct scintigram. Circulation 56:335, 1977.

32. Massie BM, Botvinick EH, Werner JA, Chatterjee K, Parmley WW: Myocardial scintigraphy with technetium-99m stannous pyrophosphate: an insensitive test for nontransmural myocardial infarction. Am J Cardiol 43:186, 1979.

33. Rude RE, Parkey RW, Bonte FJ, Lewis SE, Twieg D, Buja LM, Willerson JT: Clinical implications of the technetium-99m stannous pyrophosphate myocardial scintigraphic doughnut pattern in patients with acute myocardial infarcts. Circulation 59:721, 1979.

34. Ahmad M, Dubiel JP, Logan KW, Verdon Ta, Martin RH: Limited clinical diagnostic specificity of technetium-99m stannous pyrophosphate myocardial imaging in acute myocardial infarction. Am J Cardiol 39:50, 1977.

35. Berman DS, Amsterdam EA, Hines HH, Salel AF, Bailey GJ, DeNardo GL, Mason DT: New approach to interpretation of technetium-99m pyrophosphate scintigraphy in detection of acute myocardial infarction: clinical assessment of diagnostic accuracy. Am J Cardiol 39:341, 1977.

36. Coleman RE, Klein MS, Roberts R, Sobel BE: Improved detection of myocardial infarction with technetium-99m stannous pyrophosphate and serum MB creatine phosphokinase. Am J Cardiol 37:732, 1976.

37. Cowley MJ, Mantle JA, Rogers WJ, Russell RO, Rackley CE, Logic JR: Technetium-99m stannous pyrophosphate myocardial scintigraphy. Reliability and limitations in assessment of acute myocardial infarction. Circulation 56:192, 1977.

38. Parkey RW, Bonte FJ, Meyer SL, Atkins JM, Currey GC, Stokely EM, Willerson JT: A new method for radionuclide imaging of acute myocardial infarction in humans. Circulation 50:540, 1974.

39. Perez LA: Clinical experience: technetium 99m labeled phosphates in myocardial imaging. Clin Nucl Med 1:2, 1976.

40. Prasquier R, Taradash MR, Botvinick EH, Shames DM, Parmley WW: The specificity of the diffuse pattern of cardiac uptake in myocardial infarction imaging with technetium 99m stannous pyrophosphate. Circulation 55:61, 1977.

41. Hisada K, Suzuki Y, Iimori M: Technetium 99m pyrophosphate bone imaging in the evaluation of trauma. Clin Nucl Med 1:18, 1976.

42. Pugh BR, Buja LM, Parkey RW, Poliner LR, Stokely EM, Bonte FJ, Willerson JT: Cardioversion and false positive technetium 99m stannous pyrophosphate myocardial scintigrams. Circulation 54:399, 1976.

43. Kim E: Calcified costal cartilage as a cause of false interpretation on myocardial imaging. Clin Nucl Med 1:159, 1976.

44. Serafini AN, Raskin MM, Zand LC, Watson DD: Radionuclide breast scanning in carcinoma of the breast. J Nucl Med 15:1149, 1974.

45. Bossuyt A, Verbeelen D: Accumulation of ^{99m}Tc pyrophosphates in the skin lesions of pseudoxanthoma elasticum. Clin Nucl Med 1:245, 1976.

46. Ahmad M, Dubiel JP, Verdon TA, Martin RH: Technetium[99m] stannous pyrophosphate myocardial imaging in patients with and without left ventricular aneurysm. Circulation 53:833, 1976.

47. Donsky MS, Curry GC, Parkey RW, Meyer SL, Bonte FJ, Platt MR, Willerson JT: Unstable angina pectoris. Clinical, antiographic and myocardial scintigraphic observations. Br Heart J 38:257, 1976.

48. Chiu CL, Roelofs JD, Go RT, Doty DB, Rose EF, Christie JH: Coronary angiographic and scintigraphic findings in experimental cardiac contusion. Radiology 116:679, 1975.

49. Go RT, Doty DB, Chiu CL, Christie JH: A new method of diagnosing myocardial contusion in man by radionuclide imaging. Radiology 116:107, 1975.

50. Righetti A, O'Rourke RA, Schelbert H, Henning H, Hardarson T, Daily PO, Ashburn W, Ross J: Usefulness of preoperative and postoperative Tc-99m (Sn)-pyrophosphate scans in patients with ischemic and valvular heart disease. Am J Cardiol 39:43, 1977.

51. Perez LA, Hayt DB, Freeman LM: Localization of myocardial disorders other than infarction with ^{99m}Tc-labeled phosphate agents. J Nucl Med 17:241, 1976.

52. Klein MS, Coleman RE, Weldon CS, Sobel BE, Roberts R: Concordance of electrocardiographic and scintigraphic criteria of myocardial injury after cardiac surgery. J Thorac Cardiovasc Surg 71:934, 1976.

53. Platt MR, Mills LJ, Parkey RW, Willerson JT, Bonte FJ, Shapiro W, Sugg WL:

346

Perioperative myocardial infarction diagnosed by technetium 99m stannous pyrophosphate myocardial scintigrams. Circulation 54:III-24, 1976.
54. Lorell B, Leinbach RC, Pohost GM, Gold HK, Dinsmore RE, Hutter AM Jr, Pastore JO, Desanctis RW: Right ventricular infarction. Clinical diagnosis and differentiation from cardiac tamponade and pericardial constriction. Am J Cardiol 43:465, 1979.
55. Sharpe DN, Botvinick EH, Shames DM, Schiller NB, Massie BM, Chatterjee K, Parmley WW: The noninvasive diagnosis of right ventricular infarction. Circulation 57:483, 1978.
56. Wackers FJ, Lie KI, Sokole EB, Res J, Van der Schoot JD, Durrer D: Prevalence of right ventricular involvement in inferior wall infarction assessed with myocardial imaging with thallium-201 and technetium 99m pyrophosphate. Am J Cardiol 42:358, 1978.
57. Lewis M, Buja LM, Saffer S, Mishelevich D, Stokely EM, Lewis S, Parkey R, Bonte F, Willerson J: Experimental infarct sizing using computer processing and a three-dimensional model. Science 197:167, 1977.
58. Singh M, Berggren MJ, Gustafson DE, Dewanjee MK, Bahn RC, Ritman EL: Emission-computed tomography and its application to imaging of acute myocardial infarction in intact dogs using Tc-99m pyrophosphate. J Nucl Med 20:50, 1979.
59. Weiss ES, Ahmed SA, Welch MJ, Williamson JR, Ter-Pogossian MM, Sobel BE: Quantification of infarction in cross sections of canine myocardium in vivo with positron emission transaxial tomography and ^{11}C-palmitate. Circulation 55:66, 1977.

14. POSTMORTEM: ANATOMIC QUANTITATION

RAYMOND E. IDEKER, DONALD B. HACKEL, and ERIC C. McCLEES

Anatomic estimation of infarct size is considered to be the standard against which other methods of estimating infarct size should be tested. In most animal studies, evaluation of techniques for estimating infarct size as well as evaluation of interventions for limiting infarct size are based upon the direct anatomic determination of infarct size as a benchmark. Clinical studies using direct anatomic estimation of infarct size are less common because, fortunately, relatively few hospitalized patients die after an infarct. Moreover, the small percentage of patients in clinical studies who are autopsied may not be representative of the entire study population, since large or complicated infarcts are probably more common in this group than in the general population of patients with infarcts. Although a larger percentage of patients with small infarcts could be studied by obtaining needle biopsies of the left ventricle during cardiac surgery [1], such studies would not enable accurate estimation of infarct size because of the limited amount of tissue sampled.

Even when the patient's heart is obtained at autopsy, it may still not be possible to quantitate the size of the infarct anatomically. For example, without the use of special histochemical techniques (see Fallon, p. 373), infarcts less than one day old cannot be sized by direct anatomic observation. Although many of these infarcts can be detected because they exhibit 'wavy fibers' or contraction bands [2], these findings do not enable the extent of an infarct to be determined. Since wavy fibers and contraction bands can be present for two weeks after an infarct [2], extension of an infarct just before the patient's death cannot always be reliably detected in standard histologic sections.

METHODS FOR ANATOMIC QUANTITATION OF INFARCT SIZE

Most methods for quantitating the amount of infarct by direct anatomic observation involve cross-sectioning the ventricles into 5–10 slices by cutting the heart perpendicular to its long axis, estimating the area of infarct from the cut surface of each slice, estimating the amount of infarct in each slice from the cross-sectional areas of infarcted tissue, and summing the amount of infarct in all of the slices to determine the total amount of infarcted tissue in the heart.

Wagner GS (ed): Myocardial Infarction: Measurement and Intervention, pp 347–371.
© 1982 Martinus Nijhoff Publishers, The Hague/Boston/London.

A few methods do not follow this general procedure. These exceptions include determining the percentage of the left ventricle infarcted (a) entirely by subjective examination of the heart [3], (b) by cutting out the infarcted tissue and weighing it [4], and (c) by ligating the left circumflex coronary artery in a constant location in an animal model and determining the area of infarct for only two or three cross sections [5]. The amount of infarct in these two or three cross sections has been shown to be representative of the entire amount of infarct [5]. The developers of this last method have more recently begun to estimate infarct size using five slices [6].

Preparation of the tissue

Although some anatomic methods use fresh or frozen [7] tissue to enable special histochemical or autoradiographic techniques, most methods employ fixation of the heart by formalin. While formalin fixation increases the thickness of right and left ventricular walls [8], marked shrinkage of tissue (30%–40%) is produced by the dehydration and infiltration steps in the preparation of histologic sections [9]. Formalin fixation also changes heart weight [8]. For this reason, some anatomic methods specify sectioning the heart while it is fresh and weighing the slices or blocks from the slices before they are placed in formalin [10]. To enable both histologic and electron-microscopic study, the heart can be fixed in 3% glutaraldehyde rather than formalin. Electron microscopy can detect early myocardial injury before light microscopy [11].

Identification of the infarct

Infarcts can be identified by gross examination alone, by gross examination after applying histochemical stains, or by microscopic examination. Although some methods use only gross examination or only microscopic examination to estimate infarct size, many methods use both. In our experience, gross examination alone will underestimate infarct size; with old infarcts, regions of slight, patchy fibrosis will be missed, while with acute infarcts, microscopic foci of necrosis just outside the grossly visible infarct border will be missed. The gross estimation of infarct size can be improved by the use of special stains (see Fallon, p. 374).

Estimation of the cross-sectional slice area of the infarct

Several different techniques have been used to estimate the area of infarct on the cut surface of each slice including (a) subjective estimation, (b) cutting and weighing photomicrographs, (c) determining the circumferential extent of the infarct, (d) point counting, and (e) computer-assisted planimetry.

Subjective estimation

These methods involve estimating the amount of infarcted tissue within each slice. With one such method [12], the ventricles are cut transversely into five slices of equal thickness and the gross involvement of each infarct is recorded on standard cross-sectional diagrams of each slice (Figure 1). Each slice is then divided into six standard blocks from which histologic sections are prepared (Figure 1). Microscopic examination of these slides is then used to correct the extent of the infarcts on the diagrams. From the corrected diagrams the percent infarct of each block of each slice is estimated to the nearest 25%. The percent infarct of each segment is multiplied by the average amount of the left and right

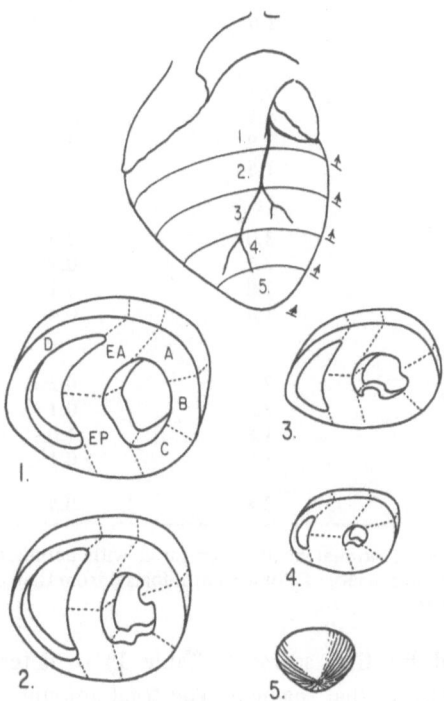

Figure 1. Diagram illustrating division of the ventricles into segments for one subjective method of estimating infarct size. The drawing of the anterior surface of the heart (*top*) shows the levels taken from the base (*1*) to the apex (*5*). The cross sections present the scheme of segmentation at each level, A, anterior; B, lateral; C, posterior; D, right ventricle; EA, anterior septum; EP, posterior septum. Reprinted with permission of the American Society of Clinical Pathologists from Hackel and Ratliff [12].

Table 1. Percentages of total heart weight accounted for by individual segments of Figure 2[a]

	Mean	± SE of mean
Section A		
1	2.8	0.2
2	2.9	0.2
3	2.5	0.1
4	1.7	0.1
Section B		
1	2.6	0.1
2	2.8	0.2
3	2.6	0.1
4	1.7	0.1
Section C		
1	2.8	0.2
2	2.6	0.1
3	2.4	0.1
4	1.6	0.1
Section D		
1	9.3	0.6
2	4.1	0.3
3	2.8	0.2
4	1.5	0.1
Section EA		
1	3.0	0.3
2	2.6	0.1
3	1.8	0.1
4	1.4	0.4
Section EP		
1	2.6	0.2
2	2.5	0.1
3	1.8	1.0
4	1.2	0.1
Apex	3.8	0.4

[a] Based on 20 normal hearts. Reprinted with permission of the American Society of Clinical Pathologists from Hackel and Ratliff [12].

ventricles represented by that segment (Table 1) to determine the percent infarct of the ventricles in that segment. The total amount of infarct for both ventricles is obtained by summing the infarct in all the segments [12]. A similar method uses seven slices instead of five [13].

Cutting and weighing photomicrographs

Quantitation of infarct size from histologic sections alone has been performed using photomicrographs of each section. Each photomicrograph is cut into infarcted and noninfarcted portions and the portions are weighed to the nearest milligram [5]. The weight of the infarcted portion divided by the weights of both portions is taken as the fraction of the cross section that is infarcted.

Determining the circumferential extent of the infarct

The infarcted fraction of the cut surface of a heart slice has been expressed as the fraction of the circumference of the slice that contains infarcted tissue [14–16]. Little difference was noted between the fraction of the endocardial and epicardial circumferences that were infarcted [14]. If the infarct is not solid and transmural, this method will overestimate infarct size. Underestimation of infarct size because of wall thinning (see below) is avoided with this method.

Point counting

These methods involve placing a grid of regularly spaced points over the gross slice or histologic section [17]. The number of points over infarcted and non-infarcted myocardium is counted. The number of points over infarcted tissue divided by the sum of the number of points over both non-infarcted and infarcted tissue is taken as the fraction of the slice that is infarcted. With one such method [18], the gross slices are stained with a solution of nitroblue tetrazolium, and each slice is covered with a transparent sheet of cellulose film in which a regular pattern of small holes has been etched, each 2 mm apart, arranged in a series of equilateral triangles; each hole represents a point. Another method uses a standard 35-mm projector to project microscopic slides onto a screen containing a point grid [19]. Many of the steps in point counting have been automated including generating the points with a graphics terminal [20], counting the points with an electronic digitizer [21], and processing the data with a microcomputer [22].

Computer-assisted planimetry techniques

In these methods [23–30], a hand-held digitizing pen is used to enter into a computer the epicardial and endocardial outlines of the left ventricle (and frequently the right ventricle) and the borders of any infarcted region from the top cut surface of the slice. The area within each traced outline is then computed from the digitized points by the trapezoid rule or, if the points are equally spaced, by Simpson's rule, Newton's three-eighths rule, or Weddle's rule [31]. The area within the epicardial outline (plus the area of the papillary muscles) minus the area within the endocardial outline is taken as the area of ventricular muscle. This figure divided into the area of infarcted tissue yields the fraction of the surface of the slice that consists of infarct. As discussed more fully below, the percent infarct of the top of each slice, together with either the weight or volume of each slice, is used to compute the total weight, volume, or percent of infarct.

The epicardial, endocardial, and infarct outlines of the gross slices have been traced from several different sources. They have been traced from 35-mm color transparencies projected either directly on the tablet of the digitization device [32] or first onto tracing paper and then planimetered [33], from 8" × 10" photographic enlargements of the top of each slice [34], and from clear Plexiglas sheets that had previously been placed over the heart slices on which the epicardial, endocardial, and infarct outlines had been traced with a grease pencil [33]. Planimetry has also been performed on photomicrographs of microscopic sections of infarcted myocardium [35].

Patchy infarcts

Infarcts are frequently patchy with regions of normal and infarcted tissue interspersed. Methods estimating the cross-sectional amount of infarct directly from histologic sections enable quantitation of each patch, but are more tedious than methods based on the gross slices. One method employing gross slices attempts to account for this patchy distribution by using the histologic sections to estimate the amount of viable muscle within the infarcted region to the nearest 25% [34]; the area of infarct planimetered from the photograph of the gross slice (Figure 2) is multiplied by this fraction by a computer program.

Wall thinning

The wall of the ventricle can be thinned in infarcted regions and the cause may differ in acute and old infarcts. Expansion of acute infarcts caused by systolic ventricular pressure can lead to stretching and thinning of the ventricular wall in the infarcted region [36]. Since the wall thinning is accompanied by circumferential stretching, the change in the area of infarct on the surface of the slice may not be large. No anatomic sizing method has yet been devised to compensate for these changes in volume of acute infarcts. Methods based on the circumferential extent of infarct will overestimate the size of these infarcts.

In old infarcts, wall thinning can be caused by phagocytosis and removal of necrotic tissue during organization of the infarct and by contraction of the fibrous scar during healing of the infarct. In this case, wall thinning represents an actual loss of myocardial tissue. One method attempts to account for this tissue loss by having the investigator estimate the thickness of the wall before infarction (Figure 2) [34]. The area of estimated tissue loss caused by wall thinning is determined by planimetry and this area is counted as part of the infarct for the top surface of the slice [34]. With the exception of the papillary muscles and the outflow tract, the thickness of the left ventricle is relatively uniform in any given cross section. For this reason, the average thickness of the wall in those portions of the slice that are free of infarct is used as an estimate of the original thickness of the infarcted portion of the wall [34]. This method cannot be used for circumferential infarcts.

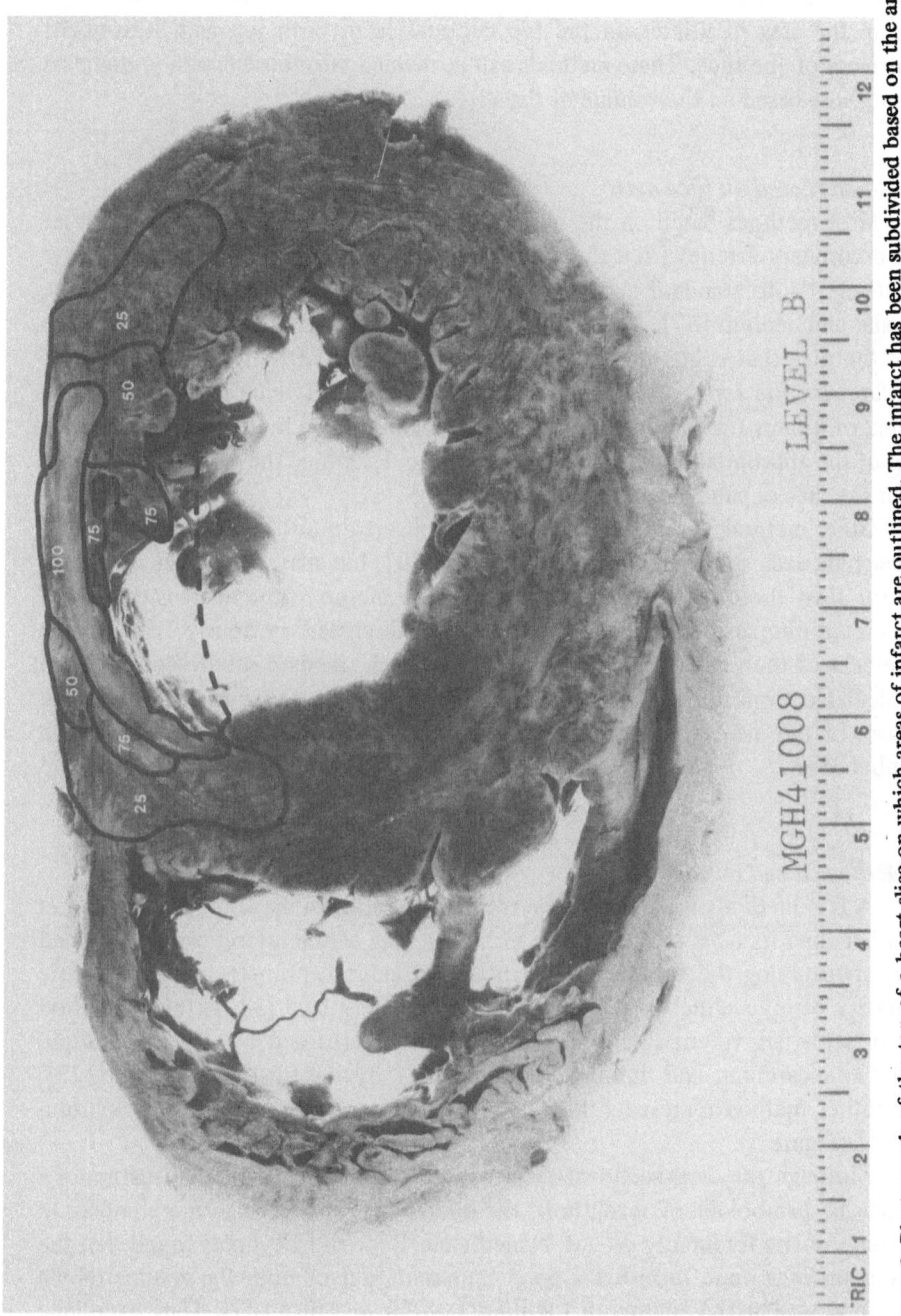

Figure 2. Photograph of the top of a heart slice on which areas of infarct are outlined. The infarct has been subdivided based on the amount of viable muscle interspersed with infarct in each subdivision. The border of each subdivision is shown by black lines. The numbers give the percent of the area within each subdivision consisting of infarct estimated to the nearest 25%. The dashed line indicates the estimated location of the endocardium before the infarction.

Estimation of infarct volume

Several methods have been used to estimate the volume of infarct within a slice from the area of infarct on the top cut surface or both top and bottom cut surfaces of the slice. These methods can be divided into those based on the mass and those based on the volume of the slice.

Methods based on slice mass

Most methods based on the mass of each slice require trimming epicardial fat and coronary arteries from the slice, and weighing the slice either intact or after cutting it into standard subdivisions such as the right and left ventricular free walls and septum [37]. The fraction of the surface area of the top cut surface of the slice that is infarcted, either alone or averaged with the fractional area of infarct for the top cut surface of the next lower slice (which is the same as the area of infarct for the bottom of the slice), is multiplied by the mass of the slice or of the appropriate subdivision of the slice to determine the mass of the infarct for the slice or subdivision.

Other methods based on the mass of the heart do not require trimming and weighing each subdivision of each slice [12, 13], but may be subject to greater error than those methods that do. With these methods, the heart is cut into a standard number of slices and subdivisions as discussed previously. The average percent of the mass of the heart occupied by each standard subdivision has been calculated from normal hearts. These average percentages are multiplied by the mass of the heart whose infarcts are being sized to estimate the mass of each subdivision.

Methods based on slice volume

A few methods use a geometric formula to estimate the volume of an infarct rather than its mass [25, 34]. The mass in grams of the infarct can be obtained by multiplying the volume of the infarct in cubic centimeters by the specific gravity of myocardial tissue which is approximately 1.05 [38, 39]. One method represents all volumes within the slice, those enclosed by the epicardium, the endocardium, and within the infarct itself, by the frustum of a cone [25]. Another method represents them by the frustum of a paraboloid of revolution [34] (Figure 3).

Although the cross-sectional slices of the ventricles resemble the frustum of a cone or paraboloid of revolution, the infarcts within the slices are complex in structure and frequently do not. Nonetheless, Boor and Reynolds found that the frustum of a cone furnishes a good representation of both the volume of the slice as well as the volume of the infarct within the slice [25]. They examined

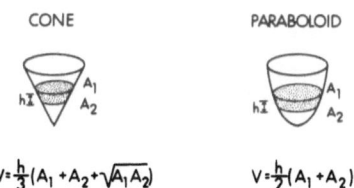

$$V = \frac{h}{3}(A_1 + A_2 + \sqrt{A_1 A_2})$$ $$V = \frac{h}{2}(A_1 + A_2)$$

Figure 3. Two geometric representations of a slice of the left ventricle: the frustum of a cone and the frustum of a paraboloid of revolution. Formulas for the volumes of the frustums are also given where V = volume of frustum, A_1 = area of top of frustum, A_2 = area of bottom of frustum, and h = height of frustum.

eight human hearts, four of which contained infarcts. The infarcted hearts were stained with triphenyl tetrazolium chloride. All areas of infarct revealed by the stain were dissected from the left ventricle. Weights of the left ventricle and the myocardial infarct for each slice were recorded and compared with the weights calculated by planimetry. Computation of volume was based on the formula for the frustum of a cone, and conversion to weight was performed by multiplying by a specific gravity of 1.05. The correlation coefficient between the calculated and actual weight for the left ventricle of all the slices of the eight hearts was 0.94 and for the myocardial infarcts in four of the hearts was 0.91. This method, however, consistently underestimated the mass of the most apical slice of the left ventricle (see their Figure 5) [25].

Although the formula for the frustum of a paraboloid of revolution yields a slightly larger volume than the formula for the frustum of a cone for the same measurements, we found that the paraboloid of revolution also underestimates the volume of the apical slice of the left ventricle. We cut ten normal human hearts into six slices, planimetered the endocardial and epicardial (including the right side of the septum) surfaces of each slice, and computed the volume of each slice based on the formula for the frustum of a paraboloid of revolution. The computed volume of each slice was compared with the volume of the slice determined by water displacement according to Archimede's principle. Besides underestimating the volume of the apical slices, the volume of the most basal slice was overestimated. This latter finding is explained by the fact that the thickness of the left ventricular wall and septum decreases near the atrioventricular groove. We found that the most basal slice of the left ventricle could be better represented by a cylinder capped by a parabolic toroid (Figure 4) [34]. To improve estimation of the size of an infarct, the values obtained for the volume of each slice and the infarct within the slice computed from the formula for the frustum of a paraboloid of revolution are multiplied by correction factors obtained by taking the ratio of the computed volume and measured volume from water displacement of the slices from the ten normal hearts (Table 2).

356

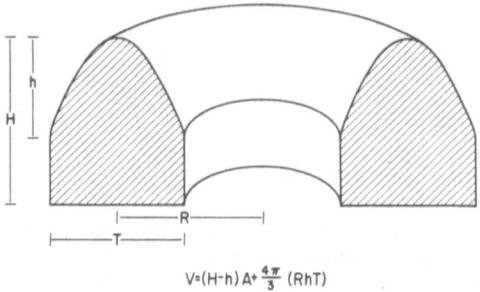

$$V = (H-h) A + \frac{4\pi}{3} (RhT)$$

Figure 4. Representation of half of the most basal slice of the left ventricle as a cylinder capped by a parabolic toroid: V = volume of slice, T = average thickness of slice, R = average distance from centroid of epicardial outline to middle of the wall at the bottom of the slice, A = area of the bottom cut surface of the slice, H = average height of slice, and h = height of parabolic portion of slice which is set equal to $0.75\ T$.

Table 2. Volume correction factors for heart slices

Slice	Factor ± SD
1	1.04 ± 0.06
2	1.02 ± 0.05
3	1.13 ± 0.09
4	1.11 ± 0.07
5	1.20 ± 0.08
6	1.42 ± 0.21

Reprinted with permission of the American Heart Association from Ideker, et al. [34].

METHODS FOR ANATOMIC QUANTITATION OF INFARCT LOCATION

Although many autopsy studies have been performed in which the presence or absence of infarct within particular locations of the ventricles has been noted [40–44], only a few studies have quantitated the amount of infarct within different subdivisions of the left ventricle [12, 23, 28, 34, 45]. One method quantitates the amount of infarct in that portion of the left ventricle seen in the RAO ventriculogram [45]. A second method divides the left ventricle into septal, posterior, and anterior thirds and quantitates the amount of infarct in each third [23].

Another method [28, 34] quantitates infarct location by dividing the left ventricle into 12, 24, or 48 subdivisions (Figure 5). The amount of infarct is quantitated within each subdivision by a computer program from planimetered heart slices. The heart is subdivided based upon a cylindrical coordinate system in

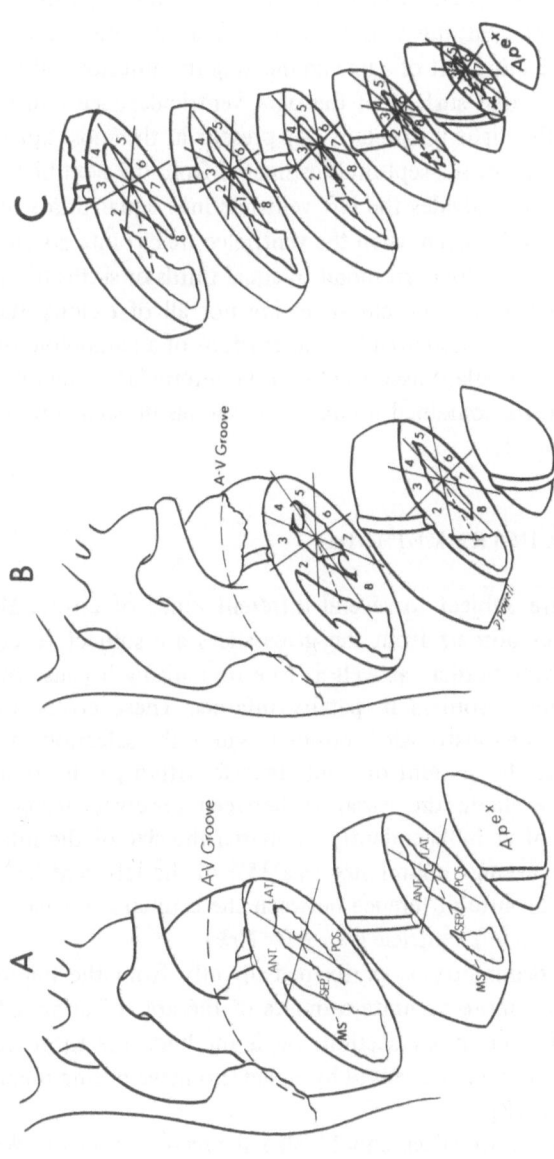

Figure 5. Partitioning of the left ventricle into 12 (*A*), 24 (*B*), and 48 (*C*) subdivisions for quantitating infarct location: C, centroid of the outline of the left ventricular epicardium and right septal border; MS, point in the midseptum half way between the anterior and posterior endocardial insertions of the right ventricle into the septum. The dashed line bisects the septal quadrant (*A*) and octant 1 (*B* and *C*).

which the z-axis roughly corresponds to the long axis of the heart. The outline of each slice of the left ventricle is divided into either four or eight equiangular sectors. The point of origin of these sectors is the centroid of the outline created by the epicardial surface of the left ventricle and the right side of the septum (Figure 5). The sectors are oriented based upon a line connecting the centroid of the epicardial outline and the middle of the septum. The middle of the septum is defined as the midpoint of a line connecting the anterior and posterior insertions of the endocardial surface of the right ventricular free wall into the septum. Occasionally the right ventricle is not present in the most apical slice. In that case, the midpoint of the septum is estimated from the next higher slice. This coordinate system also divides the left ventricle into equal thirds or sixths from base to apex (Figure 5). Even when the ventricles are cut into six slices, the levels of the cuts do not exactly correspond to equal thirds or sixths of the total base to apex distance because the cut slices are not all of exactly the same thickness. Each cut slice is represented by the frustum of a paraboloid of revolution, and a geometric formula is used to obtain the interpolated fraction of the volume of the slice and its contained infarct that belongs in each third or sixth of the left ventricle [28, 34].

SOURCES OF ERROR IN THE METHODS

All of the methods are subject to several different kinds of errors. Methods based on tracing infarct borders from the gross slices are subject to errors in recognition of the infarct borders as well as to errors arising because of viable muscle within the infarct borders in patchy infarcts. These errors are only partially decreased by using histologic sections to guide the selection of infarct borders and to estimate the amount of viable muscle within patchy infarcts to the nearest 25%. To evaluate the variation between observers using such a method, two or more of us independently estimated the size of the infarcts in 12 human hearts. The average infarct size was 35% of the left ventricle (range 6%–56%). The mean absolute difference between the estimates for each of the infarct sizes was 4% of the left ventricle (range 0–10%).

Methods in which planimetry is performed directly from the microscopic sections probably yield a more accurate estimate of the area of infarcted tissue within the surface of each cross section. Such methods are more tedious, however, and are subject to errors caused by tissue shrinkage during preparation of the histologic sections [8].

Increasing the number of slices should also decrease the error. We have examined the effect of using different numbers of slices on estimated infarct size in seven hearts that had been cut into nine slices plus the base. Infarct size was estimated from all slices as well as from only five slices by planimetering every other slice. Average infarct size was 18% (range 7%–39%) of the left ventricle. The mean absolute difference between the two estimates of infarct size for the seven hearts was only 0.6% (range 0–2.4%) of the left ventricle.

While methods based on the weight of each slice require trimming epicardial fat and the coronary arteries from each slice and weighing it, methods based on slice volume require only measuring the thickness of each slice. Even when cut with a motorized meat slicer, however, slices may not be of uniform thickness, especially if the heart is cut before fixation. The mass of a slice can be measured more accurately than can its thickness.

Methods based on volume computed from a geometric model lend themselves more readily to quantitation of infarct location. If a purely histologic method is to be used and quantitation of infarct location is also desired, then either (a) whole mounts of each cross section must be made; (b) the tissue blocks must be cut in a standard, predetermined way; or (c) a computer program must be developed to orient each planimetered section in its proper place in space.

Methods for quantitating infarct location are also subject to several types of errors. The midpoint of the septum is not a fixed reference point because the septum spirals slightly from base to apex (Figure 6) [46]. The centroid of the outline of the cut surface of a cross section will be in error if the heart contains

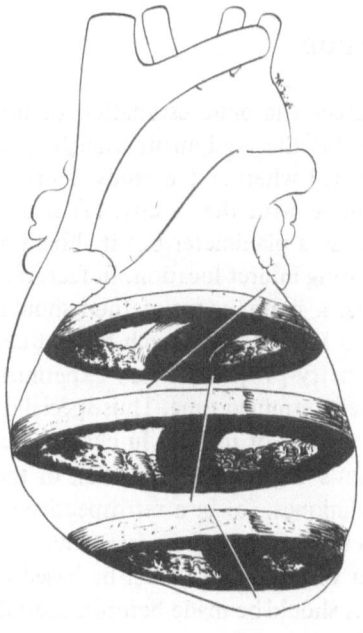

Figure 6. Anterior view of the human heart showing the compound curves of the interventricular septum. Reprinted with permission of Harper and Row from James [46].

an aneurysm, if the heart was distorted during fixation, or if the cross section was not cut perpendicular to the long axis of the heart. Infarct expansion will increase the circumferential extent of the infarct by stretching of the infarcted wall [36], thus complicating the quantitation of infarct location.

The greatest reduction in the error of a particular method for estimating infarct size can be achieved by decreasing the largest source of error in the method. For example, if a method has two independent sources of error that cause errors of 10% and 5% (expressed as a standard deviation) in estimated infarct size, then the overall error will be 11.2% (the square root of the sum of the squares of each error, $\sqrt{10^2 + 5^2}$) [47]. If efforts are made to decrease the smaller error by 2%, from 5% to 3%, the overall error is decreased only to 10.4%. If instead efforts are made to decrease the larger error by 2%, from 10% to 8%, the overall error is decreased to 9.4%.

Another consideration is the expense in time or equipment necessary to reduce each error. For example, although a complex geometric model may furnish an estimate of infarct size that is only slightly better than a much simpler geometric model, once the computer programs are developed, the method using the complex geometric model requires no more work than the other method, since after planimetry all of the arithmetic is performed by the computer.

SELECTION OF A METHOD

The best method for direct anatomic estimation of infarct size depends upon several factors including (a) the equipment available, (b) whether the study is clinical or experimental, (c) whether the study is prospective or retrospective, and (d) what is to be done with the results. (a) If a computer is available, it should not just be used as a planimeter but it should also be utilized for data analysis and for quantitating infarct location. In fact, if a computer is only to be used to planimeter areas, a point count method should be used instead. Point count methods have been shown to be much faster than and just as accurate as computer-assisted planimetry [48]. (b) In an experimental study, the animals will be sacrificed at a predetermined time. Thus special histologic techniques can be used to identify the regions of infarct. In clinical studies, the relatively long time between the patient's death and acquisition of the heart effectively rules out the use of such techniques. (c) In a retrospective clinical study, the hearts have already been dissected according to a particular protocol, and the method for anatomic estimation of infarct size must be based on the manner in which they were cut. (d) Efforts should be made before undertaking a study to estimate the precision required for the anatomic estimation of infarct size. For example, it makes no sense to cut the heart into 200 cross sections and planimeter directly from the microscopic sections for all of these cross sections to achieve a precision of 0.1% infarct of the left ventricle if the purpose of the study is to test a clinical method for estimating infarct size which is a priori expected to have an accuracy of no more than ± 5% infarct of the left ventricle. Because of the large variation among different patients or animals, in general it is better to spend time studying a larger group of cases rather than to spend time to determine the amount of infarct in each slice with great precision [49, 50].

QUANTITATIVE MORPHOLOGIC ASPECTS OF INFARCTS

Direct anatomic estimation of infarct size has been used to study the clinical significance of infarct size, the ability of numerous clinical methods to estimate infarct size (see the remaining chapters in Part II, 'Methods for determining infarct size'), and the usefulness of pharmacologic methods of limiting infarct size (see Part III, 'Interventions for limiting infarct size,' p. 387). Direct anatomic methods have also supplied quantitative morphologic information about the differences and similarities among infarcts in different portions of the left ventricle. One series of studies quantitated the size and location of single uncomplicated infarcts in 66 patients, each of whom exhibited no signs of left or right ventricular hypertrophy, right or left bundle branch block, or anterior or posterior fascicular block in the electrocardiogram and whose heart did not exhibit an aneurysm or rupture of the wall [28–30]. The left ventricle was divided into equiangular thirds and the infarcts were grouped according to which third of the left ventricle contained the largest amount of infarct in each case (Figure 7); 26 infarcts predominated in the anterior third of the left ventricle [28], 26 in the inferior third [29], and 14 in the posterolateral third [30]. Infarcts predominating in the posterolateral third of the left ventricle were smaller and more heterogeneous in both location and arterial supply than were the anterior or inferior infarcts. Infarcts predominating in the anterior third of the left ventricle (Figure 8) averaged 21% (range 1%–57%) of the left ventricle [28], infarcts predominating in the inferior third (Figure 9) averaged 16% (range 4%–41%) [29], and infarcts predominating in the posterolateral third (Figure 10) averaged 7% (range 1%–21%) [30]. Infarcts predominating in the anterior third were all within the distribution of the left anterior descending coronary artery or one or more of its branches [28]; infarcts predominating in the inferior third were in the distribution of the posterior descending coronary artery, and sometimes other branches arising from the vessels supplying the posterior descending coronary artery [29]; while infarcts predominating in the posterolateral third were sometimes in the distribution to the distal portion of the left circumflex coronary artery, and occasionally in the distribution of an optional diagonal branch arising from the left main coronary artery [30]. Anterior infarcts frequently involved relatively little of the base of the left ventricle but were frequently circumferential at the apex [28].

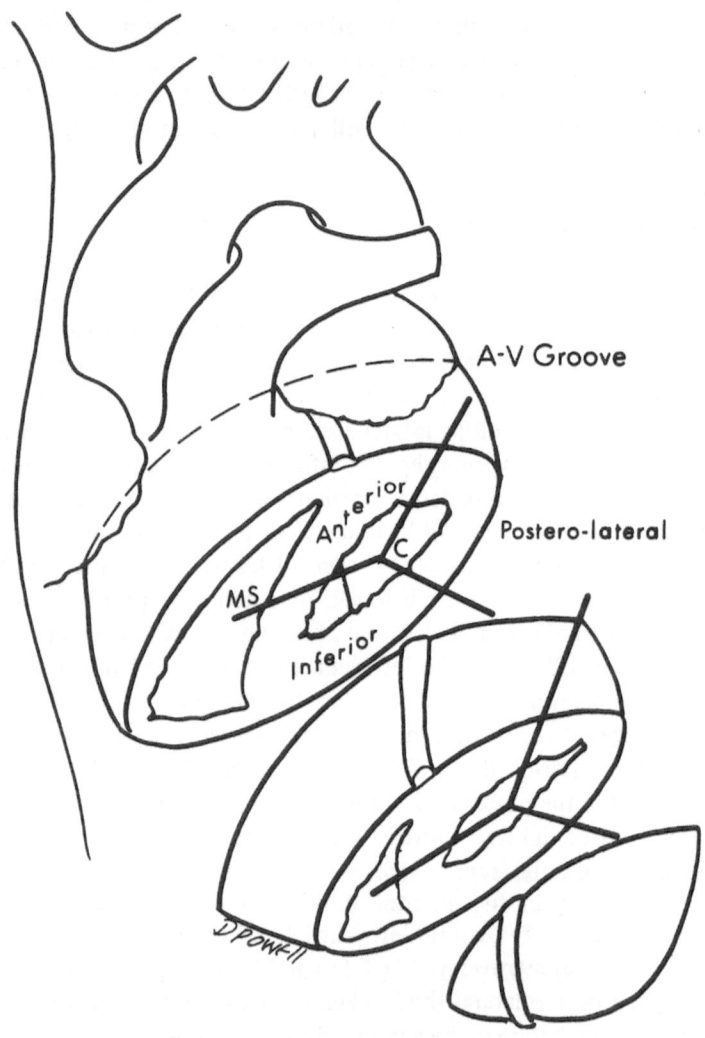

Figure 7. Division of the left ventricle into thirds (see Figure 5).

The opposite was true for inferior infarcts, which generally involved little of the apex but much of the base of the left ventricle [29]. The basal to apical location of posterolateral infarcts was more variable; four infarcts centered in the base of octants 4 or 5 (Figure 5B), six infarcts ran straight down from base to apex centered about octant 6, and four infarcts spiraled downward from octant 4 or 5 in the base to octant 6 in the middle and apex [30].

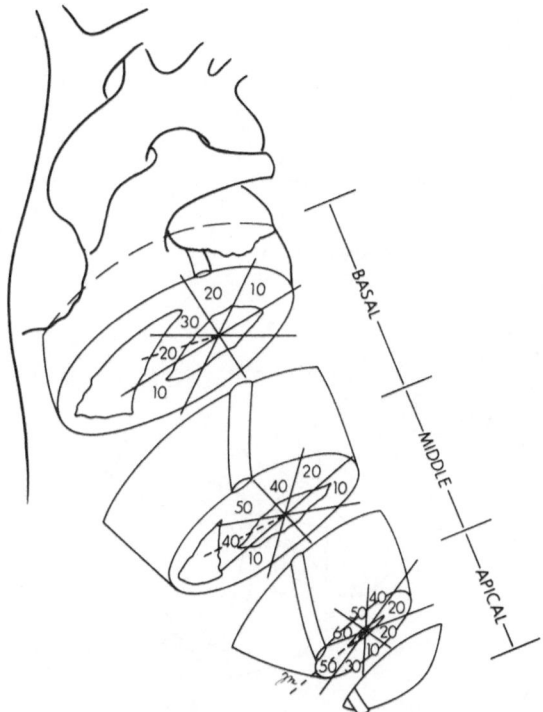

Figure 8. Average percent infarct within basal, middle, and apical octants for 26 infarcts predominantly in the anterior third of the left ventricle.

MYOCARDIAL ISCHEMIA

Only a few studies have attempted to identify regions of chronic ischemia by direct anatomic observation [51–53]. Subendocardial areas that microscopically exhibit vacuolated fibers, patchy fibrosis, and foci of coagulation necrosis in the presence of severe coronary atherosclerosis are thought to represent regions of chronic, severe ischemia (Figure 11). As opposed to an acute infarct, in which the myocardial cells all die within a few hours or days, these morphologic changes are thought to indicate a slow, continuous progression to cell death extending over months to years. The myofibers are thought to become vacuolated because of loss of cellular organelles, to become necrotic without inducing a neutrophil reponse, and finally to be replaced by fibrous connective tissue. These morphologic findings are found in regions of the subendocardium with a persistent, diffuse uptake of technetium-99 m stannous pyrophosphate [54]. No

364

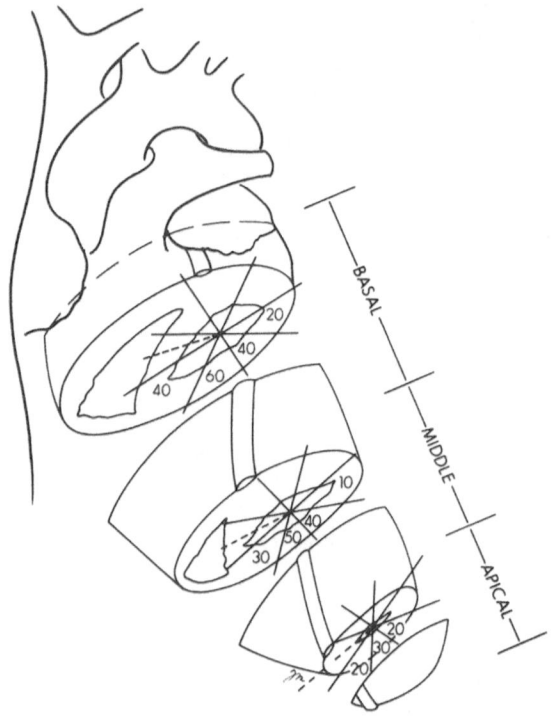

Figure 9. Average percent infarct within basal, middle, and apical octants for 26 infarcts predominantly within the inferior third of the left ventricle.

one has yet attempted to quantitate the amount of ischemic myocardium based on these morphologic findings, and it is not known what degree of ischemia is necessary to produce these changes. The presence of these morphologic findings is not related to the amount of coronary artery disease in patients with myocardial infarcts [55]. Also, these changes are not specific for ischemia but are thought to occur as a result of metabolic imbalance caused by many different disorders [56].

FUTURE DEVELOPMENTS IN ANATOMIC QUANTITATION OF INFARCT SIZE

Much additional work is needed. A better geometric model for the volume methods can be found. For example, an ellipsoid might better represent the apex of the left ventricle. While manual methods exist to estimate the amount of

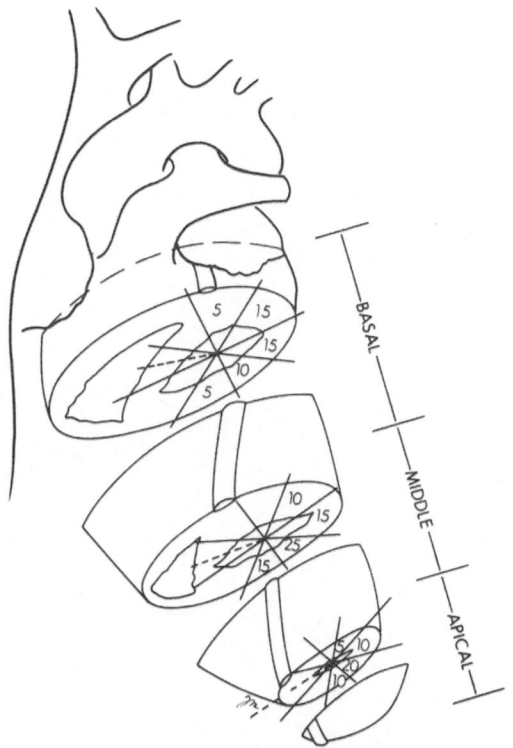

Figure 10. Average percent infarct within basal, middle, and apical octants for 16 infarcts predominantly within the posterobasal third of the left ventricle.

infarct in the endocardial, intramural, and epicardial thirds of the left ventricle [6, 19], a computerized method is needed to quantitate the transmural extent of an infarct similar to the computerized methods to quantitate the circumferential and basal to apical extent of an infarct.

The effects on cardiac function and patient survival of other morphologic characteristics of infarcts besides just their size should be examined. The basal to apical location of the infarct, its circumferential extent [57], its transmural extent, and whether it is patchy or solid may all be important. For example, all of the infarcts shown in Figure 12 are the same size, but each may have a different effect on patient mortality, cardiac function, and the incidence of arrhythmias.

To evaluate interventions to limit infarct size, an anatomic method is needed that can estimate what the size of the infarct would have been in the absence of the intervention. A first step toward developing such a method has been made by showing that the primary determinant of infarct size is the amount of left

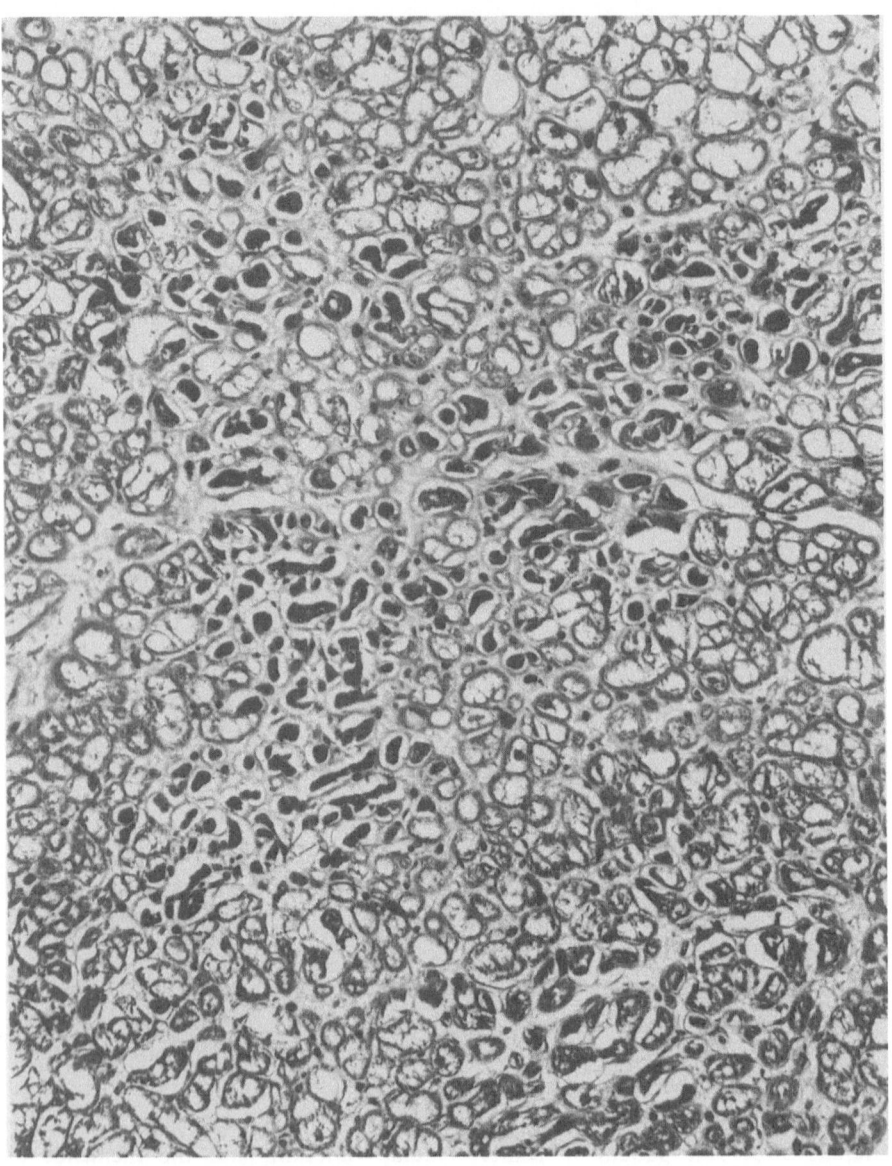

Figure 11. Subendocardial myocardium showing vaculated fibers, coagulation necrosis, and patchy fibrosis thought to be caused by chronic ischemia. (Masson, X 175).

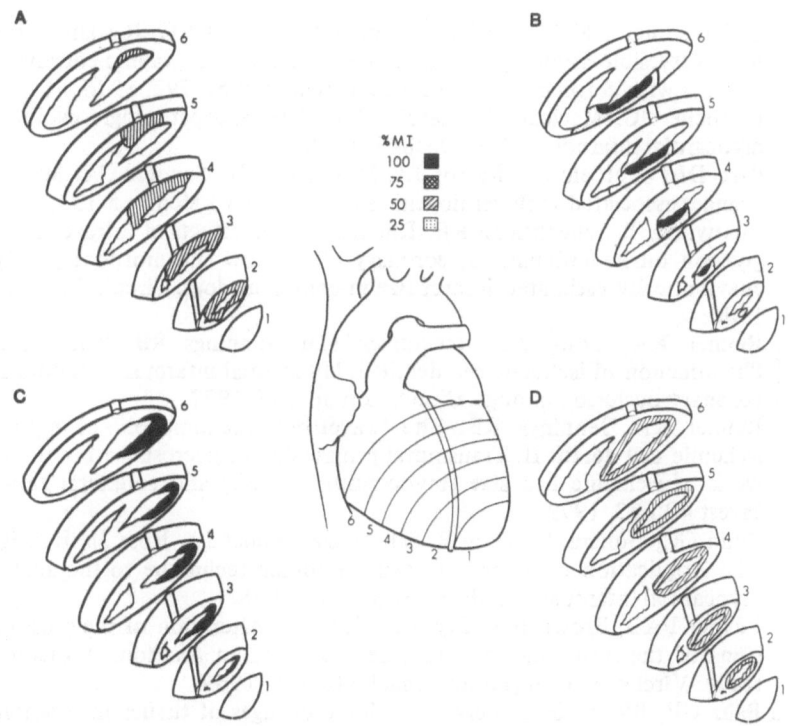

Figure 12. Four infarcts that each occupy 20% of the left ventricle, demonstrating marked differences in location and patchiness.

ventricle within the vascular bed of the coronary artery that supplies the infarcted region [6, 58, 59]. Thus an infarct that was 10% of the left ventricle in a vascular bed supplying 30% of the left ventricle might indicate limitation of the infarct size by an intervention while another infarct that was 10% of the left ventricle but was in a vascular bed supplying only 15% of the left ventricle might indicate no effect by the intervention. The size of the vascular bed can be quantitated by injecting the coronary arteries post mortem with a radio-opaque solution and planimetering the bed roentgenograms of the heart slices [59].

Acknowledgments. Supported in part by Research Grant HL-17670 from the National Heart, Lung and Blood Institute. R.E.I. is the recipient of Research Career Development Award HL-00546 and D.B.H. is the recipient of Research Career Award HL-K6-14188 from the National Heart, Lung and Blood Institute.

REFERENCES

1. Bodenheimer MM, Banka VS, Hermann GA, Trout RG, Rasdar H, Helfant RH: Reversible asynergy. Histopathologic and electrographic correlations in patients with coronary artery disease. Circulation 53:792, 1976.
2. Fishbein MC, Maclean D, Maroko PR: The histopathologic evolution of myocardial infarction. Chest 73:843, 1978.
3. Page DL, Caulfield JB, Kastor JA, DeSanctis RW, Sanders CA: Myocardial changes associated with cardiogenic shock. N Engl J Med 285.133, 1971.
4. Fukuyama T, Schechtman KB, Roberts R: The effects of intravenous nitroglycerin on hemodynamics, coronary blood flow and morphologically and enzymatically estimated infarct size in conscious dogs. Circulation 62:1227, 1980.
5. Reimer KA, Lowe JE, Rasmussen MM, Jennings RB: The wavefront Phenomenon of ischemic cell death: I. Myocardial infarct size vs duration of coronary occlusion in dogs. Circulation 56:786, 1977.
6. Reimer KA, Jennings RB: The 'wavefront phenomenon' of myocardial ischemic cell death: II. Transmural progression of necrosis within the framework of ischemic bed size (myocardium at risk) and collateral flow. Lab Invest 40:633, 1979.
7. Budd GC, Gohara A, White P, Schott DR, Kooel JA, Ross JN Jr, Leighton RF: Application of a serial frozen sectioning technique to the analysis of myocardial infarct size. Lab Invest 38:533, 1978.
8. Eckner FAO, Brown BW, Overll E, Glgov S: Alteration of the gross dimensions of the heart and its structures by formalin fixation. A quantitative study. Virchows Arch [Pathol Anat] 346:318, 1969.
9. Bahr GF, Bloom G, Friberg U: Volume changes of tissues in physiological fluids during fixation in osmium tetroxide or formaldehyde and during subsequent treatment. Exp Cell Res 12:342, 1957.
10. Poliner LR, Buja LM, Parkey RW, Stokely EM, Stone MJ, Harris R, Saffer SW, Templeton GH, Bonte FJ, Willerson JT: Comparison of different noninvasive methods of infarct sizing during experimental myocardial infarction. J Nucl Med 18:517, 1977.
11. Ferrans VJ: Morphological methods for evaluation of myocardial protection. Ann Thorac Surg 20:11, 1975.
12. Hackel DB, Ratliff NB Jr: A technic to estimate the quantity of infarcted myocardium post mortem. Am J Clin Pathol 61:242, 1974.
13. Alonso DR, Scheidt S, Post M, Killip T: Pathophysiology of cardiogenic shock: quantification of myocardial necrosis, clinical, pathologic, and electrocardiographic correlations. Circulation 48:588, 1973.
14. Maclean D, Fishbein MC, Maroko PR, Braunwald E: Hyaluronidase-induced reductions in myocardial infarct size. Science 194:199, 1976.
15. Virmani R, Roberts WC: Quantification of coronary arterial narrowing and of left ventricular myocardial scarring in healed myocardial infarction with chronic, eventually fatal, congestive cardiac failure. Am J Med 68:831, 1980.
16. Spadaro J, Fishbein MC, Hare C, Pfeffer MA, Maroko PR: Characterization of myocardial infarcts in the rat. Arch Pathol Lab Med 104:179, 1980.
17. Weibel ER: Stereological methods, vol 1: Practical methods for biological morphometry. London, New York: Academic Press, 1979.

18. Hanarayan C, Bennett MA, Brewer DN, Pentecost BL: Study of infarcted myocardium in cardiac shock. Br Heart J 32:555, 1970.
19. Cheitlin MD, Robinowitz M, McAllister H, Hoffmann JIE, Bharati S, Lev M: The distribution of fibrosis in the left ventricle in congenital aortic stenosis and coarctation of the aorta. Circulation 62:823, 1980.
20. DiBona DR, Powell WJ Jr: Quantitative correlation between cell swelling and necrosis in myocardial ischemia in dogs. Circ Res 47:653, 1980.
21. White FC, Sanders M, Peterson T, Bloor CM: Ischemic myocardial injury after exercise stress in the pressure-overloaded heart. Am J Pathol 97:473, 1979.
22. Gil J, Sailage DA: Morphometry of pinocytotic vesicles in the capillary endothelium of rabbit lungs using automated equipment. Circ Res 47:384, 1980.
23. Smith LR, Zissermann D, Cunningham W, Wixson SE, Bishop SP, Hood WP Jr, Mantle JA, Rogers WJ, Russell RO Jr, Logic JR, Rackley CE: Measurement of cardiac parameters from cardiovascular images. In: Computers in cardiology. Long Beach, CA: IEEE Computer Society, 1976, p 49.
24. Savage RM, Wagner GS, Ideker RE, Podolsky SA, Hackel DB: Correlation of postmortem anatomic findings with electrocardiographic changes in patients with myocardial infarction: retrospective study of patients with typical anterior and posterior infarcts. Circulation 55:279, 1977.
25. Boor PJ, Reynolds ES: A simple planimetric method for determination of left ventricular mass and necrotic myocardial mass in postmortem hearts. Am J Clin Pathol 68:387, 1977.
26. Schuster EH, Bulkley BH: Expansion of transmural myocardial infarction: a pathophysiologic factor in cardiac rupture. Circulation 60:1532, 1979.
27. Schuster EH, Bulkley BH: Ischemic cardiomyopathy: a clinicopathologic study of fourteen patients. Am Heart J 100:506, 1980.
28. Ideker RE, Wagner GS, Ruth WK, Alonso DR, Bishop SP, Bloor CM, Fallon JT, Gottlieb GJ, Hackel DB, Phillips HR, Reimer KA, Roark SF, Rogers WJ, Savage RM, Selvester RH: Evaluation of a QRS scoring system for estimating myocardial infarct size. II. Correlation with quantitative anatomic findings for anterior infarcts. (Submitted for publication.)
29. Roark SF, Ideker RE, Wagner GS, Alonso DR, Bishop SP, Bloor CM, Fallon JT, Gottlieb GJ, Hackel DB, Phillips HR, Reimer KA, Rogers WJ, Ruth WK, Savage RM, Selvester RH: Evaluation of a QRS scoring system for estimating myocardial infarct size. III. Correlation with quantitative anatomic findings for inferior infarcts. (Submitted for publication.)
30. Ward RM, Ideker RE, Wagner GS, Alonso DR, Bishop SP, Bloor CM, Fallon JT, Gottlieb GJ, Hackel DB, Phillips HR, Reimer KA, Roark SF, Rogers WJ, Ruth WK, Savage RM, Selvester RH: Evaluation of a QRS scoring system for estimating myocardial infarct size. IV. Correlation with quantitative anatomic findings for postero-lateral infarcts. (Submitted for publication)
31. James G, James RC (eds) Mathematics dictionary. New York: Van Nostrand Reinhold, 1976.
32. Laxer C, Ideker RE, Smith WM, German LD, Harrison L, Pilkington TC: Computer acquisition of a database for relating myocardial infarct geometry to cardiac electrical potentials. In: Computers in cardiology. Los Angeles, CA: IEEE Computer Society, 1980, p 339.
33. Roberts AJ, Cipriano PR, Alonso DR, Jacobstein JG, Combes JR, Gay

WA Jr: Evaluation of methods for quantification of experimental myocardial infarction. Circulation 57:35, 1978.

34. Ideker RE, Behar VS, Wagner GS, Starr JW, Starmer CF, Lee KL, Hackel DB: Evaluation of asynergy as an indicator of myocardial fibrosis. Circulation 57:715, 1978.

35. Stokely EM, Buja LM, Lewis SE, Parkey RW, Bonte FJ, Harris RJ Jr, Willerson JT: Measurement of acute myocardial infarcts in dogs with ^{99m}Tc-stannous pyrophosphate scintigrams. J Nucl Med 17:1, 1976.

36. Hutchins GM, Bulkley BH: Infarct expansion versus extension: two different complications of acute myocardial infarction. Am J Cardiol 41:1127, 1978.

37. Rivas F, Cobb FR, Bache RJ, Greenfield JC Jr: Relationship between blood flow to ischemic regions and extent of myocardial infarction. Serial measurement of blood to ischemic regions in dogs. Circ Res 38:439, 1976.

38. Bardeen CR: Determination of the size of the heart by means of the X-rays. Am J Anat 23:423, 1918.

39. Rackley CE, Dodge HT, Coble YD Jr, Hag RE: A method for determining left ventricular mass in man. Circulation 29:666, 1964.

40. Barnes AR: Correlation of initial deflections of ventricular complex with situation of acute myocardial infarction. Am Heart J 9:728, 1934.

41. Sayen JJ, Sheldon WF: The heart muscle and the electrocardiogram in coronary disease. II. Difficulties of description and illustration of ventricular muscle lesions, with a method for their graphic representation in a myocardial map. Am Heart J 38:688, 1949.

42. Burch GE, Horan LG, Ziskind J, Cronvich JA: A correlative study of post-mortem, electrocardiographic, and spatial vectorcardiographic data in myocardial infarction. Circulation 18:325, 1958.

43. Horan LG, Flowers NC, Johnson JC: Significance of the diagnostic Q wave of myocardial infarction. Circulation 43:428, 1971.

44. Richman HG, Yokoi M, Gleason D, Nishijima K, Simonson E: Reliability of the vectorcardiographic diagnosis of myocardial infarction. In: Vectorcardiography II. Amsterdam: North-Holland, 1971, p 343.

45. Baltaxe HA, Alonso DR, Lee JG, Prat J, Husted JW, Stakes JW III: Impaired left ventricular contractility in ischemic heart disease: angiographic and histopathologic correlations. Radiology 113:581, 1974.

46. James TN: Anatomy of the coronary arteries. New York: Harper and Row, 1961.

47. Bevington PR: Data reduction and error analysis for the physical sciences. New York: McGraw-Hill, 1969.

48. Mathieu O, Cruz-Orive LM, Hoppeler H, Weibel ER: Measuring error and sampling variation in stereology: comparison of the efficiency of various methods for planar image analysis. J Microsc 121: 75, 1981.

49. Gundersen HJG, Østerby R: Optimizing sampling efficiency of stereological studies in biology: or 'Do more less well!' J Microsc 121:65, 1981.

50. Shay J: Economy of effort in electron microscope morphometry. Am J Pathol 81:503, 1975.

51. Geer JC, Crago CA, Little WC, Gardner LL, Bishop SP: Subendocardial ischemic myocardial lesions associated with severe coronary atherosclerosis. Am J Pathol 98:663, 1980.

52. Baroldi G: Different types of myocardial necrosis in coronary heart disease:

a pathophysiologic review of their functional significance. Am Heart J 89:742, 1975.

53. Sulkin NM, Sulkin DF: An electron microscopic study of the effects of chronic hypoxia on cardiac muscle, hepatic, and autonomic ganglion cells. Lab Invest 14:1523, 1965.

54. Buja LM, Poliner LR, Parkey RW, Pulido JI, Hutcheson D, Platt MR, Mills LJ, Bonte FJ, Willerson JT: Clinicopathologic study of persistently positive technetium-99 m stannous pyrophosphate myocardial scintigrams and myocytolytic degeneration after myocardial infarction. Circulation 56:1016, 1977.

55. Silver MD, Baroldi G, Mariani F: The relationship between acute occlusive coronary thrombi and myocardial infarction studied in 100 consecutive patients. Circulation 61:219, 1980.

56. Schlesinger MJ, Reiner L: Focal myocytolysis of the heart. Am J Pathol 31:443, 1955.

57. Ratshin RA, Massing GK, James TN: The clinical significance of the location of acute myocardial infarction. In. Corday E, Swan HJC (eds) myocardial infarction: new perspectives in diagnosis and management. Baltimore: Williams and Wilkins, 1973, p 77.

58. Lowe JE, Reimer KA, Jennings RB: Experimental infarct size as a function of the amount of myocardium at risk. Am J Pathol 90:363, 1978.

59. Lee JT, Ideker RE, Reimer KA: Myocardial infarct size and location with respect to the coronary vascular bed at risk in man. Circulation 64:526, 1981.

15. POSTMORTEM: HISTOCHEMICAL TECHNIQUES

JOHN T. FALLON

Gross anatomic observation can be used to accurately diagnose, locate, and size myocardial infarcts at autopsy when the infarct is sufficiently developed (see Ideker, p. 347), i.e., at least 18–24 h old, and its borders are clearly defined. Similarly, histologic approaches to infarct identification and quantification are reliable only after 12–18 h of in vivo development, and are time consuming, expensive, and tedious. This chapter is concerned with macroscopic techniques for quantifying myocardial infarcts in experimental and human hearts; it is specifically concerned with the use of tetrazolium dyes. These techniques have the major advantage of identifying myocardial necrosis due to ischemic injury routinely by 3–6 h and experimentally as early as 1 h after the onset of myocardial infarction.

The accurate pathologic identification of early myocardial infarction is often helpful in diagnosing acute myocardial infarction in cases of sudden or unexpected death in man, for validating many of the newly developed 'noninvasive' infarct imaging techniques, and for evaluating experimental protocols of intraoperative and postinfarction myocardial preservation. Histochemical techniques, utilizing one of the tetrazolium salts, have many advantages over either direct macroscopic or microscopic techniques. Tetrazolium staining of the myocardium is both reliable and accurate not only for demonstrating infarct location but also as a basis for quantitative determination of myocardial infarct size. Furthermore, the use of this technique enables macroscopic identification of evolving experimental infarcts as early as 1 h old, long before the classic gross or histologic changes diagnostic of myocardial infarction [1, 2] become apparent.

THEORETICAL CONSIDERATIONS

The theoretical basis for the tetrazolium staining of myocardium derives from the observation that when viable tissue is exposed to a tetrazolium salt, a colored formazan is deposited at the site where the following reduction reaction is taking place:

Wagner GS (ed): Myocardial Infarction: Measurement and Intervention, pp 373–384.
© 1982 Martinus Nijhoff Publishers, The Hague/Boston/London.

$$\left[\begin{array}{c} RC = N \\ \diagdown \\ \quad\quad NAr \\ \diagup \\ N = N^+ \\ \diagdown \\ \quad Ar' \end{array} \right] Cl^- \quad ----\text{---}\rightarrow \quad \begin{array}{c} RC = NNHAr \\ | \\ N = NAr' \end{array}$$

$$\text{Reduction}$$

Tetrazolium salt   Colored formazan

This reduction reaction depends on the availability of an appropriate substrate and an intact oxidative enzyme system, e.g., succinate dehydrogenase, within the myocyte. Oxidation of the substrate, e.g., succinate, produces a reduced coenzyme that then passes electrons to the tetrazolium, causing its reduction to the formazan. The rate of this reaction depends on the concentration of substrate and coenzyme present as well as on the local pH and temperature. In the absence of active enzyme, the tetrazolium salt is not converted to the colored formazan and the infarcted myocardium remains unstained. It is important to note that by definition, 'ischemic' tissue contains active enzyme and therefore will stain. However, 'infarcted' or necrotic tissue does not contain active oxidation enzymes and therefore remains unstained. Furthermore, this reaction is not appreciably affected, i.e., decreased, by autolysis at room temperatures until about 24 h post mortem. After this time, the reaction becomes unreliable unless substrate and coenzyme are added. If the tissue is maintained at 4°C, however, the staining is reliable for up to 72 h post mortem and frozen tissues can be reliably stained several months post mortem.

TECHNIQUES

Several tetrazolium salts and staining procedures are suitable for the histochemical delineation of myocardial infarcts. These are outlined in Tables 1 and 2, respectively.

The least expensive salt is triphenyltetrazolium chloride (TTC). Reduction of TTC produces a monoformazan that is deep red or bright purple. The formazan of TTC is soluble in lipids and alcohol and is therefore removed from tissues during parafin-embedding procedures. TTC is light sensitive, both in crystalline form and in solution, and therefore should be light protected at all times. This does not pose a great technical problem when used experimentally. Blue tetrazolium (BT) is approximately ten times the cost of TTC. BT produces a dark blue diformazan within tissues that is also lipid and alcohol soluble. It is not as light sensitive as TTC and is therefore an excellent reagent for routine autopsy studies. Nitro-blue tetrazolium (NBT) is relatively expensive, costing

Table 1. Tetrazolium salts commonly used for histochemical staining

Common name	Chemical name	Cost per gram
Tetrazolium red (TTC)	2, 3, 5 triphenyltetrazolium chloride	0.29
Blue tetrazolium (BT)	3, 3'-(3, 3'-dimethoxy [1, 1'-biphenyl]-4, 4' diyl) bis [2, 5-diphenyltetrazolium] dichloride	3.90
Nitro-blue tetrazolium (NBT)	2, 2'-di-p-nitrophenyl-5, 5'-diphenyl-3, 3'-(3, 3'-dimethoxy-4, 4'-biphenylene) ditetrazolium chloride	36.00

100 times the equivalent amount of TTC. It produces a dark blue to deep purple diformazan that is not lipid or alcohol soluble. Its major advantage is that the formazan remains in tissue sections after histologic preparation. When used in conjunction with a perfusion procedure of staining, NBT produces a specimen in which an objective cell-to-cell differentiation of viability versus necrosis can be made. Although NBT is widely used for routine autopsy staining of myocardium, its expense is not often justified.

Two basic staining procedures are widely used: slice incubation and post-mortem perfusion. The slice incubation technique is easy to perform and requires little technical expertise. It has the disadvantage of staining only the surface of the slice so that, even if NBT is used, only the superficial layer of myocytes will contain formazan granules in histologic sections. It also has disadvantages for infarct sizing since fresh hearts are difficult to slice accurately and smoothly (even when chilled or frozen) and therefore difficult to accurately measure and planimeter. However, for routine diagnostic work, it is rapid and efficient. The postmortem perfusion procedure results in a completely stained specimen that can be fixed and sliced to provide a basis for precise infarct sizing. It requires equipment for constant and controlled pressure perfusion of the coronaries and the technical expertise and time necessary to do this. In experimental studies this procedure works well, but for human hearts the perfusion often results in nonstaining artifacts that are difficult to interpret as discussed below. A modification of the perfusion procedure for experimental studies is the in vivo infusion of the tetrazolium. This latter technique results in a

Table 2. Procedures for histochemical staining of myocardial infarcts

Technique	Staining solution(s)	Use
Slice incubation	PO_4-buffered BT or NBT with substrate	Human/experimental
Postmortem perfusion	PO_4-buffered BT or TTC with substrate Tris-buffered NBT with substrate and NAD	Experimental Human
In vivo infusion	2% TTC in normal saline	Experimental

completely stained specimen without the expense, time, or equipment needed for the postmortem perfusion.

HISTORICAL SURVEY

The slice incubation technique originated in Germany in 1957 with Sandritter and Jestädt [3, 4], who first used a solution of TTC and exogenous substrate to macroscopically demonstrate infarcts in guinea pig and human hearts as early as 4 h after experimental myocardial infarction or the onset of clinical symptoms in patients who died. In 1963, Nachlas and Shnitka [5, 6] introduced a solution of NBT made in Sorensen's phosphate buffer (0.1M, pH 7.4) for staining slices of canine and human myocardium. Their studies showed that NBT was more sensitive than TTC, NBT provided better color contrast than TTC owing to the presence of hemoglobin, and the formazan pigment of NBT was not extracted from tissues, as was TTC's formazan, during paraffin-embedding procedures. They found that infarcts could be identified as early as 2 h after experimental coronary occlusion; for human hearts, 8 h had to intervene between the onset of symptoms and death if consistent results were to be obtained. The addition of substrate, coenzymes, and inhibitors can shorten this time interval considerably. Ramkisson [7] had similar results using this method for staining human heart slices.

Brody et al. [8], McVie [9], and Anderson and Hansen [10] showed the usefulness of the NBT solution in identifying myocardial infarcts that could not be seen by gross inspection of unstained slices of human heart. The earliest infarcts that were demonstrated by Brody et al. [8] using NBT were 18 h old by history. They found that the addition of substrate (0.1M lactate) enhanced the reaction when the postmortem interval was 12 h or longer. On the other hand, Anderson and Hansen [10] reported several examples of infarcts less than 8 h old that were demonstrated by histochemical staining.

In 1975, Lie et al. [11] described a slice incubation method for macroscopic enzyme mapping of experimental canine myocardial infarcts based on a modification of the Sandritter and Jesdädt technique [3, 4] using TTC without an exogenous substrate. This method used a 1% solution of TTC made in phosphate buffer (pH 8.5–8.6). Staining was carried out at 37°–40°C for 30–40 min. Using this technique, experimental canine infarcts 1 h old were undetectable, 2-h infarcts were slightly pale, but 4-h and older infarcts showed striking contrast between the pale, unstained infarct zones and the TTC-stained, dark red, noninfarcted myocardium surrounding the infarcts. In addition to clearly demonstrating an early infarct that was otherwise invisible in the unstained ventricular slice, the TTC staining provided a useful substrate for quantifying infarct size by using the estimation method of Hackel and Ratliff [12].

This TTC slice incubation technique was successfully applied in studies of human myocardial infarcts by Mittleman and co-workers [13] and by Boor and Reynolds [14]. The latter investigators stained multiple 1-cm-thick ventricular slices of fresh autopsy hearts for 20–30 min at room temperature in a 1% TTC solution buffered with $0.2M$ Tris (pH 7.8). None of the infarcts were less than three days old. Color transparencies of the stained slices were used for planimetry measurements to obtain infarct size calculated from a mathematical model previously described by these same investigators [15]. Histologic studies showed acute left ventricular infarction in each case that correlated with the TTC staining pattern. Three of the hearts also showed areas of nonstaining by TTC in the right ventricle; two proved histologically to represent recent infarction but the third showed no definite histologic evidence of infarction.

The postmortem perfusion method of histochemical staining was initially reported in 1973 [16] but was not fully evaluated until 1976 by Feldman et al. [17]. They stained canine and human hearts by a retrograde aortic perfusion at a controlled pressure of 100 mmHg for 40 min with a 37°C solution containing 0.5 mg/ml NBT and 0.05 mg/ml nicotinamide adenine nucleotide (NAD) in $0.1M$ Sorenson's phosphate buffer (pH 7.4) with added substrate. Substrates included $0.1M$ alpha-hydroxybutyrate, $0.1M$ lactate or $0.1M$ succinate. Each substrate showed good results, but staining was most intense with hydroxybutyrate. In canine hearts subjected to in vivo coronary ligation, infarcts were demonstrated as early as 6 h after ligation. However, all the canine hearts showed small, randomly scattered zones of nonstaining throughout the myocardium that became stained when the slices were incubated in the NBT-substrate solution. Although Feldman at al. [17] believed these staining defects represented myocardial ischemic injury rather than obstruction to flow of the perfusate, our own work suggests that they are perfusion artifacts that can be eliminated by heparinization of the experimental animal just prior to sacrifice and by initial coronary perfusion with buffered saline before perfusing with the tetrazolium staining solution (Figure 1).

Feldman et al. [17] also examined the results of perfusion of human hearts by NBT as part of a standardized protocol for the evaluation of coronary artery disease. They found good correlation between the distribution of nonstaining myocardium and both clinical data and histologic results. However, as in their canine studies, small, poorly delineated foci of nonstaining myocardium were noted. Roesch et al. [18], in an independent evaluation of the Feldman method, also found such nonstaining areas that stained when the slices were reexposed to NBT by the slice incubation technique. They concluded that the perfusion technique was not suitable for analysis of acute or recent infarcts in human hearts but that the usual incubation method proved useful and accurate for macroscopic localization. However, recent unpublished studies (T. Schaffner,

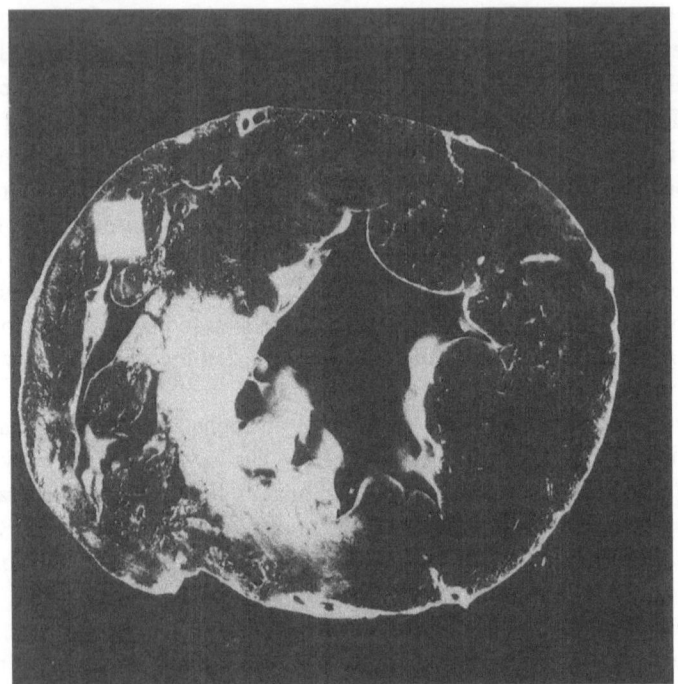

Figure 1. Ventricular slice from canine heart subjected to in vivo ligation of the left anterior descending artery. At 6 h after ligation, the heart was removed and TTC perfusion staining was performed. A well-defined area of nonstaining (white) is apparent in the anterior septal region of the left ventricle.

R.W. Wissler, S. Glagov, personal comunication) suggest that these bothersome nonstaining areas are diminished by pre-perfusing human hearts with Tris-buffered saline (pH 7.6) and by using an NBT solution made in 0.1 M Tris (pH 7.6) and containing NAD and beta-hydroxybutyrate (see Table 3).

The reliability of tetrazolium staining of human autopsy hearts was further supported by the work of Sakurai [19] and of Derias and Adams [20]. The

Table 3. Recommended procedure for postmortem perfusion of human hearts

A) Cannulate aorta with tubing of similar OD. Aortic valve must be positioned closed.

B) Perfusion at room temperature and under controlled pressures of 80–100 mmHg with:
   1) 7 liters 0.03 M Tris-buffered (pH 7.6) saline
   2) 2 liters 0.1 M Tris-buffered (pH 7.6) solution containing 1 g NBT, 200 mg NAD, and 25 g butyric acid (collect perfusate and perfuse for total of 45 min).

C) Continue perfusion with 5% neutral buffered formalin for 30 min or infuse heart with postmortem angiographic dyes and then fix by immersion in formalin.

D) *Result*: All viable myocardium stains dark blue while infarcted areas remain unstained. Frequently, small nonstaining areas are encountered.

latter workers studied 81 cases of clinically suspected myocardial infarction by an NBT slice incubation method. Slices of fresh myocardial tissue were incubated at 37°C for 20–30 min in a solution of 50 mg/100 ml NBT in 0.2 M Tris–HCl at pH 7.4 alone or with beta-hydroxybutrate (12.7 g/100 ml) as substrate. Sodium cyanide (500 mg/100 ml), to inhibit electron use by the cytochrome oxidase system, and NAD (100 mg/100 ml) were added to the incubation solution and the final pH was adjusted to 7.1 with 0.2 M Tris without HCl. The NBT test was positive in 20 of 30 cases in which infarction could not be seen with the naked eye and where no definite histologic evidence of infarction was found. Of 17 cases studied with apparent infarcts of only 1 h duration, 10 showed evidence of regional infarction by NBT staining. These studies provide good evidence that the NBT method is of diagnostic use in the gross detection of infarcts 1 h old and older. Tetrazolium staining was not appreciablly diminished by postmortem intervals of up to 72 h even when the tissue was maintained at room temperatures.

RECOMMENDATIONS AND CONCLUSIONS

Although the accurate recognition of acute myocardial infarction at autopsy has always been a major problem to pathologists, many still seem reticent to use the tetrazolium technique. One reason may be the not so insignificant expense of the NBT methods, especially those using added NAD and done by the perfusion technique. Our own experience suggests that the NBT methods are indeed prohibitively expensive for routine autopsy work. However, we have found the method outlined in Table 4 using a phosphate buffered solution (pH 7.6) of BT (1%) containing succinate, to be quite satisfactory for daily autopsy use (Figures 2 and 3). These solutions are reliable, inexpensive, easy

Table 4. Slice incubation procedure for routine histochemical staining of human hearts

A) Solutions (kept at 4°C, made fresh every two weeks):
1) 500 mg BT in 500 ml distilled water
2) 54 g Na-succinate in 1 liter distilled water
3) 2.28 g NaH_2PO_4 and 21.8 g Na_2HPO_4 in 1 liter distilled water (pH 7.4).

B) Mix 20 cc solution 1, 50 cc solution 2, and 50 cc solution 3. Prewarm to 37°C.

C) After removing epicardial coronary arteries, cut multiple transverse sections of ventricles. Examine slices for gross features of infarction. Incubate slice(s) in prewarmed staining solution for 30–45 min with constant agitation.

D) *Results*: Viable myocardium stains dark blue, indicating presence of dehydrogenase activity. Infarcted areas remain unstained as do areas of fibrosis. Subsequent fixation in formalin further enhances differentiation, but prolinged storage will result in loss of dye from tissue.

380

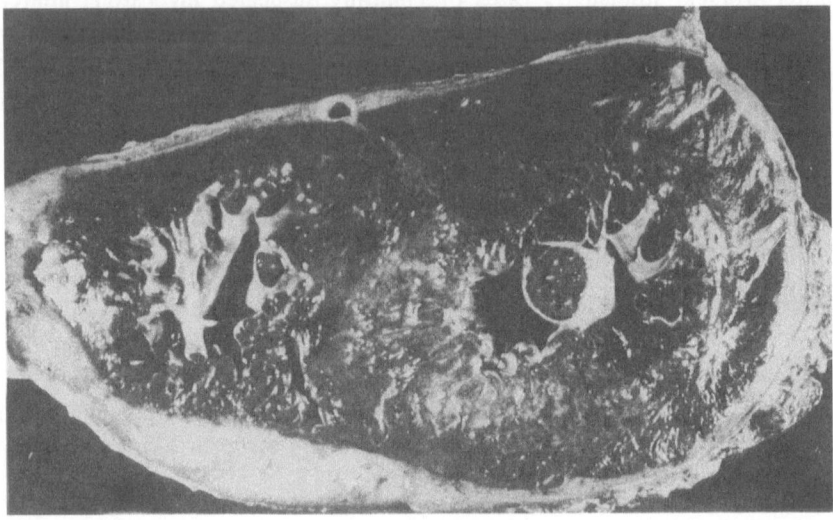

Figure 2. Slice of ventricular myocardium from a patient with onset of clinical signs and symptoms of myocardial infarction 5 h prior to death. The infarct delineated here (pale, nonstained anterior-septal area) by the BT slice incubation technique was not grossly apparent.

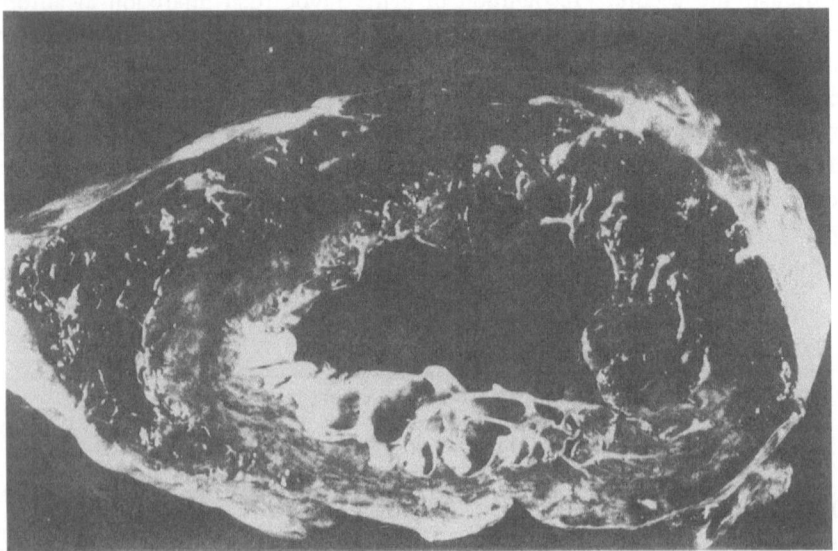

Figure 3. BT-slice from heart of patient who had an ECG and enzyme documented 24-h-old myocardial infarct. Although the central region of this large anterior infarct was grossly visible in the unstained slice, the full extent of the infarct was not appreciated until the slice was histochemically stained.

to make, and provide a stained ventricular slice within 1 h by incubation at 37° C. We and others [21] have found that this method provides macroscopic identification of infarcts that is readily correlated with microscopic findings and can serve as a basis for infarct sizing by planimetric [15] or stereologic techniques [22].

Another possible reason for the reticence of pathologists to use these techniques may be the lack of histologic correlation in the early infarction period. However, our own studies as well as those of Fishbein et al. [23] and Kloner and co-workers [24, 25] have demonstrated that although these histochemical techniques delineate myocardial infarcts before definitive histologic changes become apparent, by electron microscopy, changes of irreversible myocardial cell injury are present and correlate well ($r = 0.9$) with unstained areas.

It is also disconcerting that many recent experimental studies designed to evaluate newly developed clinical techniques for infarct imaging and sizing or protocols to test the efficacy of various drugs to reduce the size of infarcts have not taken advantage of the tetrazolium methods for infarct sizing [26]. We and others [27–30] have found that the original tetrazolium incubation methods are superior to unaided gross observation in such clinical studies. Perfusion of experimental hearts with a Tris-buffered solution of TTC without added substrate provides an excellent specimen for sizing of early infarcts [31, 32].

Recently, we have developed a simplified method of staining experimental myocardial infarcts by using an in vivo technique of tetrazolium staining [33]. For canine experiments, the following protocol was used [34, 35]. A 2% solution of TTC was made in normal saline without addition of substrate. The dog was heparinized and the solution of TTC (250 ml) was given intravenously over a period of 15–20 min. The TTC was given only to a fully anesthesized animal, on mechanical ventilation, with the chest open, since its administration often induced ventricular fibrillation or cardiac arrest. In such an event, the heart was manually massaged to enable the complete administration of the TTC staining solution. The heart was then removed and immediately cut to obtain tissue samples for electron microscopy, immunofluorescence, diffusible ion studies, or counting of rapid-decay radioisotopes by using the TTC staining pattern as a guide to tissue sampling. For infarct size determinations or other studies when immediate tissue procurement was not necessary, the excised heart was incubated in saline at 37°C for 30 min to further enhance the differential staining. Fixation was then performed by immersion in 5% buffered formalin overnight. This in vivo infusion technique will outline infarcts as early as 1 h after coronary ligation (Figure 4).

The various methods of tetrazolium staining of myocardial infarcts each produce a specimen with a well-outlined infarct that is readily perceived by the unaided eye. We are presently devising a system whereby images of slices of

382

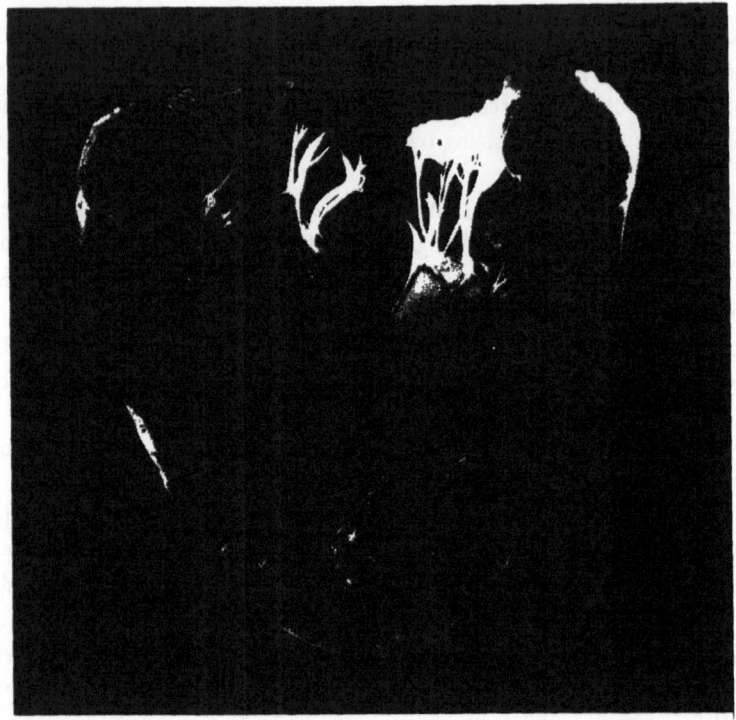

Figure 4. 1-h-old infarction of the tips of the posterior papillary muscles are well delieated (nonstaining white areas) in this sagitally cut slice of canine myocardium stained by the in vivo infusion of TTC. The infarct was produced by ligation of the distal left circumflex artery.

TTC-infusion-stained experimental hearts are digitized using a TV camera, the images assessed quantitatively by a computer with the aid of an operator to outline the infarcts, and a three-dimensional reconstruction made of the ventricle and infarct. The computer image of the heart is then used for comparison with images obtained of the same heart in vivo by imaging techniques such as [201]thallium gamma imaging, positron imaging, or NMR imaging; images that are already digitally stored in a computer and readily accessible for direct comparison either visually or statistically [36, 37].

REFERENCES

1. Mallory GK, White PD, Salcedo-Salgar J: The speed of healing of myocardial infarction. A study of the pathologic anatomy in seventy-two cases. Am Heart J 18:647–671, 1939.
2. Fishbein MC, Maclean D, Maroko PR: The histopathologic evolution of myocardial infarction. Chest 73:843–849, 1978.

3. Sandritter W, Jestädt R: Triphenylterazoliumchlorid (TTC) als Reduktionsindikator zur makrokopischen Diagnose des frischen Herzinfarktes. Zentralbl Allg Pathol 97:188–189, 1957–1958.

4. Jestädt R, Sandritter W: Erfahrungen mit der TTC (Triphenyltetrazoliumchlorid) Reaktion für die pathologisch-anatomische Diagnose des frischen Herzinfarktes. Kreislaufforsch 48:802–809, 1959.

5. Nachlas MM, Shnitka TK: Macroscopic identification of early myocardial infarcts by alterations in dehydrogenase activity. Am J Pathol 42:379–405, 1963.

6. Shnitka TK, NachlasMM: Histochemical alterations in ischemic heart muscle and early myocardial infarction. Am J Pathol 42:507–527, 1963.

7. Ramkissoon RA: Macroscopic identification of early myocardial infarction by dehydrogenase alterations. J Clin Pathol 19:479–481, 1966.

8. Brody GL, Belding A, Belding RM, Feldman SA: The identification and delineation of myocardial infarcts. Arch Pathol 84:312–317, 1967.

9. McVie JG: Postmortem detection of inapparent myocardial infarction. J Clin Pathol 23:203–209, 1970.

10. Anderson JA, Hansen BF: The value of the nitro-BT method in fresh myocardial infarction. Frequency and location of fresh myocardial infarction in a consecutive series of autopsies. Am Heart J 85:611–619, 1973.

11. Lie JT, Pairolero PC, Holley KE, Titus JL: Macroscopic enzyme-mapping verification of large, homogeneous, experimental myocardial infarcts of predictable size and location in dogs. J Thorac Cardiovasc Surg 69:599–605, 1975.

12. Hackel DB, Ratliff NB Jr: A technic to estimate the quantity of infarcted myocardium postmortem. Am J Clin Pathol 61:242–246, 1974.

13. Mittleman R, Szabo S, Heinsimar J, Reynolds ES, von Lichtenberg F: Macroscopic histochemical detection of myocardial necrosis in the heart at autopsy by the triphenyl tetrazolium chloride (TTC) technique. Clin Res 23:198A, 1975.

14. Boor PJ, Reynolds ES: Myocardial infarct size: clinicopathologic agreement and discordance. Human Pathol 8:685–695, 1977.

15. Boor PJ, Reynolds ES: A simple planimetric method for determination of left ventricular mass and necrotic myocardial mass in postmortem hearts. Am J Clin Pathol 68:387–392, 1977.

16. Lichtig C, Glagov S, Feldman S, Wissler RW: Myocardial ischemia and coronary artery atherosclerosis: a comprehensive approach to postmortem studies. Med Clin North Am 57:79–91, 1973.

17. Feldman S, Glagov S, Wissler RW, Hughes RH: Postmortem delineation of infarcted myocardium. Coronary perfusion with nitro blue tetrazolium. Arch Pathol Lab Med 100:55–58, 1976.

18. Roesch LH, Kuch J, Knieriem HJ: Vergleichende fermenthistochemische Untersuchungen am normalen Herzmuskel, bei Koronarinsuffizienz und Herzinfarkt. Virchows Arch [Pathol Anat] 370:21–39, 1976.

19. Sakurai I: Pathology of acute ischemic myocardium. Special references to (I) evaluation of morphological methods for detection of early myocardial infarcts, and (II) lipid metabolism in infarcted myocardium. Acta Pathol Jpn 27:587–603, 1977.

20. Derias NW, Adams CW: Nitroblue tetrazolium test: early gross detection of human myocardial infarcts. Br J Exp Pathol 59:254–258, 1978.

384

21. Schaper W, Frenzel H, Hort W, Winkler B: Experimental coronary artery occlusion. II. Spatial and temporal evolution of infarcts in the dog heart. Basic Res Cardiol 74:233–239, 1979.
22. Hansen BF: Heart autopsy in ischemic heart disease. An autopsy protocol. Acta Pathol Microbiol Scand 86:241–244, 1978.
23. Fishbein MC, Meerbaum S, Rit J, Lando U, Kanmatsuse K, Mercier JC, Corday E, Ganz W: Early phase acute myocardial infarct size quantification: validation of the triphenyl tetrazolium chloride technique. Am Heart J 101:593–600, 1981.
24. Kloner RA, Darsee JR, DeBoer LW, Carlson N: Can tetrazolium stains reliably identify myocardial infarction prior to definite histological necrosis? [abstr] Circulation [Suppl 3] 62:III-246, 1980.
25. Darsee JR, Kloner RA, Braunwald E: Demonstration of lateral and epicardial border zone salvage by flurbiprofen using an in vivo method for assessing myocardium at risk. Circulation 63:29–35, 1981.
26. Boor PJ: Infarct size measurement. Circulation 60:966–967, 1979.
27. Reimer KA: Myocardial infarct size. Measurements and predictions. Arch Pathol Lab Med 104:225–230, 1980.
28. Schaper W, Frenzel H, Hort W: Experimental coronary artery occlusion. I. Measurement of infarct size. Basic Res Cardiol 74:46–53, 1979.
29. Roberts AJ, Cipriano PR, Alonso DR, Jacobstein JG, Combes JR, Gay WA Jr: Evaluation of methods for the quantification of experimental myocardial infarction. Circulation 57:35–41, 1978.
30. Wackers FJ, Becker AE, Samson G, Sokole EB, van der Schoot JB, Vet AJ, Lie KI, Durrer D, Wellens H: Location and size of acute transmural myocardial infarction estimated from thallium-201 scintiscans. A clinico-pathological study. Circulation 56:72–78, 1977.
31. Khaw BA, Gold HK, Leinbach RC, Fallon JT, Strauss W, Pohost GM, Haber E: Early imaging of experimental myocardial infarction by intra-coronary administration of ^{131}I-labelled anticardiac myosin $(Fab')_2$ fragments. Circulation 58:1137–1142, 1978.
32. Khaw BA, Fallon JT, Beller GA, Haber E: Specificity of localization of myosin-specific antibody fragments in experimental myocardial infarction. Histologic, histochemical, autoradiographic and scintigraphic studies. Circulation 60:1527–1531, 1979.
33. Fallon JT: Simplified method for histochemical demonstration of experimental myocardial infarct [abstr]. Circulation [Suppl 2] 59 and 60:II-42, 1979.
34. Frame L, Fallon JT, Khaw B, Haber E, Powell WJ: Radiolabelled anticardiac myosin $(Fab')_2$: detection of membrane damage during reflow following coronary occlusion [abstr]. Circulation [Suppl 3] 62:III-81, 1980.
35. Khaw BA, Gold H, Strauss HW, Fallon JT, Locke E, Haber E: Fibrin deposition in ischemic myocardium and its prevention by propranolol: studies with ^{99m}Tc-DPTA-fibrinogen [abstr]. Circulation [Suppl 3] 62:III-290, 1980.
36. Budinger TF, Cahoon JL, Derenzo SE, Gullberg GT, Moyer BR, Yano Y: Three-dimensional imaging of the myocardium with radionuclides. Radiology 125:433–439, 1977.
37. Lewis M, Buja LM, Saffer S, Mishelevich D, Stokely E, Lewis S, Parkey R, Bonte F, Willerson J: Experimental infarct sizing using computer processing and a three-dimensional model. Science 197:167–169, 1977.

III. INTERVENTIONS FOR LIMITING INFARCT SIZE

16. OVERVIEW OF POTENTIAL MECHANISMS

KEITH A. REIMER

The potential benefits of limiting infarct size in man have been inferred primarily from clinical and experimental studies that have demonstrated a direct relationship between infarct size and the incidence and severity of arrhythmic and hemodynamic complications of a myocardial infarct [1]. For example larger infarcts in dogs have been associated with a greater loss of contractility [2, 3] and a greater decrease in the ventricular fibrillation threshold [4]. Large infarcts in man, as estimated from serial measurements of serum creatine kinase (CK), have been associated with worse cardiac function [5, 6], a higher frequency of ventricular ectopic beats [7, 8], and higher initial mortality [5]. In 20 autopsies of patients who died in cardiogenic shock, all infarcts involved at least 40% of the left ventricle [9].

The idea that human infarct size could potentially be limited [10–12] received early support from the frequent observation, at autopsy, of infarcts that were smaller than the myocardial region supplied by the occluded coronary artery. The apparently patchy admixture of necrotic and viable myocytes forming the boundaries between infarcted and viable regions suggested that a broad border zone of myocardium existed in which jeopardized myocytes were tenuously balanced on the line between life and death, such that their outcome could be determined by hemodynamic or pharmacologic modifications.

Some recent studies have cast doubt on the existence of a meaningful salvageable border zone at the lateral boundaries of myocardial infarcts. Apparently isolated islands of necrotic myocardium on two-dimensional histologic sections of completed infarcts have been shown by three-dimensional analysis to be peninsulas extending out from the central mass of the infarct [13]. Thus, infarct boundaries are irregular but sharp. In addition, although the transmural extent of experimental or human infarcts is variable, the lateral boundaries of an infarct show a relatively constant relationship to the boundaries of the vascular bed [14, 15]. Thus, whether any therapeutic intervention can limit the lateral (as opposed to transmural) dimension of a myocardial infarct is controversial at this time.

The postulate that overall infarct size can be limited is firmly based on the early observations of Jennings et al. [16] that the onset of myocardial ischemia is not immediately followed by cell death. Ischemic cells first enter a *reversible* phase of injury, during which time reperfusion could prevent infarct. Later, ischemic cells enter a phase of *irreversible* injury such that cell death occurs even if myocardial blood flow is restored.

PREREQUISITES FOR EFFECTIVE INTERVENTION TO LIMIT INFARCT SIZE

If any therapy is to limit infarct size, two prerequisites [12, 17] must be fulfilled: (a) Intervention must occur while ischemic cells are still present that are reversibly injured but eventually destined to die. (b) The intervention itself, or its beneficial effects, must be continued until ischemia can be alleviated by either lysis of thrombi, revascularization, or growth of collateral connections between occluded and nonoccluded arteries. Although these prinicples seem obvious, they are emphasized here because they have too often been ignored in clinical or animal studies of the effect of drugs on indices of ischemic injury or infarct size. Adherence to the first principle also has been hampered by uncertainty of the time frame in which cell death occurs in a myocardial infarct.

The duration of coronary occlusion required to kill ischemic myocardium has been evaluated in open-chest dogs by comparing infarcts produced by various periods of temporary occlusion followed by reperfusion with infarcts produced by permanent ligation of the circumflex artery [14, 16, 18]. In these studies, cell death was quantitated, using histologic techniques, 2–4 days after the acute event. No necrosis develops after a 15-min period of coronary occlusion, but confluent subendocardial necrosis develops after 40 min of ischemia. With longer periods of ischemia, a transmural wavefront of cell death spreads from the subendocardial to the subepicardial region so that, by 3–6 h, the infarct reaches its maximum transmural extent (Figure 1). The mechanism of this transmural progression of ischemic cell death may be related to the transmural distribution of collateral flow in the ischemic region. In addition, variation in the final transmural extent of an infarct is closely related to the amount of collateral flow available to the subepicardial region during the first few hours after the onset of ischemia (Figure 2).

The timing of ischemic cell death cannot be studied directly in man, but must be inferred from indirect clinical evidence or from experimental studies. Clearly the potential for effective therapy to limit myocardial infarct size in man exists only if the process of infarction is slower in man than in open-chested dogs, because the delay between the onset of symptoms and access to medical therapy is often three or more hours. Theoretical consideration [17] plus some indirect clinical data support the hope that some human infarcts develop more slowly than experimental infarcts defined in the open-chested animal preparation

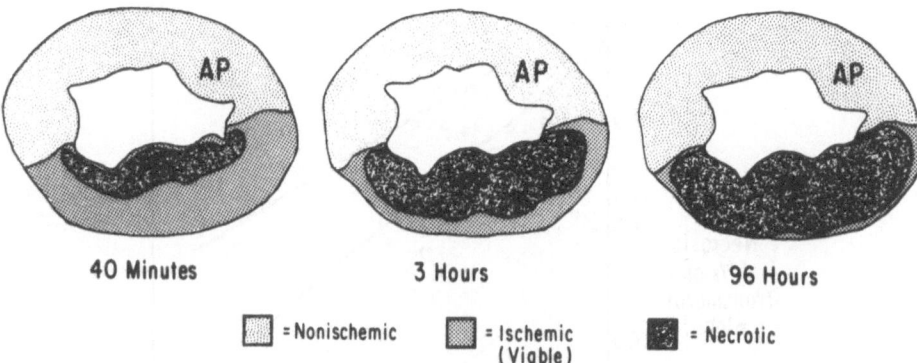

40 Minutes   3 Hours   96 Hours

▨ = Nonischemic   ▨ = Ischemic   ▨ = Necrotic
(Viable)

Figure 1. Progression of cell death *versus* time after occlusion of the circumflex artery (LCC) in open-chest dogs. Necrosis occurs first in the subendocardial myocardium. With longer occlusions, a wavefront of cell death moves from the subendocardial zone across the wall to involve progressively more of the transmural thickness of the ischemic zone. Thus, there is typically a large zone of subepicardial myocardium in the ischemic bed that is salvageable by early reperfusion but that dies in the absence of such an intervention. In contrast, the lateral margins in the subendocardial region of the infarct are established as early as 40 min after occlusion and are sharply defined by the anatomic boundaries of the ischemic bed. Reprinted from Reimer et al. [14] by permission of the publishers.

(see Becker, p. 440). Unlike experimental infarcts, human infarcts seldom result from the sudden occlusion of a previously normal artery, but rather occur as a final complication of longstanding atherosclerotic disease; thus, the acute event is often preceded by a chronic or intermittent stimulus for the development of collateral connections.

The evolution of an acute infarct in man also may be modified by the precipitating events. For example, thrombotic occlusion of a coronary artery may cause a solid and transmural infarct, similar to infarcts produced experimentally in dogs by sudden coronary ligation. On the other hand, thrombotic coronary occlusions cannot always be implicated in human infarcts, particularly in patients with smaller, subendocardial infarcts [19]. It seems likely that some of these infarcts may be caused by less severe ischemia induced by subtotal coronary narrowing, perhaps associated with transient episodes of coronary spasm. Ischemic cell death may be delayed in such infarcts.

The possibility that myocardial infarction in man may be a relatively slow and perhaps intermittent process has been suggested by the time course of myoglobin and CK release from evolving infarcts (see Roberts, p. 112). Myoglobin release is frequently intermittent, and myoglobinemia may persist for 2–3 days after the onset of symptoms [20]. The duration of CK release has also been shown to range from 16 to 60h [21]. Elevation of the ST segment of the ECG also frequently persists for one or more days after a myocardial infarct (see Arnsdorf, p. 91), and may indicate the persistence of ischemic but still viable

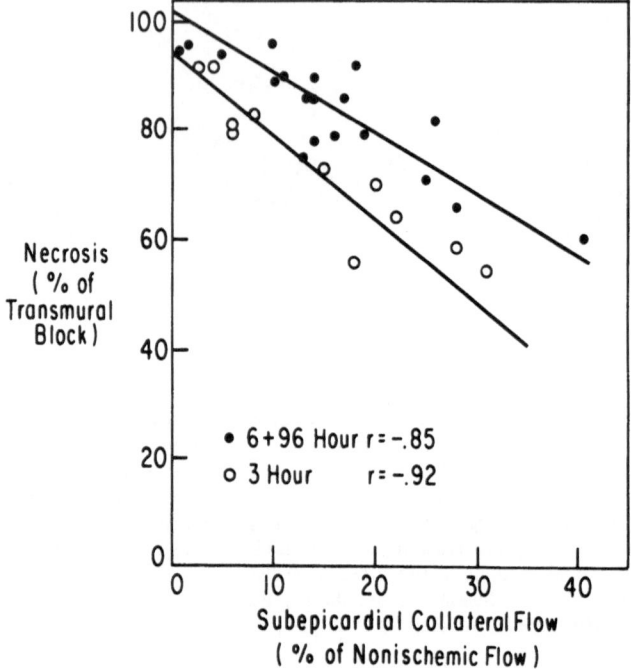

Figure 2. Relation between transmural necrosis and subepicardial collateral flow in dogs with circumflex artery occlusions is illustrated. Permanent infarcts and infarcts reperfused at 6 h formed the same line and were combined (•). Infarcts reperfused at 3 h are indicated by the open circles. In both groups, the transmural extent of necrosis measured at four days was inversely related to subepicardial collateral flow measured at 20 min after LCC occlusion. Thus, in each group, necrosis could be predicted from early collateral flow. However, the 3-h line was below the line defined by the 6-h and permanent infarcts. Thus, reperfusion at 3 h resulted in less necrosis than expected from the level of collateral flow. Reprinted from Reimer et al. [14] by permission of the publishers.

myocardium [22]. However, all of these indices are indirect measurements that must be interpreted with caution. The timing of enzyme or myoglobin release from necrotic myocardium may reflect poor or absent perfusion of the infarct center rather than continuing cell death. Prolonged elevation of the ST segment may reflect postinfarct pericarditis or an aneurysm rather than persistent ischemic injury. Although infarct 'extension' (based on clinical criteria of new chest pain, new changes in the ST-T segment, secondary enzyme release, or increased cardiac failure) occurs in up to 80% of patients [23], postmortem examination of such infarcts shows a low frequency of new and quantitatively important necrosis [24]. Thus, the duration of the evolution of a myocardial infarct, and therefore the period in which therapeutic intervention could potentially limit the size of an infarct, has not been established in man.

The time required for collateral vessels to enlarge in response to an acute ischemic event in man also is not well documented. In dogs, in which the pattern of collateral anastomoses is similar to that in man, collateral blood flow increases considerably during the first four days after an acute coronary occlusion [25]. The only direct data available from man is the report of one patient who sustained a traumatic fistula between the right coronary artery and the right atrium [26]. Nine days after the initial trauma, an angiogram showed collateral connections to the distal segment of the artery. Thus, collateral enlargement in man may not vary greatly from that observed in the dog. In some patients, however, the diffuse nature of atherosclerotic disease might limit the amount of flow that could be provided through these connections.

MECHANISTIC APPROACH TO THERAPEUTIC INTERVENTIONS

The most logical approach to the development of therapy to limit infarct size would be to first identify the critical subcellular step(s) that dictate(s) the transition from reversible to irreversible ischemic cell injury [12]. Therapy could then be developed to reverse the most critical step(s) in the ischemic process. To date, however, although several subcellular events have been temporally associated with the onset of irreversible injury, the proximate cause of cell death has not been established. As a consequence, a large variety of potential therapies with widely differing postulated mechanisms have been under study. These agents could be classified according to drug category, e.g., β-blocking agents, steroids, and vasodilators. An alternative approach, which is being followed in this section of this book, is to attempt to classify potential mechanisms of infarct limitation (Table 1). This classification is useful in that it provides a rational means for attacking the problem of protecting ischemic myocardium and for selecting new and as yet untested modes of therapy. The major drawback to a mechanistic classification is that individual drugs often do not conveniently fall into a single mechanistic category. Many potential therapies have several potentially beneficial pharmacologic effects or a combination of beneficial and detrimental effects.

The classification of therapeutic mechanisms in Table 1 is based on the most common definition of ischemia, i.e., an inequality between oxygen supply and demand. In more precise terms, ischemia can be defined as insufficient energy production relative to the energy utilization of the cell. Based on this definition, the severity of ischemia could be alleviated in one of two general ways, i.e., by either (a) reducing the energy utilization of the ischemic cell, or (b) improving the capacity of the cell to produce energy. A third general approach to protective therapy, irrespective of the balance between energy production and utilization, would be to mount a direct attack against one or more of the subcellular consequences of ischemia, i.e., to prevent the damage caused by ischemia.

Table 1. Potential ways to limit acute necrosis (minimize infarct size) or prevent subsequent necrosis (prevent infarct extention)

(A) Decrease energy utilization
    (1) Reduce hemodynamic work
        (a) Reduce heart rate – β blockade, carotid sinus stimulation
        (b) Reduce contractility – β blockade, Ca^{++} flux inhibition (verapamil), prostaglandins
        (c) Reduce afterload – intraaortic balloon counterpulsation
        (d) Reduce preload – nitrates – digitalis (in the failing heart)
    (2) Reduce cell metabolism directly
        (a) Reduce Ca^{++} influx – β blockade, verapamil, nifedipine
        (b) Induce hypothermia

(B) Increase the potential for energy production
    (1) Restore or preserve existing perfusion of ischemic myocardium
        (a) Do emergency revascularization
        (b) Alter coagulation
            (1) Lyse existing thrombi – streptokinase
            (2) Prevent microthrombi – aspirin, prostaglandins
        (c) Improve or preserve collateral blood flow
            (1) Increase diastolic blood pressure
                (a) Balloon counterpulsation
                (b) α-Adrenergic stimulation – methoxamine, norepinephrine
            (2) Use vasodilators – verapamil, nifedipine, nitrates, α-adrenergic blockade, prostaglandins, dipyridamole
            (3) Decrease diastolic wall tension (reduce preload) – nitrates
            (4) Prevent myocardial edema – osmotic agents (mannitol), hyaluronidase
    (2) Increase blood oxygen or substrate content despite persistent ischemia
        (a) Increase oxygen – correct hypoxemia and anemia, hyperbaric oxygen
        (b) Increase substrates – GIK, hypertonic glucose, ATP
        (c) Enhance tissue diffusion – hyaluronidase

(C) Reduce catabolism, stabilize cell structure
    (1) Inhibit adenine nucleotide catabolism
    (2) Inhibit lipolysis – β pyridyl carbinol, prostaglandins
    (3) Reduce electrolyte shifts/prevent cell swelling – β blockade, Ca^{++} flux inhibition (verapamil, nidedipine), osmotic agents (mannitol)
    (4) Stabilize cell membranes (plasmalemma, lysosomes) – steroids, prostaglandins

This table presents a classification of mechanisms that could protect ischemic myocardium (see text for explanation). The drugs or classes of drugs listed are included for illustrative purposes. Thus this table is not meant to be a compendium of all drugs that may have beneficial effects on ischemic myocardium. In addition, inclusion of a therapy on this list does not necessarily imply that direct tests of efficacy have been done or that positive results have been obtained. In fact, no therapy has yet been accepted for general clinical use. Note that many drugs, e.g., β blockers or calcium antagonists, have more than one potentially beneficial effect.

(A) In general terms, the energy utilization of the ischemic cell might be decreased either by reducing the hemodynamic determinants of myocardial energy utilization or by directly inhibiting those reactions within the ischemic cell that continue to consume high-energy phosphates. Reduction of energy utilization will be considered further in the following chapter.

(B) On the other side of the energy production/utilization equation, a large number of suggested therapies have actions that might increase the potential for energy production. In general terms, the potential for energy production could be increased either by increasing blood flow to the ischemic region (see Becker, p. 416) or by increasing the oxygen or substrate delivery to the region despite persistent ischemia. Perfusion could be restored directly by emergency revascularization or by lysis of thrombi (see Griggs, p. 457). Collateral perfusion also might be improved by interventions that either increased diastolic blood pressure, dilated collateral anastomoses, or decreased external compression of the microvasculature. The capacity of ischemic cells to produce energy could be increased despite persistent ischemia if the blood oxygen or substrate content were increased or if interstitial diffusion of oxygen or substrates could be increased (see Swain, p. 479).

(C) Irrespective of the balance between energy production and utilization, some potential therapies are pertinent because they might slow or reverse one or more of the effects of ischemia on the structural or internal milieu of the cell. A complete review of the metabolic and structural consequences of ischemia that are known to occur in association with the transition to irreversibility is beyond the scope of this chapter. However, metabolic effects of ischemia, in addition to depletion of high-energy phosphates, include degradation of adenine nucleotides, intracellular acidosis [2, 8], accumulation of lactate via anaerobic glycolysis [27, 29], and accumulation of free fatty acids [27] via accelerated lipolysis [30]. Energy depletion also inhibits ion transport, which eventually leads to cell swelling [31] and calcium overload [32]. Plasmalemmal damage is an early structural feature of ischemic injury and may be the lethal event [27, 33]. Lysosomal [34] and mitochondrial [33] damage also have been observed in ischemia. Thus, agents that could inhibit catabolism, prevent cell swelling or calcium overload, or stabilize cell membranes have been of interest relative to protection of ischemic myocardium (see Swain, p. 479).

REFERENCES

1. Sobel BE: Infarct size, prognosis, and causal contiguity. Circulation 53:I-146–149, 1976.
2. Bakshandeh K, Kaiser GA, Bolooki H: Hemodynamic correlates of the size of myocardial infarct. Surg Forum 23:152–153, 1974.
3. Opherk D, Finke R, Mittmann U, et al: The influences of the size of acute ischemic myocardial lesions on coronary reserve and left ventricular function in the dog. Basic Res Cardiol 72:402–410, 1977.
4. Bloor CM, Ehsani A, White FC, Sobel BE: Ventricular fibrillation threshold in acute myocardial infarction and its relation to myocardial infarct size. Cardiovasc Res 9:468–472, 1975.
5. Sobel BE, Bresnahan GF, Shell WE, Yoder RD: Estimation of infarct size in man and its relation to prognosis. Circulation 46:640–648, 1972.

6. Mathey D, Bleifeld W, Hanrath P, Effert S: Attempt to quantitate relation between cardiac function and infarct size in acute myocardial infarction. Br Heart J 36:271–279, 1974.
7. Roberts R, Husain A, Ambos HD, Oliver GC, Cox JR Jr, Sobel BE: Relation between infarct size and ventricular arrhythmia. Br Heart J 37:1169–1175, 1975.
8. Cox JR Jr, Roberts R, Ambos HD, Oliver GC, Sobel BE: Relations between enzymatically estimated myocardial infarct size and early ventricular dysrhythmia. Circulation 53:I-150–155, 1976.
9. Page DL, Caulfield JB, Kastor JA, DeSanctis RW, Sanders CA: Myocardial changes associated with cardiogenic shock. N Eng J Med 285:133–137, 1971.
10. Maroko PR, Kjekshus JK, Sobel BE, Watanabe T, Covell JW, Ross J Jr, Braunwald E: Factors influencing infarct size following experimental coronary artery occlusion. Circulation 43:67–82, 1971.
11. Maroko PR, Braunwald E: Modification of myocardial infarction size after coronary occlusion. Ann Intern Med 79:720–733, 1973.
12. Jennings RB, Reimer KA: Salvage of ischemic myocardium. Mod Concepts Cardiovasc Dis 43:125–130, 1974.
13. Factor SM, Sonnenblick EH, Kirk ES: The histologic border zone of acute myocardial infarction – islands or peninsulas? Am J Pathol 92:111–124, 1978.
14. Reimer KA, Jennings RB: The 'wavefront phenomenon' of myocardial ischemic cell death: II. Transmural progression of necrosis within the framework of ischemic bed size (myocardium at risk) and collateral flow. Lab Invest 40:633–644, 1979.
15. Lee JT, Ideker RE, Reimer KA: Myocardial infarct size and location with respect to the coronary vascular bed in man. Circulation 64:526–534, 1981.
16. Jennings RB, Sommers HM, Smyth GA, Flack HA, Linn H: Myocardial necrosis induced by temporary occlusion of a coronary artery in the dog. Arch Pathol 70:68–78, 1960.
17. Reimer KA, Jennings RB: The changing anatomic reference base of evolving myocardial infarction. Underestimation of myocardial collateral blood flow and overestimation of experimental anatomic infarct size due to tissue edema, hemorrhage and acute inflammation. Circulation 60:866–876, 1979.
18. Reimer KA, Lowe JE, Rasmussen MM, Jennings RB: The wavefront phenomenon of ischemic cell death: I. Myocardial infarct size vs duration of coronary occlusion in dogs. Circulation 56:786–794, 1977.
19. Roberts WC: Coronary artery pathology in fatal ischemic heart disease. In: Braunwald E (ed) The myocardium: failure and infarction. New York: HP Publishing Co, 1974, ch 18.
20. Kagen L, Scheidt S, Butt A: Serum myoglobin in myocardial infarction: the 'staccato phenomenon'. Is acute myocardial infarction in man an intermittent event? Am J Med 62:86–92, 1977.
21. Mathey D, Bleifeld W, Buss H, Hanrath P: Creatine kinase release in acute myocardial infarction: correlation with clinical electrocardiographic, and pathological findings. Br Heart J 37:1161–1168, 1975.
22. Mills RM Jr, Young E, Gorlin R, Lesch M: Natural history of S-T segment elevation after acute myocardial infarction. Am J Cardiol 35:609–614, 1975.

23. Reid PR, Taylor DR, Kelly DT: Myocardial-infarct extension detected by precordial ST-sgement mapping. N Engl J Med 290:123–128, 1974.
24. Hutchins GM, Bulkley BH: Infarct expansion vs extension: two different complications of acute myocardial infarction. Am J Cardiol 41:1127–1132, 1978.
25. Bloor CM, White FC: Functional development of the coronary collateral circulation during coronary artery occlusion in the conscious dog. Am J Pathol 67:483–500, 1972.
26. Siepser SL, Kaltman AJ, Mills N, Pughkem T, Fox AC: Coronary collateral flow after traumatic fistula between right coronary artery and right atrium. N Engl J Med 287:754–756, 1972.
27. Jennings RB, Hawkins HK, Lowe JE, Hill ML, Klotman S, Reimer KA: Relation between high energy phosphate and lethal injury in myocardial ischemia in the dog. Am J Pathol 92:187–214, 1978.
28. Gevers, W: Generation of protons by metabolic processes in heart cells [editorial]. J Mol Cell Cardiol 9:867–873, 1977.
29. Braasch W, Gudbjarnason S, Puri PS, Ravens KG, Bing RJ: Early changes in energy metabolism in the myocardium following acute coronary artery occlusion in anesthetized dogs. Circ Res 23:429–438, 1968.
30. Neely JR, Rovetto MJ, Whitmer JT: Rate-limiting steps of carbohydrate and fatty acid metabolism in ischemic hearts. Acta Med Scand [Suppl] 587:9–13, 1976.
31. Leaf A: Regulation of intracellular fluid volume and disease. Am J Med 49:291–295, 1970.
32. Shine KI, Douglas AM, Ricchiuti NV: Calcium, strontium, and barium movements during ischemia and reperfusion in rabbit ventricle. Implications for myocardial preservation. Circ Res 43:712–720, 1978.
33. Jennings RB, Ganote CE, Reimer KA: Ischemic tissue injury. Am J Pathol 81:179–198, 1975.
34. Decker RS, Wildenthal K: Sequential lysosomal alterations during cardiac ischemia. II. Ultrastructural and cytochemical changes. Lab Invest 38:662–673, 1978.

17. DECREASING MYOCARDIAL ENERGY UTILIZATION

KEITH A. REIMER and ROBERT B. JENNINGS

ENERGY DEPLETION AND LETHAL ISCHEMIC CELL INJURY

The onset of myocardial ischemia is followed by the rapid depletion of residual oxygen in the tissues; mitochondrial respiration is inhibited and, within the first 15–30 s, the energy metabolism of the cell converts to anaerobic glycolysis [1]. In areas of milder ischemia, some blood glucose may be available as a substrate and the available oxygen may support a reduced level of mitochondrial oxidative metabolism [2]. In areas of severe ischemia, however, the conversion of glycogen to lactate becomes the only meaningful source of high-energy phosphate production. Although the complete oxidation of 1 μmol glucose nets 38 μmol ATP, conversion of glycogen to lactate nets only 3 μmol ATP per μmol glucosyl units consumed. Thus, anaerobic glycolysis cannot meet the normal energy needs of the working myocardium.

The major pathway for myocardial energy consumption, i.e., mechanical work, also is inhibited at the onset of anaerobic metabolism [3]. Nevertheless, ATP utilization continues (Figure 1) [4]. Continued electrical and minimal mechanical activity utilize some high-energy phosphate (HEP). Continued maintenance of trans-sarcolemmal gradients of Na^+ and K^+ occurs via a Na^+/K^+ ATPase [5]. As much as one-third of the basal energy requirements of a cell may be devoted to this process [6]. Other potential drains on HEP include Ca^{++} accumulation by the sarcoplasmic reticulum and various other ATPases of the cell. In addition, minor utilization would occur from the activity of fatty acid CoA synthetase and adenyl cyclase [7].

In areas of severe ischemia, these basal sources of ATP utilization must be fueled either by the preexisting HEP stores of the tissue or by ATP production from anaerobic glycolysis. The reserve stores of HEP in left ventricular myocardium of the dog include a mean of 8 μmol creatine phosphate, 5.6 μmol ATP, and 1.5 μmol ADP per gram left ventricle [1, 8]. However, each μmol ATP contributes 2 μmol HEP. Thus, a reserve store of 20–22 μmol HEP per gram is present [9, 10]. In addition, the glycogen content of dog left ventricle varies from 27 to 47 μmol glucosyl units. Anaerobic glycolysis could thus produce 81–141 μmol/g HEP from glycogen [11]. Both the reserve supply of HEP and anaerobic glycolysis together could provide roughly 100–162 μmol HEP per gram ischemic heart if all of the reserve glycogen was fully utilized [9].

Wagner GS (ed): Myocardial Infarction: Measurement and Intervention, pp 397–414.
© 1982 Martinus Nijhoff Publishers, The Hague/Boston/London.

398

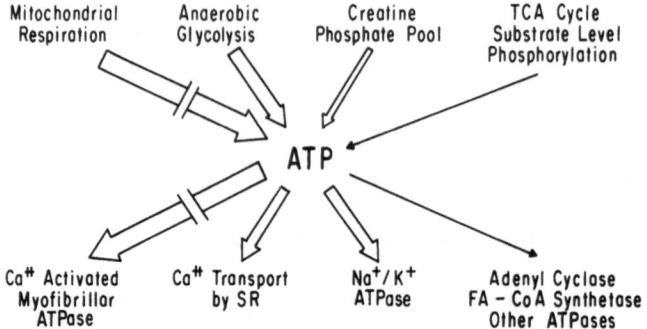

Figure 1. The principal reactions producing and utilizing HEP in ischemic tissue. In severe ischemia, aerobic respiration is abolished. The preexisting stores of HEP, in the form of creatine phosphate or ATP, are relatively small. Thus, anaerobic glycolysis becomes the principal source of energy, producing 80%–90% of the high-energy phosphate bonds that can be utilized by ischemic tissue. Energy utilization also is markedly reduced during ischemia. Cardiac contraction, which is mediated by the Ca^{++}-activated myofibrillar ATPase, consumes much of the ATP produced in aerobic myocardium. Although contraction is abolished or severely depressed in areas of severe ischemia, ATP continues to be required to remove Na$^+$ from the cell, to keep Ca^{++} sequestered in the sarcoplasmic reticulum, and for a variety of other cellular processes that may continue to compete for the remaining ATP. Reprinted from Jennings and Reimer [4] with permission of the publishers.

Thus, 80%–90% of the energy reserves of ischemic myocardium are in the form of glycogen. Although there is a rapid burst of anaerobic glycolysis immediately after the onset of ischemia, flux through the glycolytic pathway subsequently slows markedly. The factors that limit the rate of glycolysis are not entirely understood but may include inhibition of glyceraldehyde-3-phosphate dehydrogenase by high levels of NADH and lactate and inhibition of phosphofructokinase by the acidic pH of ischemic cells [12–15].

Thus, although both HEP utilization and production are markedly reduced during ischemia, production always lags behind utilization (Figure 2) and there is a progressive depletion of the HEP reserves (Figures 3 and 4) [9]. In fact, most of the creatine phosphate content of the myocardium is gone within the first 1–3 min of severe ischemia in dogs [1, 7]. By 15 min, when the injury is still reversible, 65% of the ATP is also gone and by 40 min, which is lethal for most of the most severely ischemic subendocardial region, 90% is gone (Figure 4) [7].

Although HEP depletion has long been recognized as an obvious consequence of ischemia, the rapidity of this depletion in areas of severe ischemia has not been fully appreciated until recently [7]. Furthermore, there has been little evidence to provide a direct link between ATP depletion per se and the onset of lethal cell injury. Metabolic consequences of ischemia, other than ATP depletion, that could lead to cell death include the deleterious effects of cellular acidosis [14, 16], lactate accumulation [17], or excessive intracellular calcium

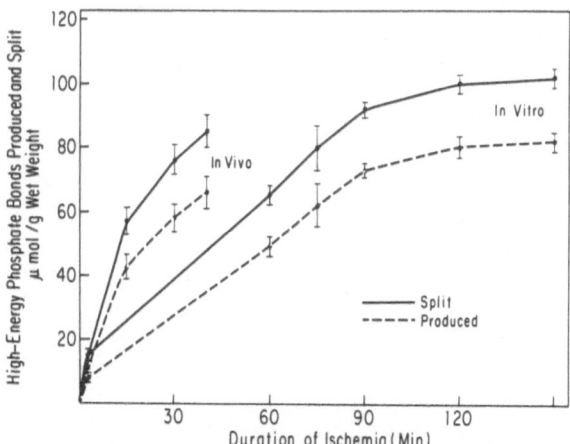

Figure 2. The rates of high-energy phosphate bond utilization (split) and production via anaerobic glycolysis (estimated from lactate accumulation) at 37°C in severe ischemia in vivo or total ischemia in vitro are plotted as a function of the duration of ischemia. The rates of both production and utilization were much higher in vivo than in vitro. Reprinted from Jennings et al. [9] with permission of the publishers.

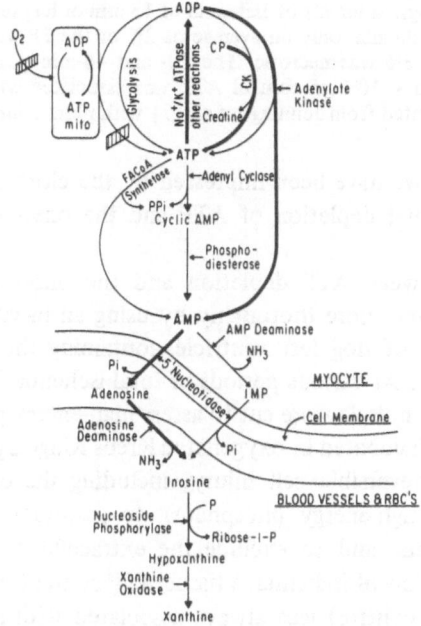

Figure 3. The major metabolic pathways of high-energy phosphate and adenine nucleotide degradation during myocardial ischemia. The quantitatively most important pathways are indicated by the solid thick arrows. Reprinted from Jennings et al. [7] with permission of the publishers.

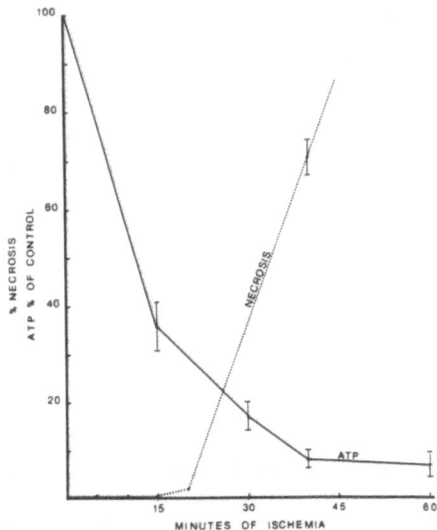

Figure 4. This graph plots the relationship between the level of ATP remaining in the severely ischemic portion of the posterior papillary muscle (PP) and the amount of irreversible injury in this muscle after various periods of ischemia induced by circumflex occlusion in open-chest dogs. Intervals of ischemia of 15 min or less result in no irreversible injury. After 20 min of ischemia, only an average of 2% of the PP was necrotic, but after 40 min of ischemia 72% ± 3% was necrotic. The 20- and 40-min points are based on 15 and 24 dogs. Depletion to < 10% of control ATP was associated with extensive necrosis within the PP tissue. Reprinted from Jennings et al. [7] with permission of the publishers.

levels [18]. However, we have been impressed by the close association in time between the almost total depletion of ATP and the onset of irreversible cell injury (Figure 4).

The association between ATP depletion and the onset of lethal ischemic injury has been evaluated more thoroughly by using an in vitro model of total ischemia [19]. Blocks of dog left ventricle containing the papillary muscles were incubated in vitro. At various periods of total ischemia from 0 to 150 min, slices of these blocks of muscle were cut to assess high-energy phosphate content. Additional slices were incubated in oxygenated Krebs Ringers phosphate medium to assess indices of irreversible cell injury, including the capacity of injured cells to resynthesize high-energy phosphates, to restore normal cell volume and electrolyte contents, and to exclude the extracellular marker, inulin. Irrespective of the duration of ischemia, a tissue ATP content of less than 5 μmol/ g dry weight (20% of control) was always associated with a lowered capacity to resynthesize creatine phosphate or ATP. Impaired cell volume regulation, sodium extrusion, and potassium accumulation were detectable in the same slices. Overt damage of the cell membrane, as indicated by an increased inulin diffusible space, was detectable in slices cut 15–30 min later, by which time the ATP content of the tissue had decreased to less than $2\,\mu mol/g$ dry weight. Thus, both in vivo and in vitro, the development of characteristic features of irreversible ischemic injury occurs concomitant with, or shortly after, ATP has been depleted to less than 20% of normal.

The close association between marked ATP depletion and cell death in the above experiments is consistent with a cause-and-effect relationship between ATP depletion and ischemic cell death. This association also provides a rational basis for the hypothesis that interventions that could delay energy utilization by ischemic myocardium might also delay the onset of cell death and limit the ultimate size of an infarct.

DECREASING MYOCARDIAL ENERGY UTILIZATION

In general theoretical terms (see Table 1 in the preceding chapter), myocardial energy utilization could be altered either by reducing residual mechanical work of the ischemic myocardium or by inhibiting energy dependent reactions of the cell per se. In aerobic working myocardium, mechanical work is the principal energy-consuming function. Heart rate, contractility, and developed wall tension (as determined by intraventricular developed pressure and volume) are the major hemodynamic indices of myocardial oxygen utilization [20]. The same hemodynamic indices of cardiac metabolism have generally been assumed to be determinants of energy utilization in ischemic myocardium. However, because contractile function is abolished in areas of severe ischemia and markedly depressed in areas of milder ischemia, hemodynamic perturbations may not have major effects on the rate of energy utilization. Nevertheless, in experimental studies, ST segment elevation has been reduced by reduction of heart rate by vagal stimulation [21], and other experimental studies have shown reduction of ST elevation or limitation of infarct size by unloading the ventricle with intra-aortic balloon counterpulsation [22-24]. If the assumption that hemodynamic work determines the energy utilization of ischemic myocardium is correct, reduction of hemodynamic work should be beneficial.

Reduction of cardiac work can also be achieved by pharmacologic interventions that reduce heart rate, contractility, afterload, or preload. Specific examples include β blockade, which has both bradycardic and negative inotropic effects. Calcium antagonists represent a second class of drugs that reduce both cardiac contractility and afterload. Preload can be reduced by vasodilators such as the nitrates. β blockade and Ca^{++} antagonists will be discussed in more detail below. For further discussion of aortic counterpulsation and the nitrates, see Becker, p. 426.

Energy utilization could be reduced directly by slowing overall metabolism by hypothermia or by inhibiting one or more of the reactions utilizing ATP in ischemic cells. Intracellular calcium is known to activate a variety of ATPases associated with myofibrillar contraction [25, 26], calcium sequestration by the sarcoplasmic reticulum [27], mitochondrial calcium accumulation [28], etc. Thus reduction of calcium influx across the sarcolemma would be expected to reduce the energy requirements of the ischemic cell [29]. The slow inward calcium current that contributes to the plateau phase of the cardiac action potential can be specifically blocked by the so-called calcium antagonists including verapamil and nifedipine [30]. β blockade also reduces intracellular Ca^{++} levels indirectly by preventing catecholamine-induced stimulation of Ca^{++} influx across the sarcolemma and release from the sarcoplasmic reticulum [31]. In the sections that follow, hypothermia, β blockade, and Ca^{++} antagonists will be considered in more detail.

HYPOTHERMIA

Recent studies of dog hearts subjected to total ischemia, in vitro, at various temperatures have demonstrated that the rate of ATP depletion in ischemia is markedly temperature dependent (Figure 5) [32]. A decrease of as little as 3°C from 37° to 34° significantly slowed the rate of ATP depletion in these studies. Successive increments of cooling in other groups of hearts to 28° further delayed ATP depletion whereas hyperthermia exacerbated ATP depletion.

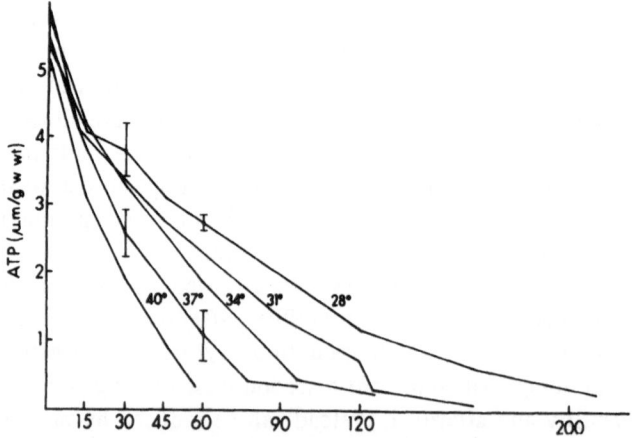

Figure 5. Tissue ATP as a function of the period of total ischemia at different temperatures. Septal tissue of dog left ventricle was excised from each of 4–6 hearts that had been arrested with 30 mM K$^+$ and were subjected to total ischemia at 28°–40°C. The bars represent the standard error of the mean. Reprinted from Jennings and Reimer [4] with permission of the publishers.

Coincident with the hypothermia-induced delay in ATP utilization, the onset of cardiac rigor and various indices of lethal cell injury including defective cell volume regulation also were delayed. Similar effects of temperature on HEP levels have been reported in isolated ischemic rat hearts [33].

Many studies conducted over the past three decades have shown beneficial effects of hypothermia on postoperative survival and cardiac function following cardiac surgical procedures. As a consequence, hypothermia has become a standard mode of cardiac preservation among many cardiac surgeons for procedures that require temporary interruption of myocardial perfusion. The well-known protective effects of hypothermia can likely be attributed to the preservation of myocardial high-energy phosphates.

Despite its widespread use in cardiac surgery, hypothermia has received relatively little attention as a means of limiting infarct size. In one study [34] of anesthetized dogs with myocardial infarct and cardiogenic shock, moderate hypothermia ($32°C$) significantly reduced the heart rate, left ventricular end-diastolic pressure, and overall myocardial oxygen consumption without significantly reducing cardiac output. Survival time was tripled in hypothermic dogs compared with controls. The effects of hypothermia on myocardial infarct size, per se, were not studied.

β BLOCKADE – ANIMAL STUDIES

Propranolol is now standard therapy in the treatment of angina pectoris and has been widely used to suppress various arrhythmias associated with myocardial infarct. Specific interest in β blockade as a means to limit infarct size began with the observation [35], confirmed by several studies [36–38], that positive inotropic agents such as isoproterenol worsened ischemic injury whereas β blockade with propranolol or practolol reduced ischemic injury as estimated by ST segment mapping techniques in dogs. Following these encouraging although indirect experimental results, the effect of propranolol on ischemic injury and infarct size was assessed directly. Propranolol was first shown to delay ischemic injury sufficiently to reduce the amount of necrosis produced by 20–40 min of temporary coronary occlusion in dogs [39–41]. Subsequently, several groups reported that propranolol decreased overall infarct size when assessed by gross or histologic techniques following coronary ligation in open-chest dogs [42–48]. In addition, the severity of ultrastructural damage both to myocytes and capillaries was reduced in propranolol-treated rats subjected to coronary ligation [49].

Not all of the experimental evidence with propranolol has been positive. Two independent studies have shown no reduction in the amount of creatine kinase lost from the infarcted regions of open-chest dogs treated with propranolol

[50, 51]. Furthermore, in recent studies, we have been unable to confirm our initial positive results with the drug, using doses ranging from 0.1 to 5.0 mg/kg in dogs with ischemic injury caused by 40 min of temporary occlusion (K. A. Reimer and R. B. Jennings, unpublished observations). The explanation for this discrepancy is not known. However, we have shown that the size of the occluded vascular bed and the amount of collateral blood flow within this bed are major determinants of infarct size in untreated dogs [52]. These two variables, which were not measured in any of the published studies from our own or other laboratories cited above, should be included in experimental models to assess the effect of drugs on infarct size. Otherwise, comparability among groups of animals cannot be assured. Because of a relatively high mortality and failure to control for ischemic bed size and/or collateral blood flow, artifactual selection of propranolol-treated dogs with relatively small infarcts may have occured in our study. Whatever the explanation, we have not been able to show protective effects with modest doses of propranolol during temporary circumflex occlusions of 40 min or 3 h when mortality has been low and comparable ischemic bed size and collateral flow have been assured.

Nevertheless, the composite experience with propranolol in experimental myocardial ischemia has been encouraging. Although the mechanism by which propranolol protects the myocardium has not been established, the prevailing view is that β blockade reduces the energy demands of the myocardium through its ability to reduce heart rate and contractility. Most studies of the effect of propranolol on collateral blood flow in open-chest dogs have shown either no effect or an actual decrease in the absolute collateral flow [53–56]. A redistribution of the available collateral flow toward the most severely ischemic subendocardial region has been observed in some studies [53, 57], but not in others [54]. Thus in the studies using open-chest dogs in which propranolol has reduced infarct size, the mechanism probably has not been improved collateral flow. On the other hand, propranolol has increased collateral blood flow during coronary occlusion in unanesthetized dogs [58]. Thus, it is possible that anesthesia could mask one beneficial effect of the drug.

The assumption that propranolol is protective via β blockade is supported by the absence of myocardial protection by d-propranolol, an isomer with direct cardiodepressant and membrane-stabilizing effects but without β-blocking activity [45]. In contrast, major reduction in experimental infarct size has been reported with dimethyl propranolol (UM-272), another analogue without β-blocking activity [59, 60] but with membrane-stabilizing effects. However, the protective effects with this drug have also been associated with decreased myocardial oxygen consumption [61].

β blockade with propranolol during experimental myocardial infarction reduces heart rate and contractility, two of the major hemodynamic determinants of the metabolic requirements of working myocardium. Arterial blood pressure is maintained. Thus, as long as congestive failure with concomitant cardiac dilatation and increased wall tension is avoided, the net effect of propranolol on metabolic requirements should be positive.

β BLOCKADE – PATIENT STUDIES

Several years before the current interest in limiting infarct size began, propranolol was considered as an antiarrhythmic agent for use in patients with acute myocardial infarcts. The drug had been found to be effective against recurrent ventricular fibrillation [62], and Snow [63] reported a marked reduction in short-term mortality among patients with acute myocardial infarcts given low doses of propranolol. However, several subsequent studies [64, 65] failed to confirm any improved survival in patients given low doses of propranolol and, indeed, the incidence of cardiac failure and hypotension was increased in some studies. Interest in propranolol temporarily waned.

Renewed interest in propranolol has been sparked in the last few years by the experimental evidence presented above, that propranolol reduced the severity of ischemic injury and thus might limit infarct size. Direct measurement of infarct size in comparable groups of treated and untreated patients obviously cannot be done. However, a number of recent studies have reported favorable effects of propranolol on various indirect indices of myocardial ischemia in patients with acute myocardial infarcts.

In several studies, β blockade with either propranolol or practolol has relieved pain immediately [66–68] and reduced ST segment elevation measured by precordial mapping techniques [67–71]. Propranolol has reduced the peak serum level of creatine kinase in patients treated during the first 4 h of myocardial infarction [72] and has reduced the incidence of subsequent Q waves and CK release in patients hospitalized with suspected myocardial infarcts [73]. These beneficial effects have been attributed in part to reduced heart rate and rate–pressure product, but direct metabolic effects may also be important. An improved balance between oxygen supply and demand has been supported by the findings of increased overall lactate extraction and reduced oxygen extraction by the myocardium of propranolol-treated patients [74, 75]. The incidence of cardiac failure has not been increased in these studies but remains an important possible complication from propranolol therapy. Bloch et al. [76] have reported increased evidence of cardiac failure in patients on chronic therapy with propranolol who subsequently developed a myocardial infarct. Because of this potential complication, some European investigators prefer a β blocker, such as practolol, which has no intrinsic negative inotropic properties [69, 71].

Although patient studies seem promising, the results must be interpreted cautiously. In the chapter by Gold and Leinbach, the dependence upon a partially patent coronary artery is demonstrated (p. 506). All these studies are limited by small numbers of patients and the absence of precise techniques of measuring infarct size. A multicenter trial of propranolol and hyaluronidase is currently underway and may provide more definitive evidence regarding the effect of early propranolol treatment on myocardial infarct size in man.

CALCIUM ANTAGONISTS

The so-called calcium antagonists [30] are a structurally diverse group of organic compounds. They have in common the effect of decreasing calcium conductance and thus decreasing the slow calcium inward current across the sarcolemma, which is responsible, at least in part, for the plateau phase of the cardiac action potential. This inhibition of the calcium channel is apparently specific; the fast Na^+ flux is not inhibited. The major cardiovascular effects of these drugs can be attributed to inhibition of Ca^{++} influx to cardiac myocytes, vascular smooth muscle, or cells of the cardiac conduction system. The effect on cardiac myocytes is primarily a dose-dependent reduction in cardiac contractility. The vascular effect is manifest as both peripheral and coronary vasodilation (see Becker, p. 436). The effect on cardiac conduction tissue includes sinus slowing of heart rate and first-degree to complete (at high doses) atrioventricular block. Verapamil is the prototype calcium antagonist and has been extensively studied. More recently nifedipine (BAY 1040) has received much attention because, while it shares with verapamil the Ca^{++} antagonist effects on cardiac myocytes and coronary vasculature, it has the advantage of only minimal effect on conduction fibers so that its administration is not complicated by atrioventricular conduction disturbances [77]. In addition, it is an even more potent coronary vasodilator than verapamil [30].

Calcium antagonists have shown beneficial effects in the treatment of stable and unstable angina pectoris [78–82]. The efficacy of calcium antagonists in angina is usually attributed to their coronary vasodilating properties. These agents reduce basal coronary tone and also can prevent or relieve coronary spasm induced by either alpha-adrenergic stimulation or ergotamine [82].

Approval of the calcium antagonists, for clinical use in the USA, has been slow, and no studies of these agents have been reported in patients with acute myocardial infarcts. However, they have been recently studied in several experimental models of myocardial ischemia or infarction. In theory, they could protect ischemic myocardium in several ways. (a) By reducing calcium influx to the myocyte, the activities of Ca^{++} activated myofibrillar and other ATPases are reduced. Thus contractility and the major routes of ATP utilization in contracting myocardium are reduced. (b) The peripheral vasodilation reduces blood pressure and thus further reduces the hemodynamic work load of the myocardium. (c) Coronary vasodilation could improve perfusion of ischemic myocardium through relief of coronary spasm or dilatation of collateral channels. (d) Ca^{++} flux inhibitors might also delay the development of calcium overload and thus could have a direct protective effect through prevention of the deleterious effects of Ca^{++} on the structure or homeostatic mechanisms of the cell.

The first studies [82, 83] in which verapamil was administered to open-chest dogs with acute coronary occlusion demonstrated that reductions in ST segment elevation, measured by epicardial mapping techniques, could be achieved without deleterious hemodynamic effects. Subsequently, we showed that verapamil reduced the amount of necrosis caused by a 40-min period of coronary occlusion when assessed directly by histologic analysis after 2–4 days of reperfusion [84]. These results have recently been confirmed in studies of comparable groups, in terms of ischemic bed size and collateral blood flow (Table 1) (K. A. Reimer and R. B. Jennings, unpublished observations). These positive results are most likely related to a reduced rate of high-energy phosphate depletion, which has been observed in several studies of myocardial injury induced by isoproterenol toxicity, ischemia or hypoxia [85–88]. This energy-sparing effect of Ca^{++} antagonists may lead to their clinical use as cardioplegic agents during surgical procedures that require periods of myocardial ischemia. In fact, preservation of cardiac function has been demonstrated with verapamil and nifedipine following periods of total ischemic arrest in vivo as well as in isolated heart preparations [88–90].

Whether the initial delay in high-energy phosphate depletion and the onset of irreversible ischemic injury would be manifest as a long-term limitation of infarct size has not been established. Karlsberg et al. have reported [91] that verapamil therapy, started 5 h after coronary occlusion in awake dogs, had no effect on subsequent creatine kinase depletion. However, it might be argued that in their study, the treatment was started too late, after most of the myocardium at risk was already irreversibly injured. On the other hand, we have found a similar lack of effect of verapamil on infarct size when therapy was begun 15 min after occlusion (K.A. Reimer and R.B. Jennings, unpublished observations). In the latter study, infarcts in open-chest dogs were produced by 3-h occlusions of the circumflex artery and followed by four days of reperfusion. Infarct size was quantitated by histologic techniques and analyzed with respect to the size of the ischemic bed at risk and the amount of collateral blood flow within the ischemic region. Although verapamil increased blood flow to nonischemic regions of the myocardium, collateral blood flow was slightly reduced, perhaps due to a concomitant decrease in diastolic blood pressure. Karlsberg [91] also reported no effect of verapamil on collateral blood flow. These results suggest that verapamil can delay cell injury during relatively brief

Table 1. Hemodynamics, collateral flow, and infarct size in verapamil-treated vs control dogs[a]

	No. of dogs	Heart rate/min	Mean blood pr. (mmHg)	Left ventric. pr. (mmHg)	LVEDP[b] (mmHg)	LAD[b] (% of	Circumflex flow[b]			Size of[b] LCC bed (% of LV)	Necrosis (% of LV)	Necrosis (% of LCC bed)
							I	M	O			
Verapamil	8	136.** ±7.4	86.** ±2.7	123. ±4.1	10.9 ±2.3	153.0 ±20.0	5.1 ±1.3	11.0 ±2.7	21.5 ±2.1	38.6 ±2.1	3.1** ±1.6	8.1** ±2.9
Control	6	174.0 ±5.0	119.0 ±9.4	147.0 ±11.0	9.3 ±2.7	102.0 ±10.1	4.6 ±1.2	11.3 ±1.5	22.5 ±3.3	39.9 ±1.8	13.0 ±2.8	34.3 ±8.0

Dogs were subjected to 40 min of left circumflex arterial occlusion, after which perfusion was restored. Hemodynamic and flow data were measured 20 min after occlusion. The dogs were sacrificed after four days of recovery and the size of the circumflex vascular bed and myocardial necrosis were measured by anatomic methods.

[a]The experiment began with 20 dogs; 12 in the verapamil and 8 in the control group. Two died of left ventricular failure and one of ventricular fibrillation in the verapamil group. One control died of ventricular fibrillation during occlusion. One dog in each group was excluded because the severe ischemia was not produced by the LCC occlusion. All values are means ± SE mean. Three dogs in the verapamil and one in the treated group were defibrillated at the time of reperfusion. Comparisons between means was by a two-tailed nonpaired t-test. The p values are: * < 0.05 and ** ± 0.01.

[b]LVEDP, end-diastolic pressure in left ventricle; the flow data is expressed as a % of flow to the same region of myocardium prior to occlusion; I, inner one-third; M, middle third; O, the outer third of the myocardium in the circumflex bed. Size of LCC bed as % of LV is the size of the left circumflex bed as a percent of the total left ventricle.

periods of ischemia but that cell death cannot be averted in the long run in the absence of improved perfusion of the ischemic myocardium. Henry et al. [92] have shown that nifedipine, given to awake dogs 30 min after coronary ligation, reduced the tissue loss of creatine kinase measured at 24 h. This apparent reduction of infarct size was associated with increased blood flow to tissue samples with initially moderately reduced flow levels. The improved flow observed with nifedipine in that study may have been a reflection of true increases in collateral flow or increased nonischemic flows in tissue samples containing both ischemic and nonischemic muscle. However, a later study by the same group indicates that collateral flow to ischemic myocardium is indeed improved with nifedipine [93]. Thus both positive and negative results have been observed in studies of the effects of various calcium antagonists on infarct size.

In summary, hypothermia, β blockade, and Ca^{++} antagonists represent three potential categories of interventions that reduce the energy utilization of ischemic myocardium. Hypothermia is routinely employed for cardiac preservation during surgical procedures but has not been widely considered in the context of myocardial infarction. β blockade has been studied extensively in experimental animals and in man with generally favorable effects on indices of ischemic injury. Ca^{++} antagonists have been shown to reduce the rate of high-energy phosphate depletion and have delayed cellular injury during ischemia. Direct studies of the effect of these agents on infarct size, however, have not yielded uniformly favorable results. Thus, additional studies will be required to prove the hypothesis that reduction of myocardial energy utilization can limit infarct size in experimental animals or in man.

REFERENCES

1. Braasch W, Gudbjarnason S, Puri PS, Ravens KG, Bing RJ: Early changes in energy metabolism in the myocardium following acute coronary artery occlusion in anesthetized dogs. Circ Res 23:429, 1968.
2. Opie LH: Metabolic regulation in ischemia and hypoxia: effects of regional ischemia on metabolism of glucose and fatty acids. Relative rate of aerobic and anaerobic energy production during myocardial infarction and comparison with effects of anoxia. Circ Res 38:1−52, 1976.
3. Katz AM, Hecht HH: The early 'pump' failure of the ischemic heart [editorial]. Am J Med 47:497−502, 1969.
4. Jennings RB, Reimer KA: Lethal myocardial ischemic injury. Am J Pathol 102:241−255, 1981.
5. Skou JC: Enzymatic basis for active transport of Na^+ and K^+ across cell membrane. Physiol Rev 45:596−617, 1965.
6. Hokin LE: The molecular machine for driving the coupled transports of Na^+ and K^+ is an ($Na^+ + K^+$)-activated ATPase. Trends Biochem Sci I:233−237, 1976.

7. Jennings RB, Hawkins HK, Lowe JE, Hill ML, Klotman S, Reimer KA: Relation between high energy phosphate and lethal injury in myocardial ischemia in the dog. Am J Pathol 92:187, 1978.

8. Allison TB, Ramey CA, Holsinger JW Jr: Transmural gradients of left ventricular tissue metabolites after circumflex artery ligation in dogs. J Mol Cell Cardiol 9:837–852, 1977.

9. Jennings RB, Reimer KA, Hill ML, Mayer SE: Total myocardial ischemia, in vitro. I. Comparison of high energy phosphate production, utilization and depletion and of adenine nucleotide catabolism in total ischemia in vitro vs. severe ischemia in vivo. Circ Res 49:892–900, 1981.

10. Neely JR, Liedtke AJ, Whitmer JT, Rovetto MJ: Relationship between coronary flow and adenosine triphosphate production from glycolysis and oxidative metabolism. In: Recent advances in studies on cardiac structure and metabolism, vol 8: Roy P-E, Harris P (eds). The cardiac sarcoplasm. Baltimore: University Park Press, 1974, p 301.

11. Scheuer J, Stezoski SW: Protective role of increased myocardial glycogen stores in cardiac anoxia in the rat. Circ Res 27:835–849, 1970.

12. Neely JR, Morgan HE: Relationship between carbohydrate and lipid metabolism and the energy balance of heart muscle. Annu Rev Physiol 36:4 13–459, 1974.

13. Gelet TR, Altschuld RA, Weissler AM: Effects of acidosis on the performance and metabolism of the anoxic heart. Circulation [Suppl] 39 and 40:IV-60, 1969.

14. Williamson JR, Safer B, Rich T, Schaffer S, Kobayaski K: Effects of acidosis on myocardial contractility and metabolism. Acta Med Scand [Suppl] 587:95, 1976.

15. Rovetto MJ, Lamberton WF, Neely JR: Mechanisms of glycolytic inhibition in ischemic rat hearts. Circ Res 37:742–751, 1975.

16. Armiger LC, Seelye RN, Phil D, Elswijk JG, Carnell VM, Gavin JB, Herdson, PB: Fine structural changes in dog myocardium exposed to lowered pH in vivo. Lab Invest 37:237–242, 1977.

17. Armiger LC, Seelye RN, Elswijk JG, Carnell VM, Benson DC, Gavin JB, Herdson PB: Mitochondrial changes in dog myocardium induced by lactate in vivo. Lab Invest 33:502–508, 1975.

18. Shine KI, Douglas AM, Ricchiuti NV: Calcium, strontium, and barium movements during ischemia and reperfusion in rabbit ventricle. Implications for myocardial preservation. Circ Res 43:712, 1978.

19. Reimer KA, Jennings RB, Hill ML: Total myocardial ischemia, in vitro. II. High energy phosphate depletion and associated defects in energy metabolism, cell volume regulation, and sarcolemmal integrity. Circ Res 49:901–911, 1981.

20. Braunwald E: Control of myocardial oxygen consumption: physiologic and clinical considerations. Am J Cardiol 27:416–432, 1971.

21. Redwood DR, Smith ER, Epstein SE: Coronary artery occlusion in the conscious dog: effects of alterations in heart rate and arterial pressure on the degree of myocardial ischemia. Circulation 46:323–332, 1972.

22. Maroko PR, Bernstein EF, Libby P, DeLaria GA, Covell JW, Ross J Jr, Braunwald E: Effects of intraaortic balloon counterpulsation on the severity of myocardial ischemic injury following acute coronary occlusion. Counterpulsation and myocardial injury. Circulation 45:1150–1159, 1972.

23. Roberts AJ, Alonso DR, Combes JR, Jacobstein JG, Post MR, Cahill PT, Shean-Lan TH, Abel RM, Subramanian VA, Gay WA Jr: Role of delayed intraaortic balloon pumping in treatment of experimental myocardial

infarction. Am J Cardiol 41:1202–1208, 1978.

24. Sugg WL, Webb WR, Ecker RR: Reduction of extent of myocardial infarction by counterpulsation. Ann Thorac Surg 7:310–316, 1969.
25. Weber A: On the role of calcium in the activity of adenosine 5'-triphosphate hydrolysis by actomyosin. J Biol Chem 234:2764, 1959.
26. Nayler WG, Merrillees NCR: Cellular exchange of calcium. In: Harris C (ed) Calcium and the Heart. London: Academic Press, 1971, pp 24–65.
27. Hasselbach W: The sarcoplasmic calcium pump – a most efficient ion translocating system. Biophy Struct Mech 3:43–54, 1977.
28. Lehninger AL: Ca^{2+} transport by mitochondria and its possible role in the cardiac contraction-relaxation cycle. Circ Res [Suppl 3] 34 and 35 III-83–90, 1974.
29. Dhalla NS, Yates JC, Proveda V: Calcium-linked changes in myocardial metabolism in the isolated perfused rat heart. Can J Physiol Pharmacol 55:925–933, 1977.
30. Fleckenstein A: Specific pharmacology of calcium in myocardium, cardiac pacemakers, and vascular smooth muscle. Ann Rev Pharmacol Toxicol 17:149–166, 1977.
31. Nayler WG: The effect of beta-adrenergic blocking drugs on myocardial function: an explanation at the subcellular level. Postgrad Med J [Suppl] 46:90–96, 1970.
32. Jones RN, Hill ML, Reimer KA, Wechsler AS, Jennings RB: Effect of hypothermia on the rate of myocardial ATP and adenine nucleotide degradation in total ischemia [abstr]. Fed Proc 39:1111, 1980.
33. Tyers GFO, Williams EH, Hughes HC, Todd GJ: Effect of perfusate temperature on myocardial protection from ischemia. J Thorac Cardiovasc Surg 73:766–771, 1977.
34. Boyer NH, Gerstein MM: Induced hypothermia in dogs with acute myocardial infarction and shock. J Thorac Cardiovasc Surg 74:286–294, 1977.
35. Maroko PR, Kjekshus JK, Sobel BE, Watanabe T, Covell JW, Ross J Jr, Braunwald E: Factors influencing infarct size following experimental coronary artery occlusion. Circulation 43:67–82, 1971.
36. Watanabe T, Shintani F, Fu L, Fujii J, Watenabe H, Kato K: Influence of inotropic alteration on the severity of myocardial ischemia after experimental coronary occlusion. Jpn Heart J 13:222–231, 1972.
37. Libby P, Maroko PR, Covell JW, Mallock CI, Ross J, Braunwald E: Effect of practolol on the extent of myocardial ischaemic injury after experimental coronary occlusion and its effects on ventricular function in the normal and ischaemic heart. Cardiovasc Res 7:167–173, 1973.
38. Wendt RL, Canavan RC, Michalak RJ: Effects of various agents on regional ischemic myocardial injury: electrocardiographic analysis. Am Heart J 87:468–482, 1974.
39. Sommers HM, Jennings RB: Ventricular fibrillation and myocardial necrosis after transient ischemia. Effect of treatment with oxygen, procainamide, reserpine, and propranolol. Arch Intern Med 129:780–789, 1972.
40. Reimer KA, Rasmussen MM, Jennings RB: Reduction by propranolol of myocardial necrosis following temporary coronary artery occlusion in dogs. Circ Res 33:353–353, 1973.
41. Reimer KA, Rasmussen MM, Jennings RB: On the nature of protection by propranolol against myocardial necrosis after temporary coronary occlusion in dogs. Am J Cardiol 37:520–527, 1976.
42. Ginks W, Ross J Jr, Sybers HD: Prevention of gross myocardial infarction in the canine heart. Arch Pathol 97:380–384, 1974.

43. Pierce WS, Carter DR, McGavran MH, Waldhausen JA: Modification of myocardial infarct volume. An experimental study in the dog. Arch Surg 107:682–687, 1973.
44. Shatney CH, MacCarter DJ, Lillehei RC: Effects of allopurinol, propranolol and methylprednisolone on infarct size in experimental myocardial infarction. Am J Cardiol 37:572–580, 1976.
45. Ergin MA, Dastgir G, Butt KMH, Stuckey JH: Prolonged epicardial mapping in myocardial infarction: the effects of propranolol and intra-aortic balloon pumping following coronary artery occlusion. J Thorac Cardiovasc Surg 72:892–899, 1976.
46. Raina S, Banka VS, Ramanathan K, Bodenheimer MM, Helfant RH: Beneficial effects of propranolol and digitalis on contraction and S-T segment elevation after acute coronary occlusion. Am J Cardiol 42:226–233, 1978.
47. Miura M, Thomas R, Ganz W, Sokol T, Shell WE, Toshimitsu T, Kwan AC, Singh BN: The effect of delay in propranolol administration on reduction of myocardial infarct size after experimental coronary artery occlusion in dogs. Circulation 59:1148–1157, 1979.
48. Rasmussen MM, Reimer KA, Kloner RA, Jennings RB: Infarct size reduction by propranolol before and after coronary ligation in dogs. Circulation 56:794–798, 1977.
49. Kloner RA, Fishbein MC, Cotran RS, Braunwald E, Maroko PR: The effect of propranolol on microvascular injury in acute myocardial ischemia. Circulation 55:872–880, 1977.
50. Jesmok GJ, Gross GJ, Hardman HF: Effect of propranolol and nitroglycerin plus methoxamine on transmural creatinine kinase activity after acute coronary occlusion. Am J Cardiol 42:769–773, 1978.
51. Peter T, Heng MK, Singh BN, Ambler P, Nisbet H, Elliot R, Norris RM: Failure of high doses of propranolol to reduce experimental myocardial ischemic damage. Circulation 57:534–540, 1978.
52. Reimer KA, Jennings RB: The 'wavefront phenomenon' of myocardial ischemic cell death: II. Transmural progression of necrosis within the framework of ischemic bed size (myocardium at risk) and collateral flow. Lab Invest 40:633, 1979.
53. Becker LC, Fortuin NJ, Pitt B: Effect of ischemia and antianginal drugs on the distribution of radioactive microspheres in the canine left ventricle. Circ Res 28:263–269, 1971.
54. Kloner RA, Reimer KA, Jennings RB: Distribution of coronary collateral flow in acute myocardial ischaemic injury: effect of propranolol. Cardiovasc Res 10:81–90, 1976.
55. Thomas M: The effect of beta-blockade on ST segment elevation after actue myocardial infarction in man with some experimental observations. Acta Med Scand [Suppl] 587:185–188, 1976.
56. Buck JD, Gross GJ, Warltier DC, Jolly SR, Hardman HF: Comparative effects of cardioselective versus noncardioselective beta blockade on subendocardial blood flow and contractile function in ischemic myocardium. Am J Cardiol 44:657–663, 1979.
57. Gross GJ, Winbury MM: Beta adrenergic blockade on intramyocardial distribution of coronary blood flow. J Pharmacol Exp Ther 187:451–464, 1973.
58. Vatner SF, Baig H, Manders WT, Ochs H, Pagani M: Effects of propranolol on regional myocardial function, electrograms, and blood flow in conscious dogs with myocardial ischemia. J Clin Invest 60:353–360, 1977.

413

59. Lucchesi BR, Burmeister WE, Lomas TE, Abrams GD: Ischemic changes in the canine heart as affected by the dimethyl quaternary analog of propranolol, UM-272 (SC-27761). J Pharmacol Exp Ther 199:310–328, 1976.
60. Ku DD, Lucchesi BR: Effects of dimethyl propranolol (UMO-272; SC-27761) on myocardial ischemic injury in the canine heart after temporary coronary artery occlusion. Circulation 57:541–548, 1978.
61. Kniffen FJ, Lomas TE, Burmeister WE, Lucchesi BR: Effects of dimethyl quaternary propranolol (UM-272) on oxygen consumption and ischemic ST segment changes in the canine heart. J Pharmacol Exp Ther 194:234–243, 1975.
62. Sloman G, Hunt D, Ross D: Propranolol in patients with acute myocardial infarction at the Royal Melbourne Hospital from 1965: a review. Postgrad Med J [Suppl 4] 52:150–152, 1976.
63. Snow PJ: Treatment of acute myocardial infarction with propranolol. Am J Cardiol 18:458–459, 1966.
64. Stephen SA: Propranolol in acute myocardial infarction. A multicentre trial. Lancet 2:1435–1438, 1966.
65. Norris RM, Caughey DE, Scott PJ: Trial of propranolol in acute myocardial infarction. Br Med J 2:398–400, 1968.
66. Waagstein F, Hjalmarson AC, Wasir HS: Apex cardiogram and systolic time intervals in acute myocardial infarction and effects of practolol. Br Heart J 36:1109–1121, 1974.
67. Waagstein F, Hjalmarson AC: Double-blind study of the effect of cardioselective beta-blockade on chest pain in acute myocardial infarction. Acta Med Scand [Suppl] 587:201–207, 1976.
68. Gold HK, Leinbach RC, Maroko PR: Propranolol-induced reduction of signs of ischemic injury during acute myocardial infarction. Am J Cardiol 38:689–695, 1976.
69. Reid DS, Pelides LJ, Shillingford JP, Thomas M: Electrocardiographic surface mapping of the heart following myocardial infarction and the influence of beta-blockade. Postgrad Med J [Suppl 4] 52:135–139, 1976.
70. Jugdutt BI, Lee SJ: Intravenous therapy with propranolol in acute myocardial infarction: effects on changes in the S-T segment and hemodynamics. Chest 74:514–521, 1978.
71. Heikkilä J, Nieminen MS: Rapid monitoring of regional myocardial ischaemia with echocardiography and ST segment shifts in man. Modification of 'infarct size' and hemodynamics by dopamine and beta blockade. Acta Med Scand [Suppl] 623:71–95, 1978.
72. Peter T, Norris RM, Clarke ED, Heng MK, Singh BN, Williams B, Howell DR, Ambler PK: Reduction of enzyme levels by propranolol after acute myocardial infarction. Circulation 57:1091–1095, 1978.
73. Norris RM, Clarke ED, Sammel NL, Smith WM, Williams B: Protective effect of propranolol in threatened myocardial infarction. Lancet 2:907–910, 1978.
74. Mueller HS, Ayres SM, Religa A, Evans RG: Propranolol in the treatment of acute myocardial infarction: effect on myocardial oxygenation and hemodynamics. Circulation 49:1078–1087, 1974.
75. Mueller H, Ayres SM: Propranolol in acute myocardial infarction in man: effects on haemodynamics and myocardial oxygenation. Postgrad Med J [Suppl 4] 52:141–148, 1976.
76. Bloch A, Beller GA, DeSanctis RW: Chronic propanolol administration and acute myocardial infarction. Am Heart J 92:121–123, 1976.

77. Narimatsu A, Taira N: Effects of atrio-ventricular conduction of calcium-antagonistic coronary vasodilators, local anaesthetics and quinidine injected into the posterior and the anterior septal artery of the atrio-ventricular node preparation of the dog. Arch Pharmacol 294:169–177, 1976.
78. Atterhög JH, Eklund LG, Melin AL: Effects of nifedipine on exercise tolerance in patients with angina pectoris. Eur J Clin Pharmacol 8:125, 1975.
79. Fagher B, Persson S, Svensson SE: Double-blind comparison of verapamil and practolol in the treatment of angina pectoris. Postgrad Med J 55: 61,1977.
80. Hosoda S, Kimura E: Efficacy of nifedipine in the variant form of angina pectoris. In: Jatene AD, Lichtlen PR (eds) New therapy of ischemic heart disease, 3rd Int Adaiat Symp, Proc. Amsterdam: Excerpta Medica (New York: Elsevier/North-Holland), 1976, p 195.
81. Livesley B, Catley PF, Campbell RC, Oram S: Double-blind evaluation of verapamil, propranolol, and isosorbide dinitrate against a placebo in the treatment of angina pectoris. Brit Med J 1:375–378, 1973.
82. Smith HJ, Singh BN, Nisbet HD, Norris RM: Effects of verapamil on infarct size following experimental coronary occlusion. Cardiov Res 9:569–578, 1975.
83. Wende W, Bleifeld W, Meyer J, Stuhlen HW: Reduction of the size of acute, experimental myocardial infarction by Verapamil. Basic Res Cardiol 70: 198–208, 1975.
84. Reimer KA, Lowe JE, Jennings RB: Effect of the calcium antagonist verapamil on necrosis following temporary coronary artery occlusion in dogs. Circulation 55:581–587, 1977.
85. Fleckenstein A, Doring HJ, Leder O: The significance of high-energy phosphate exhaustion in the etiology of isoproterenol-induced cardiac necrosis and its prevention by iproveratril, compound D 600 or prenylamine. In: Drugs and metabolism of myocardium and striated muscle. Nancy: Symposium International, 1969, pp 11–22.
86. Nayler WG, Grau A, Slade A: A protective effect of verapamil on hypoxic heart muscle. Cardiovasc Res 10:650–662, 1976.
87. Weishaar R, Ashikawa K, Bing RJ: Effect of diltiazem, a calcium antagonist, on myocardial ischemia. Am J Cardiol 43:1137–1143, 1979.
88. Robb-Nicholson C, Currie WD, Wechsler AS: Effects of verapamil on myocardial tolerance to ischemic arrest. Comparison to potassium arrest. Circulation [Suppl] 58:I-119–124, 1978.
89. Magee PG, Flaherty JT, Bixler TJ, Glower D, Gardner TJ, Bukley BH, Gott VL: Comparison of myocardial protection with nifedipine and potassium. Circulation 60:151–157, 1979.
90. Clark RE, Ferguson TB, West PN, Shuchleib RC, Henry PD: Pharmacological preservation of the ischemic heart. Ann Thorac Surg 24:307–314, 1977.
91. Karlsberg RP, Henry PD, Ahmed SA, Sobel BE, Roberts R: Lack of protection of ischemic myocardium by verapamil in conscious dogs. Eur J Pharmacol 42:339–346, 1977.
92. Henry PD, Shuchleib R, Borda LJ, Roberts R, Williamson JR, Sobel BE: Effects of nifedipine on myocardial perfusion and ischemic injury in dogs. Circ Res 43:372–380, 1978.
93. Henry PD, Shuchleib R, Clark RE, Perez JE: Effect of nifedipine on myocardial ischemia: analysis of collateral flow, pulsatile heat and regional muscle shortening. Am J Cardiol 44:817–824, 1979.

18. INCREASING CORONARY BLOOD FLOW

LEWIS C. BECKER

Few would question the desirability of increasing blood flow to jeopardized ischemic tissues. Since an infarct is the direct result of an insufficient blood supply, it is almost self-evident that increasing flow should provide a potent means for reducing cell damage, by both increasing the supply of oxygen and metabolic substrates and enhancing the washout of toxic products of anaerobic metabolism. Complete protection should theoretically be possible if blood flow can be increased to a level compatible with cell survival before irreversible injury begins.

In this chapter, we will examine the issue of whether flow can be increased to regions of ischemic myocardium in the setting of acute myocardial infarct, and whether the increase achieved can be meaningful with respect to myocardial salvage. The first section outlines the hemodynamic determinants of collateral flow in order to provide a conceptual framework for understanding the effects of drugs and other interventions. The second section presents a detailed review of the results that have been obtained in experimental animals and humans with acute myocardial infarct using (a) mechanical methods, (b) vasodilator and other drugs, and (c) reperfusion to increase flow. The final section discusses the issue of whether sudden complete restoration of flow may be injurious in some situations and lead to extension rather than limitation of infarct.

DETERMINANTS OF COLLATERAL BLOOD FLOW

Since a number of excellent reviews have appeared on this topic [1–3], this section will deal only with the major concepts involved in collateral blood flow.

Perfusion pressure

Perfusion pressure has long been recognized as the most important determinant of flow through collateral vessels. For many years, it was considered the *only* determinant of collateral flow since resistance was thought to be fixed at a

Wagner GS (ed): Myocardial Infarction: Measurement and Intervention, pp 415–456.
© *1982 Martinus Nijhoff Publishers, The Hague/Boston/London.*

minimal level. Collaterals were viewed as passive thin-walled tubes incapable of vasomotion and vessels located within the ischemic region were considered to be maximally dilated by metabolic stimuli. As we will see, this concept is an oversimplification that has not been confirmed using newer and more sensitive methods for measuring collateral flow.

Although perfusion pressure is commonly thought of as mean aortic root pressure, there are a number of reasons why this is not accurate. Since most of the coronary blood flow occurs in diastole, mean diastolic pressure might be considered a better first approximation. However, it is unclear whether flow through collateral vessels is apportioned between diastole and systole in a fashion similar to total coronary flow [4–7]. Quite possibly the diastolic/systolic proportion varies with the transmural location of the collateral anastomoses. Intramural and subendocardial collaterals may carry flow mainly in diastole since they are subject to compressive forces during systole. Those on the epicardial surface, on the other hand, may be able to carry flow throughout the cardiac cycle. The concept of perfusion pressure implies a pressure drop between the perfusion vessel and the tissue being perfused, i.e., a pressure over and above a back pressure generated at tissue level. In actuality, the collateral circulation has three major sites for pressure gradients: (a) the arteries supplying collateral flow, i.e., between aortic root and the point of origin of collaterals, (b) the collateral channels, and (c) the ischemic bed (between epicardial vessels and tissue level).

Even with normal coronary arteries, intracoronary pressure measured at the prearteriolar level, the point of origin of most collaterals, is slightly lower than aortic root pressure. Gradients of about 5 mmHg have been measured along the course of the large epicardial arteries [8, 9], and additional pressure drops almost certainly occur in the intramural perforating vessels that feed collaterals located intramurally and subendocardially. With obstruction in the epicardial coronary arteries, pressure gradients are accentuated and effective collateral perfusion pressure may be much less than aortic root pressure. Stenoses have additional effects on collateral perfusion pressure via changes in systolic/diastolic flow patterns (relative increase in systolic component) or regional delays in pressure transmission, although these are probably of lesser importance. Thus, while collateral perfusion pressure may be thought of simply as intracoronary pressure at the origin of the collaterals, in actuality it is a more complex function that varies with the location of the collaterals (proximal versus distal in the coronary tree, superficial versus deep in the ventricular wall), the presence of coronary obstructive disease, and the proportion of coronary flow that occurs in diastole.

The pressure gradient across the collaterals represents the major force for the opening and enlargement of preexisting collateral channels. This pressure gradient, termed 'collateral driving pressure,' is the difference between perfusion pressure and intravascular pressure within the ischemic bed ('peripheral coronary pressure') [10]. Right atrial or coronary venous pressure is usually ignored, since it is less than peripheral coronary pressure. However, when right atrial pressure becomes elevated, for example with pulmonary hypertension, constrictive pericardial disease or tricuspid insufficiency, collateral flow may be inhibited. Peripheral coronary pressure is sometimes viewed as a determinant of collateral flow, but it is far more useful to think of it as a measure or index of flow [11]. When a coronary artery is abruptly occluded in the dog, small native collaterals provide the only source of perfusion of the ischemic bed; flow is reduced to about 10%–20% of normal and peripheral coronary pressure is generally about 20 mmHg [6, 11–13]. However, when the artery is slowly occluded over a period of weeks by using an ameroid constrictor, the collateral circulation enlarges, and resting flow and pressure may become equal to that in the nonischemic coronary bed [2, 14–15]. Peripheral coronary pressure may also be a function of factors other than flow, such as the vascular capacity of the ischemic bed and extravascular transmitted forces, but the importance of these is uncertain. In addition to providing an index of overall collateral flow, peripheral coronary pressure appears to represent an important determinant of the transmural distribution of flow. Lower pressures are associated with lesser total flows and disproportionately severe ischemia of the subendocardium [2, 16–18].

Vascular resistance

In a normal coronary bed, about 90% of the total vascular resistance occurs distally at the level of the arterioles, while the proximal large epicardial arteries account for only about 10% [8, 9, 19]. With coronary obstructive disease, however, the distal arterioles dilate to maintain baseline flow and proximal resistance may become the major component of total resistance. Under these circumstances, small increases in the caliber of the epicardial arteries can produce dramatic reductions in total coronary vascular resistance.

In the case of collateral flow, the major source of vascular resistance is usually the collateral vessel itself. Although collaterals are commonly thought of as passive thin-walled tubes similar to venules, Schaper has shown that native collaterals in dogs, pigs, and humans are actually anatomically similar to arterioles [3]. As they enlarge, they dilate and develop a thick muscular coat, becoming indistinguishable from small arteries [20]. Schaper has demonstrated growth of collaterals via cell replication and considers tangential wall stresses, related to transcollateral pressure gradients, to provide the stimulus for collateral enlargement [3, 21].

Figure 1 illustrates the multiple sites at which vascular resistance can

418

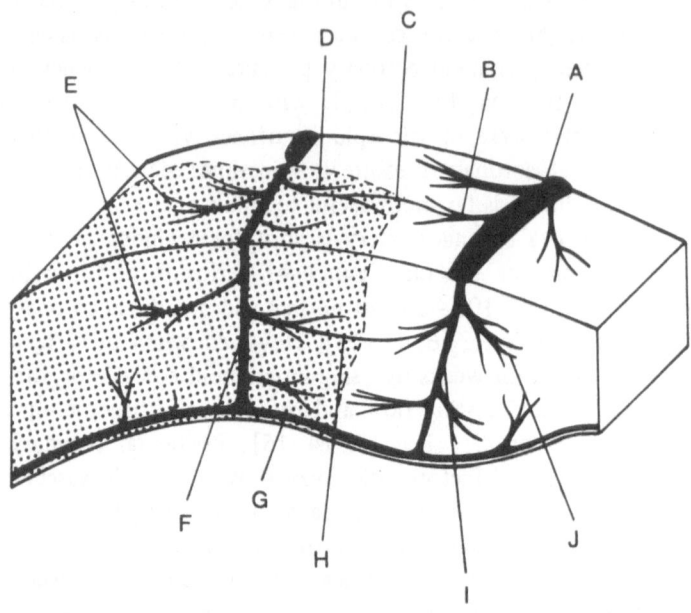

Figure 1. Collateral flow: sites of vascular resistance. Schematic cross section of left ventricular wall showing different types of vessels present in normal regions (white) and ischemic regions (dotted). Sites of vascular resistance that may influence collateral flow include large and small epicardial arteries (A, B, D), collateral vessels (C, H), intramural perforators (F, I), arterioles (E, J), and vessels in the subendocardial plexus (G).

influence the amount of collateral flow. The collateral vessels themselves, located either superficially on the epicardial surface (C) or deeper in the ventricular wall (H), provide the major source of resistance, at least in the native state. Within nonischemic areas, resistance is provided by the 'feeding' vessels, including large epicardial arteries (A) and small subepicardial (B) and intramural (I) arteries. Dilatation of these vessels by vasodilator drugs would be expected to reduce resistance and increase collateral flow, provided that perfusion pressure does not fall appreciably. A greater effect might be expected when predrug resistance in these vessels is high, as with atherosclerotic vessels. Within the ischemic area, resistance to flow is provided by small epicardial and intramural arteries (D and F, respectively). These vessels, about 200 μm in diameter, are located in the ischemic milieu, but are not believed to autoregulate. They are therefore potential candidates for dilatation with drugs. Arterioles within the ischemic region (E) are probably maximally dilated and therefore do not offer a significant source of resistance. The distribution of vascular resistances within the ischemic bed (i.e., D vs F) may influence the regional apportionment of available collateral flow, although extravascular forces are likely to be more important (see below). Arterioles in normally perfused areas (J) dilate and constrict in response to local metabolic needs. As flow changes in these beds, the pressure gradients existing along the associated epicardial arteries may be altered, thereby affecting collateral perfusion pressure. Fulton and others [22–24] have described an abundant subendocardial vascular plexus (G) in human hearts that represents the major site of intercoronary anastomoses in man. The amount of resistance supplied by these vessels and their capacity for vasomotion are unknown.

The coronary arteries possess anatomic neural connections and can be shown to change caliber in response to stimulation of sympathetic and parasympathetic nerves. Physiologic studies have shown that both α and β receptors exist in the coronary arteries, leading to constriction and dilatation, respectively [1]. Parasympathetic stimulation or infusion of acetylcholine results in dilatation of the coronary arteries, but the effects are rather minor. In intact animals, the effects of sympathomimetic agents on coronary vascular resistance are complex since there are both direct effects on coronary vascular smooth muscle and indirect effects related to changes in myocardial oxygen demands. Coronary reflexes also influence coronary vascular resistance: baroreceptor and chemoreceptor reflexes both result in cholinergically mediated coronary vasodilatation. Intercoronary reflexes, i.e., changes in resistance in one coronary artery caused by reflexes originating in an adjacent artery, were believed to be important in the 1960s but their existence has not been conclusively proven [1]. Schaper has recently shown that myelinated and nonmyelinated neural connections can be found in the collateral vessels themselves, although the physiologic role of this innervation remains obscure [3].

Extravascular resistance

During cardiac contraction, left ventricular blood flow is throttled by an increase in pressure around the intramural vessels. Greater retardation of flow has been identified in the deeper layers of the left ventricular wall and has been attributed to a vascular waterfall phenomenon with partial collapse of the downstream (venous) bed rather than kinking or pinching of arterioles [25]. It has been estimated that about 30% of overall coronary resistance is related to systolic compressive forces arising from left ventricular fiber shortening or pressure development [26].

During diastole, extravascular forces may also influence left ventricular blood flow. The perfusion pressure at which coronary flow stops has been measured to be about 20 mmHg in a number of studies [25, 27–29] and in one study pressures as high as 50 mmHg were measured [30]. The pressure associated with zero flow represents a 'back pressure' that must be subtracted from apparent perfusion pressure to obtain the effective 'pressure head' [27, 29].

Diastolic tissue pressures do not appear to be evenly distributed through the ventricular wall. Subendocardial pressures are believed to normally exceed those in the subepicardium, resulting in greater subendocardial vascular dilatation to maintain equal flow [25–29]. Further, subendocardial pressures are closely tied to left ventricular diastolic cavity pressures [29]. Under normal conditions, this is not important since intravascular perfusion pressures are much higher than tissue and cavity pressures. However, in coronary occlusive disease, distal coronary pressures may fall markedly, concomitant with an increase in left ventricular filling pressure, causing collapse of the subendocardial vessels.

It is unclear whether the conditions described above for normal myocardium also pertain to infarcting or severely ischemic regions. Diastolic forces should be at least equal to those in the rest of the heart and could even be higher because of local hemorrhage, edema and/or myofibrillar contracture. Systolic compressive forces might be expected to be low because of impaired local contractile function, but this is more than balanced by the transmission of systolic pressure to the akinetic or dyskinetic ischemic regions [31, 31]. Further, the ischemic segment may display grossly distorted systolic geometry, which could serve to greatly increase tissue pressure. Increased contraction of adjacent normal areas would be expected to exaggerate this problem.

Collateral vessels themselves may also be squeezed by systolic or diastolic extravascular forces [31, 33]. Greater effects would be expected in those species with collaterals located primarily in the subendocardium, for example, humans or pigs. In animals with predominantly epicardial collaterals, such as the dog, there should be little direct effect of tissue pressure on collateral anastomoses.

INCREASING COLLATERAL FLOW BY RAISING PERFUSION PRESSURE

Mechanical methods

Increasing perfusion pressure by mechanical means can augment collateral blood flow, with consequent reduction in the severity of ischemia. In a frequently cited study, Kattus and Gregg [6] found that retrograde flow from the distal end of a ligated circumflex coronary artery was directly related to changes in perfusion pressure produced by constriction of the descending aorta, hemorrhage, or raising and lowering a perfusion reservoir. In a similar type of study, Angell et al. [34] found that elevating coronary pressure from a reservoir led to a reduction in epicardial ST segment height and an increase in intramyocardial oxygen tension within an ischemic region.

Intraaortic counterpulsation is a clinically applicable means for mechanically raising perfusion pressure. Following coronary artery ligation in the dog, intra-aortic balloon pumping can increase flow [4, 35–36] and tissue pO_2 [37], and reduce epicardial ST segment elevation [38] in the ischemic zone for up to several hours after ligation. Shaw et al. [39] found that the increase in collateral flow was related to the extent of preexisting collateralization: when collateral flow was low before aortic pumping, the increase was very small or nonexistent, while increases were impressive when preexisting flow was high. Blood flow to areas outside the coronary ligation tends to rise if the animal is hypotensive, but in normotensive preparations, nonischemic flow does not change, or falls concordant with a reduction in myocardial oxygen demands [36]. Sugg et al. [40] using the NBT (nitro-blue tetrazolium) method, found reduced ischemic damage to myocardial tissues after 2 h of counterpulsation.

In man, the intraaortic balloon has generally been used to treat cardiogenic shock because of its ability to augment cardiac output. Mueller et al. [41] documented an improvement in total coronary blood flow related to increased mean aortic pressure, and a shift from lactate production to lactate extraction in shocked patients, while Leinbach et al. [42] found that total coronary flow was correlated with changes in overall myocardial oxygen requirements. The effect of counterpulsation on *collateral* flow was not measured in either study. Because of the invasive nature of the balloon and the lack of methods to document improved regional flow in man, there has been a reluctance to use it for the purpose of limiting infarct size in normotensive nonshocked patients. Recently, however, Leinbach et al. [43] reported results in 11 patients with acute anterior infarct less than 6 h old who were not in shock. Five of the 11 had impressive reductions in precordial ST segment elevations with less reduction subsequently in R wave voltage and good preservation of left ventricular function. The other six patients had a poor response to counterpulsation. Coronary arteriography indicated that a good response was associated with an incomplete occlusion of the left anterior descending coronary artery and a poor response with a complete occlusion. This finding suggests that increased antegrade flow through the anterior descending artery might have been a more important factor than increased collateral flow in these patients. However, the study was uncontrolled and a better outcome in the group with incomplete occlusions might have occurred without the use of aortic counterpulsation.

A limited number of studies in patients with acute myocardial infarct have utilized an external counterpulsation device in which the legs are compressed during diastole. Improved systemic hemodynamics and a reduction of both mortality rate and clinical complications have been noted [44, 45]. However, these studies did not measure effects on regional myocardial blood flow or infarct size.

Drugs to increase perfusion pressure

Sympathomimetic agents are commonly used to increase blood pressure by means of peripheral vasoconstriction, increased myocardial contractility, or both. Unlike diastolic counterpulsation, the increase in pressure is not confined to diastole and the overall cardiovascular effects may be complex. Alpha-adrenergic drugs increase systolic as well as diastolic pressure, which may impede left ventricular emptying and cause an increase in filling pressure. Reflex changes in heart rate, contractility, and coronary vascular resistance may occur as well. Beta-adrenergic agents elevate systolic pressure by increasing contractility, but diastolic pressure may fall due to peripheral dilatation; in addition, heart rate may increase significantly, reducing the diastolic time available for coronary flow.

When alpha-adrenergic agents like methoxamine are given to dogs after coronary artery occlusion, collateral flow usually increases and signs of myocardial ischemia are diminished [5, 46–49]. Beta-adrenergic agents usually have harmful effects since diastolic blood pressure falls and heart rate increases [46, 50–54]. Undoubtedly, an important factor is the level of blood pressure prior to treatment. Hypotension severe enough to limit total coronary blood flow would also limit collateral flow and should obviously be reversed. Unfortunately, the animal studies available do not specifically address the issue of whether these drugs reduce ischemic injury in shock, since they deal with well-compensated normotensive animals. An exception is the study of Watanabe et al. [55], in which the left anterior descending coronary artery was occluded after severe pharmacologic depression of the left ventricle. Elevating blood pressure with phenylephrine or aortic constriction produced an adverse rather than a beneficial effect on epicardial ST segment elevation. Myocardial oxygen demands may have increased out of proportion to collateral flow, or left ventricular dilatation may have compromised collateral function despite the increase in perfusion pressure. In either event, the results in this model may be closer to what occurs in the human infarct situation, where depression of left ventricular function is the rule, and left ventricular filling pressure is highly afterload-dependent.

What human data are available suggest that increasing blood pressure improves myocardial perfusion for infarct patients in shock [41, 56], and decreasing blood pressure is helpful for those with hypertension [57, 58]. Although no measurements of myocardial blood flow have been made in hypertensive infarct patients, systemic hemodynamics are improved with short-term phentolamine administration [57], and treatment with trimethaphan (Arfonad) diminishes the expected rise of serum creatine kinase, suggesting a limitation of infarct size [58]. It is likely that the reduction in left ventricular filling pressure that accompanies the use of these agents leads to reduced compression of subendocardial vessels, and enables improved collateral blood flow and perfusion of the subendocardium. This mechanism is less likely to be important in the dog, where collaterals are primarily epicardial in location and where only minor increases in filling pressure accompany coronary artery ligation.

VASODILATORS AND COLLATERAL FLOW

Types of vasodilators

Coronary artery dilators are commonly divided into two types: those that predominantly affect arterioles and those that primarily dilate the larger conductance vessels on the surface of the heart (Table 1). The naturally occurring

Table 1. Types of coronary artery dilators

Small vessel	Large vessel	Mixed
Adenosine*	Nitroglycerin	Verapamil
Dipyridamole	Isosorbide Dinitrate	Nifedipine
Inosine*	PGE_1^* PGI_2^*	Nitroprusside
Lidoflazine		
Carbochromen		
Papaverine		

*Naturally occurring compounds.

small-vessel dilators, such as adenosine, are believed to mediate normal autoregulatory responses. The relative potency of these different vasodilators on large and small vessels has been tested in vivo by comparing pressure gradients along the large epicardial arteries with those across the whole vascular bed [8, 9, 19]. More recently, in vivo microscopy of the epimyocardial microcirculation has been used to study responsiveness of large and small vessels [59]. Muscle strips from appropriately sized vessels have been utilized for in vitro testing [60]. The classification scheme derived from these studies agrees nicely with recent observations by Harder et al. on the membrane electrical properties of isolated large (>1 mm) and small ($<500 \mu$m) canine coronary arteries [61]. They found that calcium-dependent action potentials of vascular smooth muscle cells, induced by addition of tetraethylammonium, were preferentially blocked in small arteries by adenosine and in large arteries by nitroglycerin. Verapamil eliminated the action potentials in both-sized arteries. These results provide a mechanism for the differential effect of vasoactive agents and suggest that specific receptors may exist in different-sized vessels.

The classification of vasodilators presented in Table 1 has unquestionably provided a useful framework for thinking about these agents and interpreting experimental results. From a number of standpoints, however, this approach is overly simplistic. For example, while most of the agents predominantly affect one type of vessel, their action is not completely selective. Thus, nitroglycerin produces prolonged dilatation of large epicardial arteries, but also causes a transient reduction in small-vessel resistance [8, 9, 19] (Figure 2). Similarly,

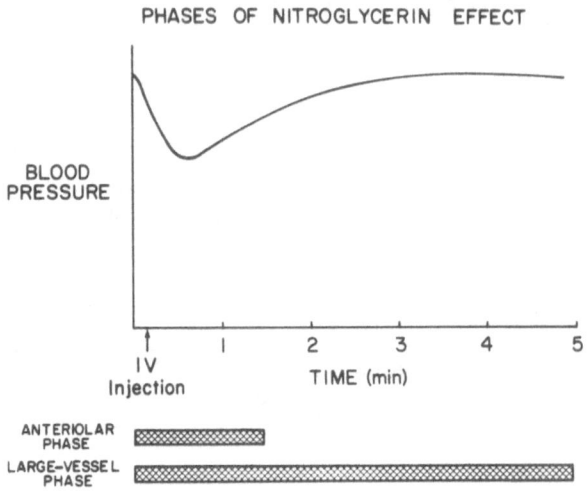

Figure 2. Depending on the time after injection, nitroglycerin may have predominant effects on either large conductive arteries or small restrictive arterioles.

adenosine can be shown to dilate large vessels during maximal vasodilation induced by low-flow coronary perfusion in the dog. [19]. Second, the response to an agent depends importantly on its mode of administration. Nitroglycerin given by i.v. bolus injection causes a transient dilatation of small vessels (1–2 min) and longer-lasting dilatation of large vessels (10–15 min) (Figure 2). As a prolonged i.v. infusion, nitroglycerin produces large vessel changes without a decrease in arteriolar resistance. With intracoronary injection, small-vessel effects tend to predominate, depending on the dose and rapidity of injection. Third, the effects of vasoactive agents may be time-dependent. Cohen and Kirk have demonstrated tachyphylaxis of *small* vessels to both nitroglycerin and angiotensin, but no waning of *large*-vessel effects with prolonged infusion of either drug [19]. Finally, since there is obviously a continuum between 'large' vessels and 'small' vessels, it is unclear where one effect stops and the other begins.

Vasodilators may also be classified by their selectivity for coronary vessels. Antihypertensive agents like hydralazine and minoxidil are potent dilators of systemic arterioles, but have only modest effects on coronary arteries [1].

In contrast, drugs like dipyridamole can increase coronary blood flow several-fold with only small changes in systemic resistance [62]. When given in small doses, nitroglycerin can be shown to increase left anterior descending and circumflex artery diameter by 20%–25% before any fall in blood pressure occurs. With higher doses there is little additional coronary effect, but increasing systemic effects occur [63].

Rationale for vasodilator use

Although for many years vasodilators were believed to be incapable of increasing flow through native collateral vessels [6, 64], more recent studies employing sensitive radiotracer techniques have conclusively shown that they can. Controversy continues, however, over the functional significance of the increases and the precise experimental conditions required. Although the literature appears to contain a number of discrepancies in this area, most of the problems can be resolved by a careful reading of the experimental details and an appropriate application of physiologic principles.

Vasodilators appear to increase collateral blood flow by two nonmutually exclusive mechanisms: (a) direct dilatation of appropriate coronary vessels leading to reduced vascular resistance to flow, and (b) indirect reduction in extravascular compressive forces due to dilatation of systemic arteries and veins. Which of the two mechanisms predominates undoubtedly depends on the experimental conditions existing at the time of drug administration and the specific agent employed.

As indicated in Figure 1, there are several potential locations for direct vasodilator action on the collateral circulation. These include (a) the collateral vessels themselves, (b) the small arteries located in nonischemic beds that 'feed' the collaterals, and (c) the small arteries in the ischemic bed that do not participate in autoregulation. In their native state, each of these vessels is believed to behave more like a conductance-type artery than a resistive arteriole although the distribution of specific receptors in these vessels has not been investigated. If this concept is correct, the dilators listed in Table 1 as predominantly large vessel or mixed in type should be better suited for increasing collateral flow. The small-vessel agents would be expected to dilate arterioles throughout the heart, but since those within the ischemic area are already more or less maximally dilated, the ones in nonischemic areas would be affected to a much greater extent. The latter are not directly in the collateral circulation pathway, and no beneficial effect on collateral flow would therefore be anticipated. As will be discussed below, dilatation of these vessels might actually produce an adverse effect by redistributing flow away from the ischemic region ('coronary steal').

The scarcity of smooth muscle fibers in native collaterals suggests that they possess only a limited degree of responsiveness to vasodilators. In contrast, transformed collaterals, developing in response to chronic ischemia, acquire a thick muscular coat and are morphologically indistinguishable from small arteries. Although the physiologic properties of chronic collaterals have not been well investigated, it is likely that these vessels exhibit a much greater direct response to large-vessel-dilator drugs [65–67].

In addition to increasing flow through collateral anastomoses, a large-vessel or mixed-type dilator could theoretically increase antegrade flow by dilating the epicardial artery responsible for the ischemic process. This is obviously not possible in an experimental animal with a ligated coronary artery, but may be important in humans, where angiography in the acute phase of infarct has demonstrated in at least some patients incomplete coronary occlusions and/or coronary spasm that can be reversed by nitroglycerin [68]. Small-vessel agents would not be expected to be effective for this purpose.

The indirect effects of vasodilators on the coronary collateral circulation stem from their action on systemic vessels. Dilatation of systemic arterioles, especially in the setting of hypertension, results in reduced afterload, better left ventricular emptying, and decreased left ventricular diastolic pressure. This in turn leads to reduced extravascular compression of subendocardial vessels, which may be of particular importance in human beings, since the subendocardium represents the major site for collateral anastomoses in man. Vasodilators can also reduce left ventricular diastolic pressure by dilatation of systemic veins, with consequent redistribution of blood volume and reduction in left ventricular filling pressure. Subendocardial perfusion in the ischemic zone might be expected to be preferentially improved by these 'extravascular' vasodilator effects. Direct vascular effects, on the other hand, might produce more complex changes in transmural flow distribution, depending on their effects on intramural vessels at various depths and the predominant location of the collaterals in the species being studied.

ACTION OF SPECIFIC VASODILATORS

Nitroglycerin

Most experimental work on nitroglycerin and collateral flow has been done in normal dogs with a single ligated coronary artery. The results have been quite conflicting, some studies showing an increase in collateral flow with nitroglycerin [48, 62, 67, 69–75], and other showing no change [6, 62, 64, 76–78]. Table 2 summarizes the methods and results of a number of these studies, in which a wide variety of techniques were used to measure flow, and

Table 2. Effect of nitrates on collateral flow and resistance (CCR)[a]

References	Method[b]	Subject[c]	Dose/route[d]	Collateral Flow[e]	CCR[e]
Wiggers and Green, 1936 [64]	BF	D, A	NaNO$_2$, i.v.	NC	D
Kattus and Gregg, 1959 [6]	BF	D, A	TNG, 0.06 mg/min, i.c.	NC	NC
Leighninger et al., 1959 [69]	BF	D, A	TNG, 0.6 mg, i.v.	I 20%	D
Fam and McGregor, 1964 [79]	BF	D, A	TNG, 0.6–0.9 mg, i.v./SL	D 16%	D
Linder and Seeman, 1967 [80]	i.c. ^{85}Kr	D, A	TNG, 0.02–0.3 mg/kg, i.v./i.c.	D 20%	D
Pasyk et al., 1971 [76]	i.c. ^{133}Xe	D, C	TNG, 0.03–0.06 mg, i.c.	NC	?
Mathes and Rival, 1971 [70]	^{86}Rb	D, A	TNG, 0.05 mg/kg, i.v.	I 25%	D
Horwitz et al., 1971 [71]	depot ^{133}Xe	M, A	TNG, 0.4 mg, SL	I 25%	D
Weisse et al., 1972 [72]	i.c. ^{85}Kr	D, A	ISD, 0.013 mg/kg/min, i.v.	I 53%	D
Goldstein et al., 1974 [77]	BF	M, A	TNG, 0.1 mg/min, i.a.	NC	D
Becker, 1976 [62]	MS	D, A	TNG, 0.4 mg, i.v., after 30 s	I 20%	D
			TNG, 0.4 mg, i.v., after 5 min	NC	D
			TNG, 0.2 mg/min, i.v.		
Chiariello et al., 1976 [73]	MS	D, A	TNG, 0.3 mg + 0.005 mg/kg/min, i.v.	I 23%	D
Capurro et al., 1976 [67]	BF	D, A f	TNG, 0.0003–0.1 mg/min, i.c.	I > 100%	D
Capurro et al., 1977 [74]	MS	D, S	TNG, 0.2–0.4 mg/min, i.v., with methoxamine	I 130%	D
Most et al., 1978 [78]	MS	P, A	TNG, 0.006–0.038 mg/kg/min, i.v.	NC	D
Bache, 1978 [48]	MS	D, C	TNG, 0.4 mg + 0.015 mg/kg/min, i.v.	I 44%	D
Jugdutt et al., 1981 [75]	MS	D, C	TNG, 0.004–0.010 mg/kg/min, i.v.	I > 100%	D

[a]Values for CCR not explicitly given in references were estimated from available arterial pressure and collateral flow data.

[b]BF, backflow; i.c., intracoronary; H, heat clearance; MS, microspheres.

[c]D, dog; M, man; P, pig; A, anesthetized; C, conscious; S, sedated.

[d]TNG, nitroglycerin; ISD, Isosorbide dinitrate; SL, sublingual; i.a., intraaortic; i.v., intravenous.

[e]NC, no change; I, increase; D, decrease.

[f]Chronic collaterals, blood pressure held constant.

Adapted from Becker, *Journal of Clinical Investigation* 58:1287–1296 1976 [62].

a number of different nitroglycerin doses and routes of administration were employed, leading to different degrees of systemic hypotension. A consistent finding, however, has been that nitroglycerin reduces collateral resistance, calculated from mean arterial pressure and collateral flow. In other words, although nitroglycerin causes the blood pressure to fall, collateral flow does not fall proportionately. When collateral resistance declines more than systemic pressure, the amount of collateral flow increases, but when the fall in pressure is excessive, collateral flow decreases.

A number of studies have examined whether nitroglycerin can improve indices of myocardial ischemia, such as epicardial ST segment elevation or regional left ventricular function (see Gold, p. 506). As with flow, the results have been divergent, with some studies showing improvement [47, 62, 66, 73, 81–86], some showing worsening [62, 78], and some showing no change [62, 66, 83, 87–89]. Interpretation of these results must take into account not only measured or assumed changes in collateral flow, but also any changes in myocardial oxygen demands that might have occurred through direct or reflex actions of the drug. Thus, reflex tachycardia, more prominent in studies using larger doses of nitroglycerin or bolus injections over short periods of time, is associated with signs of worsening ischemia [62, 78, 82, 90]. Other studies, using slower infusion rates or allowing several minutes to elapse after a bolus injection, report little tachycardia and generally a beneficial effect on ischemia. Similarly, most human studies show a reduction in ST segment elevation with nitroglycerin, although certain patients exhibiting a precipitous fall in blood pressure and associated reflex tachycardia may have adverse electrocardiographic effects [73, 91–93]. The effects of nitroglycerin on regional ventricular function in man are even more complex, since they depend on changes in loading conditions and shape in addition to changes in collateral flow and regional oxygen demands [86, 94]. An ischemic region may exhibit improved wall motion if systolic load is reduced, even if the severity of ischemia is unchanged.

Based on the reasoning that nitroglycerin's effect on collateral flow represents a balance between decreasing blood pressure and decreasing collateral resistance, a number of studies have utilized alpha-adrenergic agents with nitroglycerin to reverse the latter's systemic effects and prevent a fall in blood pressure. This approach has been very successful in canine studies using well-compensated animals. Addition of methoxamine or phenylephrine has either reversed an adverse effect [62] or augmented a beneficial effect of nitroglycerin alone [47, 48, 82]. However, addition of phenylephrine failed to produce any net benefit in pigs after coronary artery ligation [78]. In man the results are controversial. Borer et al. [93] demonstrated further reduction in ST segment elevation when phenylephrine was added to nitroglycerin in patients with acute anterior infarct. Come et al. [92], however, found that phenylephrine eliminated the beneficial hemodynamic effects of nitroglycerin as well as the reduction in ST segment elevations. The apparent discrepancy in these results is best explained by differing methods of nitroglycerin administration. Borer used sublingual tablets, while Come used a slow intravenous infusion. The tablets more often caused excessive hypotension and reflex tachycardia, reversal of which by the alpha-agonist was beneficial. In the absence of these side effects, phenylephrine increased afterload and left ventricular filling pressure, thereby increasing oxygen demands and possibly causing reduced subendocardial collateral flow. The experimental results in the pig may be explained in a similar way and may be more analogous to human infarct that the dog studies.

An important question to be asked is whether the increase in collateral flow produced by nitroglycerin is sufficient to result in long-term myocardial salvage. Most studies have shown a maximum increase in flow of 20%–50% with nitroglycerin. In absolute terms, this increase is sizable in regions with moderate flow, but very small in ischemic central core regions. Evidence suggests that salvage occurs if flow can be increased to about 50% of normal before the onset of irreversible necrosis [95–99]. Thus, when flow is only moderately reduced, i.e., to 25%–50% of normal, nitroglycerin may produce striking long-term salvage since flow can be brought above the '50% threshold' necessary for survival. However, when large areas of very low flow exist, the results may be disappointing, and salvage may be seen only at the higher flow lateral edges and subepicardial areas [75, 100, 101]. Although there have been few studies of the long-term effect of nitroglycerin in myocardial ischemia, there is little question that nitroglycerin can produce significant long-term salvage in the dog [75, 81]. We have recently completed a study in which a 6-h infusion

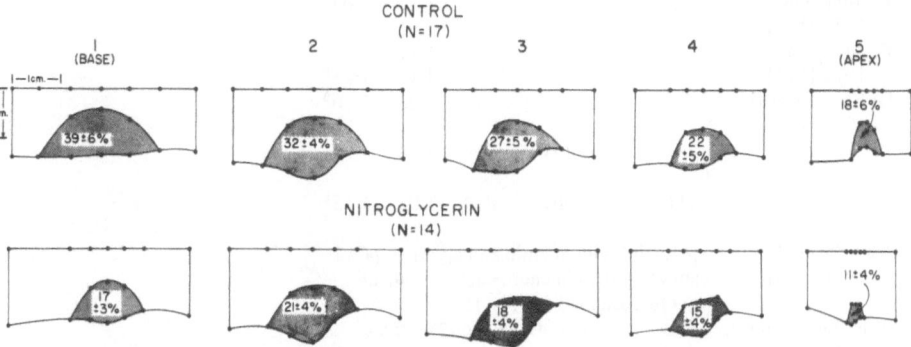

Figure 3. Effect of nitroglycerin on infarct size in conscious dogs. Diagrams represent scaled maps of average occluded coronary bed (white box) and infarct (stippled), for each ring (*1–5*) in control and treatment groups. Numbers indicate percent of occluded bed infarcted in that ring (mean ± SEM). Infarcts in nitroglycerin-treated dogs are clearly smaller – less wide, and less transmural – in all rings. Adapted from Jugdutt et al., *Circulation* 63:17–28, 1981 [75].

430

Table 3. Nitroglycerin and transmural flow distribution

References	Flow in nonischemic region			Flow in ischemic region	
	Endo	Epi	Endo/Epi	Endo	Epi
Becker et al., 1971 [13]			$1.05 \to 1.16^a$		
Bache et al., 1975 [104]				$74 \to 82^a$	$79 \to 64^a$
	$85 \to 87$	$68 \to 67$	$1.25 \to 1.30$	$13 \to 18$	$15 \to 19$
Becker, 1976 [62]	$93 \to 85$	$84 \to 81$	$1.11 \to 1.05$	$11 \to 10$	$21 \to 18$
	$93 \to 102$	$84 \to 92$	$1.11 \to 1.11$	$11 \to 13^a$	$21 \to 26^a$
	$70 \to 109^a$	$63 \to 86^a$	$1.11 \to 1.27$	$10 \to 12$	$20 \to 19$
	$70 \to 75$	$63 \to 71$	$1.11 \to 1.06$	$10 \to 12$	$10 \to 24^a$
Chiariello et al., 1976 [73]	$90 \to 89$	$85 \to 82$	$1.01 \to 1.02$	$27 \to 34^a$	$34 \to 44^a$
Capurro et al., 1977 [74]			$1.37 \to 1.37$	$7\% \to 21\%^{ab}$	$32\% \to 50\%^{ab}$
Bache, 1978 [48]		$123 \to 96^a$	$1.33 \to 1.38$	$9 \to 13^a$	
		$123 \to 157^a$	$1.33 \to 1.48$	$9 \to 19^a$	
Most, 1978 [78]	$156 \to 145$	$140 \to 136$	$1.13 \to 1.07$	$3 \to 2$	$2 \to 2$
	$156 \to 172$	$140 \to 154$	$1.13 \to 1.11$	$3 \to 2$	$2 \to 2$
Becker et al., 1969 [107]					
Forman and Kirk, 1973 [108]					
Mathes and Rival, 1971 [70]			$1.09 \to 1.06$		
Nakamura et al., 1973 [109]	NC	NC	$1.01 \to 1.07$	NC	NC
Fortuin et al., 1971 [110]			$1.12 \to 1.04$		
Paradise et al., 1976 [111]			$1.11 \to 1.13$		
			$1.11 \to 1.48^a$		
Gross and Warltier, 1977 [112]			$1.23 \to 1.10^a$		
		$93 \to 121^a$	$1.28 \to 1.25$		
	$111 \to 92$	$105 \to 81^a$	$1.05 \to 1.15^a$		
Winbury et al., 1971 [113]	$pO_2 \downarrow$ initially in endo and epi; then $pO_2 \uparrow$ above control in endo, back to control in epi; sustained for 12–15 min				
Weiss and Winbury, [114]	Endo $pO_2 \uparrow$, epi pO_2 NC, for 31–158 s post injection				

Flows in ml/min/100 g; Endo, subendocardium; Epi, subepicardium; NC, no change; D, dog; P, pig; IDH, isolated dog heart; A, anesthetized; C, conscious; BP, blood pressure; i.c., intracoronary; i.v., intravenous; RH, reactive hyperemia; [a] significant difference (p 0.05); [b] flows as percent of nonischemic region.

Endo/Epi	Subject	Coronary occlusion	Dose, route, timing of flow measurement
0.84 → 1.01[a]	D, A	30 s	5 min after 0.4 mg i.v. bolus
0.94 → 1.28[a]	D, C	Stenosis during RH	5 min after 0.015 mg/kg i.v. bolus
0.87 → 0.95	D, C	60 s	5 min after 0.015 mg/kg i.v. bolus
0.52 → 0.56	D, A	1 h	0.4 mg i.v. bolus, then 0.2 mg/min infusion
0.52 → 0.50	D, A	1 h	as above, plus methoxamine to support BP
0.50 → 0.63	D, A	1 h	0.4 mg i.v. bolus, during max hypotension
0.50 → 0.50	D, A	1 h	5 min after 0.4 mg i.v. bolus
0.57 → 0.69[a]	D, A	30 min	0.3 mg i.v. bolus, then 0.005 mg/kg/min infusion
0.29 → 0.5[a]	D, C	70 min	0.2–0.4 mg/min i.v. infusion plus methoxamine to maintain BP
0.29 → 0.47[a]	D, C	6.5 min	5 min after 0.4 mg i.v. bolus plus 0.015 mg/kg/min infusion
0.29 → 0.33	D, C	6.5 min	during 0.015 mg/kg/min infusion plus phenylephrine to increase BP 60 mm above control
1.23 → 1.00	P, A	Perm	during 0.006–0.038 mg/kg/min i.v. infusion (systolic BP down 20–30 mm)
1.23 → 1.04	P, A	Perm	during above infusion plus phenylephrine (0.02–1.0 µg/kg/min) to restore BP
1.21 → 1.38[a]	D, C	Ameroid occl (No infarct)	5 min after 0.4 mg i.v. bolus
0.82 → 0.62[a]	D, A	Stenosis	0.18 mg i.v. bolus, during max hypotension
1.07 → 0.68[a]	D, A	Stenosis	0.012 mg bolus i.c.
0.89 → 1.07[a]	D, A	Stenosis	during norepi plus 0.005 mg/kg i.v. bolus (max hypotension)
	D, A	None	0.005 mg/kg i.v. bolus, during max hypotension
0.67 → 0.86[a]	D, A	Stenosis	0.003 mg/kg/min i.v. infusion
	D, A	None	0.4 mg i.v. bolus, during max hypotension
	D, A	None	0.4 mg i.v. bolus, during max hypotension
	D, A	None	0.4 mg i.v. bolus with Ao const. to restore BP
	IDH	None	0.010 mg/min i.c. infusion during constant coronary flow
	IDH	None	0.010 mg/min i.c. infusion during constant coronary perfusion pressure
	D, A	None	5 min after end of 2 min infusion i.v. of 0.01 mg/kg/min
	D, A	None	0.005–0.02 mg/kg i.v. over 1 min
	D, A	None	0.002–0.006 mg i.c. bolus

of nitroglycerin produced a 50% reduction in infarct size and a large increase in collateral flow in the conscious dog [75, 102] (Figure 3). Nitroglycerin was begun 5 min after coronary occlusion in a dose sufficient to decrease mean arterial pressure by 10%, and no reflex tachycardia occurred. Another recent study in the conscious dog by Fukuyama and Roberts failed to find a benefit from nitroglycerin [103]. However, no increase in collateral flow occurred in their study, apparently due to an excessive decrease in blood pressure. Myocardial salvage would therefore not have been expected.

Nitroglycerin has been said to produce a disproportionate improvement in subendocardial compared with subepicardial collateral flow [9, 13, 104–106]. An examination of the literature, however, is confusing because of the number of different preparations and methods of nitroglycerin administration (Table 3). For example, Becker et al. found an increase in subendocardial flow relative to subepicardial flow in areas of transient ischemia 5 min after an intravenous bolus injection of nitroglycerin [13]. Bache et al. similarly found a relative increase in subendocardial flow 5 min after intravenous nitroglycerin during reflow through a partial stenosis [104]. On the other hand, more straight-forward preparations involving simple coronary ligation have given mixed results [48, 62, 73, 74, 78]. The changes observed in transmural flow distribution appear to depend on a complex interaction of factors. Factors favoring an increase in subendocardial flow are: (a) dilatation of intramural perforating arteries, (b) decreased tissue pressure in the subendocardium during diastole, due to diminished left ventricular filling, and (c) decreased subendocardial systolic pressure related to reduced afterload. Factors adversely affecting subendocardial flow are: (a) decreased blood pressure, which is critical for subendocardial perfusion, and (b) reduced diastolic time per minute related to reflex tachycardia. In addition, arteriolar effects of nitroglycerin could be responsible for a subendocardial-to-subepicardial 'steal' of blood flow [112]. Since subendocardial arterioles are normally more dilated, dilatation of overlying epicardial vessels may cause a redistribution of flow, especially if the total flow available is fixed. This probably explains the results of Forman et al., who found reduced subendocardial flow distal to a coronary stenosis after intracoronary nitroglycerin [108].

Dipyridamole

Dipyridamole (Persantine) is a small-vessel-type dilator that is believed to act by reducing the cellular uptake of adenosine, thereby inhibiting its metabolic degradation by adenosine deaminase, and increasing the concentration of adenosine at active vascular receptor sites. Although the drug has been popular for several years in Europe and South America for treating myocardial ischemia, it has not gained the universal acceptance of nitroglycerin. In fact, in experimental studies dipyridamole has frequently been used as a contrast to nitroglycerin [8, 9, 62, 79, 80, 113, 114].

Unlike nitroglycerin, which causes a small transient increase in coronary blood flow, dipyridamole produces a marked and prolonged increase in flow. Although considerable variability is found from animal to animal, increases of three- to fourfold are common. Following ligation of a single coronary artery in dogs, dipyridamole is found to increase flow to nonischemic regions, but have inconsistent effects on collateral flow to ischemic tissue. Table 4 lists some of

Table 4. Effect of dipyridamole on collateral flow and resistance

References	Method	Subject	Dose/route	Collateral flow	CCR
Kiese et al., 1960 [115]	H	D, A	0.4 mg/kg/min, i.v.	I 30%	D
Fam and McGregor, 1964 [79]	BF	D, A	5–10 mg, i.v.	D	NC
Linder and Seeman, 1967 [80]	i.c. ^{85}Kr	D, A	0.25–1.5 mg/kg, i.v./i.c.	I 30%	D
Rees and Redding, 1967 [116]	i.c. ^{133}Xe	D, A	0.5 mg/kg, i.v.	I[a]	D[a]
Pasyk et al., 1971 [76]	i.c. ^{133}Xe	D, C	0.5–1.0 mg, i.c., 3–5 mg, i.v.	NC	?
Grayson et al., 1971 [117]	H	D, A	0.25 mg/kg, i.v.	I	D
Cibulski et al., 1972 [118]	i.c. ^{85}Kr	D, A	0.5 mg/kg, i.v.	I 90%[b]	D[b]
Becker, 1976 [62]	MS	D, A	1 mg/kg, i.v.	NC	NC
			1 mg/kg, i.v., plus methoxamine to restore BP	I 72%	D

Values for CCR not explicitly given in references were estimated from available arterial pressure and collateral flow data. Abbreviations: see Table 3; H, heart clearance; [a]changes seen from 24 h to 10 days after coronary artery ligation but not at 2 h; [b]changes seen in animals with chronic but not acute ischemia. Adapted from Becker, *Journal of Clinical Investigation* 58:1287–1296, 1976 [62].

the studies available in this area. Despite the different methods and preparations used, there appears to be a fairly consistent reduction in coronary collateral resistance, similar to that seen with nitroglycerin (Table 2). The change in collateral flow that occurs reflects a balance between the decrease in blood pressure and the diminution in collateral resistance.

What is the mechanism of this reduction in resistance if dipyridamole is purely a small-vessel dilator? The answer is probably that dipyridamole is not completely selective. A number of studies have shown that dipyridamole has a direct dilatory action on large arteries as well as small ones, although the small-vessel effect is clearly predominant [8, 9, 19, 119, 120]. A direct coronary vascular effect is also suggested by the finding that dipyridamole has a greater effect on well-developed collaterals than on small native collaterals [65]. Indirect effects are unlikely since the drug produces minimal changes in left ventricular filling pressure and heart rate [62].

Inconsistent effects have been found on endocardial/eipcardial flow distribution with dipyridamole. In areas dependent on collateral perfusion, relative subendocardial flow has been found to increase [62], decrease [121], or not change [113]. There is probably a complex interaction of factors similar to that described for nitroglycerin. In the setting of a partial coronary stenosis, however, the effects of dipyridamole are striking and predictable. The velocity of flow across the stenosis increases as a result of downstream arteriolar dilatation. This, in turn, leads to marked accentuation of the pressure gradient due to increased turbulence at the stenosis exit [120]. The resulting fall in distal coronary pressure produces relative or absolute subendocardial ischemia [121, 122]. A similar effect is seen with other small-vessel-dilating drugs [123, 124] or with other interventions that produce downstream vascular dilatation, such as atrial pacing [7, 125].

Dipyridamole has been said to produce a 'coronary steal' by diverting flow from collateralized areas toward nonischemic regions. This is viewed as arising from its small-vessel-dilating properties and is considered an important limitation to its clinical use. Animal studies have suggested that 'steal' is a real phenomenon, and have helped to clarify the mechanisms involved [122–124, 126, 127] (Figure 4). Coronary steal appears to be caused by a fall in coronary pressure at the point of origin of the collateral vessels. This pressure most closely represents collateral perfusion pressure and is a direct determinant of collateral flow. When the upstream vessel is normal, pressure at this point is similar to aortic root pressure; even a large increase in flow does not cause an appreciable pressure gradient or reduction in distal coronary pressure. However, when a stenosis is interposed, dipyridamole produces a marked reduction of downstream pressure [122]. This in turn leads to a reduction in collateral flow and subendocardial ischemia in the region perfused by the stenotic vessel (Figure 4). Under certain conditions, steal may occur without a stenosis being present in the vessel supplying collateral flow. Schaper and colleagues used ameroid constrictors to produce chronic occlusions of the right and circumflex coronary arteries in dogs. Because of the gradual nature of the occlusions, no infarct occurred and the anterior descending artery became the source of blood flow for the entire left ventricle. In this setting, carbochromen and lidoflazine, drugs similar in action to dipyridamole, caused a coronary steal in the distribution of the occluded circumflex artery, evidently due to the development of a significant pressure gradient along the patent anterior descending vessel [123, 124].

Relatively few studies have examined the effect of dipyridamole on indices

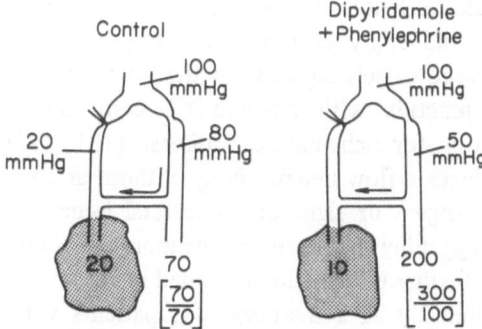

Figure 4. Schematic diagram of coronary circulation showing proposed mechanism for dipyridamole-induced coronary steal. Coronary artery divides into two branches, one completely occluded, the other stenosed but providing collaterals to the first. In the control situation on the *left*, distal pressure is low in the occluded arterial bed and there is a small gradient in mean pressure across the stenosis. Flow in the ischemic region (dotted area) is 20 ml/min/100 g and is determined by the collateral driving pressure, or the difference between distal pressures in the bed supplying collaterals (80 mmHg) and the ischemic bed (20 mmHg). Flow in the distribution of the stenoic vessel is normal at 70 ml/min/100 g and is evenly distributed between subendocardium (lower value in bracket) and subepicardium (upper value). During dipyridamole, with blood pressure maintained constant by phenylephrine, flow increases in the nonischemic bed to 200 ml/min/100 g, but becomes maldistributed between subendocardium and subepicardium. In addition, pressure distal to the stenosis falls to 50 mmHg, causing a reduction in collateral driving pressure. As a result, flow to the ischemic region decreases to 10 ml/min/100 g, interpreted as a coronary steal. From Becker, *Circulation* 57:1103–1110, 1978 [122].

of ischemia or on long-term salvage of ischemic tissue. Changes in epicardial ST segment height have been variable, although this is not surprising considering the complex interaction of factors that may exist [62, 127–128]. Recently, Roberts et al. [129] showed that 3 mg/kg dipyridamole given intravenously for 45 min to anesthetized dogs with permanent anterior descending coronary artery ligation resulted in significant limitation of infarct size. A 56% reduction in infarct mass was found at 24 h using nitro-blue tetrazolium staining to mark the irreversibly damaged tissue. Our own group has found increased collateral blood flow and striking myocardial salvage (77%) in conscious dogs treated with 6-h infusions of dipyridamole, beginning 5 min after left circumflex occlusion. The average reduction in mean arterial pressure was only 10% in our animals, indicating a significant fall in coronary collateral resistance (130). Since necrosis was not measured until 48 h post occlusion, it appears that dipyridamole actually prevented rather than delayed necrosis.

It is difficult to know, however, whether these encouraging results can be directly translated to man. Most patients with a myocardial infarct have multivessel coronary disease rather than occlusion of a single vessel. Dipyridamole would be more likely to produce steal with multivessel stenosis and could cause subendocardial ischemia in the distribution of vessels with incomplete occlusions. This would apply both to the artery responsible for the infarct as well as to diseased vessels adjacent to the infarct zone. Dipyridamole has been used in conjunction with thallium-201 perfusion imaging in patients undergoing evaluation for ischemic heart disease [131, 132]. Unlike exercise, dipyridamole produces a flow heterogeneity without an increase in myocardial oxygen demands. Angina or signs of myocardial ischemia occur in less than 10% of patients, suggesting that steal may be more a theoretical than a practical issue. In any event, further information is needed in this area before dipyridamole can be utilized clinically as a treatment for patients with acute myocardial infarct.

Slow channel calcium blockers

A class of drugs that block the cellular uptake of calcium has recently been described. These compounds, which include the agents nifedipine, verapamil, and diltiazem, have antiarrhythmic properties and variable effects on myocardial contractility (see Reimer and Jennings, p. 406). They have also been shown to dilate coronary arteries and relieve coronary spasm in patients with Prinzmetal's angina [133–135]. Experimentally, both large and small coronary vessels are affected (Table 1), and although coronary effects predominate, there is also a modest effect on systemic arteries.

The relatively limited information available suggests that these drugs have a beneficial effect on myocardial ischemia. Nifedipine, an agent with strong coronary-dilating properties but little effect on AV nodal conduction or contractility, has been shown by Henry et al. [136] to increase collateral flow and reduce ischemic necrosis in conscious dogs with left anterior descending coronary artery occlusion. Nifedipine was begun 30 min after occlusion and continued for 24 h using a constant infusion at a dose sufficient to reduce mean pressure only 5%. Flow to nonischemic myocardium also increased, in part as a response to increased heart rate and in part due to direct dilatation of coronary vessels. In experiments in anesthetized dogs, Henry et al. [137] showed that nifedipine improved myocardial segment shortening in ischemic zones. An electromagnetic flowmeter around a branch vessel in the ischemic bed recorded increased retrograde (collateral) flow after nifedipine along with reduced peripheral coronary pressure, suggesting a reduction in resistance of vessels within the ischemic bed. Other studies by the same group [138] showed reduced myocardial necrosis in isolated ischemic rabbit hearts and in dogs with 2 h of hypothermic global ischemia, indicating a direct protective effect independent of collateral blood flow. Selwyn et al. [139] showed that the benefit of nifedipine could be reversed by an excessive fall in blood pressure.

Using the [81m]Kr technique in anesthetized dogs with left anterior descending coronary artery occlusion, they showed that low-dose nifedipine (1 μg/kg over 15 min) caused a 12% decrease in blood pressure and an increase in collateral flow, while high-dose nifedipine (13 μg/kg) caused a 30% decrease in pressure and a concomitant decrease in flow. Over a 5-h period, the flow changes were associated with concordant effects on electrocardiographic R wave loss and Q wave appearance, and on creatine kinase release into the draining coronary vein.

Less information is available concerning verapamil. This drug is considered to cause greater slowing of AV nodal conduction and greater depression of myocardial function than nifedipine. Smith et al. [140] showed that verapamil reduced epicardial ST segment elevations in open-chested dogs after left anterior descending coronary artery ligation. Reimer et al. [141] demonstrated a reduction in posterior papillary muscle necrosis with verapamil treatment in dogs with 40 min of temporary circumflex artery occlusion and 2–4 days of reprefusion. Flow was not measured in either study. In another report, verapamil failed to alter infarct size in conscious dogs when it was begun 5 h after coronary occlusion [142]. More recently, Ribeiro et al. [143] have shown myocardial preservation by verapamil in anesthetized dogs with a 1-h delay in treatment.

Using diltiazem, another agent in the calcium antagonist group, Weishaar et al. [144] showed myocardial protection 1 h after coronary occlusion in anesthetized dogs. Compared with control animals, there was diminished breakdown of ATP in the ischemic region, improved glycolytic flux, increased contractility of isolated heart muscle fibers, and lowered tissue levels of lactate and free fatty acids. These effects were associated with 15% fall in blood pressure, and a significant reduction in heart rate (157 vs 127 at 30 min). Flow was not measured.

Although more work is needed with these calcium-blocking agents, including studies in patients with acute myocardial infarct, early experimental results are promising. Myocardial salvage clearly seems achievable and may occur through a number of different mechanisms, including (a) increased flow through collateral vessels, (b) increased flow by relief of coronary spasm, (c) reduction in myocardial oxygen demands, and (d) direct effects on myocardial energy utilization.

Sodium nitroprusside

Sodium nitroprusside has been widely used for left ventricular unloading in patients with impaired left ventricular function. By reducing myocardial oxygen demands and increasing cardiac output, myocardial ischemia should theoretically be ameliorated. In addition, reduction in left ventricular filling pressure should improve left ventricular subendocardial perfusion.

Two recent studies have compared the effects of nitroglycerin and nitroprusside on collateral flow in dogs. Chiariello et al. found that nitroprusside had adverse effects, including reduced flow in ischemic zones and increased ST segment elevation, while nitroglycerin gave beneficial results [73]. The drugs were given to produce an equal fall in blood pressure of about 15%. Unfortunately, all animals received nitroprusside first and nitroglycerin second rather than having the order of the drugs randomized. Capurro et al. produced gradual anterior descending coronary artery occlusion with formation of large collateral anastomoses [145]. Given by intracoronary injection, both drugs produced similar increases in retrograde flow. Intravenously, however, nitroglycerin increased retrograde flow over the entire dose range from 3 to 300 μ/min, while nitroprusside increased flow only at high doses (100–300 μg/min). Although blood pressure was held constant in these experiments, nitroprusside was observed to have greater effects on systemic resistance and therefore less selectivity for the coronary circulation. On the basis of these studies, nitroglycerin would appear to be the better drug for limiting infarct size in patients with acute myocardial infarction, although nitroprusside may be better for unloading the left ventricle and increasing cardiac output.

Prostaglandins

There has been intense interest recently in prostaglandins (PGs) and their possible protective effects on ischemic myocardium [146–148]. Certain prostaglandins act as vasodilators and are capable of reducing ischemia by increasing collateral blood flow. However, several flow-independent actions have also been identified which may be additively beneficial.

Prostaglandins are synthesized by the enzyme prostaglandin synthetase and are released locally during ischemia. Indomethacin, a nonsteroidal anti-inflammatory agent and potent inhibitor of the synthetic enzyme, has been shown in dogs to increase epicardial ST segment elevations [149] and double infarct size, without changes in collateral flow and with only minor increases in heart rate and blood pressure [150]. A related agent, ibuprofen, has been found to have opposite effects, with significant salvage found in the rat [151], cat [152–154], and anesthetized and conscious dog [143, 155], again independent of flow and myocardial oxygen demands. In addition to prostaglandin inhibition, nonflow factors such as lysozome stabilization, inhibition of leukocyte migration, and/or inhibition of platelet aggregation may be important in explaining these results. Although complete inhibition of synthesis is assumed to occur with both drugs, the precise patterns of PG release have not been examined.

Infusions of prostaglandin E_1 (PGE$_1$), an important end-product of the PG synthetic pathway, have been shown to increase collateral flow and reduce ischemic damage in cats and dogs [156–161]. We have compared PGE_1 and PGE_2 in conscious dogs after coronary artery ligation [161]. Both agents produced similar decreases in blood pressure and left atrial pressure, but the coronary effects were markedly dissimilar. Only PGE_1 increased collateral flow and reduced infarct size, suggesting that increased flow was the principal factor resulting in myocardial protection.

The pattern of flow increase with PGE_1 was similar to that seen with nitroglycerin: collateral flow was increased but flow to nonischemic areas was unchanged. Recent studies suggest that nitroglycerin in fact may work through the PG system [162]. Coincident with its hemodynamic effects, nitroglycerin causes release of PGE into coronary venous blood, while indomethacin blocks both its PGE-releasing and hemodynamic effects, systemic as well as coronary.

Prostacyclin (PGI_2) is a newly discovered prostaglandin with potent vasodilator and antiplatelet-aggregating properties manufactured by vascular endothelium. Ogletree et al. have shown in the cat that prostacyclin represents a potent myocardial salvaging agent [163]. We have similarly found that in the conscious dog 6-h infusions of prostacyclin increase collateral blood flow and reduce myocardial necrosis measured two days later [164]. These effects were produced by reducing blood pressure only 5%; with larger falls in blood pressure, no effect [165] or even adverse effects [166] on flow may occur. In our study, a few dogs demonstrated myocardial salvage with only small increases in collateral flow. This has suggested to us that direct effects, such as stabilization of lysozomes or inhibition of platelet clumping, may also be important with this agent.

Other agents

Mannitol has been shown in some, but not all, studies to protect ischemic myocardium [167–170] (see Swain, p. 483). As an osmotic agent, it reduces swelling of injured myocardial tissues and damaged capillary and arterial endothelial cells. The 'no reflow' phenomenon may thereby be averted and a late increase in collateral flow may occur via normal collateral enlargement and growth. In addition, mannitol appears to be a direct coronary vasodilator, producing increased flow to both ischemic and nonischemic zones in anesthetized dogs [167]. Hyaluronidase is another agent that experimentally produces myocardial salvage [171–175] (see Swain p. 485). Diffusion of substrates is facilitated to jeopardized tissues, but collateral blood flow may also be preserved or augmented [172].

Propranolol is believed to protect ischemic myocardium by reducing myocardial oxygen demands. In some studies, however, propranolol has increased collateral flow and/or improved subendocardial perfusion of ischemic zones, possibly through constriction of arterioles in nonischemic areas [13, 176—177].

CORONARY REPERFUSION

The most straightforward method for increasing flow to ischemic myocardium is to reestablish its blood supply. Experimentally, this usually entails removal of a constricting ligature, but in patients, emergency coronary bypass surgery or intravascular catheter dilatation is required. Although any increase in blood flow should be welcome, some studies have suggested that sudden reflow after a period of ischemia may produce local myocardial hemorrhage and infarct extension.

The effects of reflow have been the subject of numerous investigations, some of which are summarized in Table 5. Most of these studies have focused on the time course of irreversible myocardial injury following coronary occlusion; the implicit assumption is that reflow merely uncovers damage that has already occurred and does not itself cause further necrosis. Death of cells begins about 20 min after occlusion of the circumflex coronary artery in anesthetized dogs [194]. At this time, the irreversibly damaged cells appear histologically normal and even by electron microscopy show only the most subtle morphologic changes. Early studies in open-chested dogs suggested that necrosis is complete by 1—2 h, i.e., that damage at this time is equivalent to that obtained with a permanent coronary occlusion and that release of the ligature after 1—2 h does not result in myocardial salvage [194]. Most studies now indicate that infarct size can be reduced if reperfusion is accomplished by 4 h (Table 5). Quantitatively, however, reports vary widely as to how much salvage can be achieved at different times. Undoubtedly this is related to marked differences in experimental conditions and in methods for measuring necrosis. The consensus is that, at 1—2 h, 50% or more of the tissue that would have died can be saved by reperfusion [96, 189, 192]. At 3—4 h, however, reports range from 12% to 84% salvage [179, 182, 190, 192]. Most studies show no significant effect at 5—6 h, although it should be recognized that a protective effect could easily have been missed, owing to both small numbers of animals and a failure to control for the amount of myocardium rendered ischemic (as well as the intensity of ischemia). The amount of damage that occurs over time appears to be a function of both the severity of ischemia and its duration, at least over the flow range of 0—50% of normal [195].

The relevance of these animal data to man is not certain. Most of the studies have been done in anesthetized animals with high heart rates and blood pressures and therefore exaggerated myocardial oxygen demands. Under these conditions,

Table 5. Effects of coronary reperfusion

References	Subject[a]	Period of coronary occlusion	Effects of reperfusion[b]
Maroko et al., 1972 [178]	D, A	3 h	Less CK depletion and histol necrosis at 24 h; better regional fx at 1 h
Ginks et al., 1972 [179]	D, A	3 h	Less CK depletion and histol necrosis and 84% decrease in IS at 1 wk
Cox et al., 1973 [180]	D, A	$\leqslant$ 6 h	Partial return of bipolar potentials
Whalen et al., 1974 [181]	D, A	40 min	Increased water, Na, Ca content at 2–10 min
Smith et al., 1974 [182]	M, A	$\leqslant$ 6 h	Less ST elevation
		$\leqslant$ 4 h	Less R wave loss, decrease in IS (59% at 1 h, 47% at 2 h, 12% at 4 h)
Bresnahan et al., 1974 [183]	D, C	5 h	Hemorrhage and increased IS (observed CK loss > predicted) in 44% of dogs, avg 42% decrease in IS in remainder
Lang et al., 1974 [184]	D, A	3 h	K loss, arrhythmias, shock in 2/7 dogs
Banka et al., 1974 [185]	D, A	$\leqslant$ 45 min	Reversal of regional fx abn
		> 1 h	Worsening of regional fx
Kane et al., 1975 [186]	P, A	2–3 h	Decreased mitochondrial fx, accelerated R wave loss
Blumenthal et al., 1975 [187]	D, A	1–3 h	Accelerated R wave loss, washout of CK
Sharma et al., 1975 [188]	D, A	$\leqslant$ 1 h	Partial restoration of CP
		1–1½ h	Loss of nucleotides, worse EM changes, washout of enzymes
Mathur et al., 1975 [189]	D, C	2 h	Arrhythmias worse, regional fx improved in 42%, IS reduced
		5 h	Arrhythmias, Q waves, regional fx worse, IS unchanged
Constantini et al., 1975 [190]	D, A	3 h	Return of regional fx, 55% decrease in IS at 7 d
Deloche et al., 1977 [191]	R, A	$\leqslant$ 6 h	Decreased IS, decreased ST elevation
Reimer et al., 1977 [192]	D, A	$\leqslant$ 3 h	Decreased IS, (55% at 40 min, 33% at 3 h)
Capone et al., 1978 [193]	P, A	1 h	Accelerated recovery of ST elevation, hemorrhage, no effect on regional fx
White et al., 1978 [96]	D, C	2 h	About 75% decrease in IS
		$\geqslant$ 6 h	No decrease in IS
Darsee et al., 1980 [201]	D, A	2–6 h	No decrease in IS
Fishbein et al., 1980 [202]	D, A	5½ h	Hemorrhage in previously necrotic areas only

[a]D, dog; M, monkey; P, pig; R, rat; A, anesthetized; C, conscious.
[b]CK, creatine kinase; CP, creatine phosphate; fx, function; EM, electron microscopic; IS, infarct size measured pathologically or histologically, unless otherwise stated.

necrosis would be expected to progress more rapidly for a given reduction in blood flow. Furthermore, patients with acute myocardial infarct may sometimes have incomplete coronary occlusions [196] or spasm [68] or may have developed large collaterals by the time infarct occurs. In either case, flow to the myocardial segment undergoing necrosis may be only moderately reduced, as opposed to the severe reductions that occur with complete occlusion of a major coronary artery in the absence of collaterals. It is therefore possible that the progression of necrosis in at least some patients may be much slower than suggested by the available animal studies.

The question of whether reperfusion itself may cause myocardial damage should be considered. The balance of studies using pathologic endpoints of tissue necrosis have concluded that reflow does not increase infarct size, although it may grossly change the appearance of the ischemic tissue. Histologically, reflow can produce a picture of widespread hemorrhage, edema, and myofibrillar contraction [197, 198]. Dense transverse eosinophilic bands are seen representing condensations of sarcomeres ('contraction band necrosis'). (see Hutchins, p. 7). Mitochondria appear swollen and fragmented and contain electron-dense bodies thought to represent calcium deposits. In the absence of reflow, necrotic myocardium presents a very different appearance, with pale relaxed myofibrils, preserved cell structure, and lack of hemorrhage ('coagulation necrosis') [197, 198].

The histopathologic changes produced by reflow are believed to result from microvascular damage with increased vascular permeability, loss of cell volume regulation, and inrush of calcium producing widespread cellular contraction. The abnormalities are greater the longer the ischemic period preceding reflow. Extravasation of erythrocytes is maximal well inside the boundaries of the ischemic zone [199] where ischemia has been most severe, although central core areas frequently do not show this phenomenon since they cannot be reperfused. In all likelihood, hemorrhage is related to microvascular disruption. Since the oxygen requirement of vessel walls must be much less than that of myocardial cells, surrounding muscle fibers are probably already irreversibly damaged before reflow occurs [200]. Thus, reperfusion in all probability merely changes the appearance of tissue that is already dead. Although hemorrhage, edema, and contracture could theoretically increase tissue pressure and reduce local blood flow, the reopening of the normal blood supply probably outweighs any potential deleterious effects in this regard [210–201].

While reperfusion may reduce ultimate infarct size, serious short-term adverse effects on ventricular arrhythmias and left ventricular function have been identified. Ventricular tachycardia and/or fibrillation are common a few minutes after reflow in anesthetized dogs and may cause a mortality rate as high as 50% [203]. The incidence of serious arrhythmias is markedly reduced when ischemic periods last for more than 2 h [204].

A number of studies have shown deterioration of regional and global left ventricular function shortly after reperfusion. Reflow converts a pliable dyskinetic ventricular segment into a stiff swollen akinetic one. Local contracture of muscle fibers probably adds to the functional problem. A similar situation has been described during cardiac surgery, where global contracture may occur during reperfusion ('stone heart') [205]. Interestingly, the deterioration in function with reflow may only be a temporary phenomenon [190, 206, 207]. Constantini et al. found that reflow after 3 h of ischemia in anesthetized dogs produced a short-term deterioration in left ventricular function, but when the animals were reexamined one week later, function was better than in control nonreperfused animals [190].

Accelerated damage after reflow has been suggested by rapid Q wave development within minutes of reflow and by release of large amounts of myocardial enzymes into the blood [183, 187, 188]. However, the Q wave changes may merely represent an 'electrical phenomenon' independent of infarct size, while the enzyme changes probably are caused by washout of enzymes from cells that are already irreversibly damaged.

A few reports have appeared of emergency revascularization or coronary artery catheter dilatation or thrombolysis infusion in patients with acute myocardial infarct [196, 208–213] (see Gold, p. 511). Although these studies demonstrate the feasibility of an early operative approach, they have been unable to show salvage of ischemic myocardium with the methods available. Comparable control groups have been difficult to obtain. Future studies may overcome these problems and provide insight into the true benefits and indications for these aggressive treatments.

REFERENCES

1. Berne RM, Rubio R: Coronary circulation. In: Berne RM, Sperelakis N (eds) Handbook of physiology: circulation; sect 2: The cardiovascular system, vol 1: Heart. Baltimore: Williams and Wilkins, 1979, pp 873–952.
2. Schaper W, Wusten B: Collateral circulation. In: Schaper W (ed) The pathophysiology of myocardial perfusion. Amsterdam, New York: Elsevier/North-Holland, 1979, pp 415)470.
3. Schaper W: Pathophysiology of coronary circulation. Prog Cardiovasc Dis 14:275–296, 1971.
4. Brown BG, Gundel WD, Gott VL, Covell JW: Coronary collateral flow following acute coronary occlusion: a diastolic phenomenon. Cardiovasc Res 8:621–631, 1974.
5. Johansson B, Linder E, Seeman T: Effects of heart rate and arterial blood pressure on coronary collateral blood flow in dogs. Acta Physiol Scand [Suppl] 68:33–46, 1946.
6. Kattus AA, Gregg DE: Some determinants of coronary collateral blood flow in the open-chest dog. Circ Res 7: 628–642, 1959.

7. Becker L: Effect of tachycardia on left ventricular blood flow distribution during coronary occlusion. Am J Physiol 230:1072–1077, 1976.
8. Fam WM, McGregor M: Effect of nitroglycerin and dipyridamole on regional coronary resistance. Circ Res 22:649–659, 1968.
9. Winbury MM, Howe BB, Hefner MA: Effect of nitrates and other coronary dilators on large and small coronary vessels: an hypothesis for the mechanism of action of nitrates. J Pharmacol Exp Ther 168:70–95, 1969.
10. Mautz FR, Gregg DE: Dynamics of collateral circulation following chronic occlusion of coronary arteries. Proc Soc Exp Biol Med 36:797–801, 1937.
11. Gregg DE, Thornton JJ, Mautz FR: The magnitude, adequacy and source of the collateral blood flow and pressure in chronically occluded coronary arteries. Am J Physiol 127:161–175, 1939.
12. Schaper W: Residual perfusion of acutely ischemic heart muscle. In: Shaper W (ed) The pathophysiology of myocardial perfusion. Amsterdam, New York: Elsevier/North-Holland, 1979, pp 345–378.
13. Becker LC, Fortuin NJ, Pitt B: Effects of ischemia and antianginal drugs on the distribution of radioactive microspheres in the canine left ventricle. Circ Res 28:263–269, 1971.
14. Elliot EC, Jones EL, Bloor CM, Leon AS, Gregg DE: Day-to-day changes in coronary hemodynamics secondary to constriction of circumflex branch of left coronary artery in conscious dogs. Circ Res 22:237–250, 1968.
15. Becker LC, Pitt B: Collateral blood flow in conscious dogs with chronic coronary artery occlusion. Am J Physiol 221:1507–1510, 1971.
16. Becker LC, Ferreira R, Thomas M: Mapping of left ventricular blood flow with radioactive microspheres in experimental coronary artery occlusion. Cardiovasc Res 7:391–400, 1973.
17. Buckberg GD, Fixler DE, Archie JP, Hoffman JIE: Experimental subendocardial ischemia in dogs with normal coronary arteries. Circ Res 30:67–81, 1972.
18. Griggs DM Jr, Nakamura Y: Effect of coronary constriction on myocardial distribution of iodoantipyrine-[131]-I. Am J Physiol 215:1082–1088, 1968.
19. Cohen MV, Kirk ES: Differential response of large and small coronary arteries to nitroglycerin and angiotensin. Autoregulation and tachyphylaxis. Circ Res 33:445–453, 1973.
20. Schaper W, Schaper J, Xhonneux R, Vandesteene R: The morphology of intercoronary anastomoses in chronic coronary artery occlusion. Cardiovasc Res 3:315–323, 1969.
21. Schaper W, De Brabander M, Lewi P: DNA synthesis and mitosis in coronary collateral vessels of the dog. Circ Res 28:671–679, 1971.
22. Fulton WFM: The coronary arteries: arteriography, microanatomy and pathogenesis of obliterative coronary artery disease. Springfield, IL: CC Thomas, 1965.
23. Estes EH Jr, Entman ML, Dixon HB, Hackel DB: The vascular supply of the left ventricular wall. Anatomic observations plus a hypothesis regarding acute events in coronary artery disease. Am Heart J 71:58–67, 1966.
24. Farrer-Brown G: Normal and diseased vascular pattern of myocardium of human heart. I. Normal pattern in the left ventricular free wall. Br Heart J 30:527–536, 1968.

25. Downey JM, Kirk ES: Inhibition of coronary blood flow by a vascular waterfall mechanism. Circ Res 36:753–760, 1975.
26. Downey JM, Downey HF, Kirk ES: Effects of myocardial strains on coronary blood flow. Circ Res 34:286–292, 1974.
27. Rouleau J, Boerboom LE, Surjadhana A, Hoffman JIE: The role of autoregulation and tissue diastolic pressures in the transmural distribution of left ventricular blood flow in anesthetized dogs. Circ Res 45:804–815, 1979.
28. Hoffman JI: Determinants and prediction of transmural myocardial perfusion. Circulation 58:381–391, 1978.
29. Munch DF, Downey JM: Prediction of regional myocardial blood flow in dogs. Am J Physiol 239:H308–H315, 1980.
30. Bellamy RF: Diastolic coronary artery pressure-flow relations in the dog. Circ Res 43:92–101, 1978.
31. Russell RE, Chagrasulis RW, Downey JM: Inhibitory effect of cardiac contraction on coronary collateral blood flow. Am J Physiol 233:H541–H546, 1977.
32. Snyder R, Downey JM, Kirk ES: The active and passive components of extravascular coronary resistance. Cardiovasc Res 9:161–166, 1975.
33. Downey JM, Chagrasulis RW: The effect of cardiac contraction on collateral resistance in the canine heart. Circ Res 39:797–800, 1976.
34. Angell CS, Lakatta EG, Weisfeldt ML, Shock NW: Relationship of intramyocardial oxygen tension and epicardial ST segment changes following acute coronary artery ligation: effects of coronary perfusion pressure. Cardiovasc Res 9:12–18, 1975.
35. Willerson JT, Watson JT, Platt MR: Effect of hypertonic mannitol and intraaortic counterpulsation on regional myocardial blood flow and ventricular performance in dogs during myocardial ischemia. Am J Cardiol 37:514–519, 1976.
36. Powell WJ Jr, Daggett WM, Magro AE, Bianco JA, Buckley MJ, Sanders CA, Kantrowitz AR, Austen WG: Effects of intra-aortic balloon counterpulsation on cardiac performance, oxygen consumption, and coronary blood flow in dogs. Circ Res 26:753–764, 1970.
37. Goldfarb D, Brown BG, Conti CR, Gott VL: Cardiovascular responses to diastolic augmentation in the intact canine circulation and after ligation of the anterior descending coronary artery. J Thorac Cardiovasc Surg 55:243–254, 1968.
38. Maroko PR, Bernstein EF, Libby P, DeLaria GA, Covell JW, Ross J Jr, Braunwald E: Effects of intraaortic balloon counterpulsation on the severity of myocardial ischemic injury following acute coronary occlusion. Counterpulsation and myocardial injury. Curculation 45:1150–1159, 1972.
39. Shaw J, Taylor DR, Pitt B: Effects of intraaortic balloon counterpulsation on regional coronary blood flow in experimental myocardial infarction. Am J Cardiol 34:552–556, 1974.
40. Sugg WL, Webb WR, Ecker RR: Reduction of extent of myocardial infarction by counterpulsation. Ann Thorac Surg 7:310–316, 1969.
41. Mueller H, Ayres SM, Conklin EF, Giannelli S Jr, Mazzara JT, Grace WT, Nealon TF Jr: The effects of intra-aortic counterpulsation on cardiac

performance and metabolism in shock associated with acute myocardial infarction. J Clin Invest 50:1885–1900, 1971.

42. Leinbach RC, Buckley MJ, Austen WG, Petschek HE, Kantrowitz AR, Sanders CA: Effects of intra-aortic balloon pumping on coronary flow and metabolism in man. Circulation [Suppl 1] 43 and 44:I-77–81, 1971.

43. Leinback RC, Gold HK, Harper RW, Buckley MJ, Austen WG: Early intra-aortic balloon pumping for anterior myocardial infarction without shock. Circulation 58:204–214, 1978.

44. Parmley WW, Chatterjee K, Charuzi Y, Swan HJC: Hemodynamic effects of noninvasive systolic unloading (nitroprusside) and idastolic augmentation (external counterpulsation) in patients with acute myocardial infarction. Am J Cardiol 33:819–825, 1974.

45. Amsterdam EA, Banas J, Criley JM, Loeb HS, Mueller H, Willerson JT, Mason DT: Clinical assessment of external pressure circulatory assistance in acute myocardial infarction. Report of a cooperative clinical trial. Am J Cardiol 45:349–356, 1980.

46. Maroko PR, Kjekshus JK, Sobel BE, Watanabe T, Covell JW, Ross J Jr, Braunwald E: Factors influencing infarct size following experimental coronary artery occlusion. Circulation 43:67–82, 1971.

47. Smith ER, Redwood DR, McCarron WE, Epstein SE: Coronary artery occlusion in the conscious dog: effects of alterations in arterial pressure produced by nitroglycerin, hemorrhage, and alpha-adrenergic agonists on the degree of myocardial ischemia. Circulation 47:51–57, 1973.

48. Bache RJ: Effect of nitroglycerin and arterial hypertension on myocardial blood flow following acute coronary artery occlusion in the dog. Circulation 57:557–562, 1978.

49. Horwitz LD, Morgan SM: Effect of methoxamine on regional myocardial perfusion in experimental myocardial infarction. Cardiovasc Med 2:863–873, 1977.

50. Furuse A, Brawley RK, Gott VL: Effects of isoproterenol, I-norepinephrine, and glucagon on myocardial gas tensions in animals with coronary artery stenosis. J Thorac Cardiovasc Surg 65:815–824, 1973.

51. Buckberg GD, Ross G: Effects of isoprenaline on coronary blood flow: its distribution and myocardial performance. Cardiovasc Res 7:429–437, 1973.

52. Becker LC, Ferreira R, Thomas M: Effect of propranolol and isoprenaline on regional left ventricular blood flow in experimental myocardial ischemia. Cardiovasc Res 9:178–186, 1975.

53. Vatner SF, Millard RW, Patrick TA, Heyndrickx GR: Effects of isoproterenol on regional myocardial function, electrogram, and blood flow in conscious dogs with myocardial ischemia. J Clin Invest 57:1261–1271, 1976.

54. Vatner SF, Baig H: Importance of heart rate in determining the effects of sympathomimetic amines on regional myocardial function and blood flow in conscious dogs with acute myocardial ischemia. Circ Res 45:793–803, 1979.

55. Watanabe T, Covell JW, Maroko PR, Braunwald E, Ross J Jr: Effects of increased arterial pressure and positive inotropic agents on the severity of myocardial ischemia in the acutely depressed heart. Am J Cardiol 30:371–377, 1972.

56. Mueller H, Ayres SM, Gregory JJ, Giannelli S Jr, Grace WJ: Hemo-dynamics, coronary blood flow, and myocardial metabolism in coronary shock; response to I-norepinephrine and isoproterenol. J Clin Invest 49:1885–1902, 1970.
57. Kelly DT, Delgado CE, Taylor DR, Pitt B, Ross RS: Use of phentolamine in acute myocardial infarction associated with hypertension and left ventricular failure. Circulation 47:729–735, 1973.
58. Shell WE, Sobel BE: Protection of jeopardized ischemic myocardium by reduction of ventricular afterload. N Engl J Med 291:481–486, 1974.
59. Tillmanns H, Steinhausen M, Leinberger H, Thederan H: Different response of the ventricular microcirculation to coronary vasodilators [abstr[. Circulation [Suppl 2] 59 and 60:II-142, 1979.
60. Schnaar RL, Sparks HV: Response of large and small coronary arteries to nitroglycerin, $NaNO_2$, and adenosine. Am J Physiol 223:223–228, 1972.
61. Harder DR, Belardinelli L, Sperelakis N, Rubio R, Berne RM: Differential effects of adenosine and nitroglycerin on the action potentials of large and small coronary arteries. Circ Res 44:176–182, 1979.
62. Becker LC: Effect of nitroglycerin and dipyridamole on regional left ventricular blood flow during coronary artery occlusion. J Clin Invest 58:1287–1296, 1976.
63. Feldman RL, Pepine CJ, Curry RC Jr, Conti CR: Coronary arterial responses to graded doses of nitroglycerin. Am J Cardiol 43:91–97, 1979.
64. Wiggers CJ, Green HD: The ineffectiveness of drugs upon collateral flow after experimental coronary occlusion in dogs. Am Heart J 11:527–541, 1936.
65. Schaper W: Effect of drugs on collateral circulation. In: Schaper W (ed) The pathophysiology of myocardial perfusion. Amsterdam, New York: Elsevier/North-Holland, 1979, pp 471–488.
66. Cohen MV, Downey JM, Sonnenblick EH, Kirk ES: The effects of nitro-glycerin on coronary collaterals and myocardial contractility. J Clin Invest 52:2836–2847, 1973.
67. Capurro N, Kent KM, Epstein SE: Effects of intracoronary and intra-venous nitroglycerin on coronary collateral function. J Pharmacol Ther 199:262–268, 1976.
68. Oliva PB, Breckinridge JC: Arteriographic evidence of coronary arterial spasm in acute myocardial infarction. Circulation 56:366–374, 1977.
69. Leighninger DS, Rueger R, Beck CS: Effect of glyceryl trinitrate (nitro-glycerin) on arterial blood supply to ischemic myocardium. Am J Cardiol 3:638, 1959.
70. Mathes P, Rival J: Effect of nitroglycerin on total and regional coronary blood flow in the normal and ischaemic canine myocardium. Cardiovasc Res 5:54–61, 1971.
71. Horwitz LD, Gorlin R, Taylor WJ, Kemp HG: Effects of nitroglycerin on regional myocardial blood flow in coronary artery disease. J Clin Invest 50:1578–1584, 1971.
72. Weisse AB, Senft A, Kahn MI, Regan TJ: Effect of nitrate infusions on the systemic and coronary circulations following acute experimental myocardial infarction in the intact dog. Am J Cardiol 30:362–370, 1972.
73. Chiariello M, Gold HK, Leinbach RC, Davis MA, Maroko PR: Comparison

between the effects of nitroprusside and nitroglycerin on ischemic injury during acute myocardial infarction. Circulation 54:766–773, 1976.

74. Capurro NL, Kent KM, Smith HJ, Aamodt R, Epstein SE: Acute coronary occlusion: prolonged increase in collateral flow following brief administration of nitroglycerin and methoxamine. Am J Cardiol 39:679–683, 1977.

75. Jugdutt BI, Becker, LC, Hutchins GM, Bulkley BH, Reid PR, Kallman CH: Effect of intravenous nitroglycerin on collateral blood flow and infarct size in the conscious dog. Circulation 63:17–28, 1981.

76. Pasyk S, Bloor CM, Khouri EM, Gregg DE: Systemic and coronary effects of coronary artery occlusion in the unanesthetized dog. Am J Physiol 220:646–654, 1971.

77. Goldstein RE, Stinson EB, Scherer JL, Seningen RP, Grehl TM, Epstein SE: Intraoperative coronary collateral function in patients with coronary occlusive disease: nitroglycerin responsiveness and angiographic correlations. Circulation 49:298–308, 1974.

78. Most AS, Williams DO, Millard RW: Acute coronary occlusion in the pig: effect of nitroglycerin on regional myocardial blood flow. Am J Cardiol 42:947–953, 1978.

79. Fam WM, McGregor M: Effect of coronary vasodilator drugs on retrograde flow in areas of chronic myocardial ischemia. Circ Res 15:355–365, 1964.

80. Linder E, Seeman T: Effects of persantin and nitroglycerin on myocardial blood flow during temporary coronary occlusions in dogs. Angiologica (Basel) 4:225–255, 1967.

81. Hirshfeld JW, Jr., Borer JS, Goldstein RE, Barrett MJ, Epstein SE: Reduction in severity and extent of myocardial infarction when nitroglycerine and methoxamine are administered during coronary occlusion. Circulation 49:291–297, 1974.

82. Myers RW, Scherer JL, Goldstein RA, Goldstein RE, Kent KM, Epstein SE: Effects of nitroglycerin and nitroglycerin-methoxamine during acute myocardial ischemia in dogs with pre-existing multivessel coronary occlusive disease. Circulation 51:632–640, 1975.

83. Banka VS, Bodenheimer MM, Helfant RH: Nitroglycerin in experimental myocardial infarction. Effects on regional left ventricular length and tension. Am J Cardiol 36:453–458, 1975.

84. Cohen MV, Sonnenblick EH, Kirk ES: Comparative effects of nitroglycerin and isosorbide dinitrate on coronary collateral vessels and ischemic myocardium in dogs. Am J Cardiol 37:244–249, 1976.

85. Theroux P, Ross J Jr, Franklin D, Kemper WS, Sasayama S: Regional myocardial function in the conscious dog during acute coronary occlusion and responses to morphine, propranolol, nitroglycerin, and lidocaine. Circulation 53:302–314, 1976.

86. Ramanathan KB, Bodenheimer MM, Banka VS, Helfant RH: Severity of contraction abnormalities after acute myocardial infarction in man: response to nitroglycerin. Circulation 60:1230–1237, 1979.

87. Bleifeld W, Wende W, Bussmann WD, Meyer J: Influence of nitroglycerin on the size of experimental myocardial infarction. Naunyn Schmiedebergs Arch Pharmacol 277:387–400, 1973.

88. Lang TW, Meerbaum S, Corday E, Davidson RM, Hashimoto K, Farcot JC, Osher J: Regional and global myocardial effects of intravenous and

sublingual nitroglycerin treatment after experimental acute coronary occlusion. Am J Cardiol 37:523–543, 1976.

89. Komer RR, Edalji A, Hood WB Jr: Effects of nitroglycerin on echocardiographic measurements of left ventricular wall thickness and regional myocardial performance during acute coronary ischemia. Circulation 59:926–937, 1979.

90. Vatner SF, McRitchie RJ, Maroko PR, Patrick TA, Braunwald E: Effects of catecholamines, exercise, and nitroglycerin on the normal and ischemic myocardium in conscious dogs. J Clin Invest 54:563–575, 1974.

91. Flaherty JT, Reid PR, Kelly DT, Taylor DR, Weisfeldt ML, Pitt B: Intravenous nitroglycerin in acute myocardial infarction. Circulation 51:132–139, 1975.

92. Come PC, Flaherty JT, Baird MG, Rouleau JR, Weisfeldt ML, Greene HL, Becker LC, Pitt B: Reversal by phenylephrine of the beneficial effects of intravenous nitroglycerin in patients with acute myocardial infarction. N Engl J Med 293:1003–1007, 1975.

93. Borer JS, Redwood DR, Levitt B, Cagin N, Bianchi C, Vallin H, Epstein SE: Reduction in myocardial ischemia with nitroglycerin or nitroglycerin plus phenylephrine administered during acute myocardial infarction. N Engl J Med 293:1008–1012, 1975.

94. Amende I, Simon R, Hood WP Jr, Lichtlen PR: The effect of the betablocker atenolol and nitroglycerin on left ventricular function and geometry in man. Circulation 60:836–848, 1979.

95. Jugdutt BI, Becker LC, Hutchins GM: Early changes in collateral blood flow during myocardial infarction in conscious dogs. Am J Physiol 237:H371–H380, 1979.

96. White FC, Sanders M, Bloor CM: Regional redistribution of myocardial blood flow after coronary occlusion and reperfusion in the conscious dog. Am J Cardiol 42:234–243, 1978.

97. Rivas F, Cobb FR, Bache RJ, Greenfield JC Jr: Relationship between blood flow to ischemic regions and extent of myocardial infarction. Serial measurement of blood flow to ischemic regions in dogs. Circ Res 38:439–447, 1976.

98. Wégria R, Segers M, Keating RP, Ward HP: Relationship between the reduction in coronary flow and the appearance of electrocardiographic changes. Am Heart J 38:90–96, 1949.

99. Scheuer J, Brachfeld N: Coronary insufficiency: relations between hemodynamic, electrical, and biochemical parameters. Circ Res 18:178–189, 1966.

100. Jugdutt BI, Hutchins GM, Bulkley BH, Becker LC: Myocardial infarction in the conscious dog: Three-dimensional mapping of infarct, collateral flow and region at risk. Circulation 60:1141–1150, 1979.

101. Goldstein RE, Davenport NJ, Bolli R, Epstein SE: Blood flow to surviving and infarcted myocardium [abstr]. Clin Res 28:174A, 1980.

102. Jugdutt B, Hutchins G, Bulkley BH, Becker L: Reduction of infarct size by intravenous nitroglycerin infusion in conscious dogs. Circulation [Suppl 2] 57 and 58:II-98, 1978.

103. Fukuyama T, Roberts R: The effect of intravenous nitroglycerin on coronary blood flow and infarct size during myocardial infarction in conscious dogs. Clin Cardiol 3:317–323, 1980.

104. Bache RJ, Ball RM, Cobb FR, Rembert JC, Greenfield JC Jr: Effects of nitroglycerin on transmural myocardial blood flow in the unanesthetized dog. J Clin Invest 55:1219–1228, 1975.
105. Winbury MM: Redistribution of left ventricular blood flow produced by nitroglycerin. An example of integration of the macro- and microcirculation. Circ Res [Suppl 2] 28 and 29:I-140–147, 1971.
106. Moir TW: Subendocardial distribution of coronary blood flow and the effect of antianginal drugs. Circ Res 30:621–627, 1972.
107. Becker L, Fortuin NJ, Pitt B: Regional myocardial blood flow in the conscious dog [abstr]. Circulation [Suppl 3] 39 and 40:III-41, 1969.
108. Forman R, Kirk ES, Downey JM, Sonnenblick EH: Nitroglycerin and heterogeneity of myocardial blood flow. Reduced subendocardial blood flow and ventricular contractile force. J Clin Invest 52:905–911, 1973.
109. Nakamura M, Eto Y, Hamanaka N, Kuroiwa A, Tomoike H, Ishihara Y: Effects of selective coronary hypotension and nitroglycerin or Bay a 1040 on the distribution of Rb86 clearance in the canine heart. Cardiovasc Res 7:777–788, 1973.
110. Fortuin NJ, Kaihara S, Becker LC, Pitt B: Regional myocardial blood flow in the dog studied with radioactive microspheres. Cardiovasc Res 5:331–336, 1971.
111. Paradise NF, Tripp MR, Burchell HB, Gerasch DA, Swayze CR, Fox IJ: Effect of nitroglycerin with and without systemic hypotension on canine regional myocardial tritiated water deposition. Cardiovasc Res 10:182–191, 1976.
112. Gross GJ, Warltier DC: Intracoronary versus intravenous nitroglycerin on the transmural distribution of coronary blood flow. Cardiovasc Res 11:499–506, 1977.
113. Winbury MM, Howe BB, Weiss JR: Effect of nitroglycerin and dipyridamole on epicardial and endocardial oxygen tension − further evidence for redistribution of myocardial blood flow. J Pharmacol Exp Ther 176:184–199, 1971.
114. Weiss HR, Winbury MM: Intracoronary nitroglycerin, pentaerythritol trinitrate and dipyridamole on intramyocardial oxygen tension. Microvasc Res 4:273–284, 1972.
115. Kiese M, Lange G, Resag K: Die Wirkung von 2, 6-bis (diathanolamino)-4, 8-dipiperidino-pyrimido (5, 4-d) pyrimidin auf die Durchblutung des experimentellen Herzinfarkts und des gesunden Herzmuskels. [The effect of 2, 6-bis [di-(2-hydroxyethyl)amino]-4, 8-dipiperidino-pyrimido-[5, 4-d] pyrimidine on the circulation of experimental myocardial infarct and healthy myocardium.] Z Ges Exp Med 132:426–435, 1960.
116. Rees JR, Redding VJ: Effects of dipyridamole on anastomotic blood flow in experimental myocardial infarction. Cardiovasc Res I:179–183, 1967.
117. Grayson J, Irvine M, Parratt JR: Effects of carbochromen and dipyridamole on blood flow and heat production in the normal and ischaemic canine myocardium. Cardiovasc Res 5:41–47, 1971.
118. Cibulski AA, Lehan PH, Timmis HH: Retrograde flow technique vs. krypton-85 clearance technique for estimation of myocardial collaterals. Am J Physiol 223:1081–1087, 1972.
119. Csik V, Szekeres L, Udvary E: Drug-induced agumentation of coronary

flow in vessels with maximum ischemic dilatation. Arch Int Pharmacodyn Ther 224:66–76, 1976.

120. Gould KL: Pressure-flow characteristics of coronary stenoses in unsedated dogs at rest and during coronary vasodilation. Circ Res 43:242–253, 1978.

121. Flameng W. Wüsten B, Schaper W: On the distribution of myocardial flow, Part II: Effects of arterial stenosis and vasodilation. Basic Res Cardiol 69:435–446, 1974.

122. Becker LC: Conditions for vasodilator-induced coronary steal in experimental myocardial ischemia. Circulation 57:1103–1110, 1978.

123. Flameng W, Schaper W, Lewi P: Multiple experimental coronary occlusion without infarction. Effects of heart rate and vasodilatation. Am Heart J 85:767–776, 1973.

124. Schaper W, Lewi P, Flameng W, Gijpen L: Myocardial steal produced by coronary vasodilation in chronic coronary artery occlusion. Basic Res Cardiol 68:3–20, 1973.

125. O'Riordan JB, Flaherty JT, Khuri SF, Brawley RK, Pitt B, Gott VL: Effects of atrial pacing on regional myocardial gas tensions with critical coronary stenosis. Am J Physiol 232:H49–H53, 1977.

126. Maseri A: Myocardial blood flow in acute ischemia, and its measurement. In: Oliver MF (ed) Modern trends in cardiology, vol 3. London: Butterworths, 1974, pp 115–153.

127. Bleifeld W, Wende W, Meyer J, Bussmann WD: Einfluss einer Vaso-Dilatation durch Dipyridamil auf die Grösse des akuten experimentellen Herzinfarktes. Z Kardiol 63:115–128, 1974.

128. Watanabe T, Shintani F, Fu L, Kato K, Koyama S: Failure of dipyridamole (Persantin) in reducing the infarct size following experimental coronary occlusion. Jpn Heart J 13:512–520, 1972.

129. Roberts AJ, Jacobstein JG, Cipriano PR, Alonso DR, Combes JR, Gay WA Jr: Effectiveness of dipyridamole in reducing the size of experimental myocardial infarction. Circulation 61:228–236, 1980.

130. Blumenthal DS, Hutchins GM, Jugdutt BI, Becker LC: Reduction of infarct size with a nonspecific vasodilator [abstr]. Clin Res 28:158A, 1980.

131. Gould KL, Westcott RJ, Albro PC, Hamilton GW: Noninvasive assessment of coronary stenoses by myocardial imaging during, pharmacologic coronary vasodilatation. II. Clinical methodology and feasibility. Am J Cardiol 41:279–287, 1978.

132. Albro PC, Gould KL, Westcott RJ, Hamilton GW, Ritchie JL, Williams DL: Noninvasive assessment of coronary stenoses by myocardial imaging during pharmacologic coronary vasodilatation. III. Clinical trial. Am J Cardiol 42:751–760, 1978.

133. Muller JE, Gunther SJ: Nifedipine therapy for Prinzmetal's angina. Circulation. 57:137–139, 1978.

134. Parodi O, Maseri A, Simonetti I: Management of unstable angina at rest by verapamil. A double-blind corss-over study in coronary care unit. Br Heart J 41:167–174, 1979.

135. Yasue H, Omote S, Takizawa A, Nagao M, Miwa K, Tanaka S: Exertional angina pectoris caused by coronary arterial spasm: effects of various drugs. Am Heart J 43:647–652, 1979.

136. Henry PD, Shuchleib R, Borda LJ, Roberts R, Williamson JR, Sobel BE: Effects of nifedipine on myocardial perfusion and ischemic injury in dogs. Circ Res 43:372–380, 1978.

137. Henry PD, Shuchleib R, Clark RE, Perez JE: Effect of nifedipine on myocardial ischemia: analysis of collateral flow, pulsatile heat and regional muscle shortening. Am J Cardiol 44:817–824, 1979.

138. Clark RE, Christlieb IY, Henry PD, Fischer AE, Nora JD, Williamson JR, Sobel BE: Nifedipine: a myocardial protective agent. Am J Cardiol 44:825–831, 1979.

139. Selwyn AP, Welman E, Fox K, Horlock P, Pratt T, Klein M: The effects of nifedipine on acute experimental myocardial ischemia and infarction in dogs. Circ Res 44:16–23, 1979.

140. Smith HJ, Singh BN, Nisbet HD, Norris RM: Effects of verapamil on infarct size following experimental coronary occlusion. Cardiovasc Res 9:569–578, 1975.

141. Reimer KA, Lowe JE, Jennings RB: Effect of the calcium antagonist verapamil on necrosis following temporary coronary artery occlusion in dogs. Circulation 55:581–587, 1977.

142. Karlsberg RP, Henry PD, Ahmed SA, Sobel BE, Roberts R: Lack of protection of ischemic myocardium by verapamil in conscious dgos. Eur J Pharmacol 42:339–346, 1977.

143. Ribeiro LGT, Yasuda T, Lowenstein E, Braunwald E, Maroko PR: Comparative effects of anatomic infarct size of verapamil, ibuprofen, and morphine-promethazine-chlorpromazine combination [abstr]. Am J Cardiol 43:396, 1979.

144. Weishaar R, Ashikawa K, Bing RJ: Effect of diltiazem, a calcium antagonist on myocardial ischemia. Am J Cardiol 43:1137–1143, 1979.

145. Capurro NL, Kent KM, Epstein SE: Comparison of nitroglycerin-, nitroprusside-, and phentolamine-induced changes in coronary collateral function in dogs. J Clin Invest 60:295–301, 1977.

146. Needleman P, Kaley G: Cardiac and coronary prostaglandin synthesis and function. N Engl J Med 298:1122–1128, 1978.

147. Gorman RR: Prostaglandins, thromboxanes, and prostacyclin. In: International review of biochemistry, vol 20: Rickenberg HV (ed) Biochemistry and mode of action of hormones II. Baltimore: University Park, 1978, pp 81–107.

148. Dusting GJ, Moncada S, Vane JR: Prostaglandins, their intermediates and abnormal circulatory systems. Prog Cardiovasc Dis 21:405–430, 1979.

149. Kirmser R, Berger HJ, Cohen LS, Wolfson S: Effect of indomethacin, a prostaglandin inhibitor, on epicardial ST elevation and myocardial blood flow after coronary occlusion [abstr]. Circulation [Suppl 2] 54:II-194, 1976.

150. Jugdutt BI, Hutchins GM, Bulkley BH, Pitt B, Becker LC: Effect of indomethacin on collateral blood flow and infarct size in the conscious dog. Circulation 59:734–743, 1979.

151. Maclean D, Fishbein MC, Blum RI, Braunwald E, Maroko PR: Long-term preservation of ischemic myocardium by ibuprofen after experimental coronary artery occlusion [abstr]. Am J Cardiol 41:394, 1978.

152. Lefer AM, Polansky EW: Beneficial effects of ibuprofen in acute myocardial ischemia. Cardiology 64:265–279, 1979.

153. Lefer AM, Crossley K: Optimal dose of ibuprofen in acute myocardial ischemia in the cat [abstr]. Circulatory Shock 6:182, 1979.

154. Flynn PJ, Becker WK, Hammerschmidt DE, Craddock PR, Weisdorf D, Lillehei RC, Jacob HS: Myocardial infarct (MI) size is reduced by inhibition of granulocyte (PMN), not platelet aggregation [abstr]. Clin Res 28:169A, 1980.

155. Jugdutt BI, Hutchins GM, Bulkley BH, Becker LC: Salvage of ischemic myocardium by ibuprofex during infarction in the conscious dog. Am J Cardiol 46:74–82, 1980.

156. Mjös OD, Oliver MF, Reimersma RA: Prostaglandin-E_1, free fatty acids and myocardial ischemia. Acta Biol Med Germany 35:1081–1082, 1976.

157. Hutton I, Parratt JR, Lawrie TDV: Cardiovascular effects of prostaglandin E_1 in experimental myocardial infarction. Cardiovasc Res 7:149–155, 1973.

158. Takano T, Vyden JK, Rose HB, Corday E, Swan HJC: Beneficial effects of prostaglandin E_1 in acute myocardial infarction [abstr]. Am J Cardiol 39:297, 1977.

159. Wolfson S, Tacket C, Good N, Kirmser RJ, Addabbo M, Cohen LS: Role of prostaglandin E during coronary occlusion [abstr]. Circulation [Suppl 3] 55 and 56:III-122, 1977.

160. Ogletree ML, Lefer AM: Prostaglandin-induced preservation of the ischemic myocardium. Circ Res 42:218–224, 1978.

161. Jugdutt BI, Hutchins GM, Bulkley BH, Becker LC: Dissimilar effects of PGE_1 and PGE_2 on myocardial infarct size after coronary occlusion in conscious dogs. In: Samuelsson B, Paoletti R (eds) Advances in prostaglandins and thromboxane research, vol 7. New York: Raven Press, 1980, pp 675–677.

162. Morcillio E, Reid PR, Dubin N, Chodgaonkar R, Pitt B: Myocardial prostaglandin E release by nitroglycerin and modification by indomethacin. Am J Cardiol 45:53–57, 1980.

163. Ogletree ML, Lefer AM, Smith JB, Nicolaou KC: Studies on the protective effect of prostacyclin in acute myocardial ischemia. Eur J Pharmacol 56:95–103, 1979.

164. Jugdutt BI, Hutchins GM, Bulkley BH, Becker LC: Infarct size reduction by prostacyclin after coronary occlusion in conscious dogs [abstr]. Clin Res 27:177A, 1979.

165. Ribeiro LGT, Reduto LA, Brandon TA, Taylor AA, Hopkins DG, Miller RR: Effects of prostacyclin on hemodynamics, regional myocardial blood flow, infarct size and mortality in experimental myocardial infarction [abstr]. Clin Res 27:199A, 1979.

166. Jentzer JH, Sonnenblick EH, Kirk ES: Specificity of prostacyclin as a coronary artery vasodilator [abstr]. Clin Res 27:177A, 1979.

167. Willerson JT, Powell WJ Jr, Guiney TE, Stark JJ, Sanders CA, Leaf A: Improvement in myocardial function and coronary blood flow in ischemic myocardium after mannitol. J Clin Invest 51:2989–2998, 1972.

168. Hutton I, Marynick SP, Fixler DE, Templeton GH, Willerson JT: Changes in regional coronary blood flow with hypertonic mannitol in conscious dogs. Cardiovasc Res 9:47–55, 1975.

169. Fixler DE, Buja LM, Wheeler JM, Willerson JT: Influence of mannitol on

454

maintaining coronary flows and salvaging myocardium during ventriculotomy and during prolonged coronary artery ligation. Circulation 56:340–346, 1977.

170. Hirzel HO, Kirk ES: The effect of mannitol following permanent coronary occlusion. Circulation 56:1006–1015, 1977.

171. Maroko PR, Libby P, Bloor CM, Sobel BE, Braunwald E: Reduction by hyaluronidase of myocardial necrosis following coronary artery occlusion. Circulation 46:430–437, 1972.

172. Askenazi J, Hillis LD, Diaz PE, Davis MA, Braunwald E, Maroko PR: The effects of hyaluronidase on coronary blood flow following coronary artery occlusion in the dog. Circ Res 40:566–571, 1977.

173. Kloner RA, Fishbein MC, Maclean D, Braunwald E, Maroko PR: Effect of hyaluronidase during the early phase of acute myocardial ischemia: an ultrastructural and morphometric analysis. Am J Cardiol 40:43–49, 1977.

174. Kloner RA, Braunwald E, Maroko PR: Long-term preservation of ischemic myocardium in the dog by hyaluronidase. Circulation 58:220–226, 1978.

175. Hofmann M, Hofmann M, Schaper W: Influence of hyaluronidase on infarct size following experimental coronary occlusion of short (90') or long (24 h) duration. Basic Res Cardiol 75:340–352, 1980.

176. Vatner SF, Baig H, Manders WT, Ochs H, Pagani M: Effects of propranolol on regional myocardial function, electrograms, and blood flow in conscious dogs with myocardial ischemia. J Clin Invest 60:353–360, 1977.

177. Buck JD, Gross GJ, Warltier DC, Jolly SR, Hardman HF: Comparative effects of cardioselective versus noncardioselective beta blockade on subendocardial blood flow and contractile function in ischemic myocardium. Am J Cardiol 44:657–663, 1979.

178. Maroko PR, Libby P, Ginks WR, Bloor CM, Shell WE, Sobel, Ross J Jr: Coronary artery reperfusion. I. Early effects on local myocardial function and the extent of myocardial necrosis. J Clin Invest 51:2710–2716, 1972.

179. Ginks WR, Sybers HD, Maroko PR, Covell JW, Sobel BE, Ross J Jr: Coronary artery reperfusion. II. Reduction of myocardial infarct size at one week after the coronary occlusion. J Clin Invest 51:2717–2723, 1972.

180. Cox JL, Daniel TM, Boineau JP: The electrophysiologic time-course of acute myocardial ischemia and the effects of early coronary artery reperfusion. Circulation 48:971–983, 1973.

181. Whalen DA Jr, Hamilton DG, Ganote CE, Jennings RB: Effect of a transient period of ischemia on myocardial cells. I. Effects on cell volume regulation. Am J Pathol 74:381–397, 1974.

182. Smith GT, Soeter JR, Haston HH, McNamara JJ: Coronary reperfusion in primates. Serial electrocardiographic and histologic assessment. J Clin Invest 54:1420–1427, 1974.

183. Bresnahan GF, Roberts R, Shell WE, Ross J Jr, Sobel BE: Deleterious effects due to hemorrhage after myocardial reperfusion. Am J Cardiol 33:82–86, 1974.

184. Land TW, Corday E, Gold H, Meerbaum S, Rubins S, Constantini C, Hirose S, Osher J, Rosen V: Consequences of reperfusion after coronary occlusion. Effects on hemodynamic and regional myocardial metabolic function. Am J Cardiol 33:69–81, 1974.

185. Banka VS, Chadda KD, Helfant RH: Limitations of myocardial revascularization in restoration of regional contraction abnormalities produced by coronary occlusion. Am J Cardiol 34:164—170, 1974.

186. Kane JJ, Murphy ML, Bissett JK, de Soyza N, Doherty JE, Straub KD: Mitochondrial function, oxygen extraction, epicardial S-T segment changes and tritrated digoxin distribution after reperfusion of ischemic myocardium. Am J Cardiol 36:218—224, 1975.

187. Blumenthal ML, Wang HH, Lui LMP: Experimental coronary arterial occlusion and release. Effects on enzymes, electrocardiograms, myocardial contractility and reactive hyperemia. Am J Cardiol 36:225—233, 1975.

188. Sharma GP, Varley KG, Kim SW, Barwinsky J, Cohen M, Dhalla NS: Alterations in energy metabolism and ultrastructure upon reperfusion of the ischemic myocardium after coronary occlusion. Am J Cardiol 36:234—243, 1975.

189. Mathur VS, Guinn GA, Burris WH III: Maximal revascularization (reperfusion) in intact conscious dogs after 2 to 5 hours of coronary occlusion. Am J Cardiol 36:252—261, 1975.

190. Constantini C, Corday E, Lang TW, Meerbaum S, Brasch J, Kaplan L, Rubins S, Gold H, Osher J: Revascularization after 3 hours of coronary arterial occlusion: effects on regional cardiac metabolic function and infarct size. Am J Cardiol 36:368—384, 1975.

191. Deloche A, Fabiani JN, Camilleri JP, Relland J, Joseph D, Carpentier A, Dubost Ch: The effect of coronary artery reperfusion on the extent of myocardial infarction. Am Heart J 93:358—366, 1977.

192. Reimer KA, Lowe JE, Rasmussen MM, Jennings RB: The wavefront phenomenon of ischemic cell death. I. Myocardial infarct size duration of coronary occlusion in dogs. Circulation 56:786—794, 1977.

193. Capone RJ, Most AS: Myocardial hemorrhage after coronary reperfusion in pigs. Am J Cardiol 41:259—266, 1978.

194. Jennings RB, Sommers HM, Smyth GA, Flack HA, Linn H: Myocardial necrosis induced by temporary occlusion of a coronary artery in the dog. Arch Pathol 70:68—78, 1960.

195. Rude RE, DeBoer LWV, Ingwall JS, Kloner RA, Hale SL, Davis M, Maroko PR, Braunwald E: Prediction of biochemical derangement in ischemic myocardium following experimental coronary artery occlusion [abstr]. Am J Cardiol 45:415, 1980.

196. DeWood MA, Spores J, Notske R, Mouser LT, Burroughs R, Golden MS, Lang HT: Prevalence of total coronary occlusion during the early hours of transmural myocardial infarction. N Engl J Med 303:897—902, 1980.

197. Herdson PB, Sommers HM, Jennings RB: A comparative study of the fine structure of normal and ischemic dog myocardium with special reference to early changes following temporary occlusion of a coronary artery. Am J Pathol 46:367—386, 1965.

198. Kloner RA, Ganote CE, Whalen DA Jr, Jennings RB: Effect of a transient period of ischemia on myocardial cells. II. Fine structure during the first few minutes of reflow. Am J Pathol 74:399—422, 1974.

199. Fishbein MC, Rit J, Lando U, Kanmatsuse K, Mercier JC, Gaz W: Localization of reperfusion hemorrhage and vascular injury in experimental myocardial infarcts [abstr]. Circulation [Suppl 2] 59 and 60:II-43, 1979.

200. Kloner RA, Rude RE, Maroko PR, Braunwald E: Microvascular damage and myocardial cell injury following coronary artery occlusion: Which comes first? [abstr]. Circulation [Suppl 2] 59 and 60:II-42, 1979.

201. Darsee JR, Kloner RA: The no reflow phenomenon: a time-limiting factor for reperfusion after coronary occlusion? Am J Cardiol 46:808–806, 1980.

202. Fishbein MC, Y-Rit J, Lando U, Kanmatsuse K, Mercier JC, Ganz W: The relationship of vascular injury and myocardial hemorrhage to necrosis after reperfusion. Circulation 62:1274–1279, 1980.

203. Sommers HM, Jennings RB: Ventricular fibrillation and myocardial necrosis after transient ischemia. Effect of treatment with oxygen, procainamide, reserpine, and propranolol. Arch Intern Med 129:780–789, 1972.

204. Reimer KA, Jennings RB: The 'wavefron phenomenon' of myocardial ischemic cell death. II. Transmural progression of necrosis within the framework of ischemic bed size (myocardium at risk) and collateral flow. Lab Invest 40:633–644, 1979.

205. Baroldi G, Milam JD, Wukasch DC, Sandiford FM, Romognoli A, Cooley DA: Myocardial cell damage in 'stone hearts'. J Mol Cell Cardiol 6:395–399, 1974.

206. Schaff HV, Flaherty JT, Goldman RA, Frederiksen JW, Gott VL: Mechanism of the elevated left ventricular end diastolic pressure following ischemic arrest and reperfusion. Am J Physiol 9:H300–307, 1981.

207. Theroux P, Ross J Jr, Franklin D, Kemper WS, Sasayama S: Coronary arterial reperfusion. III. Early and late effects of regional myocardial function and dimensions in conscious dogs. Am J Cardiol 38:599–606, 1976.

208. Bolooki H, Kotler MD, Lottenberg L, Dresnick S, Andrews RC, Kipnis, S, Ellis RM: Myocardial revascularization after acute infarction. Am J Cardiol 36:395–406, 1975.

209. DeWood MA, Spores J, Notske RN, Lang HT, Shields JP, Simpson CS, Rudy LW, Grunwald R: Medical and surgical management of myocardial infarction. Am J Cardiol 44:1356–1364, 1979.

210. Mathey OG, Kuck KH, Tilsner V, Kiebber HJ, Bleiseld W: Nonsurgical coronary artery recanalization on acute transmural myocardial infarction. Circulation 63:489–497, 1981.

211. Ganz W, Buchbinder N, Marcus H, Mondkar A, Maddahi J, Charuzi Y, O'Connor L, Shell W, Fishbein MC, Kass R, Mihamoto A, Swan HJC: Intracoronary thrombolysis in evolving myocardial infarction. Am Heart J 101:4–13, 1981.

212. Rentrop P, Blanke H, Karsch KR, Kaiser H, Köstering H, Leitz K: Selective intracoronary thrombolysis in acute myocardial infarction and unstable angina pectoris. Circulation 63:307–317, 1981.

213. Markis JE, Malagold M, Parker JA, Silverman KJ, Barry WN, Als AV, Paulin S, Grossman W, Braunwald E: Myocardial salvage after intracoronary thrombolysis with streptokinase in acute myocardial infarction. Assessment with intracoronary thallium-201. N Engl J Med 305:777–782, 1981.

19. ALTERATIONS IN THE COAGULATION SYSTEM

THOMAS R. GRIGGS

Since the first description of coronary thrombosis as a related event in the pathogenesis of myocardial infarct, physicians have suspected that inhibiting the thrombotic process might limit or prevent the development of myocardial necrosis in patients with acute myocardial infarct. After the introduction of coumarin anticoagulants in 1943, many clinical trials were conducted to test the effects of anticoagulation on the mortality and morbidity of acute myocardial infarct. Unfortunately the interpretation of the results of these trials continues to be a focus of disagreement. To this date, no antithrombotic agent has been generally accepted as beneficial in this clinical setting. Nevertheless, there has been a recent resurgence of interest in the study of the role of thrombosis, and especially platelet-mediated events, in the pathogenesis of myocardial ischemia and infarct.

At least three elements of the thrombotic process might increase coronary vascular resistance and thereby precipitate or aggravate an acute myocardial infarct: (a) the development of a platelet-fibrin thrombus, (b) the presence of a platelet plug with or without associated platelet microembolism to small coronary arteries, and (c) the spasm-producing influence of thromboxane A_2 and possibly other factors that are released when platelets are 'activated.' These elements may be operative with and without the presence of atherosclerotic plaque. However, since atherosclerotic plaque is present in the vast majority of patients with ischemic heart disease, a major effort must be made to understand the possible interactions between the pathophysiologic effects of atherosclerotic vascular disease and the effects of the elements of the thrombotic process.

FIBRIN-PLATELET CORONARY THROMBOSIS

Since before the turn of this century, pathologists have demonstrated that most patients who come to autopsy following a clinical myocardial infart have coronary thrombosis [1, 2]. When thrombus is present, it is almost always found in the epicardial coronary artery that provides blood to the infarcted area of myocardium. The thrombus is usually about 1 cm in length, and it is commonly attached to the vessel wall in an area that is severely narrowed by atherosclerotic

Wagner GS (ed): Myocardial Infarction: Measurement and Intervention, pp 457–477.
© *1982 Martinus Nijhoff Publishers, The Hague/Boston/London.*

plaque [3]. A large majority of recently formed coronary thrombi are associated with ulceration, erosion, or rupture of this underlying plaque [4]. This disruption of the vascular endothelium is thought by some to be the event that initiates the thrombogenic process.

A fresh thrombus is composed of platelets, red blood cells, and fibrin (Figures 1 and 2). Judging from histologic markers, the coronary thrombus probably begins as a small nidus of platelets at a site of disruption of endothelium. This nidus probably grows over some variable period of time to form a partially occlusive platelet plug. As the plug grows, fibrin and red and white blood cells are incorporated. The thrombus grows by the addition of cellular and fibrinous material proximally in the vessel [3].

While there is general agreement among pathologists about the morphology of coronary thrombosis, there is controversy about the temporal and causal relationship of the thrombus to acute myocardial infarct [5, 6]. Early investigators tended to relate the presence of thrombosis to myocardial infarct as causal [1, 2]. Subsequently, cases were described in which thrombosis had occurred without infarct [7]. The protection from infarct in these hearts was thought to be collateral blood vessels. Other investigators showed that infarct could be demonstrated in hearts where no coronary thrombosis was present. These hearts tended to show patchy, nontransmural infarct and severe, multiple-vessel atheroscerotic disease [8]. As a result of these studies and others [9] a feeling evolved, which is now widely held by pathologists, that transmural myocardial infarcts are usually the result of coronary occlusion by thrombus and that nontransmural infarcts are usually due to hypoperfusion not related to coronary thrombosis. Unfortunately, again, this feeling is not consensus. Several groups of investigators have shown that the rate of demonstration of thrombosis with myocardial infarct is very high. On the other hand, other groups have found the rate of thrombosis in patients with myocardial infarct who come to autopsy to be as low as 20%–50%. This discrepancy probably results in part from differences in case selection and definition. For instance, the term 'large' to describe an infarct has been applied to areas that measure more than 3 cm in diameter and to areas determined by three-dimensional mapping to be more than 40% or 50% of the ventricular myocardium. These two methods would probably select slightly different groups of patients.

Other differences in case selection probably stem from inadequate comparability of clinical markers. Thrombus in a coronary artery is more easily identified if the thrombus is fresh rather than partially or completely organized. Therefore the duration of time between clinical infarct and autopsy must be comparable if two groups of cases are to be compared. Moreover, the clinical circumstances of the deaths seem to be important variables in the selection of groups of patients with and without coronary thrombosis at autopsy. Patients who die very suddenly are unlikely to have coronary thrombosis, while patients who die after

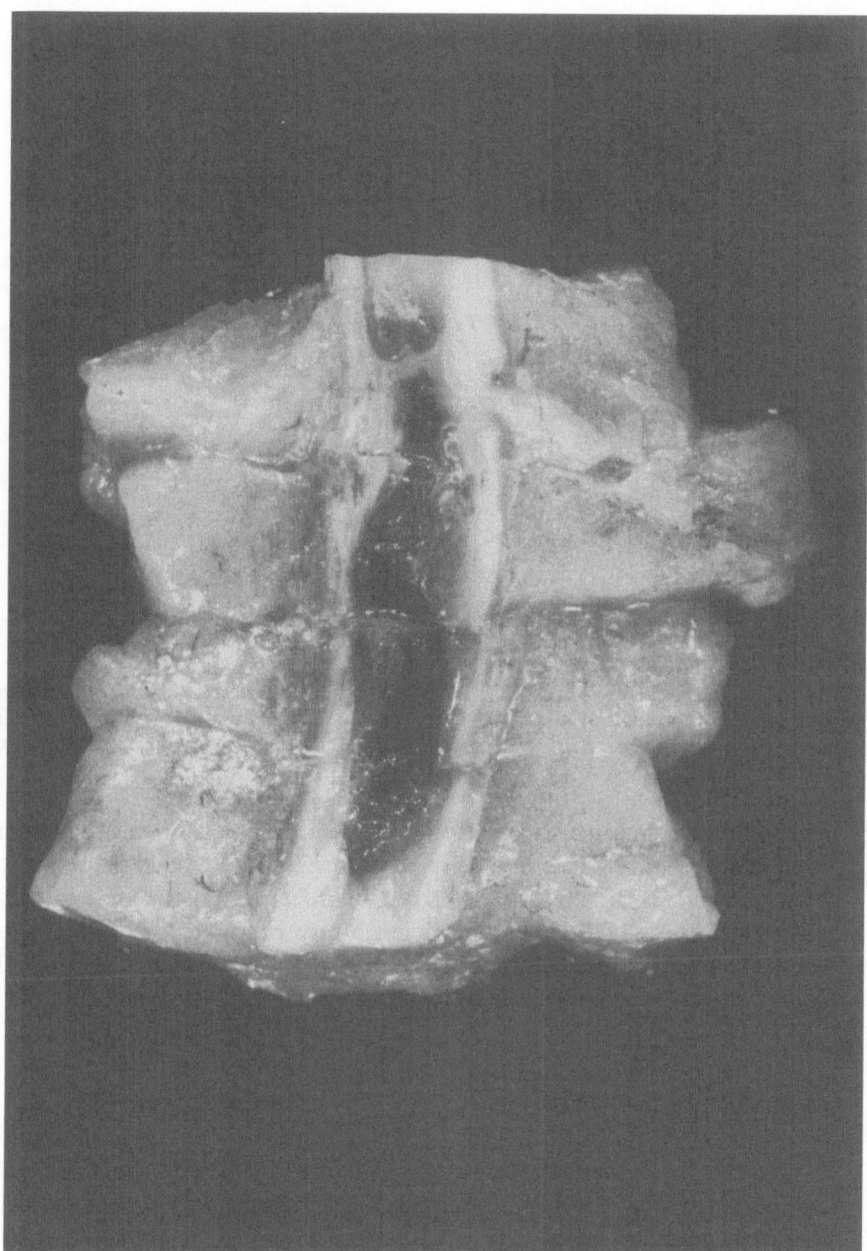

Figure 1. Coronary thrombosis. The coronary artery was cut along its length from proximal above to distal below. Atherosclerotic stenoses are present in the artery at both ends of the thrombosis. The patient died from myocardial rupture 8 h after the onset of chest pain.

460

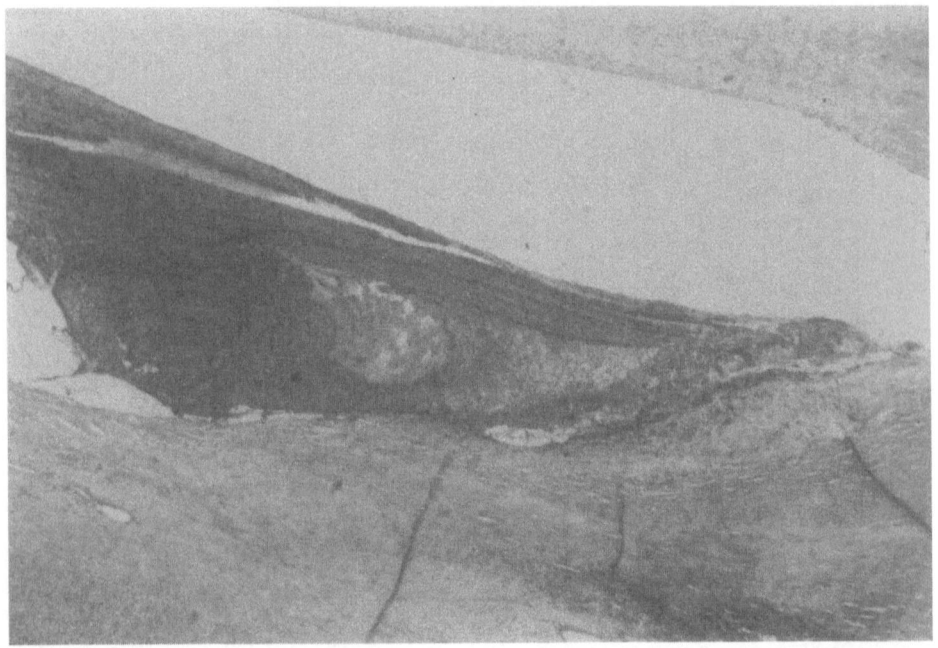

Figure 2. A platelet-fibrin coronary thrombus. Note the platelet head at the point of attachment of the thrombus to the wall of the vessel and the fibrin-red blood cell tail. The streaming effect is associated with layering of platelets and fibrin. Phosphotungstic acid hematoxylin stain, × 60.

a period of cardiogenic shock have a greater likelihood of having coronary thrombosis [3]. This latter point has been used as evidence that the thrombosis results from stasis in the coronary artery after infarct and therefore results from, rather than causes, the infarct. This controversy continues, and the problems with case selection and definitions are unresolved. It appears now, in fact, that the controversy is unlikely to be solved by studies of autopsy material.

ANTICOAGULANT DRUGS

In spite of the continuing disagreement among pathologists about the causal relationship between coronary thrombosis and myocardial infarct, many attempts have been made to show that inhibition of some aspect of the coagulation process would prevent, reduce, or remove coronary thrombosis and limit the evolution of acute myocardial infarct. Only very recently has the ability to inhibit platelet function been available. Therefore most of the studies have employed heparin or warfarin anticoagulants or fibrinolytic agents. The effects of these agents were assessed primarily by comparing morality between treated and untreated groups. No study has demonstrated the ability of one of these agents to reduce the size of myocardial infarct in humans.

The efficacy of heparin during the early stage of myocardial infarct has been considered to be no better than oral anticoagulation [10, 11]. However, Griffin and Boggs have claimed, without supporting evidence, that chest pain may be reduced by the early use of heparin [12]. More recently, Saliba et al. have shown that large doses of heparin administered to dogs after coronary ligation reduce the degree of epicardial ST segment elevation, the degree of myocardial creatine kinase depletion, and the extent of histologically determined myocardial necrosis [13]. There was no known component of thrombosis in their acute model, so the mechanism of these effects may well have been unrelated to thrombosis. Although no similar study has been done in humans, there are data from studies of patients with preinfarct angina that suggest that the rate of infarct and subsequent death is reduced by the use of anticoagulating doses of heparin [14, 15]. The design of these studies has been questioned, however, and the use of high-dose heparin in treatment of unstable angina pectoris has largely been replaced by use of vasodilators, beta-adrenergic-blocking agents and calcium-binding agents.

The use of oral anticoagulant drugs, with or without heparin, to inhibit evolution of acute myocardial infarct has also been intensively studied. These agents probably have a beneficial effect on mortality, but the mechanism is as likely to be prevention of the thromboembolic complications of myocardial infarct as inhibition of the development of coronary thrombosis. Since the first big clinical trial of anticoagulant therapy in myocardial infarct in 1948 [16], an enormous number of studies have been done that either confirm or deny an effect of anticoagulation on mortality and morbidity after acute myocardial infarct. Chalmers et al. critically reviewed 32 such trials in 1977 [17]. Data from these trials showed a significantly lower rate of thromboembolism and mortality in the treated group (15.4% mortality) compared with the untreated group (19.6% mortality). The authors pointed out that the demonstrated effect on mortality was possible only because the data from multiple trials were pooled; they also argued that the well-controlled, randomized trials included in the review had failed to show significant differences because of the inadequate numbers of patients studied. The mechanisms by which anticoagulation might have brought about the observed reduction in mortality were not discussed. It seems highly probable that a major part of the patient salvage was the result of reduced thromboembolism. There are no data from these trials to suggest that the mass of infarcted myocardium was reduced in patients treated with anticoagulant drugs. Further, these trials provide no evidence that patients treated with anticoagulation suffered less heart failure or fewer immediately recurrent myocardial infarcts than the nontreated group.

462

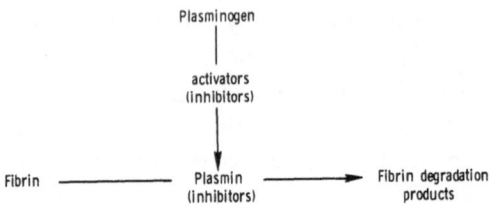

Figure 3. Fibrin clot is lysed by the enzymatic action of plasmin. Plasmin is a product of the cleavage of a precursor, plasminogen, by a number of activators. Among these activators are streptokinase and urokinase, two agents that have been used to stimulate the therapeutic lysis of clot. There are circulating inhibitors to both the activation of plasminogen and the action of plasmin. However, inhibitors are less active within the clot matrix than the activators, a situation that is thought to account for the fact that lysis of formed clot can occur without simultaneous uncontrolled systemic fibrinogenolysis.

The effect of anticoagulation on prevention of recurrent myocardial infarct has also been argued. Several clinical trials have shown slightly reduced rates of recurrent infarct in treated patients. The improvement in most studies was usually demonstrable only within the first two years [18]. The better-controlled studies, however, failed to show significant differences in mortality or incidence of recurrent myocardial infarct [19].

In summary, coronary platelet-fibrin thrombosis seems to occur frequently after acute myocardial infarct, especially in hearts with large, transmural infarcts. However, the causal relationship between the thrombosis and the infarct is still hotly debated [20]. Data from numerous clinical trials have failed to show conclusively that anticoagulant agents will prevent myocardial infarct, will alter mortality from recurrent or expanded myocardial infarct, or will reduce the morbidity from heart failure after myocardial infarct.

FIBRINOLYTIC AGENTS

The notion that myocardial infarct may be caused or aggravated by thrombosis precipitated thoughts about the possible benefits of fibrinolytic agents as early as 1959 [21]. Subsequently, many studies examined the feasibility of the use of systemic fibrinolytic agents in patients with myocardial infarcts, and the results from a number of controlled clinical studies are now available. Although these results are tainted to some degree by problems with study design, they can be used in a limited fashion to provide some information about the possible relationship between the hemostatic system and the evolution of myocardial infarct. The clinical experience with intracoronary thrombolytic therapy during the early hours of acute infarction is discussed in the chapter by Gold and Leinbach (p. 511).

Fibrinolysis involves a complicated system of enzymatic activators and inhibitors (Figure 3). The key element in this system is plasmin, a proteolytic enzyme that can cleave peptides from fibrin. Plasmin, in turn, is the product of proteolysis of a precursor, plasminogen. There are probably several enzymatic activators of plasminogen. Plasminogen activator can be released from vessel walls at the time of an injury, for instance. Additionally, there are circulating plasminogen activators that will become active upon the exposure of factor XII to a surface. Under normal circumstances, these activators are controlled by circulating inhibitors. Within a fibrin clot matrix, however, the inhibitors of plasminogen activation, as well as inhibitors of plasmin function, are excluded or diluted, and fibrin degradation progresses. Fibrinolytic agents used for therapeutic purposes act by cleaving plasminogen to produce plasmin.

There are two plasminogen activators that have been used extensively in humans: streptokinase and urokinase. Streptokinase is a protein secreted by hemolytic streptococci. It is easily produced and relatively inexpensive. Since streptokinase is a foreign protein in humans, however, it is immunogenic. Antibodies produced in a patient as a result of previous treatment with streptokinase or because of previous infection with streptococci can cause both resistance to the fibrinolytic effects of the drug and systemic allergic reactions. Fortunately, most of the systemic reactions involve simply chills and fever. Further, the inhibitory effects of antibodies have been shown to be satisfactorily overcome by use of a loading dose for the purpose of blocking the antibodies.

Urokinase is a trace protein secreted by human kidneys and by human kidney cells in culture. The major problem with this agent in the past has been the expense of extracting it from human urine. The use of cell culture systems, however, has reduced the cost somewhat. Urokinase has been used in just one controlled clinical trial in patients with myocardial infarct. However, there is extensive clinical experience with the use of this agent in this country because of the Urokinase Pulmonary Embolism trial [22].

Fibrinolytic agents could work by several mechanisms to limit the evolution of an acute myocardial infarct. It might be assumed that the lysis of an occluding thrombus in a major coronary artery would allow reperfusion of infarcted myocardium (see Gold and Leinbach, p. 511).

A second therapeutic effect of fibrinolysis in myocardial infarct involves the microcirculation around the area of infarct. It is assumed that the cellular dysfunction and edema in the area of myocardium adjacent to an infarct disrupt normal flow in the microcirculation and thereby promote deposition of platelets and fibrin. This coagulation process, in turn, further embarrasses flow of nutrients and oxygen to, and removal of toxins from, myocardial cells in the area around the infarct. There is the possibility, therefore, that fibrinolytic removal of the products of coagulation in the microcirculation would help preserve blood flow to cellular elements in periinfarct areas. The result of successful maintenance of flow to these areas would be preservation of myocardium. This mechanism might be equally effective whether or not the infarct is precipitated by a coronary artery thrombosis.

Nydick et al. have studied the effects of fibrinolysis on the microcirculation [23]. They studied dogs by occluding a diagonal branch of the left anterior descending coronary artery for 3 h. Animals treated with an infusion of plasmin starting 2 h after the occlusion and lasting 5 h were compared with control animals. The extent of gross infarct was estimated, and microscopic sections of myocardium were examined for presence of microthrombi. The investigators noted confluent transmural myocardial infarct in 11 of 13 control dogs as compared with two of 15 treated dogs. Hearts from treated dogs showed predominantly small focal and subendocardial infarcts. Microthrombi were noted in 10 of the 13 control animals as compared with two of 15 treated animals. Therefore, the fibrinolytic treatment was associated with a marked reduction in the incidence of microthrombi, which in turn was associated with reduction in the extent of myocardial necrosis. These findings suggest, but do not prove, the contention that fibrinolytic therapy limits infarct size by preventing or destroying microthrombi in periinfarct vessels.

Effects of fibrinolysis on both the rheologic properties of flowing blood and the determinants of myocardial oxygen demand have been demonstrated. Removal of the fibrinogen and other proteins by lysis reduces the viscosity of the plasma. This reduced viscosity can result in improved flow via microcirculation to ischemic areas. There are no direct data to support a major role of this mechanism in altering perfusion to threatened areas of myocardium after myocardial infarct.

There are data to suggest an effect of streptokinase on myocardial oxygen demand. Patients with acute myocardial infarct who had no evidence of heart failure have been shown to experience a decrease in systemic vascular resistance after treatment with streptokinase [24]. The fall in systemic vascular resistance was associated with a small fall in arterial blood pressure and a significant increase of cardiac output. Patients receiving heparin showed no change in any of these hemodynamic parameters. Similarly, patients in the European Cooperative Study Group [25] who received streptokinase had a greater decrease in arterial blood pressure and pulmonary artery pressure than did control patients. The mechanism for this effect of streptokinase is not known, nor is it known that urokinase would cause similar hemodynamic changes in patients with myocardial infarct. The possibility that streptokinase may cause a decreased demand of myocardium for oxygen deserves further study.

An effect by any of these mechanisms, or by any combination of the mechanisms, would result in preservation of periinfarct myocardium. Several controlled clinical trials have used death as the primary endpoint. If reduction in infarct size is reflected in decreased mortality, then death from pump failure or from arrhythmia associated with left ventricular dysfunction should be noticably reduced. This information is not clearly identified in many of the clinical trials, but some indications of an effect of treatment on ventricular dysfunction can be distinguished among the data from those trials.

Table 1. Controlled clinical trials of systemic fibrinolytic agents in patients with acute myocardial infarcts

References	Patients Treated No.	Control No.	Mortality Treated %	Control %	Observation Period Days[b]	Effect on Heart failure Reported
Schmutzler et al. [26]	297	261	14.1[a]	21.7	40	+
Schmutzler et al. [27]	138	131	14.5[a]	26.0	40	+
Amery et al. [28]	83	84	24.1	17.9	H	−
European Working Party [29]	373	357	18.5[a]	26.3	H	+
Heikinheimo et al. [30]	219	207	9.2	9.0	42	−
Breddin et al. [31]	102	104	12.7[a]	27.9	H	−
Dioguardi et al. (CCU)[c] [32]	164	157	11.6	11.5	40	−
Burkart et al. [33]	159	158	17.0	13.9	21	−
Bett et al. (CCU)[c] [34]	321	332	15.3	17.5	365	−
Aber et al. (CCU)[c] [35]	302	293	15.9	17.8	180	−
European COOP (CCU) [25]	155	157	15.6[a]	30.6	180	+

[a] $p < 0.01$.
[b] H, hospital stay.
[c] (CCU), most patients treated in coronary units.

The key elements of the studies and results are shown in Table 1 [25–35]. All of the studies except that of Burkart [33] used systemic streptokinase. The dose was usually 250,000 units for a loading effect followed by a 12- to 24-h infusion of 100,000 units per hour. An important exception to this general protocol was that used in the Frankfurt study [31] where the infusion was continued for only 3 h. These authors showed a significant reduction in mortality among patients treated with this short infusion. The rate of complications was said to be acceptable by the authors of each of the studies. There seemed to be little increased bleeding associated with the fibrinolytic agents over that caused by heparin or warfarin. The one exception to this statement was the bleeding from recent puncture sites and around indwelling catheters. The bleeding associated with fibrinolysis usually stopped shortly after infusion was discontinued.

While the risks of the systemic fibrinolytic therapy were low, the benefits were not well documented. Results of the trials usually showed some trend toward improved mortality among treated patients, but this trend failed to achieve statistical significance in most of the better-designed studies. There were also strategic differences between the studies that make pooling data or even comparing the results difficult [36, 37]. However, bits of data from several studies support the notion that fibrinolytic agents might affect the extent of an evolving myocardial infarct. The study reported by the European Working Party [29] demonstrated a significantly reduced mortality among treated patients compared with controls (19.0% vs 27.4%). Heart failure was the cause of death in 4.3% of the treated patients compared with 10.6% of the control patients. This difference was significant. Heart failure was the only cause of death that differed in incidence between the two groups of patients. Similarly, the incidence of heart failure was significantly less among treated patients compared with the controls in the second German—Swiss trial [27]. A lower incidence of ventricular dysfunction among treated patients was also suggested in the latest report from the European Cooperative Study Group [25]. Their data showed a significantly greater incidence of cardiomegaly among control patients. Perhaps more importantly, the European Cooperative Study, uniquely among the more recent studies, showed a reduction of mortality associated with streptokinase treatment in a subgroup selected for moderate and high risk [25]. The criteria for increased risk included hypotension, tachycardia, tachypnea, elevated central venous pressure, arrhythmia, heart block, and second or subsequent infarct. Most of these criteria represent ventricular dysfunction. Additionally, the reduced mortality was most apparent during the period starting three weeks after the acute infarct and continuing for six months. The delayed benefit from an infusion administered during the first 24 h after an acute infarct would conceivably be derived from preservation of myocardium during the evolutionary phase of the infarct.

In summary, fibrinolytic agents administered systemically at the time of an acute myocardial infarct may exert several effects that could improve the clinical course of the patient. Intracoronary administration as presented in the chapter by Gold and Leinbach may facilitate lysis of the acute coronary thrombosis. Preliminary studies indicate that this route of administration may achieve reperfusion and therefore limitation of infarct size without significant systemic side effects.

PLATELET-MEDIATED EFFECTS IN MYOCARDIAL INFARCT

As noted above, the inception of a coronary artery thrombosis probably occurs when platelets begin to adhere at a site of endothelial injury. In humans, the injury in the endothelium is associated with an atherosclerotic plaque. There is a void in our understanding of the events surrounding the injury, the platelet and plasma responses to the injury, and the subsequent clinical events that transpire as a result of these responses. However, enthusiasm exists in the scientific and clinical communities for hypotheses that suggest that the interaction between

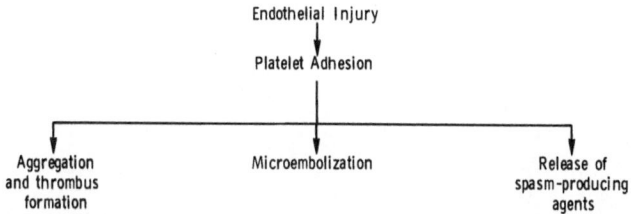

Figure 4. The activation of platelets after endothelial injury in a stenotic coronary artery might lead to myocardial ischemia by one of at least three mechanisms: (a) platelet adhesion at the point of injury might stimulate formation of platelet aggregation and thrombosis, (b) there may be obstruction in myocardial microvasculature by small platelet emboli, and (c) there may be coronary artery spasm as a response to vasoactive agents released from the activated platelets.

the platelet and the vessel wall might initiate a series of events that can create and modulate myocardial ischemia, myocardial infarct, and even sudden death.

The information about the process of platelet response to endothelial injury is based almost entirely upon studies in animal models (Figure 4–6). After removal of arterial endothelium in almost any animal preparation, there is an immediate deposition of adherent platelets on the subendothelial surface. The platelets are either individually attached to some component of the subendothelium and intact with demonstrable organelles; spread across the surface of the subendothelium with most of the organelles missing; or part of an aggregate, only a part of which is in contact with the subendothelium. The layer of spread platelets is the most consistent finding, while there is some disagreement about the presence and quantity of platelet aggregates and nonadherent platelets. It appears, in fact, that platelet thrombi are a transient phenomenon [38]. This process of platelet adhesion to the subendothelium is affected by numerous variables including the number and functional state of the platelets, the concentration of other cellular elements of the blood, flow rates, vessel geometry, von Willebrand factor, coagulability, and divalent cations [39].

There are also many variables that influence the development of platelet aggregation in an artery [40]. Aggregation probably involves a cascade of events starting with adhesion. Mediators that play a major role in the aggregation processes include von Willebrand factor, arachidonic acid metabolites, especially thromboxane A_2, adenosine diphosphate (ADP), and thrombin. Injury of the vessel wall and adhesion of platelets result in generation of small amounts of thrombin and contact between platelets and collagen. Collagen stimulates platelet-to-platelet aggregation. Aggregation, in turn, leads to the release of ADP, a potent aggregating agent, which, in turn, liberates arachidonic acid from the platelets. Metabolism of the arachidonic acid by enzymatic processes leads to the production of thromboxane A_2, another highly potent aggregating agent. Thrombin also can stimulate arachidonic acid metabolism and is itself, either by

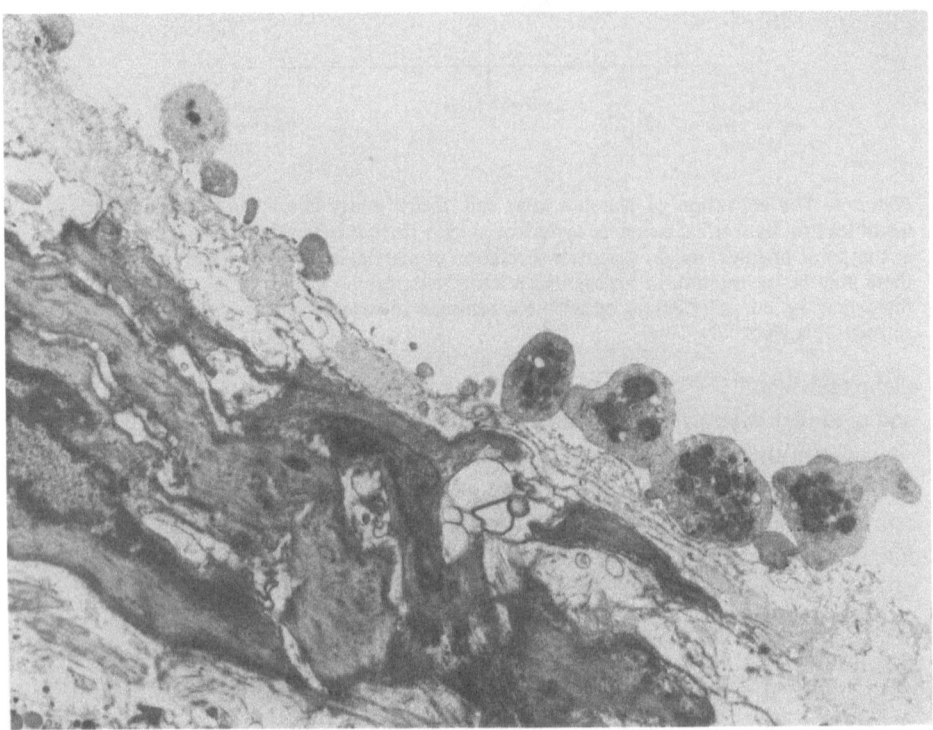

Figure 5. Porcine coronary artery after balloon denudation of endothelium. Nondegranulated platelets cover a portion of the vessel wall where the endothelium has been denudated. Platelet pseudopods are present but are short and broad. In this area, the platelets do not appear to be in contact with collagen but are instead adjacent to the laminated basement membrane present in swine coronary arteries. Smooth muscle cells are present deep to these areas. X 7200.

this mechanism or others, a potent aggregator of platelets. These interacting mediators and the control mechanisms that are related to them may well contribute to coronary or microvascular obstruction and therefore to clinical myocardial ischemia. The obstruction to flow in the coronary vascular system after platelet activation may also involve vascular spasm. This possibility is suggested by the results of experiments that show that thromboxane A_2 is a potent stimulator of arterial smooth muscle contraction [41, 42].

The clinical data linking platelet activation to myocardial ischemia and infarction are few and indirect [43, 44]. They demonstate slightly greater incidence and number of platelet microthrombi in the myocardial microvasculature of people with coronary disease who died suddenly than in people who died of other causes. Jørgensen et al. [45] have shown that injection of the aggregating

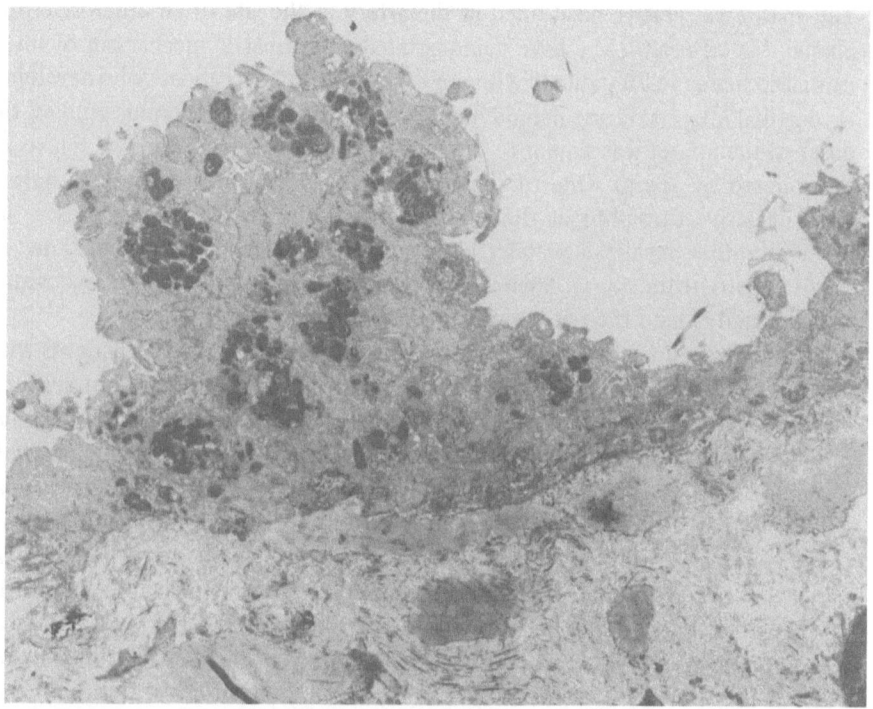

Figure 6. Porcine coronary artery after balloon denudation of endothelium. A small platelet thrombus is present in an area of complete endothelial denudation. Degranulated platelets and platelets with centralized granules make up the thrombus. The elastica is fragmented and the clump of platelets is in contact with both the elastica and collagen present in the subendothelium. X 6000.

agent, ADP, into the coronary arteries and left ventricles of experimental pigs precipitates myocardial infarct and, occasionally, sudden ventricular fibrillation. In recent studies in humans, it has been shown that circulating platelet aggregates are increased after acute myocardial infarct [46], that a platelet-derived clotting factor (platelet factor 4) is elevated in the plasma of patients with acute coronary ischemic syndromes [47], and that platelet factor 4 is elevated in patients with exercise-induced angina pectoris [48].

Of particular interest in a discussion of limitation of infarct size are some of the studies that indirectly implicate platelet activation in the relationship between coronary spasm and myocardial infarct. Hillis and Braunwald have reviewed the subject of coronary artery spasm [49]. It is now accepted that variant angina pectoris can occur spontaneously and without a preceding change in myocardial oxygen demand. These spontaneous episodes have been directly associated with angiographically documented coronary artery spasm. Spasm in coronary arteries has been demonstrated in 40% of patients with acute myocardial infarcts [50]. The spasm was always positioned in the artery at the site of an atherosclerotic plaque. Maseri et al. [51] have demonstrated a vasospastic mechanism of myocardial ischemia in 76 patients with angina at rest. In two patients who developed myocardial infarcts during hemodynamic monitoring or angiographic studies, the onset of the infarct was similar to the previous onset of angina and was felt to be precipitated by spasm. One of these patients was shown at autopsy to have a fresh occlusive thrombus at the site of previous spasm. The authors raised the possibility that localized platelet aggregation and release of thromboxane A_2 might potentiate the spasm. Such an effect might serve to prolong the myocardial ischemia and extend the potential area of the infarct.

In a similar clinical experiment, angiography was performed in patients with acute coronary insufficiency, who commonly demonstrated severe but subtotal stenosis of a major coronary artery [52]. Patients who experienced myocardial infarcts usually were shown to have complete occlusion at follow-up angiographic examination. Key findings in this study included the lack of evidence that collateral circulation improved after the acute episode of unstable angina pectoris resolved. Additionally, there was no difference in tolerance to atrial pacing in patients who were tested before and after the episode of unstable angina pectoris. These findings supported the contention that the angina at rest was associated with temporary, high-grade stenosis of the coronary artery. The authors propose that the unstable period is caused by platelet activation, aggregation and, perhaps, some related spasm. They feel that the subsequent infarct results from failure of the platelet activation process to be resolved.

There is evidence, therefore, that platelet aggregation can precipitate myocardial ischemia in animals, that coronary ischemic events in humans are associated with evidence of platelet activation, and that changes in coronary vessels that precede myocardial infarcts in some circumstances might be precipitated by platelet activation. These findings have engendered an interest in the possibility that the use of antiplatelet agents might alter the course of acute coronary syndromes. This interest has stimulated a number of excellent reviews on the pharmacology of antiplatelet drugs [40, 53–56]. Unfortunately there are no acceptable studies that show an effect of antiplatelet drugs in patients with acute myocardial infarcts.

ANTIPLATELET AGENTS

A number of antiplatelet agents have been shown to modify the evolution of myocardial infarct in animals. Folts et al. [57] have developed a model with cyclic reductions in coronary flow that are probably related to recurrent platelet aggregate formation at the site of a partial coronary occlusion. In their model, aspirin abolishes the cyclic reductions in flow. In one set of experiments, the reduced flow phase precipitated electrocardiographic changes in 24 of 35 dogs, including sudden death in six of the 24. This model is reminiscent of the hypothesis proposed by Neill et al. [52] that temporary high-grade or complete stenosis at a point of an atherosclerotic lesion is a mechanism responsible for the acute coronary insufficiency syndrome.

Other authors have highlighted the possible effects of aspirin on occlusive platelet aggregation in the myocardial microcirculation. Moschos et al. [58] produced an occlusive thrombus in the coronary arteries of dogs by administering a low-amperage electrical current to the coronary endothelium. Radiolabeled platelets were used to monitor the extent of microembolization to the ischemic and infarcted area. Aspirin, dipyridamole, and a crude thrombolytic agent all reduced the extent of the distribution of the radiolabel, and aspirin significantly reduced the incidence of ventricular fibrillation. Subsequently, in an experiment using nonthrombotic occlusion of the artery, Vik-Mo [59] showed that aspirin reduces ST segment elevations but does not affect the concentration of platelet aggregates in the coronary sinus blood. This raises the possibility that the aspirin might affect the ischemic myocardium by a mechanism that is not related to platelet aggregation.

An effect by aspirin on myocardial ischemia other than or in addition to the antiplatelet mechanism would probably involve an antiinflammatory action related to prostaglandin inhibition. Ibuprofen, a prostaglandin inhibitor with an antiplatelet effect, has been shown to reduce the size of an evolving myocardial infarct in a subacute dog model [60]. Recurrent injections of radiolabeled microspheres and postmortem angiography showed that the salvage of myocardium with ibuprofen was associated with no detectable preservation of periinfarct collateral circulation. The authors postulated that the ibuprofen was effective because of a membrane-stabilizing mechanism but that an antiplatelet mechanism could not be excluded. Lefer and Polansky [61] have also shown that ibuprofen will reduce the extent of a myocardial infarct.

Another antiplatelet agent that will reduce the size of an experimental myocardial infarct is dipyridamole [62]. Experiments with this drug highlight the multiplicity of possible mechanisms by which a single agent may work. The mean aortic blood pressure and the heart rate fell significantly in cats with experimental myocardial infarcts. The changes effected a significant fall in the tension-time index. Therefore, the demonstrated beneficial effect on infarct size might well have been related to decreased myocardial oxygen demand. Further, it has been well known for years that dipyridamole is a potent coronary vasodilator. Of course, there is a great possibility that that drug functions because of the combined effect of these actions. There is a comprehensive discussion of the possible mechanisms of action of dipyridamole in a paper by Feinberg et al. [63].

At this time, the most obvious test of a platelet function inhibitor in myocardial infarction would involve the intracoronary infusion of prostacyclin. Prostacyclin is a product of the enzymatic conversion of prostaglandin H_2. The enzyme that catalyzes this reaction is produced by endothelial cells. Prostacyclin is a potent inhibitor of platelet aggregation and a vasodilator [40], and has been used in the treatment of peripheral vascular disease [64]. Additionally, several groups are performing animal studies with the agent in anticipation of further human use. The drug, as it is now used, produces profound hypotension in animals and humans, a problem that has limited its use. However, an effort is underway to develop a similar agent with specific coronary vasodilatory and antiplatelet effects.

While there are no studies that examine the effects of antiplatelet agents in patients with acute myocardial infarcts, two studies of antiplatelet agents in patients in the recovery and chronic phases after a myocardial infarct have recently been published. The first is the sulfinpyrazone trial [65], which showed a reduction in the incidence of sudden death during the period between one month and six months after an acute myocardial infarct. The incidence of nonfatal reinfarction in the treated group was not reduced. The mechanism of the effect is unknown.

The second secondary prevention study examined the efficacy of aspirin [66]. It involved patients who were entered as late as five years after their infarct. The results showed no differences between treated and placebo groups in either mortality or incidence of reinfarct. There was significantly more gastrointestinal symptomatology in the treated group.

CONCLUSIONS

The bulk of the published evidence would support a conclusion that thrombosis is involved in the pathophysiology of an acute myocardial infarct [67] and probably accounts in part for the size of an infarct. The experimental and pathologic evidence suggests strongly that the platelet plays an important part in the process since it is involved in the initiation of the response to vascular injury. The modern literature suggests that platelet activation might be involved in vascular spasm as well as in the thrombus formation. There have been studies in humans with acute myocardial infarcts [68, 69] that indicate that antithrombotic agents will influence the evolution of the infarct (see Gold, p. 511). Finally, while there are no studies of antiplatelet agents in patients with acute myocardial infarcts there is great interest in the multiple roles that platelets play in the arterial thrombosis process. Experimental data demonstrate that aggregation can precipitate ischemic events. Additionally, a vast amount of new data has shown key metabolic events related to platelet function that could play a role in myocardial ischemia and infarct. Pharmacologic manipulation of some of these metabolic events may well make it possible to significantly limit the extent of an evolving acute myocardial infarct.

REFERENCES

1. Herrick JB: Clinical features of sudden obstruction of the coronary arteries. JAMA 59:2015–2020, 1912.
2. Herrick JB: Thrombosis of the coronary arteries. JAMA 72:387–390, 1919.
3. Roberts WC, Buja LM: The frequency and significance of coronary arterial thrombi and other observations in fatal acute myocardial infarction: a study of 107 necropsy patients. Am J Med 52:425–443, 1972.
4. Ridolfi RL, Hutchins GM: The relationship between coronary artery lesions and myocardial infarcts: ulceration of atherosclerotic plaques precipitating coronary thrombosis. Am Heart J 93:468–486, 1977.
5. Chandler AB, Chapman I, Erhardt LR, Roberts WC, Schwartz CJ, Sinapius D, Spain DM, Sherry S, Ness PM, Simon TL: Coronary thrombosis in myocardial infarction. Report of a workshop on the role of coronary thrombosis in the pathogenesis of acute myocardial infarction. Am J Cardiol 34:823–833, 1974.
6. Roberts WC: Coronary artery pathology in fatal ischemic heart disease. In: Braunwald E, Selwyn A (eds) The myocardium: failure and infarction. New York: HP Publishing Co, 1974, pp 192–204.
7. Blumgart HL, Schlesinger MJ, Davis D: Studies on the relation of the clinical manifestations of angina pectoris, coronary thrombosis, and myocardial infarction to the pathologic findings with particular reference to the significance of the collateral circulation. Am Heart J 19:1–91, 1940.
8. Friedberg CK, Horn H: Acute myocardial infarction not due to coronary artery occlusion. JAMA 112:1675–1679, 1939.
9. Miller RD, Burchell HB, Edwards JE: Myocardial infarction with and without acute coronary occlusion. A pathologic study. Arch Intern Med 88:597–604, 1951.
10. Nordöy S, Benestad AM: Evaluation of the effect of heparin in addition to oral anticoagulant therapy in acute myocardial infarction. Acta Med Scand 174:627–634, 1963.
11. Eastman GL, Cook ET, Shinn ET, Dutton RE, Lyons RH: A clinical study of anticoagulants in acute myocardial infarction with particular reference to early heparin therapy. Am J Med Sci 233:647–653, 1957.
12. Griffith GC, Boggs RP: The clinical usage of heparin. Am J Cardiol 14:39–46, 1964.
13. Saliba MJ Jr, Covell JW, Bloor CM: Effects of heparin in large doses on the extent of myocardial ischemia after acute coronary occlusion in the dog. Am J Cardiol 37:599–604, 1976.
14. Nichol ES, Phillips WC, Casten GG: Virtue of prompt anticoagulant therapy in impending myocardial infarction: experiences with 318 patients during a 10-year period. Ann Intern Med 50:1158–1173, 1959.
15. Wood P: Acute and subacute coronary insufficiency. Br Med J 1:1779–1782, 1961.
16. Wright IS, Marple CD, Beck DF: Report of the committee for the evaluation

474

of anticoagulants in the treatment of coronary thrombosis with myocardial infarction (A progress report on the statistical analysis of the first 800 cases studied by this committee). Am Heart J 36:801–815, 1948.

17. Chalmers TC, Matta RJ, Smith H Jr, Kunzler AM: Evidence favoring the use of anticoagulants in the hospital phase of acute myocardial infarction. N Engl J Med 297:1091–1096, 1977.

18. Ebert RV: Anticoagulants in acute myocardial infarction. Results of a cooperative clinical trial. JAMA 225:724–729, 1973.

19. Seaman AJ, Griswold HE, Reaume RB, Ritzmann L: Long-term anticoagulant prophylaxis after myocardial infarction. N Engl J Med 281:115–119, 1969.

20. Silver MD, Baroldi G, Mariani F: The relationship between acute occlusive coronary thrombi and myocardial infarction studied in 100 consecutive patients. Circulation 61:219–227, 1980.

21. Fletcher AP, Sherry S, Alkjaersig N, Smyrniotis FE, Jick S: The maintenance of a sustained thrombolytic state in man. II. Clinical observations on patients with myocardial infarction and other thromboembolic disorders. J Clin Invest 38:1111–1120, 1957.

22. Sasahara AA, Hyers TM, Cole CM, Ederer F, Murray JA, Wenger NK, Sherry S, Strengle JM (eds): The urokinase pulmonary embolism trial. A national cooperative study. New York: The American Heart Association, 1973.

23. Nydick I, Ruegsegger P, Bouvier C, Hutter RV, Abarquez R, Cliffton EE, LaDue JS: Salvage of heart muscle by fibrinolytic therapy after experimental coronary occlusion. Am Heart J 61:93–100, 1961.

24. Neuhof H, Hey D, Glaser E, Wolf H, Lasch HG: Hemodynamic reactions induced by streptokinase therapy in patients with acute myocardial infarction. Eur J Intensive Care Med 1:27–30, 1975.

25. European Cooperative Study Group for Streptokinase Treatment in Acute Myocardial Infarction: Streptokinase in acute myocardial infarction. N Engl J Med 301:797–802, 1979.

26. Schmutzler R, Heckner F, Kortge P, van de Loo J, Pezold FA, Poliwoda H, Praetorius F, Zekorn D: Zur thrombolytischen Therapie des frischen Herzinfarktes. I. Einfuhrung, Behandlungspläne, allgemeine klinische Ergebnisse. Dtsch Med Wochenschr 91:581–587, 1966.

27. Gillmann H, Colberg K, Keller HP, Orth HF, Borner W, Fritze E, Gebauer D, Grosser KD, Heckner F, Kortge P, van de Loo J, Pezold FA, Poliwoda H, Praetorius F, Schmutzler R, Schneider B, Zekorn D: Zur fibrinolytischen. Behandlung des akuten Herzinfarktes. II. Deutsch-schweizerische Gemeinschaftsstudie. 2. Ergebrisse der elektrokardiographischen Untersuchungen. Z Kardiol 62:193–214, 1973.

28. Amery A, Roeber G, Vermeulen HJ, Verstraete M: Single-blind randomised multicentre trial comparing heparin and streptokinase treatment in recent myocardial infarction. Acta Med Scand [Suppl 505] 187:5–35, 1969.

29. European Working Party: Streptokinase in recent myocardial infarction: a controlled multicentre trial. Br Med J 3:325–331, 1971.

30. Heikinheimo R, Ahrenberg P, Honkapohja H, Iisalo E, Kallio V, Konttinen Y, Leskinen O, Mustaniemi H, Reinikainen M, Siitonen L: Fibrinolytic treatment in acute myocardial infarction. Acta Med Scand 189:7–13, 1971.

31. Breddin K, Ehrly AM, Fechler L, Frick D, König H, Kraft H, Krause H, Krzywanek HJ, Kutschera J, Lösch HW, Ludwig O, Mikat B, Rausch F, Rosenthal P, Sartory S, Voigt G, Wylicil P: Die Kurzzeitfibrinolyse beim akuten Myokardinfarkt. Dtsch Med Wochenschr 98:861–873, 1973.

32. Dioguardi N, Lotto A, Levi GF, Rota M, Proto C, Mannucci PM, Rossi P, Lomanto B, Mattei G, Fiorelli G, Agostoni A: Controlled trial of streptokinase and heparin in acute myocardial infarction. Lancet 2:891–895, 1971.

33. Burkart F, Duckert F, Straub PW, Frick PG, Schweizer W, Koller F: Die fibrinolytische Therapie beim akuten Myokardinfarkt. Schweiz Med Wochenschr 103:1814–1816, 1973.

34. Bett JHN, Castaldi PA, Hale GS, Isbister JP, McLean KH, O'Sullivan EF, Biggs JC, Chesterman CN, Hirsh J, McDonald IG, Morgan JJ, Rosenbaum M: Australian multicentre trial of streptokinase in acute myocardial infarction. Lancet 1:57–60, 1973.

35. Aber CP, Bass NM, Berry CL, Cardon PHM, Dobbs RJ, Fox KM, Hamblin JJ, Haydu SP, Howitt G, MacIver JE, Portal RW, Raftery EB, Rousell RH, Stock JPP: Streptokinase in acute myocardial infarction: a controlled multicentre study in the United Kingdom. Br Med J 2:1100–1104, 1976.

36. Simon TL, Ware JH, Stengle JM: Clinical trials of thrombolytic agents in myocardial infarction. Ann Intern Med 79:712–719, 1973.

37. Sullivan JM: Streptokinase and myocardial infarction. N Engl J Med 301:836–837, 1979.

38. Baumgartner HR: The role of blood flow in platelet adhesion, fibrin deposition, and formation of mural thrombi. Microvasc Res 5:167–719, 1973.

39. Baumgartner HR: The subendothelial surface and thrombosis. Throm Diath Haemorrh [Suppl] 59:91–105, 1974.

40. Smith JB: The prostanoids in hemostasis and thrombosis. A review. Am J Pathol 99:743–804, 1980.

41. Ellis EF, Oelz O, Roberts LJ II, Payne NA, Sweetman BJ, Nies AS, Oates JA: Coronary arterial smooth muscle contraction by a substance released from platelets: evidence that it is thromboxane A_2. Science 193:1135–1137, 1976.

42. Needleman P, Kulkarni PS, Raz A: Coronary tone modulation: formation and actions of prostaglandins, endoperoxides, and thromboxanes. Science 195:409–412, 1977.

43. Haerem JW: Platelet aggregates in intramyocardial vessels of patients dying suddenly and unexpectedly of coronary artery disease. Atherosclerosis 15:199–213, 1972.

44. Haerem JW: Mural platelet microthrombi and major acute lesions of main epicardial arteries in sudden coronary death. Atherosclerosis 19:529–541, 1974.

45. Jørgensen L, Rowsell HC, Hovig T, Glynn MF, Mustard JF: Adenosine diphosphate-induced platelet aggregation and myocardial infarction in swine. Lab Invest 17:616–644, 1967.

46. Wu KK, Hoak JC: A new method for the quantitative detection of platelet aggregates in patients with arterial insufficiency. Lancet 2:924–926, 1974.

47. Handin RI, McDonough M, Lesch M: Elevation of platelet factor four in acute myocardial infarction: measurement by radioimmunoassay. J Lab Clin Med 91:340–349, 1978.

48. Green LH, Seroppian E, Handin RI: Platelet activation during exercise-induced myocardial ischemia. N Engl J Med 302:193–226, 1980.
49. Hillis LD, Braunwald E: Coronary-artery spasm. N Engl J Med 299:695–702, 1978.
50. Oliva PB, Breckinridge JC: Arteriographic evidence of coronary arterial spasm in acute myocardial infarction. Circulation 56:366–374, 1977.
51. Maseri A, L'Abbate A, Baroldi G, Chierchia S, Marzillia M, Ballestra AM, Severi S, Parodi O, Biagini A, Distante A, Pesola A: Coronary vasospasm as a possible cause of myocardial infarction. A conclusion derived from the study of 'preinfarction' angina. N Engl J Med 299:1271–1277, 1978.
52. Neill WA, Wharton TP Jr., Fluri-Lundeen J, Cohen IS: Acute coronary insufficiency – coronary occlusion after intermittent ischemic attacks. N Engl J Med 302:1157–1202, 1980.
53. Weiss HJ: Antiplatelet drugs – a new pharmacologic approach to the prevention of thrombosis (A review). Am Heart J 92:86–102, 1976.
54. Weiss HJ: Antiplatelet therapy (Part I: Properties of platelets). N Engl J Med 298:1344–1406, 1978.
55. Schafer AI, Handin RI: The role of platelets in thrombotic and vascular disease. Prog Cardiovasc Dis 22: 31–52, 1979.
56. Moncada S, Vane JR: Arachidonic acid metabolites and the interactions between platelets and blood-vessel walls. N Engl J Med 300:1142–1147, 1979.
57. Folts JD, Crowell EB Jr, Rowe GG: Platelet aggregation in partially obstructed vessels and its elimination with aspirin. Circulation 54:365–370, 1976.
58. Moschos CB, Lahiri K, Lyons M, Weisse AB, Oldewurtel HA, Regan TJ: Relation of microcirculatory thrombosis to thrombus in the proximal coronary artery: effect of aspirin, dipyridamole, and thrombolysis. Am Heart J 86:61–68, 1973.
59. Vik-Mo H: Effects of acute myocardial ischaemia on platelet aggregation in the coronary sinus and aorta in dogs. Scand J Haematol 19:68–74, 1977.
60. Jugdutt BI, Hutchins GM, Bulkley BH, Becker LC: Salvage of ischemic myocardium by ibuprofen during infarction in the conscious dog. Am J Cardiol 46:74–82, 1980.
61. Lefer AM, Polansky EW: Beneficial effects of ibuprofen in acute myocardial ischemia. Cardiology 64:265–279, 1979.
62. Roberts AJ, Jacobstein JG, Cipriano PR, Alonso DR, Combes JR, Gay WA Jr: Effectiveness of dipyridamole in reducing the size of experimental myocardial infarction. Circulation 61:228–236, 1980.
63. Feinberg H, Levitsky S, Coughlin TR, Merchant F, Holland CH, O'Donaghue M: Effect of dipyridamole on ischemia-induced changes in cardiac performance and metabolism. J Cardiovasc Pharmacol 2:299–307, 1980.
64. Szczeklik A, Skawinski S, Gluszko P, Nizankowski R, Szczeklik J, Gryglewski RJ: Successful therapy of advanced arteriosclerosis obliterans with prostacyclin. Lancet 1:1111–1114, 1979.
65. The Anturane Reinfarction Trail Research Group: Sulfinpyrazone in the prevention of sudden death after myocardial infarction. N Engl J Med 302:250–256, 1980.
66. Aspirin Myocardial Infarction Study Research Group: A randomized, controlled trial of aspirin in persons recovered from myocardial infarction. JAMA 243:661–669, 1980.

67. DeWood MA, Spores J, Notske R, Mouser LT, Burroughs R, Golden MS, Lang HT: Prevalence of total coronary occlusion during the early hours of transmural myocardial infarction. N Engl J Med 303:897–902, 1980.
68. Ganz W, Buchbinder N, Marcus H, Mondkar A, Maddahi J, Charuzi Y, O'Conner L, Shell W, Fishbein MC, Kass R, Miyamoto A, Swan HJC: Intra-coronary thrombolysis in evolving myocardial infarction. Am Heart J 101:4–13, 1981.
69. Rentrop P, Blanke H, Karsch KR, Kaiser H, Köstering H, Leitz K: Selective intracoronary thrombolysis in acute myocardial infarction and unstable angina pectoris. Circulation 63:307–317, 1981.

20. ALTERATIONS OF THE METABOLIC AND CELLULAR RESPONSES

JUDITH L. SWAIN

This chapter examines the interventions available to limit the extent of a myocardial infarct. Interventions that are thought to directly affect cellular metabolism and/or cellular response to ischemia can be divided into three broad categories: (a) interventions that decrease myocardial energy and substrate demand, (b) interventions that increase oxygen and/or substrate delivery, and (c) interventions that inhibit the inflammatory response and stabilize cell membranes (Table 1). The conclusions about the efficacy of various interventions depend not only on the model of infarction used, but more importantly on the method chosen to quantify the extent of an infarct. The greatest deterrant to evaluating the data regarding a specific intervention is the variety of experimental methods used by different investigators.

INTERVENTIONS DESIGNED TO DECREASE ENERGY AND SUBSTRATE DEMAND

Energy use in the aerobic heart can be equated with myocardial oxygen consumption. Since the amount of energy necessary for the myocardial cell to carry out vital cell processes is only a small percentage of the energy requirements of working muscle, the major determinants of myocardial oxygen consumption result from myocardial contractile activity. The three major determinants of myocardial oxygen consumption in the working heart are: (a) heart rate, (b) left ventricular developed wall tension, and (c) the inotropic state or contractility of the left ventricle [1]. Interventions designed to decrease one or more of the determinants of oxygen consumption include administering beta-blocking agents, stimulating the carotid sinus nerve, reducing afterload with agents such as sodium nitroprusside, using digoxin in the failing heart to decrease wall tension, and treating hypermetabolic disorders such as hyperthyroidism to reduce oxygen demand (see Reimer, Figure 1, p. 398). These interventions act indirectly on the myocardial cell by altering the amount of work the entire organ must carry out. Another intervention to be considered in the overall reduction of myocardial oxygen demand is hypothermia (see Reimer and Jennings, p. 402). With moderate hypothermia (32°C), overall oxygen consumption is directly reduced by

Wagner GS (ed): Myocardial Infarction: Measurement and Intervention, pp 479–501.
© 1982 Martinus Nijhoff Publishers, The Hague/Boston/London.

Table 1. Interventions designed to alter the metabolic and cellular responses to ischemia

I.	Decrease energy and substrate demand Hypothermia
II.	Increase oxygen and/or substrate delivery Oxygen Mannitol Hyaluronidase Glucose—insulin—potassium Purine nucleotide precursors
III.	Decrease inflammatory response and stabilize cell membranes Corticosteroids Cobra venom factor

one-third, and is further reduced secondary to a decrease in heart rate [2]. In a study of dogs in which acute left ventricular failure was produced, elevated left ventricular end-diastolic pressures were decreased by cooling to 32°C and reverted to abnormal levels with rewarming [3]. The evidence suggests that hypothermic treatment may decrease oxygen consumption and therefore possibly salvage ischemic myocardium. Hypothermia has not yet been tested in humans in the setting of acute myocardial infarcts; because of its complexity, it would be expected to be reserved for gravely ill patients.

INTERVENTIONS DESIGNED TO INCREASE OXYGEN AND/OR SUBSTRATE DELIVERY TO THE CELL

This section encompasses three general types of interventions: (a) interventions designed to increase oxygenation, (b) interventions designed to increase perfusion and thereby increase delivery of oxygen and substrates, and (c) interventions designed to increase the cellular content of substrates necessary for energy synthesis.

Oxygen therapy

Hypoxemia is common in patients with acute myocardial infarct. The degree of hypoxemia has been correlated with the severity of infarct as well as with inhospital mortality [4–7]. The effects of hypoxemia on the extent of myocardial necrosis was examined by performing coronary occlusions in two groups of dogs, one ventilated with 10% oxygen [8]. The occlusion produced greater ST segment elevation, greater myocardial creatine kinase depletion, and greater histologic abnormalities in the group breathing 10% oxygen, leading to the conclusion that hypoxemia substantially increased myocardial damage after a coronary occlusion.

Since hypoxemia has been shown to have a deleterious effect on the extent of myocardial necrosis, the correction of this condition should be beneficial. Low-flow oxygen therapy can promptly correct hypoxemia in most patients [4, 5], but is often accompanied by other hemodynamic changes. In patients with acute myocardial infarct, hemodynamic changes during oxygen therapy include a slight increase in arterial blood pressure, a fall in cardiac output, an increase in peripheral vascular resistance, and an increase in both left ventricular end-diastolic pressure and stroke work. These hemodynamic changes tend to increase myocardial oxygen demand. Thus, the increase in oxygen transport is offset by an increase in oxygen demand. Oxygen therapy has been studied in patients with acute myocardial infarct who had mild ($SaO_2 > 90\%$) or severe ($SaO_2 < 90\%$) hypoxemia [4]. Of the 13 mildly hypoxemic patients, 11 exhibited a decrease in cardiac output and stroke volume and an increase in peripheral vascular resistance with oxygen therapy, but did not show a significant increase in oxygen transport. In the group with severe hypoxemia, cardiac output and oxygen transport both increased after oxygen therapy. The authors concluded that oxygen therapy can be beneficial in the face of significant hypoxemia, but may be deleterios in normoxic or mildly hypoxic patients.

The effect of oxygen therapy on oxygen transport in the setting of normoxia and an adequate hemoglobin concentration can be calculated [9]. The binding of oxygen to hemoglobin accounts for the largest portion of oxygen transport. Because of low solubility, only a small amount of oxygen is normally dissolved in blood, with the amount dissolved dependent upon the partial pressure of oxygen. With a pO_2 of 100 mmHg and a normal hemoglobin content, approximately 20 ml oxygen is transported by hemoglobin in 100 ml arterial blood, and only 0.3 ml oxygen is in solution. If the oxygen delivered is increased to 100%, the amount of dissolved oxygen available to the tissues increases to only 1.8 ml/100 ml arterial blood. When the pO_2 was increased in anesthetized dogs from 83 to 435 mmHg by the administration of 100% oxygen, the tissue pO_2 rose by 7 mmHg [10]. Increasing the pO_2 above the normal range under normal atmospheric pressure in the absence of anemia does not appreciably alter delivery of oxygen to tissues.

The effects of oxygen therapy on the extent of myocardial infarct in dogs was studied by Maroko et al. [11], who found that inhalation of 40% oxygen reduced epicardial ST segment elevation in the area distal to the coronary occlusion, and myocardial creatine kinase depletion was decreased 24 h after coronary occlusion. No additional benefits were seen when the oxygen concentration was increased to 100%. It is difficult to explain the beneficial effects of 40% oxygen on the basis of improved oxygen content since this only added approximately 0.3 ml oxygen per 100 cc blood. If the beneficial effects were due to increased oxygen content, then 100% oxygen should have decreased the ischemic area further. The results may be explained by alterations in coronary vascular resistance produced by oxygen therapy. The effect of 100% oxygen on the distribution of myocardial blood flow has been investigated by several groups, Rivas et al. [12] administered 100% oxygen to dogs and examined its effects on regional blood flow in both ischemic and nonischemic regions 45 s after coronary occlusion. They found a uniform decrease in transmural blood flow to all regions of the heart after oxygen administration, and concluded that excessive oxygen inhalation may be deleterious to patients with myocardial ischemia. This conclusion was supported by the work of Malm et al. [13], who studied the effects of 100% oxygen on the area of myocardial ischemia 60 min after coronary occlusion. They found an increase in ischemic area as assessed by thermography in eight of ten dogs after oxygen was given. After cessation of oxygen therapy, the size of the ischemic area decreased. The authors concluded that inhalation of high concentrations of oxygen may be harmful following an acute myocardial infarct. A different result was obtained by Ribeiro et al. [14], who found that oxygen therapy augmented perfusion of the ischemic region. The discrepancy between these findings may be explained by differences in the experimental model and the method of determining ischemic area.

Several studies have been performed to assess the effects of oxygen administration on patients with acute myocardial infarct. Neill [15] assessed the effects of 100% oxygen on global myocardial metabolism in patients with and without coronary artery disease. He found no change in the ratio of lactate to pyruvate in coronary sinus blood. Bourassa et al. [16] found that myocardial lactate levels increased in some patients during therapy with 100% oxygen. Horvat et al. [17] found an increase in lactate extraction during oxygen therapy in patients undergoing pacing-induced angina. The heart rate at which angina occurred increased even though cardiac output was lowered during oxygen administration. Madias et al. [18] administered oxygen to patients during acute anterior myocardial infarct. They produced a fourfold increase in arterial pO_2 and demonstrated a reduction in ST segment elevation during therapy; these changes reverted to baseline after oxygen therapy was discontinued. Rowles and Kenmure [19] studied the effects of oxygen therapy in a double-blind study involving 157 patients with uncomplicated myocardial infarcts. They found no difference in mortality, incidence of arrhythmias, or analgesic use for chest pain between those patients treated with oxygen for 24 h and the control group, but they did find that sinus tachycardia was more common in the patients treated with oxygen.

The use of hyperbaric oxygen during acute myocardial infarct has also been investigated. The volume of oxygen dissolved in the blood at increased pressures can significantly increase oxygen transport. Oxygen administered at 2 atmospheres of pressure would be expected to increase the arterial pO_2 to approximately 1500 mmHg, increasing the oxygen carrying capacity by 4.5 ml/100 cc blood. Results of a randomized clinical trial of hyperbaric oxygen therapy in

208 patients with acute myocardial infarct suggested that mortality in high-risk patients treated with oxygen at 2 atmospheres could be significantly reduced compared with patients treated with oxygen at 6l/min under normal atmospheric pressure [20].

The effects of oxygen therapy on patients with acute myocardial infarct vary depending on the respiratory and cardiovascular status of the patient. Conclusions drawn concerning the benefits or hazards of oxygen therapy depend greatly upon the parameters used to assess the extent of myocardial ischemia and/or infarct.

Interventions designed to increase delivery of oxygen and substrates to ischemic tissue

A previous chapter by Becker (p. 422) has considered pharmacologic interventions designed to increase myocardial blood flow to ischemic tissue. Drugs such as nitroglycerin, nifedipine, and other vasodilators have been shown to directly affect coronary vascular resistance and thus alter myocardial perfusion. Two other agents designed to increase the delivery of oxygen and substrates to ischemic tissue are mannitol and hyaluronidase. These two interventions do not act directly on coronary vascular resistance, but rather affect perfusion by altering the composition of the intervascular space.

Mannitol

The interest in mannitol as an agent to salvage ischemic myocardium began with the observation that cellular edema appeared early after the onset of ischemia in several organ systems. Leaf [21] first proposed the use of hyperosmotic agents such as mannitol to prevent intracellular edema and preserve tissue viability during ischemia.

There are several reasons why a hyperosmotic agent such as mannitol might reduce tissue injury. In experimental animal models, endothelial cells of small vessels have been shown to swell shortly after the onset of ischemia [22]. The resulting narrowing of the vascular lumen may well decrease blood flow, exacerbating the effects of an ischemic insult. By increasing serum osmolarity with mannitol, this encroachment on the vascular lumen may decrease, preserving flow in an ischemic area.

Another possible mechanism of action of mannitol is the reduction or prevention of myocardial cell swelling that occurs after ischemic injury. Cellular edema is a feature of both reversible and irreversible cell injury. It may cause an alteration in internal cellular spatial relationships, displacing enzyme systems that require close proximity; this in turn might inhibit myocardial metabolism. Also, cell swelling might produce permeability changes by stretching the membrane and thus results in changes in cofactor, substrate, and/or electrolyte concentrations.

A third possibility is that mannitol may directly influence coronary vascular resistance and/or ventricular function. The effects of mannitol on regional myocardial blood flow and ventricular performance were studied in awake dogs after 48 h of coronary occlusion [23]. An infusion of 25% mannitol at 0.1 ml/min for 40 min caused a significant increase in blood flow to an area supplied by an occluded coronary artery, as well as an increase in flow to the nonischemic areas of the heart. Significant increases in cardiac output and mean aortic pressure as well as dp/dt were produced, however. Therefore increased myocardial blood flow could be accounted for, at least in part, by changes in ventricular performance.

The next question to be investigated was whether mannitol infusion could reduce myocardial ischemia and necrosis. In one study [24], coronary occlusion was produced for 40 min in two groups of dogs, then reperfusion was instituted for 2–4 days before sacrificing the animals. One group received saline infusion prior to, during, and after occlusion, and the other group received hypertonic mannitol to increase serum osmolarity to at least 330 mosm during occlusion. Saline-treated dogs had 62% necrosis of the posterior papillary muscle, while those receiving mannitol had only 27% necrosis of the papillary muscle. Mannitol did not favorably influence mortality rate from ventricular fibrillation after coronary occlusion, but on the contrary seemed to slightly increase the occurrence of lethal arrhythmias.

A study of the effect of mannitol on cell swelling and the extent of myocardial necrosis found that mannitol significantly reduced the amount of myocardial edema found in the papillary muscle after 45–60 min of ischemia followed by 15–45 min of reperfusion [25]. There was also a decrease in swelling of the capillary endothelial cells. In a second group of animals, the extent of myocardial necrosis produced by 40–60 min of coronary occlusion followed by a 12 hour period of reperfusion was examined. Papillary muscle necrosis was significantly less in animals treated with mannitol during occlusion and early reperfusion, compared with a control group receiving only saline.

Previous studies examined the effect of mannitol on myocardial necrosis during short periods of coronary occlusion. More recent studies have questioned the efficacy of infusing mannitol during prolonged periods of myocardial ischemia. Hirzela and Kirk [26] examined the effect of mannitol infusion on coronary occlusion lasting for 24 h without reperfusion. A group of animals received 25% mannitol at 2 ml/min during the first 4 h of coronary occlusion, and a second group received saline. The only change in hemodynamic parameters noted with mannitol infusion was a slight increase in dp/dt. Qualitative estimation of myocardial necrosis was similar in the two groups but the extent of necrotic damage was not quantified. Myocardial creatine kinase activity of the ischemic region was examined and no preservation of this cellular enzyme could be demonstrated in animals treated with mannitol compared with the control group. Mannitol did not produce significant differences in regional myocardial flow to either nonischemic or ischemic tissue during the time course of occlusion or reperfusion. Collateral flow was measured by assessing aortic pressure and retrograde flow from the ischemic region. The animals treated with mannitol exhibited a smaller increase in collateral flow over the 24h after coronary occlusion than did the control group. The experimental design of this study differed from previous studies in that mannitol infusion was not initiated until 15 min after the onset of ischemia whereas in other studies the intervention was initiated prior to the onset of ischemia. This may account for some of the discrepancies seen. The efficacy of mannitol infusion was also questioned in a study by Fixler et al. [27]. They produced 2h coronary occlusions followed by 24h of reperfusion. Mannitol was infused for a 2h period starting 30 min after the initiation of coronary occlusion. Mannitol was found to slightly increase regional flow in both the ischemic and nonischemic regions during the initial 30 min of administration, but these increases were not sustained by continued infusion. The decrease in myocardial flow during the period of mannitol infusion could not be accounted for by a change in hemodynamic parameters. No difference in the extent of myocardial necrosis could be demonstrated between the control group and the group treated with mannitol.

In summary, the protective effect of hypertonic mannitol in reducing myocardial injury and increasing coronary blood flow appears to be short-lived and may require initiation of mannitol therapy *prior* to the onset of severe ischemia. Since hypertonic mannitol administration produces a significant increase in serum osmolarity, large shifts in intravascular fluid and electrolytes may occur. These shifts, together with the profound diuresis produced, can lead to adverse clinical effects and thus further reduce the efficacy of mannitol administration during myocardial infarct. Potential use may exist in the setting of repetitive ischemic episodes without infarct prior to definitive surgical treatment.

Hyaluronidase

This enzyme, which depolymerizes and hydrolyzes hyaluronic acid, has undergone extensive testing as an agent to limit myocardial necrosis after coronary occlusion. In the first animal studies to assess the effect of hyaluronidase on myocardial necrosis [28], permanent coronary occlusions were produced in dogs, and epicardial electrocardiograms, myocardial creatine kinase content, hemodynamic parameters, and histologic appearance were examined. One group of dogs served as controls and the other group received 225 mg/kg hyaluronidase 30 min after coronary occlusion. Both the sum of ST elevation and the number of sites with ST elevation were significantly decreased after hyaluronidase administration. No change in ST segments occurred in the control group over the same time period. In the control group of animals, the relationship between changes in the ST segment and depletion of CK was established. The hyaluronidase-treated dogs showed less CK depletion than expected, indicating preservation of ischemic myocardium. In a third group of animals, coronary occlusion was carried out and ST segment elevation was quantified. The occlusion was released, the animals were given hyaluronidase, and a second occlusion was performed. ST segment elevation was significantly less during the occlusion produced after hyaluronidase administration. Histologic sections from animals after 24 h of coronary occlusion were stained with Alcian green to detect hyaluronic acid. The control group exhibited Alcian-positive material in the arterial walls and perivascular space; much less stain was present in comparable samples from the hyaluronidase-treated animals.

A second study was then carried out to determine the time interval following coronary occlusion during which the administration of hyaluronidase could exert a significant protective effect on ischemic myocardium [29]. Hyaluronidase (500 NF units/kg) was administered to dogs after 20 min, 3 h, 6 h, or 9 h of coronary occlusion. Epicardial electrograms were obtained prior to, 15 min after, and 24 h after coronary occlusion. Myocardial tissue samples were analyzed for CK activity and histologic appearance 24 h after occlusion. When hyaluronidase was given 20 min, 3 h, or 6 h after coronary occlusion, myocardial salvage was reflected in significantly less myocardial CK depletion for any given ST segment elevation, and less histologic evidence of infarct. There was a progressive reduction in tissue salvage as the time interval between occlusion and drug administration lengthened. Hyaluronidase administration after 9 h of coronary occlusion did not produce demonstrable tissue salvage.

Since the previous studies examined myocardial necrosis after 24 h of occlusion, the next question addressed was whether hyaluronidase produced long-term preservation of ischemic myocardium. In another study [30], dogs were separated into either a control group or a hyaluronidase-treated group. Epicardial electrocardiograms were recorded and coronary ligation was performed. The treated group received 500 NF units/kg hyaluronidase 15 min, 2 h, and 24 h after coronary occlusion. The dogs were allowed to recover, and 21 days later underwent repeat epicardial mapping and then histologic sectioning to determine myocardial infarct size. The authors found that infarct size, expressed as a percentage of the left ventricle, was significantly less in the group treated with hyaluronidase. The number of animals with complete transmural infarct was also less in this group. The treated dogs developed fewer Q waves and demonstrated greater preservation of R waves compared with the control group. Hyaluronidase thus resulted in long-term preservation of ischemic myocardium.

The role of hyaluronidase in preserving ischemic tissue over both short- and long-term has been confirmed in rats [31], but no beneficial effect on ST segment changes or wall motion was seen in a pig model [32]. The negative result found in pigs may be due to the lack of collateral flow during occlusion, preventing pharmacologic agents from effectively reaching the ischemic area.

The effects of hyaluronidase on electrocardiographic evidence of necrosis in patients with acute myocardial infarct has been studied [33]. Patients with acute anterior infarct were randomized to either a control group or a group to whom hyaluronidase (55 NF units/kg) was given after the first electrocardiogram and every 6 h for 48 h thereafter. Precordial electrocardiographic maps were obtained on admission and again seven days later. The patients treated with hyaluronidase preserved more R waves and developed fewer Q waves than the control group, suggesting that hyaluronidase reduced the frequency of electrocardiographic signs of myocardial necrosis.

The effects of hyaluronidase on the ultrastructural and morphometric changes that occur during the early phases of acute myocardial ischemia have been investigated in an attempt to determine its mechanism of action [34]. Coronary occlusions were produced in rats and the animals either were treated with hyaluronidase 5 min after occlusion or were not treated. The hearts were excised 1 or 3 h after occlusion, and light- and electron-microscopic examination was performed to assess ischemic damage. The treated animals had fewer myocardial cells and vessels with evidence of ischemic damage. The ischemically damaged cells in the treated group were like those in the untreated group except that more glycogen granules were present. This suggests that hyaluronidase protects ischemic myocardium by preserving the glycogen content of the cell. Since hyaluronidase is an enzyme that is known to depolymerize hyaluronic acid, it has been postulated that by depolymerizing mucopolysaccharides in the cardiac interstitium, hyaluronidase increases substrate transport through the extravascular space and augments the cellular supply of glucose and other nutrients. This theory is supported by the finding of decreased hyaluronic acid in the interstitial tissue of hearts treated with hyaluronidase [28]. The preservation of glycogen granules in a population of ischemically injured cells in rats treated with hyaluronidase [34] is also consistent with the postulate that the drug improves substrate delivery, but this finding does not differentiate between improved interstitial transport and improved collateral flow.

The effect of hyaluronidase on regional myocardial blood flow after coronary occlusion has been examined by Askenazi et al. [35]. Coronary occlusions were performed in dogs, and regional blood flow was measured 15 min later. One-half of the animals received hyaluronidase 20 min after occlusion, and regional blood flow was again measured in all animals 6 h after occlusion. In the control group, blood flow to the ischemic area decreased during the period between 15 min and 6 h after occlusion, whereas it did not change in the treated group. Therefore hyaluronidase administration appeared to improve collateral flow in ischemic tissue, which might explain the beneficial effect on tissue salvage. It is possible though that the increase in flow is a secondary effect, and that the primary action results from depolymerization of polysaccharides, which would increase interstitial nutrient supply leading to increased tissue salvage.

Interventions designed to increase the cellular content of substrates

Two categories of agents are available for use in increasing the cellular content of substrates necessary for energy production. Glucose or glucose–insulin–potassium infusion is thought to work by providing a source of substrate to enhance the rate of anerobic glycolysis. The other class of agents includes allopurinol, ribose, and adenosine deaminase inhibitors. These compounds are designed to increase the rate of purine nucleotide synthesis and therefore increase ATP content directly.

Glucose–insulin–potassium

The first proponents of the use of glucose–insulin–potassium in heart disease were Sodi-Pallares et al. [36]. They believed that a loss of potassium was central to the derangements seen with ischemia, and was associated with 'depolarization' of the myocardial cell. They hypothesized that the loss of intracellular potassium resulted in dysrhythmias and possible cell death due to abnormalities in mitochondrial respiration. Infusion of glucose–insulin–potassium was thought to return potassium ion to the ischemic cells and to help 'repolarize' the cells, thereby minimizing a deleterious effect of ischemia. They coined the term 'polarizing solution' for the glucose–insulin–potassium mixture.

There are other reasons why an infusion of glucose–insulin–potassium might be beneficial during myocardial ischemia. Under conditions of normal myocardial oxygenation, circulating free fatty acids are a major source of energy and can exert control over the rate at which glucose is utilized [37]. During the ischemic state, aerobic glycolysis is slowed; but because of residual blood flow and dissolved tissue oxygen, it does not stop completely [38]. The rate of anaerobic glycolysis increases during ischemia, which may be an important factor in cell viability. Thus measures to promote glucose utilization should enhance survival of the heart during limited oxygen availability. The infusion of glucose, accompanied by insulin and potassium, might be expected to enhance anerobic glycolysis and thus improve cellular energy production.

Glucose alone may be beneficial during myocardial ischemia. There is evidence that increased extracellular glucose concentration diminished the changes produced by anoxia in the transmembrane action potential in isolated papillary muscles [39]. Glucose infusion might also act through its hypertonic effect. Increased serum osmolarity may decrease cellular edema and thus improve the survival of myocardial tissue during ischemia. Glucose may act by decreasing the level of circulating fatty acids in the blood after coronary occlusion [40].

Insulin also may play a role in salvaging ischemic myocardium. In acute myo-cardial infarct, there is evidence of insulin resistance and a circulating insulin level inappropriately low in relation to the elevated blood sugar [41, 42]. There-fore adequate transport of glucose into the cell may depend on exogenous administration of insulin. Insulin may have functions other than its effects on glucose transport. Insulin has been shown to enhance membrane polarization in skeletal muscle [43], to inhibit lysosomal activity in hypoxic heart tissue [44], and possibly to reduce postocclusion arrhythmias [45].

Because of the theoretical advantages of glucose—insulin—potassium adminis-tration, several experimental and clinical trials have been carried out to assess its effects on myocardial preservation in the setting of acute ischemia. Maroko et al. [46] recorded epicardial electrocardiograms before and after producing coronary occlusion in dogs. Beginning 30 min after coronary occlusion, the animals were infused with saline, glucose (20 gm/kg), or glucose (20 gm/kg) plus potassium (8.3 meq/kg) and insulin (4.2 units/kg) for 24 h. The hearts were then excised and myocardial creatine kinase content was measured at the sites of the epi-cardial electrode recordings. Sections from the hearts were examined histologi-cally to determine the presence of myocardial necrosis. The study demonstrated that both glucose and glucose—insulin—potassium infusions preserved myocardial creatine kinase content and lessened myocardial necrosis in areas exhibiting ST elevation after coronary occlusion. Glucose—insulin—potassium produced a greater protective effect than glucose alone.

The effect of glucose—insulin—potassium infusion on the metabolic par-ameters of tissue was studied in dogs undergoing coronary ligation [47]. After a 6 h infusion of glucose—insulin—potassium that began 30 min after coronary occlusion, the dogs were found to exhibit greater extraction of glucose and decreased uptake of free fatty acids compared with untreated controls. Glucose—insulin—potassium infusion also increased the content of glycogen in the peripheral area of the infarct and increased the content of ATP in the endo-cardium of the infarcted region. The results of the study suggested that glucose—insulin—potassium infusion not only increased anerobic glycolysis but also increased aerobic energy production, decreased extraction of free fatty acids, and increased tissue glycogen content.

The metabolic effects of glucose—insulin—potassium infusion during coronary occlusion have been studied in nonhuman primates [48]. Coronary ligation was produced in baboons, and glucose—insulin—potassium infusion was started within 3 min after the onset of ischemia and continued for 60 min. These animals were compared with a control group and were found to have increased contents of creatine phosphate, ATP, and glycogen in the ischemic zone. In the nonischemic and peripheral infarct zones the content of both glycogen and lactate rose. This study demonstrated a protective effect of glucose—insulin—potassium solution on myocardial tissue early after the onset of ischemia. The animal models of myocardial ischemia and infarct generally support the contention that administration of glucose—insulin—potassium solution promotes salvage of ischemic tissue after coronary artery occlusion.

A number of studies have been carried out in humans to examine the effect of glucose—insulin—potassium administration after acute myocardial infarct. Sodi-Pallares et al. [36], the first to use glucose—insulin—potassium infusions to treat patients with acute myocardial infarct, noted qualitative improvement in the electrocardiogram of many patients after treatment, and concluded that the infusions were effective in lessening ischemia. Mittra [49] reported on 170 patients with acute myocardial infarct who were randomized to either a control group or a group treated with oral potassium and glucose together with subcutaneous insulin. He found a short-term mortality of 28.2% in the control group and 11.7% in the treated group. He concluded that the administration of subcutaneous insulin together with oral potassium and glucose produced few side effects and significantly decreased mortality from acute myocardial infarct. The Medical Research Council of Great Britain conducted a multicenter controlled clinical trial of potassium, glucose, and insulin in acute myocardial infarct [50]. Potassium and glucose were given orally unless vomiting forced i.v. administration. Insulin was given subcutaneously. After a 28-day follow-up period, no difference was detected in either mortality rate or incidence of cardiac arrhythmias between the control and the treated groups.

Heng et al. [51] initiated a clinical trial using saline, or glucose, or glucose—insulin—potassium infusion for acute myocardial infarct. They found that glucose, and to a greater extent glucose—insulin—potassium, increased cardiac index, mean arterial pressure, pulmonary artery diastolic pressure, and stroke work index. These changes in hemodynamic parameters were not associated with what the authors felt to be a favorable trend in the serum creatine kinase profile. Serious clinical complications occurred in both the glucose- and the glucose—insulin—potassium-treated groups whereas no serious complications occurred in the saline-treated group. On the basis of these findings the trial was discontinued before completion.

The largest clinical trial of glucose—insulin—potassium to date has been reported from the University of Alabama [52—57]. A solution of 300 g glucose, 50 units regular insulin, and 80 meq potassium chloride in 1 liter of sterile water was administered at a rate of 1.5 ml/kg/h to a series of 70 patients with acute myocardial infarct within 15 h after the onset of symptoms. A control group consisted of 64 patients. The solution was infused into the right atrium for 48 h, and hemodynamic and metabolic measurements were recorded for 96 h. There was a significant reduction in inhospital mortality among the patients receiving glucose—insulin—potassium. The mortality was reduced in all four Killip categories of patients. Ventricular function curves, which were developed using the pulmonary artery end-diastolic pressure and cardiac index, suggested that mechanical performance was improved in the patients receiving glucose—insulin—potassium. These same patients also had a reduction in the frequency of PVCs, the number of episodes of ventricular tachycardia, and the amount of lidocaine they required. Infusion of glucose—insulin—potassium was also found to reduce the elevated levels of free fatty acids seen in the serum of patients with myocardial infarct. Since elevated free fatty acid concentration may cause cardiac depression [58] and increased cardiac irritability [59], the decrease in serum concentration was seen as a beneficial effect of glucose—insulin—potassium infusion. Complications included volume overloading, hyperglycemia, and hyperkalemia. Because of the length of the infusions, a central line was necessary to decrease irritation to peripheral veins. Glucose—insulin—potassium infusion should be tapered slowly in patients with unstable angina, since abrupt termination was occasionally associated with rapid clinical deterioration.

In summary, experimental and clinical evidence tends to support the contention that the administration of glucose—insulin—potassium solutions has beneficial effects on patients with acute myocardial infarct. The mechanism of action whereby the solution exerts these effects is as yet unresolved.

Alteration of purine nucleotide synthesis

ATP, a purine nucleotide, is the chief energy source for myocardial contraction, and is also necessary for metabolic functions that preserve cellular viability. There is evidence that a critical cellular content of ATP exists, below which cell death occurs [60, 61], and that even short periods of ischemia may cause prolonged derangements in cellular energy stores. In a study by Swain et al. [62], 12 min coronary occlusions were produced in open-chested dogs, and repetitive myocardial biopsies were taken during the reperfusion period from the previously ischemic area. During coronary occlusion, ATP content fell to 51% of control and after 1 h of reperfusion had only recovered to 74% of control. The results indicate that short periods of ischemia may cause prolonged depletion of adenine nucleotide compounds necessary for cellular function and viability. Therefore, interventions designed to increase ATP synthesis through increased purine biosynthesis might be expected to preserve cell viability and limit the extent of tissue death.

The synthesis of ATP takes place through two different pathways [63]. ATP can be generated through the de novo pathway in which a purine compound is synthesized from glycine and then phosphorylated; or ATP can be generated from the salvage pathway of purine synthesis. In the salvage pathway, hypoxanthine and possibly adenosine can be taken up and used to synthesize ATP.

Several interventions have been tested in an attempt to increase cellular ATP content. Allopurinol has been administered in an attempt to increase salvage pathway synthesis by blocking the degradation of hypoxanthine to xanthine through inhibition of the enzyme xanthine oxidase. It was postulated that by stopping the irreversible loss of purine precursors, an increase in ATP content would occur through an increase in salvage pathway synthesis. Arnold et al. [64] produced coronary occlusions in dogs and 2h later measured infarct size by fluorescein-dye injection into the left ventricle. They found that dogs pretreated with allopurinol prior to the onset of ischemia had significantly smaller infarcts than either a group not treated or a group that received allopurinol beginning immediately after coronary occlusion. Coronary anteriograms were performed on several hearts after termination of the experiment. Animals pretreated with allopurinol had a qualitative increase in collateral vasculature. The mechanism of the reduction in infarct size with allopurinol was not evident. Its effect could have been secondary to either increased myocardial blood flow through the demonstrable collaterals, or due to an increase in the salvage pathway synthesis of ATP. Shatney et al. [65] found no decrease in infarct size when allopurinol was given 15 min after coronary occlusion. No clinical studies have been performed on patients with acute myocardial infarct.

Another method of increasing salvage pathway synthesis that has been attempted in the animal model is the administration of inosine. Inosine is readily converted to hypoxanthine by purine nucleoside phosphorylase, and hypoxanthine can then be taken up and eventually converted to ATP. In a study by Devous and Jones [66], inosine (0.5 nmol/min) was infused into dogs for 5 min starting 15 min after LAD occlusion; 5h later, the extent of myocardial infarct was quantitated using nitro-blue tetrazolium staining. Inosine appeared to increase coronary blood flow directly, independent of its positive inotropic effect. Inosine produced a significant decrease in the percent of the left ventricle infarcted compared with a group of animals not receiving inosine after coronary ligation. The authors attributed the decrease in infarct size to an increase in myocardial blood flow produced by inosine. Simultaneous adenine nucleotide determinations were not carried out, and therefore it was not possible to determine whether inosine acted through an increase in purine nucleotide synthesis.

Other interventions to increase synthesis of high-energy phosphate compounds have been considered, but no animal or patient studies have yet been performed. The use of an adenosine deaminase inhibitor to increase adenine nucleotide content has been suggested [67]. Adenosine deaminase inhibitors block the deamination of adenosine to inosine. The resulting increase in adenosine concentration may result in an increase in the synthesis of ATP. An increase in adenosine content might also preserve ischemic myocardium through its potent vasodilatory effect. Ribose has been infused in rats and has been found to abolish the ATP-depleting effect of isoproterenol treatment [68]. Ribose is thought to increase ATP content through an increase in phosphoribosylpyrophosphate, an intermediate in both de novo and salvage pathway synthesis of purine nucleotides. Amino-imidazole-carboxamide ribonucleoside

(AICAR), an intermediate in the de novo pathway of purine synthesis, has been shown to increase nucleotide levels in tissue culture [69]. The effect of these compounds on ATP content in the setting of myocardial infarct has yet to be investigated.

INTERVENTIONS DESIGNED TO INHIBIT THE INFLAMMATORY RESPONSE AND STABILIZE CELL MEMBRANES

The third category of interventions to be discussed is the group of agents thought to act through modification of the inflammatory response. Following the initiation of anoxic injury, changes occur in membrane permeability, leukotaxis, and phagocytosis. Changes in membrane permeability alter the fluid and electrolyte balance of the cell and result in the release of lysosomal enzymes injurious to the cell. Increases in leukotaxis and phagocytosis may produce further injury to potentially salvageable tissue. Attempts to alter the inflammatory response have been made using corticosteroids and also using agents that alter activation of the complement system.

Corticosteroids

In the 1950s, a number of investigators examined the effect of corticosteroids on myocardial infarct. No quantitative estimates of infarct size were made, and the results conflicted [70–73]. In 1973, Libby et al. [74] examined the effect of hydrocortisone on ST segment elevation, creatine kinase content, and histologic appearance of ischemic tissue after coronary occlusion. They found that hydrocortisone administration (50 mg/kg i.v.) either 30 min or 6 h after coronary occlusion resulted in a decrease in ST segment elevation, an increase in myocardial creatine kinase content at 24 h, and a decrease in the extent of myocardial necrosis.

This beneficial effect was confirmed by Spath and Lefer [75]. They demonstrated a decrease in ST segment elevation in cats with dexamethasone administration 60 min after coronary occlusion. Administration of dexamethasone 30 min prior to occlusion did not favorably alter ST segments. Myocardial creatine kinase was preserved by administration of dexamethasone either prior to or after coronary occlusion. Shatney et al. [65] used an intracellular lactic dehydrogenase stain to measure the extent of myocardial infarct. Dogs received methylprednisolone sodium succinate (30 mg/kg) 15 min after coronary occlusion, and the hearts were incubated in nitro-blue tetrazolium solution 6 h later. They found that corticosteroid treatment reduced myocardial necrosis by 21%. The long-term effects of corticosteroid administration have been evaluated in rats [76]. Coronary occlusion was produced and either hydrocortisone or methylprednisolone was administered. Three weeks later, infarct size was assessed by both histologic examination and myocardial creatine kinase content. Hydrocortisone reduced infarct size by an average of 14% and methyl-prednisolone by 21% compared with untreated animals, thus indicating long-term preservation of ischemic myocardium.

There are three possible mechanisms for the demonstrated reduction in myocardial infarct size: (a) alteration of hemodynamic state, (b) increase in myocardial blood flow, (c) stabilization of cell membranes. Vyden et al. [77] found that methylprednisolone administration in the cat produced an immediate decrease in heart rate and mean arterial pressure, a slight but not significant decrease in left ventricular end-diastolic pressure, and no change in contractility. These effects resulted in a net decrease in myocardial oxygen consumption. They also demonstrated a significant increase in coronary blood flow with methylprednisolone treatment. Other investigators also found an increase in blood flow in ischemic myocardium, but no alteration in hemodynamic variables [75, 78]. The membrane-stabilizing effects of corticosteroids have been demonstrated in vitro. Weissman [79] incorporated corticosteroids into liposomes (lipid spheres) and demonstrated increase stability of the lipid membrane in the setting of both pharmacologic and mechanical insults. Spath and Lefer [75] found that myocardial lysosomal hydrolase activity was preserved in the ischemic region of animals treated with corticosteroids and concluded that dexamethasone stabilizes myocardial cellular or subcellular membranes within areas of ischemia.

Other investigators have been unable to demonstrate a beneficial effect of corticosteroid administration in experimental models. Osher et al. [80] administered methylprednisolone (50 mg/kg) to dogs 1 h after coronary occlusion and measured ST segment elevation for another 2 h. They found that ST segment elevation in treated animals actually increased after 3 h of occlusion compared with animals undergoing coronary occlusion without drug treatment. They concluded that corticosteroid administration did not improve the extent of myocardial ischemia early after coronary occlusion. Vogel et al. [81] measured creatine kinase and LDH enzyme activity in myocardium. Enzyme levels were measured 24 h after either a 90 min temporary occlusion or a permanent occlusion. They could not demonstrate a reduction in enzyme depletion with corticosteroid treatment either prior to or after the onset of coronary occlusion.

A potential complication of steroid therapy is delayed healing of the ventricle after myocardial infarct. Rats treated with large amounts or repetitive doses of methylprednisolone exhibited significant thinning of the infarct area three weeks after coronary occlusion, producing ventricular aneurysms [76]. Kloner et al. [82] examined the mechanism of delayed healing. They found that corticosteroid administration resulted in the presence of a large number of 'mummified' necrotic cells in the infarcted tissue. In control animals, necrotic cells were generally degraded and phagocytized rapidly. They concluded that multiple doses of corticosteroids preserved dead myocardial cells and hence prevented the normal breakdown processes and healing of the infarct. This effect appeared to be unique for high doses of glucocorticosteroids and was not due to the antiinflammatory effect per se, since other antiinflammatory agents did not produce mummification.

The effect of corticosteroid administration in patients with myocardial infarct has been investigated. Morrison et al. [83] measured creatine kinase release in patients early in the course of myocardial infarct to predict subsequent infarct size. A subset of patients then received either one or two 2 g infusions of methylprednisolone. Completed infarct size was then calculated with all serum creatine kinase samples obtained during the course of the infarct, and compared with predicted size. Their results indicated that corticosteroid treatment produced smaller infarcts than predicted from creatine kinase release. Welman et al. [84] administered methylprednisolone to ten patients within 4 h after the onset of chest pain. They found a significant delay in the release of both creatine kinase, a cytosolic enzyme, and N-acetyl-B-glucosamidase, a lysosomal enzyme. They concluded that corticosteroid administration resulted in membrane stabilization, but could not determine whether the final extent of necrosis was reduced.

Other studies do not support the contention that corticosteroid administration is beneficial in the setting of acute myocardial infarct. Roberts et al. [85] examined the effect of methylprednisolone on infarct size as assessed by serum creatine kinase determinations. They found that infarct size was increased over predicted levels by corticosteroid treatment, and concluded that this treatment was deleterious for patients with acute myocardial infarct. Peters et al. [86] also examined creatine kinase enzyme release in patients undergoing myocardial infarct. They found no difference in enzyme release in patients treated with corticosteroids compared with an untreated control group. They concluded that high intravenous doses of steroids given early in the course of myocardial infarct have neither deleterious nor beneficial effects.

Although experimental evidence suggests a protective effect of corticosteroids following acute myocardial infarct, reduction of the extent of infarct in patients has not been conclusively demonstrated. Corticosteroids have been implicated in impairment of myocardial healing, leading to ventricular aneurysm and myocardial rupture.

Alteration of complement activation

Neutrophilic infiltration begins within several hours after the onset of myocardial necrosis. This inflammatory response, which may promote further tissue damage, is modified in part by activation of the complement system of serum proteins. Pinckard et al. [87] measured complement levels in man during acute myocardial infarct, and examined the possible mechanism of complement activation. They found a significant decrease in the complement components C1, C3, and C4 during the first 72 h after myocardial infarct. No changes were noted in patients with chest pain without infarct. The consumption of these components of complement was attributed to activation of the complement pathways. This activation was felt to be responsible in part for the neutrophilic infiltration seen in myocardial infarct. The activation of completment in this setting was shown to be independent of antimyocardial antibodies, and due to interaction of heart and mitrochondrial membranes with C1. The same group also demonstrated localization of C3 in injured areas within 12h after the onset of ischemia in nonhuman primates.

Alteration of complement activation may decrease inflammatory change caused by neutrophilic infiltration. The chemotactic activity of complement activation can be abated by activation of the alternative pathway and subsequent consumption of C3. Cobra venom factor exhibits this anticomplement effect and has been used in attempts to decrease infarct size through a decrease in the inflammatory response. Maroko et al. [88] infused cobra venom factor into dogs after coronary occlusion. They analyzed epicardial ST segment changes and creatine kinase depletion, and demonstrated a decrease in predicted infarct size. This effect was accompanied by a decrease in the components of complement, but not by changes in cardiac performance, collateral blood flow, or the clotting system. Decreased neutrophilic infiltration into the infarcted area was observed. These results were similar to those obtained by Hartmann et al. [89].

REFERENCES

1. Braunwald E: Control of myocardial oxygen consumption: physiologic and clinical considerations. Am J Cardiol 27:416–432, 1971.
2. Blair E: Clinical Hypothermia. New York: McGraw-Hill, 1964, pp 88–90.
3. Salisbury PF, Cross CE, Rieben PA: Integrative study of the circulation in moderate hypothermia. Am J Cardiol 12:184–193, 1963.
4. Sukumalchantra Y, Levy S, Danzig R, Rubins S, Alpern H, Swan HJC: Correcting arterial hypoxemia by oxygen therapy in patients with acute myocardial infarction. Am J Cardiol 24:838–852, 1969.
5. Sukumalchantra Y, Danzig R, Levy SE, Swan HJC: The mechanism of arterial hypoxemia in acute myocardial infarction. Circulation 41:641–650, 1970.
6. Davidson RM, Ramo BW, Wallace AG, Whalen RE, Starmer CF: Blood-gas and hemodynamic responses to oxygen in acute myocardial infarction. Circulation 47:704–711, 1973.
7. Helmers C, Hofvendahl S, Lundman T, Mogensen L, Nyquist O, Sawe U, Wester P: Arterial oxygen and carbon-dioxide tension in patients with acute myocardial infarction. Cardiology 58:335–346, 1973.
8. Radvany P, Maroko PR, Braunwald E: Effects of hypoxemia on the extent of myocardial necrosis after experimental coronary occlusion. Am J Cardiol 35:795–800, 1975.
9. Saltzman HA: Efficacy of oxygen enriched gas mixtures in the treatment of acute myocardial infarction [editorial]. Circulation 52:357–359, 1975.

10. Moss AJ, Johnson J: Effects of oxygen inhalation on intramyocardial oxygen tension. Cardiovasc Res 4:436–440, 1970.
11. Maroko PR, Radvany P, Braunwald E, Hale SL: Reduction of infarct size by oxygen inhalation following acute coronary occlusion. Circulation 52:360–368, 1975.
12. Rivas F, Rembert JC, Bache RJ, Cobb FR, Greenfield JC Jr: Effect of hyperoxia on regional blood flow after coronary occlusion in awake dogs. Am J Physiol 238:H244–H248, 1980.
13. Malm A, Arborelius M, Bornmyr S, Lilja B, Gill RL: Effects of oxygen on acute myocardial infarction: a thermographic study in the dog. Cardiovasc 11:512–518, 1977.
14. Ribeiro LGT, Louie EK, Davis MA, Maroko PR: Augmentation of collateral blood flow to the ischaemic myocardium by oxygen inhalation following experimental coronary artery occlusion. Cardiovas Res 13:160–166, 1979.
15. Neill WA: Effects of arterial hypoxemia and hyperoxia on oxygen availability for myocardial metabolism: Patients with and without coronary heart disease. Am J Cardiol 24:166–171, 1969.
16. Bourassa MG, Campeau L, Bois MA, Rico O: The effects of inhalation of 100 per cent oxygen on myocardial lactate metabolism in coronary heart disease. Am J Cardiol 24:172–177, 1969.
17. Horvat M, Yoshida S, Prakash R, Marcus HS, Swan HJC, Ganz W: Effect of oxygen breathing on pacing-induced angina pectoris and other manifestations of coronary insufficiency. Circulation 45:837–844, 1972.
18. Madias JE, Madias NE, Hood WB Jr: Precordial ST-segment mapping: 2. Effects of oxygen inhalation on ischemic injury in patients with acute myocardial infarction. Circulation 53:411–417, 1976.
19. Rawles JM, Kenmure ACF: Controlled trial of oxygen in uncomplicated myocardial infarction. Br Med J 1:1121–1123, 1976.
20. Thurston JGB, Greenwood TW, Bending MR, Connor H, Curwen MP: A controlled investigation into the effects of hyperbaric oxygen on mortality following acute myocardial infarction. Q J Med 42:751–770, 1973.
21. Leaf A: Cell swelling: a factor in ischemic tissue injury. Circulation 48:455–458, 1973.
22. Armiger LC, Gavin JB: Changes in the microvasculature of ischemic and infarcted myocardium. Lab Invest 33:51–56, 1975.
23. Hutton I, Curry GC, Templeton GH, Willerson JT: Influence of hypertonic mannitol on regional myocardial blood flow and ventricular performance in awake, intact dogs with prolonged coronary artery occlusion. Cardiovasc Res 9:409–419, 1975.
24. Kloner RA, Reimer KA, Willerson JT, Jennings RB: Reduction of experimental myocardial infarct size with hyperosmolar mannitol. Proc Soc Exp Biol Med 151:677–683, 1976.
25. Powell WJ JR, DiBona DR, Flores J, Leaf A: The protective effect of hyperosmotic mannitol in myocardial ischemia and necrosis. Circulation 54:603–615, 1976.
26. Hirzel HO, Kirk ES: The effect of mannitol following permanent coronary occlusion. Circulation 56:1006–1015, 1977.
27. Fixler DE, Buja LM, Wheeler JM, Willerson JT: Influence of mannitol on maintaining coronary flows and salvaging myocardium during ventriculotomy and during prolonged coronary artery ligation. Circulation 56:340–346, 1977.

498

28. Maroko PR, Libby P, Bloor CM, Sobel BE, Braunwald E: Reduction by hyaluronidase of myocardial necrosis following coronary artery occlusion. Circulation 46:430–437, 1972.
29. Hillis LD, Fishbein MC, Braunwald E, Maroko PR: The influence of the time interval between coronary artery occlusion and the administration of hyaluronidase on salvage of ischemic myocardium in dogs. Circ Res 41:26–34, 1977.
30. Kloner RA, Braunwald E, Maroko PR: Long-term preservation of ischemic myocardium in the dog by hyaluronidase. Circulation 58:220–226, 1978.
31. Maclean D, Fishbein MC, Maroko PR, Braunwald E: Hyaluronidase-induced reductions in myocardial infarct size. Science 194:199–200, 1976.
32. Most AS, Capone RJ, Mastrofrancesco PA: Failure of hyaluronidase to alter the early course of acute myocardial infarction in pigs. Am J Cardiol 38:28–33, 1976.
33. Maroko PR, Hillis LD, Muller JE, Tavazzi L, Heyndrickx GR, Ray M, Chiariello M, Distante A, Askenazi J, Salerno J, Carpentier J, Reshetnaya NI, Radvany P, Libby P, Raabe DS, Chezov EI, Bobba P, Braunwald E: Favorable effects of hyaluronidase on electrocardiographic evidence of necrosis in patients with acute myocardial infarction. N Engl J Med 296:898–903, 1977.
34. Kloner RA, Fishbein MC, Maclean D, Braunwald E, Maroko PR: Effect of hyaluronidase during the early phase of acute myocardial ischemia: an ultrastructural and morphometric analysis. Am J Cardiol 40:43–49, 1977.
35. Askenazi J, Hillis LD, Diaz PE, Davis MA, Braunwald E, Maroko PR: The effects of hyaluronidase on coronary blood flow following coronary artery occlusion in the dog. Circ Res 40:566–570, 1977.
36. Sodi-Pallares D, Testelli MR, Fishleder BL, Bisteni A, Medrano GA, Friedland C, De Micheli A: Effects of an intravenous infusion of a potassium–glucose–insulin solution on the electrocardiographic signs of myocardial infarction. Am J Cardiol 9:166–181, 1962.
37. Shipp JC, Opie LH, Challoner D: Fatty acid and glucose metabolism in the perfused heart. Nature 189:1018–1019, 1961.
38. Hearse DJ: Oxygen deprivation and early myocardial contractile failure: a reassessment of the possible role of adenosine triphosphate. Am J Cardiol 44:1115–1121, 1979.
39. Macleod DP, Daniel EE: Influence of glucose on the transmembrane action potential of anoxic papillary muscle. J Gen Physiol 48:887–899, 1965.
40. Gupta DK, Jewitt DE, Young R, Hartog M, Opie LH: Increased plasma-free-fatty-acid concentrations and their significance in patients with acute myocardial infarction. Lancet 2:1209–1213, 1969.
41. Allison SP, Chamberlain MJ, Hinton P: Intravenous glucose tolerance, insulin, glucose, and free fatty acid levels after myocardial infarction. Br Med J 4:776–778, 1969.
42. Vetter NJ, Adams W, Strange RC, Oliver MF: Initial metabolic and hormonal response to acute myocardial infarction. Lancet 1:284–288, 1974.
43. Zierler KL: Effect of insulin on membrane potential and potassium content of rat muscle. Am J Physiol 197:515–523, 1959.
44. Wildenthal K: Inhibition by insulin of cardiac cathepsin D activity. Nature 243:226–227, 1973.
45. Hiatt N, Sheinkopf JA, Warner NE: Prolongation of survival after circumflex

artery ligation by treatment with massive doses of insulin. Cardiovasc Res 5:48–53, 1971.

46. Maroko PR, Libby P, Sobel BE, Bloor CM, Sybers HD, Shell WE, Covell JW, Braunwald E: Effect of glucose–insulin–potassium infusion on myocardial infarction following experimental coronary artery occlusion. Circulation 45:1160–1175, 1972.

47. Opie LH, Owen P: Effect of glucose–insulin–potassium infusions on arteriovenous differences of glucose and of free fatty acids and on tissue metabolic changes in dogs with developing myocardial infarction. Am J Cardiol 38:310–321, 1976.

48. Opie LH, Bruyneel K, Owen P: Effects of glucose, insulin and potassium infusion on tissue metabolic changes within first hour of myocardial infarction in the baboon. Circulation 52:49–57, 1975.

49. Mittra B: Potassium, glucose, and insulin in treatment of myocardial infarction. Lancet 2:607–609, 1965.

50. Medical Research Council of Great Britain: Potassium, glucose, and insulin treatment for acute myocardial infarction. Lancet 2:1355–1360, 1968.

51. Heng MK, Norris RM, Singh BN, Barratt-Boys C: Effects of glucose and glucose–insulin–potassium on haemodynamics and enzyme release after acute myocardial infarction. Br Heart J 39:748–757, 1977.

52. Stanley AW Jr, Moraski RE, Russell RO Jr, Rogers WJ, Mantle JA, Kreisberg RA, McDaniel HG, Rackley CE: Effects of glucose–insulin–potassium on myocardial substate availability and utilization in stable coronary artery disease. Studies on myocardial carbohydrate, lipid and oxygen arterial-coronary sinus differences in patients with coronary artery disease. Am J Cardiol 36:929–937, 1975.

53. Russell RO Jr, Rogers WJ, Mantle JA, McDaniel HG, Rackley CE: Glucose–insulin–potassium, free fatty acids and acute myocardial infarction in man. Circulation [Suppl 1] 53:I–207, 1976.

54. Prather JW, Russell RO Jr, Mantle JA, McDaniel HG, Rackley CE: Metabolic consequences of glucose–insulin–potassium infusion in treatment of acute myocardial infarction. Am J Cardiol 38:95–99, 1976.

55. Rogers WJ, Stanley AW Jr, Breinig JB, Prather JW, McDaniel HG, Moraski RE, Mantle JA, Russell RO Jr, Rackley CE: Reduction of hospital mortality rate of acute myocardial infarction with glucose–insulin–potassium infusion. Am Heart J 92:441–454, 1976.

56. Rogers WJ, Segall PH, McDaniel HG, Mantle JA, Russell RO Jr, Rackley CE: Prospective randomized trial of glucose–insulin–potassium in acute myocardial infarction: effects on myocardial hemodynamics, substrates and rhythm. Am J Cardiol 43:801–809, 1979.

57. Rackley CE, Russell RO Jr, Rogers WJ, Mantle JA, McDaniel HG: Glucose–insulin–potassium infusion in acute myocardial infarction: review of clinical experience. Postrad Med 65:93–99, 1979.

58. Henderson AH, Most AS, Parmley WW, Gorlin R, Sonnenblick EH: Depression of myocardial contractility in rats by free fatty acids during hypoxia. Circ Res 26:439–494, 1970.

59. Oliver MF, Kurien VA, Greenwood TW: Relation between serum free fatty-acids and arrhythmias and death after acute myocardial infarcion. Lancet 1:710–714, 1968.

60. Schaper J, Mulch J, Winkler B, Schaper W: Ultrastructural, functional, and histochemical criteria for estimation of reversibility of ischemic injury: a

study on the effects of global ischemia on the isolated dog heart. J Mol Cell Cardiol 11:521—541, 1979.

61. Jennings RB, Hawkins HK, Lowe JE, Hill ML, Klotman S, Reimer KA: Relation between high energy phosphate and lethal injury in myocardial ischemia in the dog. Am J Pathol 92:187—214, 1978.

62. Swain JL, Sabina RL, McHale PA, Greenfield JC Jr, Holmes EW: Prolonged myocardial ATP depletion after brief ischemia in the open-chested dog. Clin Res 28:473A, 1980.

63. Wyngaarden JB, Kelley WN: Purine biosynthesis and metabolism. In: Gout and hyperuricemia. New York: Grune and Stratton, 1976, pp 67—77.

64. Arnold WL, DeWall RA, Kezdi P, Zwart HHJ: The effect of allopurinol on the degree of early myocardial ischemia. Am Heart J 99:614—624, 1980.

65. Shatney CH, Maccarter DJ, Lillehei RC: Effects of allopurinol, propranolol and methylprednisolone on infarct size in experimental myocardial infarction. Am J Cardiol 37:572—580, 1976.

66. Devous MD, Jones CE: Effect of inosine on ventricular regional perfusion and infarct size after coronary occlusion. Cardiology 64:149—161, 1979.

67. Foker J, Wang T, Einzig S, Nicoloff D: Adenosine catabolism during myocardial ischemia and recovery [abstr]. Circulation [Suppl 2] 60:II—115, 1979.

68. Zimmer HG, Ibel H, Steinkopff G, Korb G: Reduction of the isoproterenol-induced alterations in cardiac adenine nucleotides and morphology by ribose. Science 207:319—321, 1980.

69. Thomas CB, Meade JC, Holmes EW: Aminoimidazole carboxamide ribonucleoside toxicity: a model for study of pyrimidine starvation. J Cell Physiol (in press).

70. Johnson AS, Scheinberg SR, Gerisch RA, Saltzstein HC: Effect of cortisone on the size of experimentally produced myocardial infarcts. Circulation 7:224—228, 1953. 7

71. Chapman DW, Skaggs RH, Thomas JR, Greene JA: The effect of cortisone in experimental myocardial infarction. Am J Med Sci 223:41—44, 1952.

72. Opdyke DF, Lambert A, Stoerk HC, Zanetti ME, Kuna S: Failure to reduce the size of experimentally produced myocardial infarcts by cortisone treatment. Circulation 8:544—548, 1953.

73. Hepper NG, Pruitt RD, Donald DE, Edwards JE: The effect of cortisone on experimentally produced myocardial infarcts. Circulation 11:742—748, 1955.

74. Libby P, Maroko PR, Bloor CM, Sobel BE, Braunwald E: Reduction of experimental myocardial infarct size by corticosteroid administration. J Clin Invest 52:599—607, 1973.

75. Spath JA Jr, Lefer AM: Effects of dexamethasone on myocardial cells in the early phase of acute myocardial infarction. Am Heart J 90:50—55, 1975.

76. Maclean D, Fishbein MC, Braunwald E, Maroko PR: Long-term preservation of ischemic myocardium after experimental coronary artery occlusion. J Clin Invest 61:541—551, 1978.

77. Vyden JK, Nagasawa K, Rabinowitz B, Parmley WW, Tomoda H, Corday E, Swan HJC: Effects of methylprednisolone administration in acute myocardial infarction. Am J Cardiol 34:677—696, 1974.

78. Masters TN, Harbold NB Jr, Hall DG, Jackson RD, Mullen DC, Daugherty HK, Robicsek F: Beneficial metabolic effects of methylprednisolone sodium succinate in acute myocardial ischemia. Am J Cardiol 37:557—563, 1976.

79. Weissmann G: Corticosteroids and membrane stabilization. Circulation [Suppl 1] 53:I–171, 1976.
80. Osher J, Lang T-W, Meerbaum S, Hashimoto K, Farcot J-C, Corday E: Methyl-prednisolone treatment in acute myocardial infarction. Effect on regional and global myocardial function. Am J Cardiol 37:564–571, 1976.
81. Vogel VM, Zannoni VG, Abrams GD, Lucchesi BR: Inability of methyl-prednisolone sodium succinate to decrease infarct size or preserve enzyme activity measured 24 hours after coronary occlusion in the dog. Circulation 55:588–595, 1977.
82. Kloner RA, Fishbein MC, Lew H, Maroko PR, Braunwald E: Mummification of the infarcted myocardium by high dose corticosteroids. Circulation 57:56–63, 1978.
83. Morrison J, Reduto L, Pizzarello R, Geller K, Maley T, Gulotta S: Modification of myocardial injury in man by corticosteroid administration. Circulation [Suppl 1] 53:I–200, 1976.
84. Welman E, Selwyn AP, Fox KM: Lysosomal and cytosolic enzyme release in acute myocardial infarction: effects of methylprednisoline. Circulation 59:730–733, 1979.
85. Roberts R, DeMello V, Sobel BE: Deleterious effects of methylprednisolone in patients with myocardial infarction. Circulation [Suppl 1] 53:I–204, 1976.
86. Peters RW, Norman A, Parmley WW, Emilson BB, Scheinman MM, Cheitlin M: Effect of therapy with methylprednisolone on the size of myocardial infarcts in man. Chest 73:483–488, 1978.
87. Pinckard RN, Olson MS, Giclas PC, Terry R, Boyer JT, O'Rourke RA: Consumption of classical complement components by heart subcellular membranes in vitro and in patients after acute myocardial infarction. J Clin Invest 56:740–750, 1975.
88. Maroko PR, Carpenter CB, Chiariello M, Fishbein MC, Radvany P, Knostman JD, Hale SL: Reduction by cobra venom factor of myocardial necrosis after coronary artery occlusion. J Clin Invest 61:661–670, 1978.
89. Hartmann JR, Robinson JA, Gunnar RM: Chemotactic activity in the coronary sinus after experimental myocardial infarction: effects of pharmacologic interventions on ischemic injury. Am J Cardiol 40:550–555, 1977.

21. THE RELATIONSHIP BETWEEN CORONARY ANGIOGRAPHIC PATTERNS AND THE EFFECTS OF INFARCT LIMITING INTERVENTIONS

HERMAN K. GOLD and ROBERT C. LEINBACH

Transmural myocardial infarct begins with a sudden reduction of flow in the distribution of a major epicardial coronary artery. This process of reversible injury, progressing to necrosis, correlates with characteristic electrocardiographic and enzyme changes. The relationship of these changes to the coronary anatomy has remained a matter of controversy because coronary angiography has seldom been performed during the early phase of myocardial infarct. Without angiographic studies, our understanding of the interrelationships between the degree of luminal narrowing, the intensity and duration of myocardial injury, and the response to therapy is limited.

Blumgart and associates showed by postmortem angiographic studies nearly 40 years ago that the site of infarct correlated with an obstructive narrowing in the artery supplying blood to the infarcted zone [1]. In the majority of cases, the degree of luminal narrowing exceeded 75% of the vessel diameter [2–4]. In some cases, however, the degree of obstruction was less severe, and in a few cases no coronary artery narrowing was demonstrated [5]. This variation in the severity of obstruction made it difficult to develop a unifying hypothesis for the pathophysiology of an infarct. Moreover, acute events, such as coronary artery spasm or abrupt thrombosis, may not be discernible at postmortem examination, since a spasm may disappear and an intraluminal thrombus may be rapidly lysed [6].

The development and refinement of coronary angiography made it possible to overcome these limitations by examining the coronary anatomy in vivo. There was early concern about the morbidity of acute angiography and the lack of a clear-cut indication for study, however, which precluded angiography in the first hours of infarct, studies done as late as three weeks after the event did not add to our understanding of the mechanisms of acute interruption of coronary flow.

In 1968, the intraaortic balloon pump was developed, enabling detailed angiographic studies to be performed safely during the acute phase of an infarct in the hope that operative intervention could be applied. Leinbach and co-workers reviewed the angiographic results of patients who were studied within 2–4 days of infarct [7] and found that the coronary artery supplying the infarcted zone was severely obstructed in all patients. Patients with anterior

Wagner GS (ed): Myocardial Infarction: Measurement and Intervention, pp 503–514.
© *1982 Martinus Nijhoff Publishers, The Hague/Boston/London.*

504

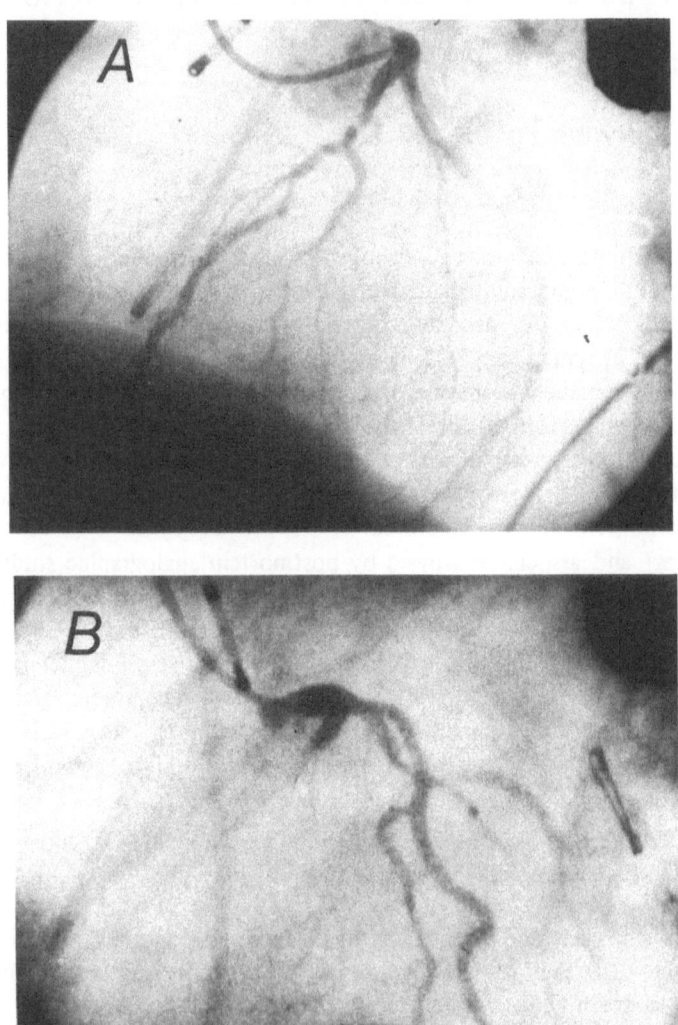

Figure 1. (*A*) The left coronary artery in the left anterior oblique view in a patient with sub-total left anterior descending obstruction. (*B*) Left coronary artery in the left anterior oblique view in a patient with complete obstruction and antegrade flow to the anterior myo-cardial wall.

transmural infarct exhibited one of two angiographic patterns: (a) the absence of identifiable flow to the anterior myocardial wall due to total obstruction of the left anterior descending coronary artery (LAD) with no collateral; (b) the presence of reduced flow to the anterior wall, either by antegrade flow through a subtotally obstructed vessel or by a collateral (Figure 1). The results of bypass

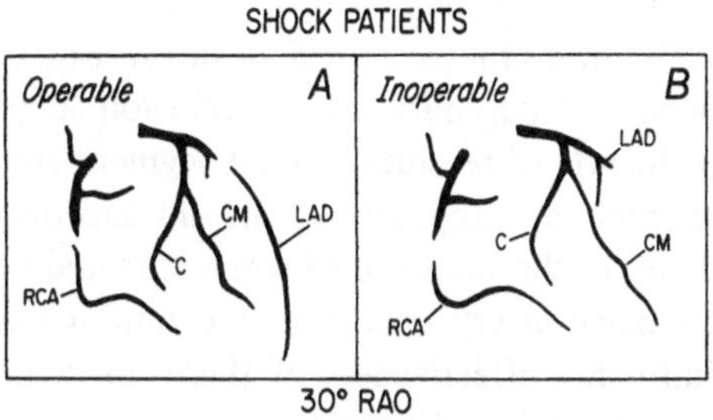

SHOCK PATIENTS

Figure 2 (*A*) Composite coronary angiographic pattern of patients with subtotal obstruction of the left anterior descending coronary artery: LAD, left anterior descending; C, circumflex; CM, circumflex marginal; RCA, right coronary artery. (*B*) Right anterior oblique projection of a composite coronary angiographic pattern in patients with complete occlusion of the left anterior descending artery.

grafting were better in the group with some residual flow into the LAD zone (Figure 2A). In patients in whom obstruction was complete and no collateral existed, the surgical mortality was 100% and the postmortem examinations showed infarct of 40% or more of the left ventricular myocardium (Figure 2B). Although these studies demonstrated that an extensive transmural infarct could result from subtotal coronary occlusion, it was not possible to determine the frequency with which complete occlusion occurred. Moreover, large transmural infarcts predispose to secondary coronary arterial thrombosis [2], obscuring the distinction between cause and effect.

Confirmation of the safety of angiography, even in patients with shock, and an awareness of the potential for interrupting ischemic injury by intervening early with nitroglycerin and propranolol led us to perform angiography during the course of studies designed to limit infarct size. Our initial studies in 1975 were performed 1–10 days after the onset of acute anterior transmural infarct in 20 patients without shock. The two angiographic patterns that have been described above were again observed (Figure 1). These patterns were equally prevalent. We subsequently studied ten patients with acute inferior infarct 7–10 days after infarct had begun. The angiographic patterns were similar to those present in anterior infarct, except that collaterals to the infarcted zone were almost always present.

FACTORS THAT INFLUENCE RESPONSE TO THERAPY

Studies during experimental infarcts have shown that propranolol and the intra-aortic balloon pump are capable of limiting myocardial injury and preventing an extensive infarct [8]. When this work was extended to clinical studies, it became clear that a significant number of patients were resistant to therapy and that clinical and electrocardiographic features did not distinguish responders from nonresponders. One hypothesis to explain this resistance to therapy is that it depends on the degree of coronary artery occlusion supplying the infarcted zone. We believe that the rate of resolution of ST segment elevation produced by various interventions such as propranolol, the intraaortic balloon pump, or nitroglycerin depends upon the presence of some antegrade flow to the zone of infarct. Complete coronary artery occlusion and minimal or absent collateral flow significantly limits the effectiveness of these interventions. In our early pilot studies of infarct limitation, 12 patients whose acute anterior myocardial infarcts were less than 8 h old received intravenous propranolol [9]. Within 30 min after the infusion was completed, the sum of ST segment elevation in the six standard precordial leads ($\Sigma\, ST_6$) decreased by an average of 40%. The effects of propranolol were more pronounced in patients with angiographically demonstrable flow to the zone of infarct. Patients who had some antegrade flow to the anterior myocardial wall showed a greater than 45% reduction of $\Sigma\, ST_6$ acutely; patients with no demonstrable flow to the zone of infarct had a less than 40% reduction in $\Sigma\, ST_6$ (Figure 3).

In a second study, the intraaortic balloon pump was used for the control of ischemic injury in patients with anterior myocardial infarct without shock. Intraaortic balloon pumping was begun within 8 h of the onset of infarct. Two

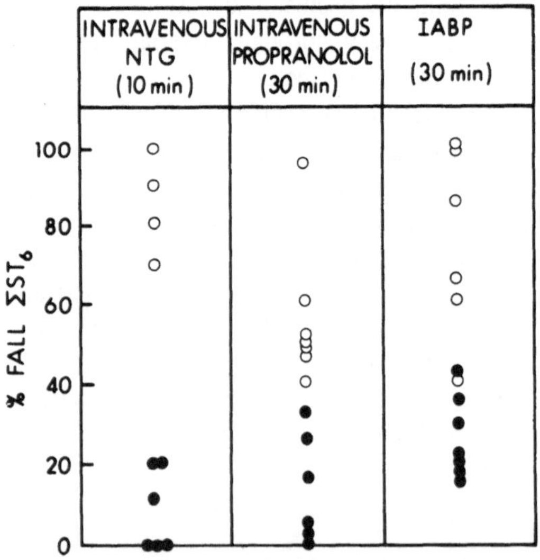

Figure 3. Relation between the degree of reduction in ST segment elevation and the presence or absence of angiographically demonstrable flow into the infarcted zone. Patients with subtotal occlusion of the left anterior descending coronary artery with antegrade flow to the infarcted zone (o) responded better to all three interventions. Patients with complete occlusion of the left anterior descending coronary artery (•) showed a less marked fall in $\Sigma\, ST_6$ following nitroglycerin, propranolol administration, or the use of the intraaortic balloon pump.

patterns of ST segment response occurred: (a) a rapid decrease in ST segment elevation, at least 50% within 30 min; (b) a gradual improvement in ST segment elevation that did not clearly differ from the natural history of ST segment resolution. The relationship between ST segment fall in response to therapy and the coronary perfusion patterns was similar to that seen in the propranolol-treated patients: patients with subtotal left anterior descending artery obstruction showed rapid resolution of ΣST_6, and patients with complete left anterior descending obstruction and poor collaterals showed incomplete resolution of $X ST_6$ [10] (Figure 3).

A similar relationship between the degree of occlusion of the left anterior descending coronary artery and response of ST segments has been observed following the intravenous infusion of nitroglycerin [11]. The ranges of response of ST segment changes were 0%–20% in the six patients with completely occluded vessels and 70%–100% in the four patients with less than complete occlusions (Figure 3).

This dependence of ST segment response upon either the partial patency of the obstructed vessel or the presence of well-developed collaterals suggests that infarct size could be limited minimally even in the absence of flow. Therefore it is important to determine the status of coronary arteries and collaterals during the early hours following onset of the infarct process when salvage of myocardium would be possible. De Wood et al. [12] have performed coronary angiography within 4 h of the onset of symptoms in 126 patients. Approximately 50% were having an anterior infarct and 50% of an inferior infarct. In 110 of the 126 patients (87%) the occlusion was 100%. From this study, one might conclude that only 13% of patients with electrocardiographic evidence of evolving anterior or inferior infarcts would have an anatomic situation that could enable limitation of infarct size, even if they were treated within 4 h of onset of symptoms.

There is a positive correlation between the rate of resolution of ST segment elevation and left ventricular ejection fraction. Patients with subtotal coronary artery obstruction, who had shown a greater than 45% fall in ΣST_6 acutely in response to propranolol demonstrated a left ventricular ejection fraction of greater than 50%. Those with total obstruction of the left anterior descending artery, who had shown less complete resolution of ST segment elevation, had an ejection fraction of less than 50% (Figure 4A). A similar relationship between the rate of resolution of ST segments acutely in response to the intraaortic balloon pump was also demonstrated (Figure 4B).

MECHANISM OF OCCLUSION: SPASM VS THROMBUS

The most likely causes of acute coronary artery occlusion are spasm, thrombosis, or plaque hemorrhage (Figure 5). Angiographically, spasm presents as a tapered

508

A

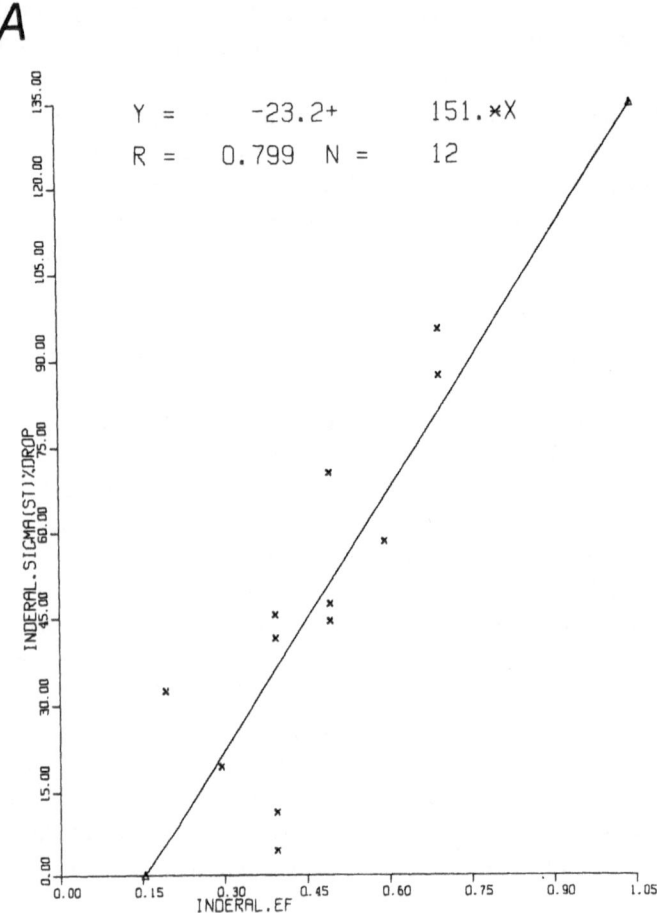

Figure 4. The relationship between the degree of reduction in ST segment elevation and the residual ejection fraction measured by gated blood pool scan or left ventriculography in patients treated with propranolol (*A*) or intraaortic balloon pumping (*B*). Patients with subtotal left anterior descending coronary artery obstruction who show a greater than 50% fall in $\Sigma\ ST_6$ acutely demonstrate a residual ejection fraction of greater than 0.5. In contrast, the patients with total left anterior descending obstruction who show less than 50% fall in $\Sigma\ ST_6$ acutely have a residual ejection fraction of less than 0.5.

occlusion that responds to nitrates by restoring flow, usually through a persistent area of stenosis. A thrombus can be identified as a filling defect, which is sometimes observed in its entirety but more often is seen as a convex defect in the angiographic stream on either the proximal or distal end of an obstructive lesion. Plaque hemorrhage may appear as an abrupt cutoff or a tapered occlusion unresponsive to nitroglycerin.

Coronary artery spasm has recently been postulated to play an important role

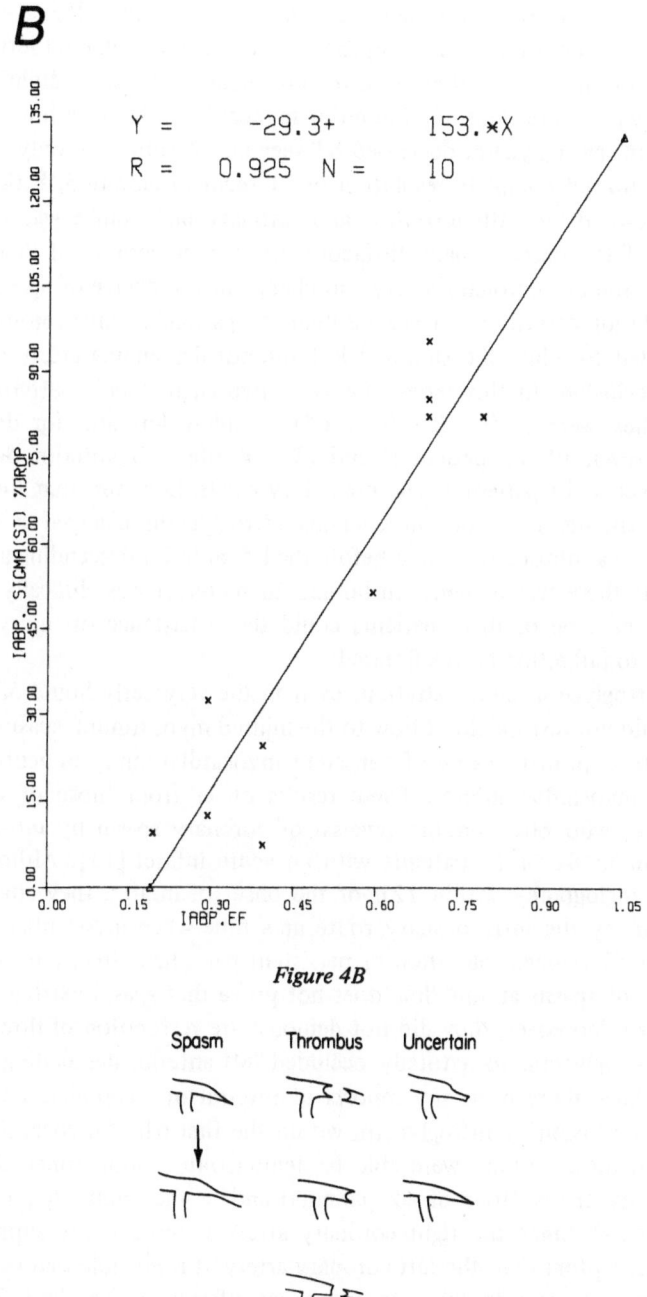

Figure 4B

Figure 5. The schematic representation of the causes of acute left anterior descending coronary artery occlusion: (*left*) coronary artery spasm; (*middle*) intraluminal thrombus; (*right*) plaque hemorrhage.

in the pathogenesis of acute transmural myocardial infarct [13, 14]. In an attempt to overcome spasm and improve antegrade and collateral left anterior descending coronary artery flow, intravenous nitroglycerin was administered to 13 patients with acute transmural anterior myocardial infarct within 2 h of the onset of pain. Nitroglycerin decreased ST segment elevation by only 5%–18%; no patient showed complete resolution of ST segment elevation. Patients were then taken directly to catheterization and coronary angiography was performed within 4 h of the onset of pain. Intracoronary nitroglycerin (200–600 μg) was infused into the left coronary artery: no change in the degree of obstruction in the left anterior descending artery resulted. In particular, intracoronary nitroglycerin failed to dilate the stenosed left anterior descending artery or reverse complete occlusion. In this series, the same two angiographic patterns seen in earlier studies were again identified: (A) complete left anterior descending occlusion (seven of 13 patients), and (B) subtotal left anterior descending occlusion (six of 13 patients). The possibility exists, however, that there was a subset of patients in whom intravenous nitroglycerin changed a complete obstruction to a subtotal occlusion before the left anterior descending artery was opacified. If there was a change in luminal diameter, it was clinically insignificant, since in none of these patients could the persistence of injury and the progression to infarction be ameliorated.

Since nitroglycerin administration, even in the very early hours of an acute infarct, could not restore blood flow to the injured myocardium, spasm does not appear to be a primary cause of persistent myocardial injury in acute anterior transmural myocardial infarct. These results differ from those of Oliva and Breckinridge, who observed the reversal of coronary spasm by intracoronary nitroglycerin in six of 15 patients with an acute infarct [13]. Although they performed angiography within 12 h of the onset of infarct, they administered nitroglycerin by the intracoronary route at a time when myocardial injury, as reflected in ST segment elevation or persistent pain, had already resolved. The observation of spasm at this time does not prove that spasm existed when the infarct began. Moreover, they did not demonstrate restoration of flow by intracoronary nitroglycerin to a totally occluded left anterior descending coronary artery nor have there been any reports of reversal of a complete left anterior descending occlusion by nitroglycerin within the first 6 h of myocardial infarct. In addition, these authors were able to demonstrate spasm principally in the right coronary artery (four of six patients) and in the circumflex artery (one of six patients). Since the right coronary artery is more richly supplied with adrenergic receptors than the left coronary artery, it is possible that spasm plays a more important role in the pathogenesis of inferior myocardial infarct [14]. Chahine et al. in 1975 reported a series of patients with either spontaneous or catheter-induced spasm and summarized the experience from the literature until that time regarding the site of spasm in the coronary arteries: 78% occurred in the right coronary artery; the remainder of instances were distributed through the left coronary (main left 11%, anterior descending 7%, and circumflex 4%).

Maseri and coworkers [15] also postulated that coronary artery spasm may initiate transmural myocardial infarct. Angiographic evidence of a spasm, however, was limited to the preinfarct period, since angiographic studies of patients who developed infarct were delayed 2–15 days. In only one patient was angiography performed during the acute infarct, and in this case sublingual and intracoronary nitroglycerin failed to reverse complete coronary artery obstruction. The observation that patients with Prinzmetal's angina may later suffer acute myocardial infarct does not prove that spasm caused their infarct.

De Wood et al. [12] have examined the obstructed coronary artery during coronary artery bypass surgery in 79 patients with acute myocardial infarcts. A Fogarty catheter was passed to recover any thrombus that contributed to the arterial occlusion. In 57 (72%) of the 79 patients, a thrombus was present consistently situated both proximal and distal to the area of atherosclerotic obstruction. Thus, an intervention directed at altering the acute thrombosis might establish sufficient flow to either limit the size of the infarct directly or facilitate the effects of other interventions (see Griggs, p. 462).

Experimental observation confirms that thrombosis-induced myocardial injury can be largely reversed by administering intracoronary streptokinase to restore flow [16]. Rentrop and co-workers have also shown that early intracoronary streptokinase administration may restore flow in some patients whose acute infarct has resulted from total obstruction in the responsible artery [17]. This restoration of flow was often associated with resolution of ST segment elevation and cessation of pain. These same workers have recently reported the results of transluminal recanalization of totally occluded coronary arteries performed by catheter techniques [18]. Late follow-up studies of these patients have shown further resolution of the obstructive lesion, suggesting that clot lysis plays an important role in restoring flow to totally occluded arteries.

We have recently analyzed the angiographic features of patients with myocardial infarcts in whom coronary angiography was completed within 3 h of the onset of infarct [19] (Table 1). We infused streptokinase (2000–6000 IU/min) into the occluded coronary artery; repeat angiograms of the 16 patients with a convex filling defect showed that streptokinase had restored antegrade flow. Chest pain was relieved and ST segments were reduced thereby in most, but not all, of these patients. After intracoronary streptokinase infusion, the residual coronary artery stenosis was greater than 60%. Despite anticoagulant therapy, the coronary arteries reoccluded in four of the 16 patients within 2–8 weeks of streptokinase therapy. These observations prove that acute thrombosis has an important causal role in patients whose infarct coexists with a convex defect in the responsible artery.

Recent reports from Mathey et al. [20], Ganz et al. [21], and Rentrop et al.

Table 1. Experience with direct intracoronary thrombolytic therapy in acute MI

Reference	No. pts with total occl	Hours post onset	Protocol	Initially opened	Remained open
Gold and Leinbach [19]	20	≤ 3	Streptokinase 2000–6000 IU/min	16/20 80%	12/16 75%
Mathey et al. [20]	37	≤ 3	Plasminogen 500 IU Streptokinase 2000 IU/min	28/37 76%	13/15 87%
Ganz et al. [21]	20	≤ 3	Thrombolysin 2000–4000 IU/min	19/20	–
Rentrop et al. [22]	29	1.5–15	Streptokinase 1000–2000 IU/min	22/29 76%	18/19 95%

[22] are summarized in Table 1. Varying amounts of streptokinase and other thrombolytic agents have been administered to more than 100 patients in whom complete arterial occlusion had been documented during the early hours following the onset of acute infarcts. Overall incidence of establishment of coronary blood flow was 80% (85 of 106) and persistence of flow at restudy after 2–8 weeks was 86% (43 of 50). Initial therapy with heparin and subsequent therapy with warfarin was instituted in all patients.

CONCLUSION

Intraoperative and angiographic studies support the hypothesis that an occlusive intracoronary thrombus is the cause of persistent myocardial injury in many patients with acute myocardial infarcts. Those patients who undergo angiography within 3 h of the onset of pain will demonstrate one of two patterns: (a) complete occlusion, or (b) high-grade stenosis with a severe reduction in antegrade flow. In a majority of cases, intraluminal thrombus identified as a convex filling defect plays an important role in the persistence of myocardial injury. The inability to restore antegrade flow in patients with complete occlusion limits the effectiveness of therapy with interventions such as nitroglycerin, propranolol, or intraaortic balloon pumping. In patients with complete left anterior descending occlusion, effective therapy can be achieved only after the obstructing intracoronary thrombus has been resolved. Further studies are required to determine whether significant differences are present in right coronary or left circumflex occlusion versus left anterior descending occlusion. Selective coronary angiography can be performed safely during the acute phase of myocardial infarction and provides important information regarding the nature of the obstructive lesion in the vessel supplying the infarct zone. Ventricular fibrillation appears to be the only complication that occurs commonly during the acute phase, and its incidence may be reduced by diminishing the number of coronary injections. The benefits of early angiography in the management of patients with myocardial infarct require further study.

Acknowledgment. This work has been supported by NIH grant IP50 HL 26215-01 (SCOR on Ischemic Heart Disease); Project II-4, Invasive Therapy of Myocardial Infarction.

REFERENCES

1. Blumgart HL, Schlesinger MJ, Davis D: Studies on the relation of the clinical manifestations of angina pectoris, coronary thrombosis, and myocardial infarction to the pathologic findings: with particular reference to the significance of the collateral circulation. Am Heart J 19:1–91, 1940.
2. Roberts WC, Buja LM: The frequency and significance of coronary arterial thrombi and other observations in fatal acute myocardial infarction. A study of 107 necropsy patients. Am J Med 52:425–443, 1972.
3. Roberts WC, Jones AA: Quantification of coronary arterial narrowing at necropsy in acute transmural myocardial infarction: analysis and comparison of findings in 27 patients and 22 controls. Circulation 61:786–790, 1980.
4. Silver MD, Baroldi G, Mariani F: The relationship between acute occlusive coronary thrombi and myocardial infarction studied in 100 consecutive patients. Circulation 61:219–227, 1980.
5. El-Maraghi NRH, Sealey BJ: Recurrent myocardial infarction in a young man due to coronary arterial spasm demonstrated at autopsy. Circulation 61:199–207, 1980.
6. O'Reilly RJ, Spellberg RD: Rapid resolution of coronary arterial emboli. Myocardial infarction and subsequent normal coronary anteriograms. Ann Intern Med 81:348–350, 1974.
7. Leinbach RC, Gold HK, Dinsmore RE, Mundth ED, Buckley MJ, Austen WG, Sanders CA: The role of angiography in cardiogenic shock. Circulation [Suppl 3] 47 and 48: III-95–98, 1973.
8. Maroko PR, Kjekshus JK, Sobel BE, Watanabe T, Covell JW, Ross J Jr, Braunwald E: Factors influencing infarct size following experimental coronary artery occlusions. Circulation 43:67–82, 1971.
9. Gold HK, Leinbach RC, Maroko PR. Propranolol-induced reduction of signs of ischemic injury during acute myocardial infarction. Am J. Cardiol 38:689–695, 1976.
10. Leinbach RC, Gold HK, Harper RW, Buckley MJ, Austen WG: Early intra-aortic balloon pumping for anterior myocardial infarction without shock. Circulation 58:204–210, 1978.
11. Harper WH, Gold HK, Leinbach RC: Acute myocardial infarction. In: Johnson RA, Haber EH, Austen WG (eds) The practice of cardiology. Boston: Little, Brown and Company, 1980, pp 310–338.
12. De Wood MA, Spores J, Notske R, Mouser LT, Burroughs R, Golden MS,

Lang HT: Prevalence of total coronary occlusion during the early hours of transmural myocardial infarction. N Engl J Med 303:897–902, 1980.

13. Oliva PB, Breckinridge JC: Arteriographic evidence of coronary arterial spasm in acute myocardial infarction. Circulation 56:366–374, 1977.

14. Chahine RA, Raizner AE, Ishimori T, Luchi RJ, McIntosh HD: The incidence and clinical implications of coronary artery spasm. Circulation 52:972–978, 1975.

15. Maseri A, L'Abbate A, Baroldi G, Chierchia S, Marzilla M, Ballestra AM, Severi S, Parodi O, Biagini A, Distante A, Pesola A: Coronary vasospasm as a possible cause of myocardial infarction: a conclusion derived from the study of 'preinfarction' angina. N Engl J Med 229:1271–1277, 1978.

16. Kanmatsuse K, Lando U, Mercier JC, Fishbein MC, Swan HJC, Ganz W: Rapid lysis of coronary thrombi by local application of fibrinolysin. Circulation [Suppl 2] 60:II–216, 1979.

17. Rentrop P, Blanke H, Karsch KR: Limitation of myocardial injury by transluminal recanalization in acute myocardial infarction. Circulation [Suppl 2] 60: II–163, 1979.

18. Rentrop KP, Blanke H, Karsch KR, Kreuzer H: Initial experience with transluminal recanalization of the recently occluded infarct-related coronary artery in acute myocardial infarction. Comparison with conventionally treated patients. Clin Cardiol 2:1–5, 1979.

19. Gold HK, Leinbach RC: Coronary flow restoration in myocardial infarction by intracoronary streptokinase [abstr]. Circulation [Part II] 62:III-161, 1980.

20. Mathey D, Kuck K-H, Tilsner V, Bleifeld W: Non-surgical coronary artery recanalization in acute myocardial infarction. [abstr]. Circulation [Part II] 62:III–160, 1980.

21. Ganz W, Buchbinder N, Marcus H, Mondkar A, Maddahi J, Charuzi Y, O'Connor L, Shell W, Fishbein MC, Kass R, Miyamoto A, Swan HJC: Intracoronary thrombolysis in evolving myocardial infarction. Am Heart J 101:4–13, 1981.

22. Rentrop P, Blanke H, Karsch KR, Kaiser H, Köstering H, Leitz K: Selective intracoronary thrombolysis in acute myocardial infarction and unstable angina pectoris. Circulation 63:307–317, 1981.

IV. AN OVERVIEW

22. CURRENT STATUS OF MEASUREMENTS AND EFFORTS TO REDUCE MYOCARDIAL INFARCT SIZE IN MAN

JAMES E. MULLER, ROBERT E. RUDE, and EUGENE BRAUNWALD

Ischemic heart disease represents the most common serious health problem of contemporary Western society. In this country alone, more than 675,000 patients die each year from ischemic heart disease and its complications, approximately 1,300,000 patients develop a myocardial infarct, and countless more suffer from congestive heart failure secondary to ischemic myocardial damage. Acute myocardial infarction thus remains the most common cause of inhospital deaths in this country, indeed in the Western world. Inhospital deaths of patients with acute myocardial infarction result mainly from primary arrhythmias and from pump failure [1]. Whereas death due to arrhythmias has been reduced by modern monitoring techniques and more vigorous prophylaxis and treatment, the death rate following mechanical failure manifested by cardiogenic shock and/or pulmonary edema is still very high. These syndromes have been found to be associated with larger infarcts than those exhibited by other patients who succumbed to myocardial infarction, but who did not die as a consequence of pump failure [2, 3]. The prognosis for patients with larger infarcts is distinctly worse than it is for those with smaller infarcts [3].

The myocardium in the vascular territory of a totally obstructed coronary artery had long been thought to rapidly become ischemic, with only a brief interval before the damage became irreversible. Clinical prognosis following infarction is now known to depend directly on the quantity of residual viable, normally functioning myocardium. If one could effectively limit tissue damage following coronary occlusion, pump failure and its consequences might be averted. Basic to any consideration of this problem is the progression of myocardial ischemic injury following coronary artery occlusion (see Hutchins, p. 11). In studies of experimentally induced infarcts in animals, myocardial tissue supplied by an occluded vessel does not show an essentially homogeneous area of necrosis. Rather, after occlusion the affected myocardium is likely to manifest a region of central necrosis surrounded in patchy fashion by a substantial amount of abnormal but still viable tissue. The ischemic zone may increase in size for some time, while the necrotic zone remains relatively small. According to some studies, the ischemic zone may continue to enlarge for up to 18 h after occlusion [4]; thereafter the region of central necrosis expands rapidly at the expense of ischemic tissue. The absence of a clear demarcation

Wagner GS (ed): Myocardial Infarction: Measurement and Intervention, pp 517–546.
© *1982 Martinus Nijhoff Publishers, The Hague/Boston/London.*

between normal and necrotic tissue on histologic examination of human hearts at autopsy has been noted repeatedly, and it appears likely that the progression from ischemic damage to necrosis follows a time course in man similar to that in experimental animals.

Death from cardiogenic shock may now be viewed as the end result of a vicious cycle [5]. Coronary obstruction leads to myocardial ischemia, which impairs myocardial contractility and ventricular performance; this, in turn, reduces arterial pressure and therefore coronary perfusion pressure, leading to further ischemia and extension of necrosis, until, in most cases, death occurs. There is some evidence that stasis in the smaller arteries and arterioles distal to a major proximal occlusion can result in secondary microvascular obstruction, further impairing myocardial perfusion.

Accordingly, a treatment that could decrease the extent of tissue death in the myocardium, and by this mechanism decrease the frequency of intractable cardiogenic shock and pulmonary edema, would be extremely useful, not only by reducing immediate mortality, but also by leaving the patient who had suffered a coronary occlusion with more viable myocardium. Such a patient would probably be less likely to develop chronic heart failure and would have a greater reserve of functioning myocardium should another coronary occlusion occur.

The above-mentioned considerations suggested to us in 1967 that the ultimate size of a myocardial infarct is not irrevocably determined by the site of coronary occlusion, but might be modified by other factors [6]. We then proposed that when coronary occlusion occurs, the survival of the cardiac tissue normally perfused by the obstructed vessel depends on the balance between oxygen available to that segment of myocardium and its oxygen requirements and that the survival of the patient with coronary occlusion could, in large measure, be dependent on the balance between myocardial oxygen supply and demand [7].

MEASUREMENT OF INFARCT SIZE

The preceding chapters in this book have described many techniques for measuring the quantity of myocardium infarcted and the effect of an infarction on ventricular function. The several available techniques, each with its own advantages and limitations, have led to development of a specialized area of activity in clinical research. Although mastery of this complex area is not essential for the routine clinical care of patients with acute myocardial infarction, clinicians not actively engaged in research on infarct size must be sufficiently informed about the techniques to evaluate the results of the many studies of limitation of infarct size that are now in progress. The clinical investigator who seeks to determine the effects of an intervention on ischemic myocardium must be thoroughly familiar with the capabilities and limitations of each of the techniques described below.

Electrocardiographic methods

The clinical use of both ST segment and QRS mapping is based on the close relationship between changes in epicardial and precordial electrical potentials (see Selvester, p. 23; and Arnsdorf, p. 66) [8]. A reduction in the ST segment elevation in precordial electrocardiograms without a simultaneous development of a Q wave can, in general, be considered a sign of a beneficial effect of an intervention on acute myocardial ischemic injury. Since patients with acute myocardial infarction ordinarily demonstrate progressive reductions of elevations of ST segments as a function of time alone, it is essential that results in a group of treated patients be compared with those in a separate group of comparable untreated controls. This approach was employed in an investigation which demonstrated that patients with acute myocardial infarction who received hyaluronidase showed a significantly more rapid fall in ST segment elevation than a control group [9].

Alternatively, the patient may be used as his own control; with this approach a control period precedes the application of the intervention under investigation. Using this method, it has been demonstrated that accelerated reductions in precordial ST segment elevation may occur following various beneficial interventions [10–13]. The results of this approach are most persuasive when a postintervention control study is reported and the ST segments revert to their previous elevations. However, since it is possible that the beneficial effect of an intervention can persist after the intervention ends, it is not essential for a demonstration of efficacy that ST segment elevation increase after cessation of treatment. Reelevation of ST segments has also been suggested as a method of detecting extensions of the original area of ischemic injury [14].

Analysis of the ST segment is of little if any value in assessing interventions in the presence of pericarditis or any other conditions that may, by themselves, alter ST segment elevation. In addition, an accelerated rate of fall of ST segment elevation may reflect accelerated progression from ischemic injury to necrosis. Only an independent assessment of actual myocardial necrosis, as can be provided by analysis of changes in the QRS complex, can confirm tissue salvage.

The following method of precordial QRS mapping has been used in patients with acute myocardial infarction: Precordial electrocardiograms are recorded from 35 sites on the patient's chest, as soon as the patient comes under observation [15]. The patient is then randomly assigned to a control or treatment group. A second precordial map is recorded one week later in order to evaluate changes in the QRS complex at the sites at risk (i.e., the sites that exhibited

ST segment elevations on the first map), and the extent of the change in the control and treatment groups is compared. Even with relatively small sample sizes, this QRS mapping technique can be used to detect protection of ischemic myocardium.

The greatest limitation of electrocardiographic mapping (ST and QRS) is its restriction to patients with transmural anterior or lateral myocardial infarct (although it has been suggested that orthogonal leads and vectorcardiograms may be used to study infarcts in other locations [16]). In addition, patients must be free of significant intraventricular conduction defects. For QRS mapping, the patient must survive one week without developing a conduction abnormality so that the post-treatment map can be obtained, but such prolonged survival is not required for ST segment mapping. QRS mapping is useful in assessing directional differences in infarct size between treated and control groups, whereas ST segment mapping can be employed in detecting short-term beneficial or deleterious effects on acute myocardial ischemia. Finally, electrocardiographic mapping in its present form does not yield quantitative results in terms of the actual amount of myocardium infarcted or salvaged. Therefore, the demonstration of a difference in QRS evolution between two groups of patients cannot be translated into an estimate of the actual quantity of myocardium preserved.

Enzymatic estimation of infarct size

An impressive documentation of the accuracy of CK release techniques for the measurement of infarct size was provided by Bleifeld and associates, who reported an excellent correlation between enzymatically (total CK) estimated and anatomically measured infarct size in 17 patients coming to autopsy soon after a transmural infarct; anatomically measured infarct size also correlated well with the level of peak serum CK when frequent determinations were made [17]. The original observations of Sobel and his associates indicated that infarct size estimated enzymatically is a good predictor of subsequent death from pump failure and of the functional disability of survivors [3]. Also, Roberts et al. have described a positive correlation between CK infarct size and the frequency of ventricular dysrhythmias in the first 20 h after hospital admission; the correlation was improved when only patients having their first infarct were analyzed [18]. More recently, Geltman et al. have confirmed the relationship between enzymatically estimated infarct size and prognosis as well as the incidence of late ventricular arrhythmias [19]. Rogers et al. have reported a good correlation of CK-MB infarct size with the number of abnormally contracting segments and an inverse correlation with ejection fraction determined by biplane left ventriculography performed approximately one month after infarct; as might be anticipated, their data showed poorer correlations in patients with prior infarcts and in those with suspected right ventricular infarct [20]. The inverse correlation between infarct size estimated enzymatically and the left ventricular ejection fraction has recently been confirmed by single-plane ventriculography performed two months after infarction [21].

Estimation of infarct size by measurement of plasma enzymes remains one of the most promising currently available methods (see Roberts, p. 113; and Cobb and Roe, p. 156). Of all techniques, it is probably the most readily applicable to infarcts of varying types (anterior and inferior, transmural and non-transmural) and sizes. However, it requires that the patient come under observation within 10—12 h of the onset of the clinical event so that the full curve of CK activity can be recorded. Although enzymatically estimated infarct size in an individual patient is generally available too late to affect acute management decisions, and may not be a better predictor of prognosis than more easily obtained clinical data (see Rogers, p. 162), the technique may prove very useful in assessing differences in infarct size between groups of patients subjected to different interventions. Before widespread acceptance of such data, however, more correlations between infarct size estimation and post-mortem findings are needed.

Scintigraphic methods

In recent years, great advances have been made in the application of radio-nuclide methods that assess the heart's global and regional wall motion and volume [22—24], the state of myocardial perfusion [25—27], and the integrity of myocardial metabolic pathways [28]. In addition, radionuclides have been developed that sequester preferentially in regions of the myocardium that are acutely injured and undergoing necrosis [29, 30]. These techniques have proved useful for measuring the size and physiologic consequences of acute myocardial infarction. Prototype techniques are myocardial imaging with infarct-avid radio-nuclides, such as technetium-99m pyrophosphate (TcPYP), so-called 'hot spot' imaging because of the positive image created by radionuclide uptake in an area of infarct; perfusion imaging with thallium-201, known as 'cold spot' imaging because of the relative lack of radionuclide uptake in areas with diminished blood flow; radionuclide angiography to assess left ventricular wall motion; X-ray imaging with computerized tomography; and 'metabolic imaging' with positron-emitting substances that demarcate regions of abnormal myocardial metabolism.

Imaging with infarct-avid radionuclides (see Marcus, p. 326)

The problems encountered in sizing infarcts in patients with TcPYP have been enumerated by Marcus and Kerber and by Willerson [31, 32]. Probably the most fundamental problem is that a two-dimensional quantity, TcPYP infarct *area* determined by planimetry of a single scintigraphic projection, is being used to estimate infarct *volume*, a three-dimensional quantity. Certain infarct locations (inferior, septal) appear to be underestimated by two-dimensional sizing techniques because their largest dimension is not viewed *en face* in standard scintigraphic projections. Three-dimensional 'reconstruction' of experimental infarcts has been attempted with some success by using two-dimensional data and a number of geometric assumptions [33]. The development of a tomographic scintillation camera for use with TcPYP scintigraphy might provide a true three-dimensional image [32]. A variety of advances currently taking place, such as augmentation of the resolution power of the scintillation cameras, gating of studies to reduce blurring of images due to cardiac motion, development of more reproducible automatic edge detection techniques, and subtraction or filtering techniques to avoid confusion of myocardial activity with that of overlying or underlying structures (particularly bone), all suggest that the accuracy of infarct size measurement by 'hot spot' myocardial imaging will be improved in the near future.

Myocardial perfusion imaging (see Okada, p. 295)

A significant problem that arises when myocardial perfusion scintigraphy is used to measure infarct size is the variability of the size of the defect, particularly early in the infarction process. Wackers et al. found ^{201}Tl perfusion defects in all patients studied within 6 h of onset of symptoms of a confirmed infarction, but noted negative or equivocal scintigrams with increasing frequency in patients studied later, especially those with smaller infarcts; repeat scintigrams in some patients confirmed decreasing size of the ^{201}Tl defect, probably due to increasing collateral blood flow to the ischemic region [34]. Redistribution of ^{201}Tl into the initially demonstrated defect has been observed in dogs with brief coronary occlusions followed by coronary perfusion, in patients with exercise-induced myocardial ischemia [35] and in patients studied within 6–12 h of the development of acute myocardial infarction [36]. These observations emphasize that ^{201}Tl scintigraphy primarily reflects the state of regional myocardial perfusion at a given instant (see Cobb and Murdock, p. 277). It does not provide specific identification and quantification of acute infarct.

Radionuclide angiography (see Wackers, p. 199)

Serial radionuclide angiograms have been reported in patients with acute myocardial infarction [37, 38]. From these studies, it has become clear that global left ventricular function (reflected in the ejection fraction) varies considerably soon after infarction. Patients with an uncomplicated clinical course or progressive improvement tend to have stable or increasing ejection fractions on serial studies, while patients with clinical deterioration have depressed ejection fractions that fail to improve and sometimes even decrease in serial studies [37, 38]. Rigo et al. observed a good correlation between global left ventricular ejection fraction and the percent of the left ventricular wall considered to be akinetic, and proposed that the latter reflects infarct size [37]. Sharpe et al. reported a correlation between the percentages of abnormally contracting segments on radionuclide angiography and the area of infarct estimated by TcPYP scintigraphy [39].

No quantitative studies relating indices of regional ventricular functional impairment and anatomically measured infarct size have been reported in experimental animals or in man, and therefore the role of radionuclide angiography in measuring infarct size is still unsettled. This technique, like ^{201}Tl perfusion scintigraphy, is more effective in revealing altered function rather than in demarcating areas of necrosis. Regional wall motion abnormalities can result from old or new infarction, ischemic dysfunction without infarction, and even from impairment of myocardial function not due to ischemic disease. Therefore other markers of acute infarction are required in conjunction with radionuclide angiography, if a specific estimate of acute infarct size is to be made. Regardless of these limitations, the results of *serial* radionuclide angiographic studies in groups of patients may prove to be of great value in assessing the impact of interventions on left ventricular function, and in indicating whether certain therapeutic interventions have favorable short- or long-term effects on ventricular function.

Computed tomography (see Whitaker, p. 261)

Since the development of computerized transverse axial tomography, this exciting technique of noninvasive reconstruction of internal anatomy has been applied to most regions of the body, including the heart. Early *in vitro* studies of canine hearts excised after experimental myocardial infarction demonstrated that infarcted myocardium exhibits an area of decreased X-ray attenuation, thought to be caused by the edema associated with the acute infarct [40–42]. Gray et al. attempted to size experimentally produced infarcts by this technique following the intravenous injection of iodinated contrast material just prior to the animal's sacrifice; a good correlation was found with infarct volume determined anatomically [43]. Unfortunately, the use of this promising technique *in vivo* has been hampered by motion artifacts associated with the beating heart. Its clinical application for infarct sizing awaits the perfection of methods for gating images to specific phases of the cardiac cycle, and of differentiating fresh from old infarcts, as well as ischemic from infarcted myocardium.

ALTERATION OF INFARCT SIZE

There is a bewildering array of interventions that have been shown in experimental animals to exert a favorable effect on ischemic myocardium (Table 1)

Table 1. Interventions that modify experimental myocardial injury following coronary occlusion

---

(1) By decreasing myocardial oxygen demand
　　Propranolol
　　Cardiac glycoside in the failing heart
　　Intraaortic balloon counterpulsation
　　Decreasing afterload in hypertensive individuals – Arfonad
　　Inhibiting calcium influx – verapamil
　　Hypothermia

(2) By increasing myocardial oxygen supply
　　(a) Directly
　　　　Coronary artery reperfusion
　　　　Elevating arterial pO_2
　　(b) Through collateral vessels
　　　　Elevation of coronary perfusion pressure by methoxamine, neosynephrine, or
　　　　　norepinephrine
　　　　Intraaortic balloon counterpulsation
　　　　By coronary vasodilatation – calcium blockers – verapamil, prostacyclin
　　(c) Reverse coronary steal or favorable redistribution of regional myocardial blood
　　　　flow – nitroglycerin

(3) By increasing plasma osmolality
　　Mannitol
　　Hypertonic glucose

(4) By augmenting anaerobic metabolism (presumed)
　　Glucose–insulin–potassium
　　Hypertonic glucose
(5) By enhancing transport to the ischemic zone of substrate utilised in energy production
　　(presumed)
　　Hyaluronidase
(6) By protecting against autolytic and heterolytic processes (presumed)
　　Glucocorticoids
　　Cobra venom factor
　　Aprotinin
　　Nonsteroidal antiinflammatory agents – Ibuprofen

---

[44]. We review here the clinical experience with the most promising and most extensively studied interventions.

Beta-adrenergic blocking agents (see Reimer and Jennings, p. 397)

Peter et al. have reported the results of a randomized trial of propranolol (0.1 mg/kg intravenously followed by 320 mg orally over the next 27 h). Patients treated within 4 h of the onset of symptoms of uncomplicated myocardial infarcts exhibited significantly lower peak serum CK levels, lower calculated CK release, and a slower rate of appearance of CK in the serum than did patients without specific therapy [45]. The same investigators have also reported that patients with suspected myocardial infarct, treated within 4 h of onset of symptoms with the same regimen of propranolol, had a significantly lower incidence of electrocardiographic evolution compatible with transmural or nontransmural infarction as well as a lower incidence of serum CK elevation, suggesting that 'threatened' myocardial intarction might actually be prevented by early beta-blockade [46]. A more recent study has been conducted in 215 patients treated acutely with the beta-blocker atenolol. The incidence of infarction was 61% in the control group versus 31% in the atenolol-treated group among patients who did not have infarction at the time of entry into the study [47]. Earlier studies had suggested a decreased incidence of myocardial infarction in patients already taking beta-blockers who were admitted to the hospital with suspected infarction [48].

In 1977, Mueller and Ayres collected 126 cases of acute myocardial infarction treated in several centers with intravenous propranolol while hemodynamic monitoring was carried out [49]. Patients were selected because of acute infarction in the absence of left ventricular failure, heart block, or other contraindications to beta-blockade, and usually received 0.1 mg/kg propranolol intravenously; hemodynamic effects included decreases in cardiac output, arterial pressure, heart rate, and myocardial oxygen consumption [50]; adverse effects of carefully monitored therapy were very rare, in contrast to earlier reports of the precipitation of heart failure by propranolol [51]. The negative chronotropic and inotropic effects of beta-blockers may be reversed by therapy with a beta-adrenergic agonist; the endogenous catecholamine, dopamine, or the synthetic sympathomimetics, dobutamine or prenalterol, may be particularly effective.

Gold et al. have demonstrated that intravenous propranolol accelerated the fall of ST segment elevation in patients with acute myocardial infarction [13]. Waagstein et al. observed a dramatic decrease in chest pain when beta-blockade was administered to patients with acute infarction [52]. These investigators have also emphasized that beta-blockade may be particularly effective in the subset of patients with markedly elevated beta-adrenergic activity [53].

In summary, beta-adrenergic blockade has beneficial effects on ischemic myocardium in both experimental animals and patients. Intravenous and oral therapy with beta-blockers is safe if patients are carefully selected; hemodynamic monitoring with a balloon catheter, arterial line, and cardiac output measurements is not always necessary. Although preliminary reports indicate that early intervention with intravenous propranolol might limit infarct size or even prevent its occurrence [45–47], these findings must be confirmed in rigorously controlled clinical trials utilizing several techniques for assessing infarct size before acute beta-blockade can be considered standard therapy for uncomplicated myocardial infarction. Beta-blockade is likely to produce symptomatic relief of unstable angina pectoris, the most likely diagnosis if infarction does not evolve. Harm may result from discontinuation of chronic beta-blocker therapy in patients who present with acute myocardial infarction, although it should be emphasized that reports of propranolol withdrawal phenomena apply to ambulatory patients [54] and do not provide information on discontinuation of beta-blockade in the patient hospitalized with acute myocardial infarction.

Counterpulsation (see Becker, p. 420)

There is preliminary evidence that intraaortic balloon counterpulsation (IABC) may limit ischemic injury in patients with uncomplicated acute myocardial infarction [55, 56]. IABC was initiated less than 6 h after the commencement of pain in 11 patients with anterior myocardial infarction without cardiogenic shock [56]. In patients with stenosis but without complete occlusion of the left anterior descending coronary artery, there was an accelerated fall of ST segment elevation during IABC. A beneficial response was also more likely if IABC was initiated soon after the onset of pain [56]. Presumably ischemia and myocardial infarct size are reduced by lowering systolic ventricular pressure (which decreases myocardial oxygen demands) and by raising arterial diastolic pressure (which improves myocardial perfusion).

These studies, together with supporting laboratory evidence, have led to the proposal that a randomized multicenter trial be conducted to determine if IABC should be routinely utilized to limit the size of a myocardial infarction [56]. The efficacy of this technique must be firmly established because its application is expensive and associated with some risk. Complication rates as high as 23% have been reported [57]. The frequency of complications increases markedly with increased duration of counterpulsation and is greatest in patients with peripheral vascular disease.

An intraaortic balloon that can be inserted percutaneously with the use of the Seldinger technique has recently been developed [58]. The reported ease of insertion and freedom from vascular complications of this new method may lead to a major increase in the use of IABC. However, even with greater ease of insertion, recommendation for the widespread use of IABC to limit infarct size must await the results of a prospective, randomized trial.

External counterpulsation (ECP) is another technique by which the aortic diastolic pressure can be augmented. The patient's legs are enclosed in chambers in which positive and negative pressures are applied during diastole and systole, respectively. The primary impetus for the development of this technique has been the desire to avoid the difficult initiation and the complications of IABC. In a comparative study, ECP produced an increase in cardiac output comparable to IABC, although the latter produced a greater increase in diastolic arterial pressure [59]. While ECP failed to show a beneficial effect on enzymatically determined infarct size in that study, counterpulsation was not initiated until 7 h after the increase in plasma CK [60]. A randomized multicenter trial of the value of ECP has been conducted in 258 patients with acute myocardial infarction. There was no significant difference in mortality between treated and control groups, although analysis of subgroups did reveal significant mortality differences [61].

In summary, ECP can produce beneficial hemodynamic changes and may well limit infarct size. Its routine use cannot be advocated until a randomized study demonstrates significant beneficial results in all randomized patients or in a prospectively identified subgroup.

Nitroglycerin and other nitrate preparations (see Becker, p. 426)

Favorable hemodynamic effects (fall in left ventricular filling pressure) have been reported following the use of sublingual nitroglycerin in patients with acute myocardial infarction [62, 63]. Come et al. studied a group of patients treated an average of 6 h after the onset of anterior transmural infarction; intravenous nitroglycerin (average dose 41 μg/min) was given to lower mean arterial blood pressure by 20 mmHg [64]. Addition of the alpha-adrenergic agonist phenylephrine to raise mean arterial pressure to control levels resulted in reelevation of precordial ST segment values to levels not significantly different from those observed before nitroglycerin therapy, and also reversed the nitroglycerin-induced fall in left ventricular filling pressure [64]. Further studies showed consistent reductions in ST segment elevations in 15 patients with anterior infarcts treated with intravenous nitroglycerin (average dose 57 μg/min for 1–3 h) given to decrease mean arterial blood pressure by 20 mmHg; this beneficial effect on ischemia was noted in patients with both normal and abnormal left ventricular filling pressure [65].

Borer et al. [66] administered nitroglycerin (1.5–2.5 mg) sublingually and observed a significant decline in precordial ST segment elevation; a further reduction in this index of ischemia was noted when phenylephrine was infused to reverse the hypotensive effects of nitroglycerin. The seven patients with normal left ventricular filling pressure had no definite or consistent fall in Σ ST with nitroglycerin alone, but a decline in Σ ST was evident with the addition of phenylephrine. In contrast, patients with initially elevated left ventricular filling pressures demonstrated a decrease in ST segment elevation with nitroglycerin alone and some reversal of this apparent beneficial effect when the arterial pressure was increased to control levels with phenylephrine. The apparent differences in the findings of Borer et al. and Come et al., emphasized by their publication in the same issue of the same journal [64, 66], highlight the fact that the response of acute myocardial ischemia to nitroglycerin is variable, depending to uncertain degrees on the route of administration, the dose, and the baseline hemodynamic state of the patient.

In addition to its effect on indices of acute myocardial ischemia, intravenous nitroglycerin has been reported to affect measurements of infarct size. Chiche, Derrida, and their associates have been conducting a randomized, though not double-blinded, trial of prolonged nitroglycerin infusion in patients with acute myocardial infarction [67, 68]. Although a detailed report of their methods and data is not yet available, approximately 95 patients (50 treated with nitroglycerin at an average infusion rate of 51 μg/min for 5–7 days, and 45 controls) have been studied; precordial ST segment mapping in those with anterior infarcts showed a 30% decrease in ΣST 30 min after the start of nitroglycerin therapy, and precordial ECG maps after seven days showed less R wave fall at initially ischemic sites in the nitroglycerin-treated group. Furthermore, in patients with heart failure, mortality was lower in the nitroglycerin group (6%) than in controls (35%); the incidence of serious arrhythmias (ventricular tachycardia and ventricular fibrillation) was lower as well. Bussmann et al. have reported the preliminary results of a prospective randomized trial of intravenous nitroglycerin in 60 patients with acute myocardial infarction [69]. They observed significantly lower values of peak serum CK, slower rates of CK release, and smaller calculated infarct size (in CK gram-equivalents). In patients treated with intravenous nitroglycerin for 48 h, followed for 72 h with nitroglycerin ointment, Becker et al. observed enhanced postinfarction improvement of myocardial perfusion measured with thallium-201 scintigraphy [70].

Although detailed information on adverse effects of therapy is not available from the many preliminary reports, a review of published studies [11, 64, 65] reveals that *intravenous* nitroglycerin infusion at rates up to approximately 50 μg/min has not caused consistent acceleration of heart rate, and that decreases in mean arterial pressure of up to 25 mmHg have been well tolerated. In fact, reports of clinically deleterious tachycardia and hypotension seem more prominent in those studies in which *sublingual* nitroglycerin is used [66, 71, 72], perhaps because of the variability in absorption of sublingual preparations and the inability to rapidly control the hemodynamic response, as is possible with skillfully monitored intravenous nitroglycerin infusion.

Bussmann et al. have recently studied the effects of variable doses of intravenous nitroglycerin on ST segment elevation in patients with acute myocardial infarction; ΣST was decreased with infusions of 50 μg/min, but this effect was partially reversed when 100 μg/min was administered [73]. This apparent adverse effect on ischemia was associated with a slight rise in the heart rate, and was more prominent in patients without heart failure, as had been noted earlier by Epstein et al. [74]. Come and Pitt have described another acute hemodynamic complication of sublingual and intravenous nitroglycerin in patients with acute myocardial infarction—severe hypotension and bradycardia, which responds to leg raising and intravenous atropine; this complication occurred in 9% of the initial experience with 54 patients treated within 24 h of the onset of infarction. Only one of the patients had inferior infarction, which is generally associated with such episodes [75]. Other investigators have recently reported an increase in the frequency of ventricular premature beats, but not in repetitive ectopy, following 24 h of therapy with intravenous nitroglycerin after the onset of infarction; in addition, no decrease in infarct size (calculated from CK-release curves) was found, and there was no difference in analgesic requirements in the treatment and control groups [75, 76].

At present, the use of nitroglycerin to reduce infarct size in patients must still be considered experimental. Although recent clinical studies have suggested that intravenous infusion, perhaps followed by sublingual or topical therapy, reduces the extent of myocardial necrosis, and perhaps even mortality, in patients with myocardial infarction and left ventricular failure, the great variability in study methods (patient selection and method of determining the dose appropriate for any given patient) and the lack of a randomized double-blind trial showing efficacy, caution against routine nitroglycerin administration to all patients with acute myocardial infarction. The reported adverse effects [66, 71, 77] demand careful scrutiny by future investigators. At the present time, the use of nitroglycerin to limit infarct size should be restricted to those centers endeavoring to determine its efficacy in a prospective fashion with structured data collection, and the drug should be used only with careful hemodynamic and electrocardiographic monitoring, for purposes of both patient safety and data acquisition.

Hemodynamic improvement in the patient with acute myocardial infarction is not necessarily accompanied by an amelioration of the ischemic process or a reduction in infarct size, and the distinction between these two possible effects of nitroglycerin and other vasodilators should be kept in mind in the interpretation of results and in considering future studies. Thus, while nitroglycerin has not been definitively proved to reduce infarct size, it does improve circulatory dynamics in normotensive patients with left ventricular failure and the reported experience indicates good short-term tolerance of the agent in most patients with acute infarction. It should be considered for the relief of postinfarction angina in patients who do not tolerate opiate analgesics.

Other vasodilators (see Becker, p. 423)

Vasodilator agents other than the nitrates have produced more variable effects on acute ischemic injury than nitroglycerin, and are therefore considered separately. In general, these agents induce more peripheral arteriolar vasodilation than do the nitrates (whose principal vasodilator action is on the venous, not the arteriolar bed), thereby decreasing arterial blood pressure and augmenting the cardiac output when administered to patients with elevated systemic vascular resistance [78–80]. Their effect on the coronary arteries and coronary blood flow is controversial [81–83]. Nitroprusside has been the most widely used drug in this group [81–85], although phentolamine [80] and trimethaphan [86] have also been employed.

Early clinical studies of vasodilators in acute myocardial infarction focused on hemodynamic changes with therapy, and usually included patients with evidence of left ventricular dysfunction or systemic hypertension complicating infarction, with therapy frequently beginning several days after the onset of the clinical event [78, 79, 84]. Although vasodilator therapy can improve the clinical course and perhaps even the short-term survival of patients with pump failure complicating infarction, the long-term outlook for these patients is poor, even with attempts at chronic nitrate therapy [85]. Shell and Sobel reported a smaller than predicted infarct size determined enzymatically in 14 hypertensive patients treated with trimethaphan to lower arterial pressure [86].

Arterial hypotension, reflex tachycardia, and resulting coronary hypoperfusion with intensification of ischemia are the major potential dangers associated with vasodilator therapy in acute myocardial infarction. Fortunately these hemodynamic effects of intravenously administered agents are reversible within minutes of discontinuation of the drug. Potential beneficial actions include decreased afterload and left ventricular volume with resultant decreases in myocardial oxygen consumption. Invasive hemodynamic monitoring for potential complications, as well as for titration of doses to the desired hemodynamic effects, is mandatory.

In summary, parenterally administered vasodilators, other than nitrates, although potentially useful for management of left ventricular failure and systemic hypertension complicating infarction, may intensify acute ischemic injury when given within hours after onset of acute infarction. The evidence that they may decrease infarct size is extremely tenuous at this time.

Reperfusion (see Gold, p. 511)

Limited clinical experience in patients suggests that, as in animal studies, reperfusion accomplished less than 3 h after coronary occlusion may result in salvage of ischemic myocardium [87, 88]. Such early reperfusion is feasible primarily in patients whose coronary occlusion occurs in the hospital. However, there is considerable controversy regarding the advisability of treating uncomplicated acute myocardial infarction with reperfusion by coronary artery bypass grafting. In one investigation, emergency coronary artery bypass grafting was performed in 96 patients with acute myocardial infarction with a 5.2%

mortality [89]. Despite the impressive nature of these results, this experience cannot be used as a basis for recommending that coronary artery bypass grafting be routinely performed for myocardial infarction since a randomized control group was not available. In another study, a low inhospital mortality (5.8%) in 187 patients in whom coronary artery bypass grafting was performed during infarction was also reported. Mortality in a medically treated control group, which was selected retrospectively and therefore in a nonrandomized manner, was 11.5%. Differences in mortality between the treated and control groups were statistically significant if patients with Killip class IV congestive heart failure were excluded or if the comparison was made between the control group and surgical patients whose CK was not elevated preoperatively. Phillips et al. also demonstrated the safety of coronary artery bypass grafting during infarction (1.3% operative mortality in 75 patients) but noted that it was not possible to know how extensive the infarct would have been had surgery not been performed [90]. The authors conclude, as do we, that a controlled randomized trial of coronary artery bypass grafting for evolving myocardial infarction is in order.

An interesting new method of reperfusion has recently been introduced. In seven of 13 patients with acute myocardial infarction Rentrop et al. were able to pass a guidewire through an obstruction (presumably a thrombus) and reestablish flow through the vessel to the previously ischemic myocardium [91]. Intracoronary nitroglycerin and streptokinase were also administered to diminish the possible contribution of spasm and thrombosis to occlusion. Angiograms performed in six patients after the acute event demonstrated continued patency of the vessel in all cases. In a control group of nine patients (not randomly selected), only four showed patency at follow-up. Although this technique is less traumatic than coronary artery bypass grafting, it too must also be evaluated in a controlled randomized trial before its widespread use is advocated.

Oxygen (see Swain, p. 490)

Two large clinical series have shown no definite beneficial effects of high-flow supplemental oxygen on the clinical course of patients with acute myocardial infarction [92, 93]. However, in a smaller study of patients with transmural anterior infarction, the magnitude and extent of precordial ST segment elevation was decreased by short-term oxygen therapy; these electrocardiographic findings returned to the pretreatment baseline values when oxygen therapy was discontinued [12]. The pretreatment arterial pO_2 was 70 mmHg or less, and oxygen therapy elevated arterial pO_2 in most cases to levels of 250 mmHg or more.

Major adverse effects have not been noted in clinical studies of oxygen therapy in acute myocardial infarction [12, 92, 93], although Rawles et al. found an increased heart rate in their oxygen-treated group [93]. Other studies have noted increased systemic vascular resistance and arterial pressure, and decreased cardiac output in patients receiving high-flow oxygen therapy [92, 94]. Although such hemodynamic changes could theoretically increase myocardial oxygen demands and thereby augment myocardial ischemia, no evidence for such a deleterious effect has been noted. In fact, it has been postulated that a slight elevation of arterial pressure might increase coronary perfusion pressure, and that oxygen-induced vasoconstriction of coronary arteries supplying non-ischemic zones could divert blood flow to the ischemic zone [95, 96]. Although pulmonary oxygen toxicity can result from prolonged inhalation of 100% oxygen, such complications are unlikely with lesser concentrations of oxygen [97].

Thus, there is some evidence that administration of oxygen to elevate arterial oxygen tensions above the normal physiologic range might decrease myocardial ischemia. Patients without arterial hypoxemia can be treated with prolonged inhalation of high concentrations of oxygen (e.g., 40%) without significant adverse effects, even though the long-term clinical effects of such therapy on ischemic injury and infarct size remain to be elucidated. Certainly patients with hypoxemia complicating myocardial infarction should be treated with supplemental oxygen to restore their blood oxygen content to the normal range. The use of hyperbaric oxygenation in attempts to limit infarct size remains an experimental, extremely costly, and cumbersome approach that is not widely available [98].

Anticoagulant and thrombolytic agents (see Griggs, p. 460)

Thrombolytic agents, such as streptokinase and urokinase, have been used both to dissolve existing coronary thrombi and to prevent further thrombus formation in patients with acute myocardial infarction [99, 100]. There is suggestive evidence of slightly decreased mortality when parenteral streptokinase therapy is compared with treatment with placebo or anticoagulants, although the results are not uniform. Evidence of faster resolution of ischemic ECG changes [101], more rapid release of enzymes from the necrotic myocardium [101, 102], and reduction in pump failure complicating infarction [103] suggest that thrombolytic therapy, initiated within 24 h of acute myocardial infarction, may also decrease infarct size. However, marked differences in drug dosage, patient populations, and concurrent therapy make these studies somewhat difficult to compare and to extrapolate to routine clinical practice [99]. Furthermore, additional data are needed on the incidence and severity of bleeding complications in patients with infarction, particularly those who may require invasive procedures, such as insertion of a pacemaker or placement of an arterial line.

More detailed study of systemic thrombolytic therapy on indices of infarct size must be performed before acceptance of the hypothesis that such treatment protects ischemic myocardium (see Gold p. 512). Experimental and early clinical studies [100, 101] have suggested that coronary thromboses can be lysed by direct intracoronary infusion of streptokinase, and that coronary artery patency can be restored, with beneficial effects on electrocardiographic ischemic changes and the clinical course of the patient. Direct intracoronary infusion of the drug avoids the need for systemically effective doses and their potential hemorrhagic complications [101]. Although these preliminary studies appear to be promising, the use of intracoronary streptokinase should be confined to protocols investigating its efficacy in a systematic fashion. If pilot studies continue to suggest favorable results, a controlled trial of this therapy is indicated.

Hyaluronidase (see Swain, p. 485)

The use of hyaluronidase in human myocardial infarction is an attractive proposition because the agent has no known deleterious hemodynamic or electrophysiologic effects, because it can be readily and easily administered, and because allergic reactions to the agent are rare [104, 105, 106]. For these reasons, studies of its efficacy were undertaken in patients with acute myocardial infarction. In an open trial of 25 patients with anterior or lateral transmural infarction, hyaluronidase was shown to reduce myocardial ischemia, as reflected by a more rapid reduction in both the number of precordial sites with ST segment elevation and the summed precordial ST elevation (ΣST) on 35-lead precordial maps in treated than in placebo-treated patients [9]. Thereafter, a randomized multicenter study with blinded endpoint analysis was undertaken to investigate the effects of hyaluronidase on electrocardiographic evidence of myocardial necrosis in patients with acute anterior infarction [106]. Hyaluronidase, 500 NF units/kg, was administered intravenously within 8 h of the onset of symptoms and then every 6 h for 48 h; 35-lead precordial maps were performed before treatment and seven days later. The sum of R wave voltages (ΣR) at initially ischemic sites (leads with ST segment elevations exceeding 0.15 mV) fell to a greater extent in the control group of 45 patients than in the 46 patients treated with hyaluronidase, and Q waves appeared in fewer initially ischemic sites, consistent with a reduction in the extent of necrosis in hyaluronidase-treated patients. Cairns et al. have reported a smaller, double-blind trial of hyaluronidase administered to patients with myocardial infarction. Although there was a trend toward smaller CK infarct size in 21 patients treated within 6 h of symptoms compared with controls, the difference did not achieve statistical significance [107].

Hyaluronidase must therefore be regarded as an agent for use in further clinical studies that seek to define its effects on infarct size; if such therapy is demonstrated to be effective in all types of infarctions, intravenous hyaluronidase, with its low incidence of side effects, may be recommended for widespread use in patients with suspected acute myocardial infarction. Its lack of effect on hemodynamics and cardiac conduction and rhythm, the simplicity of its mode of administration, and lack of adverse effects make the agent quite promising for use in patients with a wide spectrum of infarction and hemodynamic complications. Presumably it can also be used in combination with other drugs, such as propranolol and/or nitroglycerin. Indeed, it has been demonstrated experimentally that the combination of these three agents reduced the severity of ischemia more than did any of those agents alone [108].

Glucose–insulin–potassium (GIK) (see Swain, p. 488)

Rogers, Rackley, Russell, and their associates have reported a series of studies of the metabolic, hemodynamic, and clinical effects of GIK therapy in patients with ischemic heart disease, especially acute myocardial infarction [109–116]. Administration of a solution containing 300 g glucose, 50 units regular insulin, and 80 meq CK^+ per liter of water at an average rate of 1.5 ml/kg/h into the central venous circulation has been shown to be a safe, well-tolerated intervention that increases myocardial utilization of glucose, diminishes the utilization of free fatty acids [110], and decreases myocardial oxygen consumption [113] without inducing major changes in left ventricular filling pressure or cardiac index. Pilot studies with 48-h infusions of GIK begun an average of 8 h after the onset of symptoms of acute myocardial infarction suggested a decreased hospital mortality in comparison with a group of retrospectively analyzed controls managed during the preceding year at the same institution [112]. Based on these preliminary findings, these investigators have begun a randomized, prospective trial of GIK in patients with acute myocardial infarction, designed to characterize the clinical course and infarct size by a variety of metabolic, hemodynamic, electrocardiographic, scintigraphic, and enzymatic techniques [109, 114]; the trial is not blinded and nitrates, which may have significant independent effects on endpoints, are used liberally [114]. Preliminary findings in 91 randomized patients include decreased ventricular ectopic activity and lower left ventricular filling pressures after GIK therapy [109, 114]; in addition, hospital mortality has been lower in GIK-treated patients with initially normal or only mildly disturbed hemodynamic function

[114]. Improvement in ventricular function in the GIK-treated group has been suggested by analysis of regional wall motion in a subgroup of patients undergoing contrast ventriculography several weeks after infarction [114, 115] as well as by ventricular function curves obtained two and three days after infarction [116]. These studies, as well as those of Reduto et al., have not shown a decrease in infarct size measured by serum CK analysis [109, 117], but the relatively small number of patients in each study would allow even a major reduction in CK release to go undetected.

Adverse effects of GIK therapy are uncommon when intravenous infusion is carefully monitored. The most common abnormalities are hyperglycemia and mild hyperkalemia, the latter tending to be most pronounced after discontinuation of a prolonged infusion [111]. Transient elevations of lactate dehydrogenase and serum glutaminoxaloacetic transaminase enzymes, presumably of hepatic origin, have also been noted [111]. Major alterations in serum osmolarity have not been a problem and adverse hemodynamic effects have not complicated slow continuous intravenous infusion of GIK, when the glucose concentration is limited to 300 g/liter. Local phlebitis has occasionally occurred following peripheral intravenous infusion and pulmonary infiltrates have complicated infusion into the pulmonary artery [118], but infusion of GIK into the right atrium has not produced local complications [109].

Thus, GIK is a relatively safe, easily administered intervention that is potentially widely applicable because of good tolerance by most patients with acute myocardial infarction. The acute effects of therapy on electrocardiographic, metabolic, and hemodynamic accompaniments of myocardial ischemia and infarction are encouraging, but the long-term consequences of therapy need to be elucidated in prospective, randomized, and appropriately blinded trials in large numbers of patients. Changes in mortality with GIK cannot be ascribed to a limitation of infarct size without independent confirmation of the latter, because of the possible effect of therapy on arrhythmias following infarction. Serum electrolytes, glucose, and osmolality must be monitored and the hazards of such therapy in patients with diabetes mellitus, renal insufficiency, and heart failure must be better defined.

Corticosteroids (see Swain, p. 493)

Early clinical studies of corticosteroid therapy in acute myocardial infarction focused on patient mortality as an endpoint [119–121]. A nonrandomized study without a concurrent control group suggested a decreased mortality in selected high-risk patients treated with a 14-day course of parenteral hydrocortisone [120], but a randomized, double-blinded trial of hydrocortisone given intramuscularly and then orally for a total of two weeks showed no difference in mortality between control and treatment groups, and no apparent effect of treatment in subgroups of patients with cardiogenic shock or arrhythmias [121]. Barzilai et al. reported a lower mortality in 446 patients treated with parenteral hydrocortisone for three days following infarction than that observed in 491 patients managed routinely on another medical service; a beneficial effect was evident only in patients having their first myocardial infarction [122]. Morrison et al. have reported a lower mortality and reduction in enzymatically estimated infarct size in 66 patients treated with one or two 2-g doses of intravenous hydrocortisone an average of 9 h after the initial serum CK rise, compared with 35 concurrently managed control patients [123]. Further suggestive evidence that corticosteroid therapy reduces infarct size has been presented by Selwyn et al., who found less Q wave development than predicted from initial precordial ST segment mapping in eight patients treated with a single dose of intravenous methylprednisolone within 6 h of onset of symptoms of anterior myocardial infarction [124].

Although the studies by Morrison et al. and Selwyn et al. cited above suggest that infarct size may be limited in man by early, short-term treatment with corticosteroids, these studies cannot be considered conclusive because of their nonrandomized, unblinded designs, the small number of patients studied, and the failure of contemporary studies to demonstrate similar effects [125, 126]. Thus, Roberts et al. have reported that multiple-dose methylprednisolone therapy resulted in an *increase* in enzymatically estimated infarct size and in ventricular dysrhythmias; in addition, two of 12 patients with multidose therapy died with rupture of the interventricular septum [125]. Multiple-dose, prolonged corticosteroid therapy for Dressler's syndrome following myocardial infarction has also been linked with a high incidence of ventricular aneurysm [127], presumably due to impaired myocardial healing. On the other hand, cardiac rupture has not been a frequent mode of death in several trials of corticosteroids in acute myocardial infarction [123, 126]. Nausea and hypotension may result from large doses of intravenous steroids and profound euphoria sometimes accompanies corticosteroid therapy; this psychotropic effect can improve both the patient's and the physician's outlook on the disease process [119, 121, 128].

In summary, some, though certainly not all clinical studies of corticosteroids in acute myocardial infarction have suggested that early therapy might reduce infarct size and patient mortality, but experimental design, small patient numbers, and conflicting results prevent these studies from being considered conclusive. In addition, prolonged corticosteroid treatment may be associated with serious adverse effects, ventricular aneurysm formation, cardiac rupture, and ventricular arrhythmias. Well-designed trials of short-term corticosteroid therapy, with appropriate safeguards for patient safety, are needed to define whether a role exists for corticosteroids in acute myocardial infarction.

Ibuprofen, a nonsteroidal antiinflammatory agent with antiplatelet properties, has been shown to be extremely effective in limiting infarct size in animals [129, 130], and should also be investigated in patients.

DIRECTIONS OF CLINICAL RESEARCH ON INFARCT SIZE

It is difficult to determine the appropriate role of the interventions discussed in this book in the routine care of patients with acute myocardial infarction. A major impediment to the needed research is the speed with which an intervention must be initiated. Research is further complicated by inadequate techniques of measuring infarct size and the variable clinical course of patients with infarction. Furthermore, even the demonstration that an intervention limits infarct size does not ensure that it will ultimately benefit the patient. It must also be shown that, after the acute event, patients do not suffer from angina or arrhythmias arising from salvaged, but poorly perfused myocardium [131].

A Multicenter Investigation of the Limitation of Infarct Size (MILIS) has been organized by the National Heart, Lung and Blood Institute to address many of the difficulties mentioned above. The study is a cooperative effort carried out in five coronary care units to determine whether hyaluronidase and propranolol are beneficial. Infarct size and ventricular function are being evaluated by CK-MB, ECG, technetium pyrophosphate, and radionuclide ventriculographic techniques; hence precise evaluation of the relationships between the various measurement methods will be possible. In addition, survivors undergo treadmill exercise tests and Holter monitor recordings performed after the acute events to determine whether the frequencies of angina or arrhythmia are increased in the treated groups. The study, which has enrolled more than 650 patients at the time of this writing, is scheduled for completion in 1984.

For the future, it is hoped that techniques for measurement of infarct size in patients will be improved. Such techniques would help with the resolution of such complex issues as the value of combinations of interventions and the time after occlusion within which an intervention must be initiated. Despite the inability, at this time, to make definitive recommendations concerning the use of interventions to limit infarct size in the routine treatment of acute myocardial infarction, the repeated demonstration of salvage of ischemic myocardium in experimental preparations, the beneficial effects observed in numerous pilot clinical studies, and the enormous medical and social importance of the problem all indicate that further clinical investigation in this field is strongly indicated.

Acknowledgments. We are grateful for the assistance of Ms. Deidre Bernard and Ms. Gail Aylmer in the preparation of this manuscript.

538

REFERENCES

1. Harnarayan C, Bennett MA, Pentecost BL, Brewer DB: Quantitative study of infarcted myocardium in cardiogenic shock. Br Heart J 32:728–732, 1970.
2. Page DL, Caulfield JB, Kastor JA, DeSanctis RW, Sanders CA: Myocardial changes associated with cardiogenic shock. N Engl J Med 285: 133–137, 1971.
3. Sobel BE, Bresnahan GF, Shell WE, Yoder RD: Estimation of infarct size in man and its relation to prognosis. Circulation 46:640–648, 1972.
4. Cox JL, McLaughlin VW, Flowers NC, Horan LG: The ischemic zone surrounding acute myocardial infarction. Its morphology as detected by dehydrogenase staining. Am Heart J 76:650–659, 1968.
5. Braunwald E (ed): Symposium on protection of the ischemic myocardium. Circulation [Suppl 1] 53:162–168, 1976.
6. Braunwald E: The pathogenesis and treatment of shock in myocardial infarction. Topic in clinical medicine. Johns Hopkins Med J 121:421–429, 1967.
7. Braunwald E, Covell JW, Maroko PR, Ross J Jr: Effects of drugs and of counterpulsation on myocardial oxygen consumption. Observations on the ischemic heart. Circulation [Suppl 4] 40:IV-220–228, 1969.
8. Muller JE, Maroko PR, Braunwald E: Evaluation of precordial electrocardiographic mapping as a means of assessing changes in myocardial ischemic injury. Circulation 52:16–27, 1975.
9. Maroko PR, Davidson DM, Libby P, Hagan AD, Braunwald E: Effects of hyaluronidase administration on myocardial ischemic injury in acute infarction: a preliminary study in 24 patients. Ann Intern Med 82:516–520, 1975.
10. Maroko PR, Kjekshus JK, Sobel BE, Watanabe T, Covell JW, Ross J Jr, Braunwald E: Factors influencing infarct size following experimental coronary artery occlusion. Circulation 43:67–82, 1971.
11. Flaherty JT, Reid PR, Kelly DT, Taylor DR, Weisfeldt ML, Pitt B: Intravenous nitroglycerin in acute myocardial infarction. Circulation 51:132–139, 1975.
12. Madias JE, Madias NE, Hood WB Jr: Precordial ST-segment mapping. 2. Effects of oxygen inhalation on ischemic injury in patients with acute myocardial infarction. Circulation 53:411–417, 1976.
13. Gold HK, Leinbach RC, Maroko PR: Propranolol-induced reduction of signs of ischemic injury during acute myocardial infarction. Am J Cardiol 38:689–695, 1976.
14. Reid PR, Taylor DR, Kelly DT, Weisfeldt ML, Humphries JO, Ross RS, Pitt B: Myocardial-infarct extension detected by precordial ST-segment mapping. N Engl J Med 290:123, 1974.
15. Madias JE, Venkataraman K, Hood WB Jr: Precordial ST-segment mapping. I. Clinical studies in the coronary care unit. Circulation 52:799, 1975.
16. Foerster JM, Vera Z, Janzen DA, Foerster SJ, Mason DT: Evaluation of precordial orthogonal vectorcardiographic lead ST-segment magnitude in the assessment of myocardial ischemic injury. Circulation 55:728, 1977.
17. Bleifeld W, Mathey D, Hanrath P, Buss G, Effert S: Infarct size estimated from serial serum creatine phosphokinase in relation to left ventricular hemodynamics. Circulation 55:303, 1977.

18. Roberts R, Husain A, Ambos HD, Oliver GC, Cox JR Jr, Sobel BE: Relation between infarct size and ventricular arrhythmia. Br Heart J 37: 1169–1175, 1975.
19. Geltman EM, Ehsani AA, Campbell MK, Schechtman K, Roberts R, Sobel BE: The influence of location and extent of myocardial infarction on long-term ventricular dysrhthmia and mortality. Circulation 60:805–814, 1979.
20. Rogers WJ, McDaniel HG, Smith LR, Mantle JA, Russell RO Jr, Rackley CE: Correlation of angiographic estimates of myocardial infarct size and accumulated release of creatine kinase MB isoenzyme in man. Circulation 56:199–205, 1977.
21. Hori M, Inoue M, Fukui S, Shimazu T, Mishima M, Ohgitani N, Minamino T, Abe H: Correlation of ejection fraction and infarct size estimated from the total CK released in patients with acute myocardial infarction. Br Heart J 41:433–440, 1979.
22. Maddox DE, Wynne J, Uren R, Parker JA, Idoine J, Siegel LC, Neill JM, Cohn PF, Holman BL: Regional ejection fraction: a quantitative radionuclide index of regional left ventricular performance. Circulation 59: 1001–1009, 1979.
23. Mason DT, Ashburn WL, Harbert JC, Cohen LS, Braunwald E: Rapid sequential visualization of the heart and great vessels in man using the wide-field anger scintillation camera: radioisotope-angiography following the injection of technetium-99m. Circulation 39:19, 1969.
24. Ashburn WL, Schelbert HR, Verba JW: Left ventricular ejection fraction. A review of several radionuclide angiographic approaches using the scintillation camera. Prog Cardiovasc Dis 20:267–284, 1978.
25. Wackers FJ, Becker AE, Samson G, Sokole EB, van der Schoot JB, Vet AJTM, Lie KI, Durrer D, Wellens H: Location and size of acute transmural myocardial infarction estimated from thallium-201 scintiscans. A clinicopathologic study. Circulation 56:72–78, 1977.
26. Cannon PJ, Dell RB, Dwyer EM Jr: Regional myocardial perfusion rates in patients with coronary artery disease. J Clin Invest 51:978, 1972.
27. Holman BL, Adams DF, Jewitt D, Eldh P, Idoine J, Cohn PF, Gorlin R, Adelstein SF: Measuring regional myocardial blood flow with ^{133}Xe and the Anger camera. Radiology 112:99, 1974.
28. Weiss ES, Ahmed SA, Welch MJ, Williamson JR, Ter-Pogossian MM, Sobel BE: Quantification of infarction in cross sections of canine myocardium in vivo with positron emission transaxial tomography and ^{11}C-palmitate. Circulation 55:66–73, 1977.
29. Bonte FJ, Parkey RW, Graham KD, Moore J, Stokeley EM: A new method for radionuclide imaging of acute myocardial infarcts. Radiology 110: 473–474, 1974.
30. Holman BL, Lesch M, Zweiman FG, Temte J, Lown B, Gorlin R: Detection and sizing of acute myocardial infarcts with [99m]Tc(Sn) tetracycline. N Engl J Med 291:159–163, 1974.
31. Marcus ML, Kerber RE: Present status of the [99m]technetium pyrophosphate infarct scintigram. Circulation 56:335, 1977.
32. Willerson JT: Can acute myocardial infarcts be sized accurately with technetium-99m stannous pyrophosphate? In: Rapaport E (ed) Current controversies in cardiovascular disease. Philadelphia: Saunders, pp 235–246. 1980.

540

33. Lewis M, Buja LM, Saffer S, Mishelevich D, Stokely E, Lewis S, Parkey R, Bonte F, Willerson JT: Experimental infarct sizing utilizing computer processing and a three-dimensional model. Science 197:167–169, 1977.
34. Wackers JF, Sokole EB, Samson G, Schoot JB, Lie KI, Liem KL, Wellens HJJ: Value and limitations of thallium-201 scintigraphy in the acute phase of myocardial infarction. N Engl J Med 295:1–5, 1976.
35. Pohost GM, Zir LM, Moore RH, McKusick KA, Guiney TE, Beller GA: Differentiation of transiently ischemic from infarcted myocardium by serial imaging after a single dose of thallium-201. Circulation 55:294–302, 1977.
36. Smitherman TC, Osborn RC Jr, Narahara KA: Serial myocardial scintigraphy after a single dose of thallium-201 in men after acute myocardial infarction. Am J Cardiol 42:177–182, 1978.
37. Rigo P, Murray M, Strauss HW, Taylor DR, Kelly D, Weisfeldt ML, Pitt B: Left ventricular function in acute myocardial infarction evaluated by gated scintiphotography. Circulation 50:678–684, 1974.
38. Schelbert HR, Henning H, Ashburn WL, Verba JW, Karliner JS, O'Rourke RA: Serial measurements of left ventricular ejection fraction by radionuclide angiography early and late after myocardial infarction. Am J Cardiol 38:407–415, 1976.
39. Sharpe DN, Botvinick EH, Shames DM, Norman A, Chatterjee K, Parmley WW: The clinical estimation of acute myocardial infarct size with ^{99m}technetium pyrophosphate scintigraphy. Circulation 57:307–313, 1978.
40. Adams DF, Hessel SJ, Judy PF, Stein JA, Abrams JL: Computed tomography of the normal and infarcted myocardium. Am J Roentgenol 126: 786, 1976.
41. Powell WJ Jr, Wittenberg J, Maturi RA, Dinsmore RE, Miller SW: Detection of edema associated with myocardial ischemia by computerized tomography in isolated, arrested canine hearts. Circulation 55:99–108, 1977.
42. Gray WR Jr, Lewis SE, Parkey RW, Buja LM, Hagler H, Twieg DB, Willerson JT: Computed tomography for localization and sizing of experimental acute anterior myocardial infarcts in dogs [abstr]. Circulation [Suppl 3] 55 and 56:III-8, 1977.
43. Gray WR Jr, Parkey RW, Buja LM, Stokely EM, McAllister RE, Bonte FJ, Willerson JT: Computed tomography: in vitro evaluation of myocardial infarction. Radiology 122:511, 1977.
44. Kloner RA, Braunwald E: Observations on experimental myocardial ischaemia. Cardiovasc Res 14:371–395, 1980.
45. Peter T, Norris RM, Clarke ED, Heng MK, Singh BN, Williams B, Howell DR, Ambler PK: Reduction of enzyme levels by propranolol after acute myocardial infarction. Circulation 57:1091–1095, 1978.
46. Norris RM, Sammel NL, Clarke ED, Smith WM, Williams B: Protective effect of propranolol in threatened myocardial infarction. Lancet 2: 907–909, 1978.
47. Yasuf S, Ramsdale D, Peto R, Furse L, Bennett D, Bray C, Sleight P: Early intravenous atenolol treatment in suspected acute myocardial infarction: preliminary report of a randomized trial. Lancet 2:273–275, 1980.
48. Fox KM, Chopra MP, Portal RW, Aber C: Long-term beta-blockade: possible protection from myocardial infarction. B Med J 1:117, 1975.

49. Mueller HS, Ayres SM: The role of propranolol in the treatment of acute myocardial infarction. Prog Cardiovasc Dis 19:405–412, 1977.

50. Mueller HS, Ayres SM, Religa A, Evans RG: Propranolol in the treatment of acute myocardial infarction: effect on myocardial oxygenation and hemodynamics. Circulation 49:1078, 1974.

51. Bay G, Lund-Larsen P, Lorentsen E, Sivertssen E: Haemodynamic effects of propranolol (Inderal) in acute myocardial infarction. Br Med J 1:141–143, 1967.

52. Waagstein F, Hjalmarson AC: Double-blind study of the effect of cardio-selective beta-blockade on chest pain in acute myocardial infarction. Acta Med Scand [Suppl] 587:201, 1976.

53. Videbaek J, Christensen NJ, Sterndorff B: Serial determination of plasma catecholamines in myocardial infarction. Circulation 46:846, 1972.

54. Miller RR, Olson HG, Amsterdam EA, Mason DT: Propranolol-withdrawal rebound phenomenon. Exacerbation of coronary events after abrupt cessation of antianginal therapy. N Engl J Med 293:416–418, 1975.

55. Maroko PR, Bernstein EF, Libby P, DeLaria GA, Covell JW, Ross J Jr, Braunwald E: Effects of intraaortic balloon counterpulsation on the severity of myocardial ischemic injury following acute coronary occlusion: counterpulsation and myocardial injury. Circulation 45:1150–1159, 1972.

56. Leinbach RC, Gold HK, Harper RW, Buckley MJ, Austen WG: Early intraaortic balloon pumping for anterior myocardial infarction without shock. Circulation 58:204–210, 1978.

57. McCabe JC, Abel RM, Subramanian VA, Gay WA Jr: Complications of intra-aortic balloon insertion and counterpulsation. Circulation 57:769–773, 1978.

58. Bregman D, Nichols AB, Weiss MB, Powers ER, Martin EC, Casarella WJ: Percutaneous intraaortic balloon insertion. Am J Cardiol 46:261–264, 1980.

59. Beckman CB, Romero LH, Shatney CH, Nicoloff DM, Lillehei RC, Dietzman RH: Clinical comparison of the intra-aortic balloon pump and external counterpulsation for cardiogenic shock. Trans Am Soc Artif Intern Organs 19:414–418, 1973.

60. Gowda SK, Gillespie TA, Byrne JD, Ambos HD, Sobel BE, Roberts R: Effects of external counterpulsation on enzymatically estimated infarct size and ventricular arrhythmia. Br Heart J 40:308–314, 1978.

61. Amsterdam EA, Banas J, Criley JM, Loeb HS, Mueller H, Willerson JT, Mason DT: Clinical assessment of external pressure circulatory assistance in acute myocardial infarction. Report of a cooperative clinical trial. Am J Cardiol 45:349–356, 1980.

62. Gold HK, Leinbach RC, Sanders CA: Use of sublingual nitroglycerin in congestive heart failure following acute myocardial infarction. Circulation 46:839–845, 1972.

63. Delgado CE, Pitt B, Taylor DR, Weisfeldt ML, Kelly DT: Role of sub-lingual nitroglycerin in patients with acute myocardial infarction. Br Heart J 37:392–396, 1975.

64. Come PC, Flaherty JT, Baird MG, Rouleau JR, Weisfeldt ML, Greene HL, Becker L, Pitt B: Reversal by phenylephrine of the beneficial effects

542

of intravenous nitroglycerin in patients with acute myocardial infarction. N Engl J Med 293:1003–1007, 1975.

65. Flaherty JT, Come PC, Baird MG, Rouleau J, Taylor DR, Weisfeldt ML, Greene HL, Becker LC, Pitt B: Effects of intravenous nitroglycerin on left ventricular function and ST segment changes in acute myocardial infarction. Br Heart J 38:612–621, 1976.

66. Borer JS, Redwood DR, Levitt B, Cagin N, Bianchi C, Vallin H, Epstein SE: Reduction in myocardial ischemia with nitroglycerin or nitroglycerin plus phenylephrine administered during acute myocardial infarction. N Engl J Med 293:1008–1012, 1975.

67. Derrida JP, Sal R, Chiche P: Effects of prolonged nitroglycerin infusion in patients with acute myocardial infarction. Am J Cardiol 41:407, 1978 (abstr).

68. Chiche P, Baligadoo SJ, Derrida JP: A randomized trial of prolonged nitroglycerin infusion in acute myocardial infarction [abstr]. Circulation [Suppl 3] 60:II-165, 1979.

69. Bussmann WD, Passek D, Seidel W, Kaltenbach M: Prospective randomized trial of intravenous nitroglycerin in acute myocardial infarction [abstr]. Circulation [Suppl 2] 60:II-164, 1979.

70. Becker LC, Bulkley BH, Pitt B, Flaherty JT, Weiss JL, Gerstenblith G, Rehn T, Pond M, Mason S, Silverman K, Wang DJ, Weisfeldt ML: Enhanced reduction of thallium 201 defects in acute myocardial infarction by nitroglycerin treatment: Initial results of a prospective randomized trial [abstr]. Clin Res 26:219A, 1978.

71. Williams DO, Amsterdam EA, Mason DT: Hemodynamic effects of nitroglycerin in acute myocardial infarction: decrease in ventricular preload at the expense of cardiac output. Circulation 51:421–427, 1975.

72. Awan NA, Amsterdam EA, Vera Z, DeMaria AN, Miller RR, Mason DT: Reduction of ischemic injury by sublingual nitroglycerin in patients with acute myocardial infarction. Circulation 54:761–765, 1976.

73. Bussmann WD, Schofer H, Kurita A, Gang W: Nitroglycerin in acute myocardial infarction. X. Effect of small and large doses of nitroglycerin on sigma ST segment deviation – experimental and clinical results. Clin Cardiol 2:106–109, 1979.

74. Epstein SE, Kent KM, Goldstein RE, Borer JS, Redwood DR: Reduction of ischemic injury by nitroglycerin during acute myocardial infarction. N Engl J Med 292:29–35, 1975.

75. Come PC, Pitt B: Nitroglycerin-induced severe hypotension and bradycardia in patients with acute myocardial infarction. Circulation 54:624–628, 1976.

76. Branconi JM, Bowen WG, Cain ME, Goldstein RA, Brodarick SA, Ambos HD, Jaffe AS, Roberts R: The effect of intravenous nitroglycerin on pain and ventricular arrhythmias in patients with acute myocardial infarction [abstr]. Clin Res 27:156A, 1979.

77. Bowen WG, Branconi JM, Goldstein RA, Cain ME, Brodarick SM, Geltman EM, Jaffe AS, Ambos HD, Roberts R: A randomized prospective study of the effects of intravenous nitroglycerin in patients during myocardial infarction. Circulation [Suppl 2] 60:II-70, 1979.

78. Chatterjee K, Parmley WW, Ganz W, Forrester JS, Walinsky P, Crexalls C,

Swan HJC: Hemodynamic and metabolic responses to vasodilator therapy in acute myocardial infarction. Circulation 48:1183–1193, 1973.

79. Kelly DT, Delgado CE, Taylor DR, Pitt B, Ross RS: Use of phentolamine in acute myocardial infarction associated with hypertension and left ventricular failure. Circulation 47:729–735, 1973.

80. Walinsky P, Chatterjee K, Forrester J, Parmley WW, Swan HJC: Enhanced left ventricular performance with phentolamine in acute myocardial infarction. Am J Cardiol 33:37–41, 1974.

81. daLuz PL, Forrester JS, Wyatt HL, Tyberg JV, Chagrasulis R, Parmley WW, Swan HJC: Hemodynamic and metabolic effects of sodium nitroprusside on the performance and metabolism of regional ischemic myocardium. Circulation 52:400–407, 1975.

82. Chiariello M, Gold HK, Leinbach RC, Davis MA, Maroko PR: Comparison between the effects of nitroprusside and nitroglycerin on ischemic injury during acute myocardial infarction. Circulation 54:766–773, 1976.

83. Mann T, Cohn PF, Holman BL, Green LH, Markis JE, Phillips DA: Effects of nitroprusside on regional myocardial blood flow in coronary artery disease. Results in 25 patients and comparison with nitroglycerin. Circulation 57:732–738, 1978.

84. Armstrong PW, Walker DC, Burton JR, Parker JO: Vasodilator therapy in acute myocardial infarction. A comparison of sodium nitroprusside and nitroglycerin. Circulation 52:1118–1122, 1975.

85. Chatterjee K, Swan HCJ, Kaushik VS, Jobin G, Magnusson P, Forrester JS: Effects of vasodilator therapy for severe pump failure in acute myocardial infarction on short-term and late prognosis. Circulation 53:797–802, 1976.

86. Shell WE, Sobel BE: Protection of jeopardized ischemic myocardium by reduction of ventricular afterload. N Engl J Med 291:481–486, 1974.

87. Cohn LH, Gorlin R, Herman MV, Collins JJ Jr: Aorta-coronary bypass for acute coronary occlusion. J Thorac Cardiovasc Surg 64:503–513, 1972.

88. Muller JE, Antman E, Green LH, Koster JK Jr: Salvage of acutely ischemic myocardium by emergency coronary artery bypass grafting. Clin Cardiol (in press).

89. Berg R Jr, Kendall RW, Duvoisin GE, Ganji JH, Rudy LW, Everhart FJ: Acute myocardial infarction. A surgical emergency. J Thorac Cardiovasc Surg 70:432–439, 1979.

90. Phillips SJ, Kongtahworn C, Zeff RH, Benson M, Iannone L, Brown T, Gordon DF: Emergency coronary artery revascularization: A possible therapy for acute myocardial infarction. Circulation 60:241–246, 1979.

91. Rentrop KP, Blanke H, Karsch KR, Kreuzer H: Initial experience with transluminal recanalization of the recently occluded infarct-related coronary artery in acute myocardial infarction – comparison with conventionally treated patients. Clin Cardiol 2:92–105, 1979.

92. Kenmure ACF, Murdock WR, Beattie AD, Marshall JCB, Cameron AJV: Circulatory and metabolic effects of oxygen in myocardial infarction. Br Med J 4:360–364, 1968.

93. Rawles JM, Kenmure ACF: Controlled trial of oxygen in uncomplicated myocardial infarction. Br Med J I:1121–1123, 1976.

94. Thomas M, Malmcrona R, Shillingford J: Haemodynamic effects of

oxygen in patients with acute myocardial infarction. Br Heart J 27:401–407, 1965.

95. Maroko PR, Radvany P, Braunwald E, Hale SL: Reduction of infarct size by oxygen inhalation following acute coronary occlusion. Circulation 52:360–368, 1975.

96. Sobol BJ, Wanlass SA, Joseph EB, Azarshahy I: Alteration of coronary blood flow in the dog by inhalation of 100 per cent oxygen. Circ Res II:791–802, 1962.

97. Wolfe WG, De Vires WC: Oxygen toxicity. Annu Rev Med 26:203–217, 1975.

98. Whalen RE, Saltzman HA: Hyperbaric oxygenation in the treatment of acute myocardial infarction. Prog Cardiovasc Dis 10:575, 1968.

99. Simon TL, Ware JH, Stengle JM: Clinical trials of thrombolytic agents in myocardial infarction. Ann Intern Med 79:712–719, 1973.

100. Kordenat RK, Kezdi P, Powley D: Experimental intracoronary thrombosis and selective in situ lysis by catheter technique. Am J Cardiol 30:640, 1972.

101. Schmutzler VR, Heckner F, Kortage P, van de Loo J, Pezold FA, Poliwoda H, Praetorius F, Zedoin D: On the thrombolytic therapy for recent myocardial infarction. Dtsch Med Wochenschr 91:581–587, 1966.

102. European Cooperative Study Group for Streptokinase Treatment in Acute Myocardial Infarction: Streptokinase in acute myocardial infarction. N Engl J Med 301:797–802, 1979.

103. Schmutzler R, Fritze E, Gebauer D: Fibrinolytic therapy in acute myocardial infarction. In: Mammen EF, Anderson GF, Barnhart MI (eds) Transactions of the nineteenth annual symposium on blood Stuttgart: F-K Schattauer, 1971, p 211.

104. Martins de Oliveira J, Carballo R, Zimmerman HA: Intravenous injection of hyaluronidase in acute myocardial infarction: preliminary report of clinical and experimental observations. Am Heart J 57:712–722, 1959.

105. Britton RC, Habif DV: Clinical uses of hyaluronidase: a current review. Surgery 33:917–942, 1953.

106. Maroko PR, Hillis LD, Muller JE, Tavazzi L, Heyndrickx GR, Ray M, Chiariello M, Distante A, Askenazi J, Salerno J, Carpentier J, Reshetnaya NI, Radvany P, Libby P, Raabe DS, Chazov EI, Bobba P, Braunwald E: Favorable effects of hyaluronidase on electrocardiographic evidence of necrosis in patients with acute myocardial infarction. N Engl J Med 296:898, 1977.

107. Cairns JA, Holder DA, Tanser PA, Missirlis E: Double blind trial of hyaluronidase for limitation of human infarct size [abstr]. Clin Res 28:159A, 1980.

108. Hillis LD, Khuri SF, Braunwald E, Kloner RA, Tow D, Barsamian E, Maroko PR: Assessment of the efficacy of interventions to limit ischemic injury by direct measurement of intramural carbon dioxide tension after coronary artery occlusion in the dog. J Clin Invest 63:99–107, 1979.

109. Rogers WJ, Segall PH, McDaniel HG, Mantle JA, Russell RO Jr, Rackley CE: Prospective randomized trial of glucose-insulin-potassium in acute myocardial infarction: effects on myocardial hemodynamics, substrates, and rhythm. Am J Cardiol 43:801–809, 1979.

110. Stanley AW, Moraski RE, Russell RO Jr, Rogers WJ, Mantle JA,

Kreisberg RA, McDaniel HG, Rackley CE: Effects of glucose-insulin-potassium on myocardial substrate availability and utilization in stable coronary artery disease. Studies on myocardial carbohydrate, lipid and oxygen arterial coronary sinus differences in patients with coronary artery disease. Am J Cardiol 36:929–937, 1975.

111. Prather JW, Russell RO Jr, Mantle JA, McDaniel HG, Rackley CE: Metabolic consequences of glucose-insulin-potassium infusion in treatment of acute myocardial infarction. Am J Cardiol 38:95–99, 1976.

112. Rogers WJ, Stanley AW Jr, Breinig JB, Prather JW, McDaniel HG, Moraski RE, Mantle JA, Russell RO Jr, Rackley CE: Reduction of hospital mortality rate of acute myocardial infarction with glucose-insulin-potassium infusion. Am Heart J 92:441–454, 1976.

113. Rogers WJ, Russell RO Jr, McDaniel HG, Rackley CE: Acute effects of glucose-insulin-potassium infusion on myocardial substrates, coronary blood flow and oxygen comsumption in man. Am J Cardiol 40:421–428, 1977.

114. Rogers WJ, Mantle JA, McDaniel HG, Russell RO Jr, Rackley CE: Prospective randomized trial of glucose-insulin-potassium in acute myocardial infarction [abstr]. Circulation [Suppl 2] 60:II-165, 1979.

115. Mantle JA, Rogers WJ, Reeves RC, Russell RO Jr, Bream PR, Rackley CE: Preservation of ischemic myocardium with glucose-insulin-potassium in patients with isolated left anterior descending stenosis [abstr]. Am J Cardiol 45:484, 1980.

116. Mantle JA, Rogers WJ, McDaniel HG, Holmes RA II, Russell RO Jr, Rackley CE: Metabolic support of mechanical performance in myocardial infarction – a randomized clinical trial of glucose-insulin-potassium [abstr]. Am J Cardiol 43:395, 1979.

117. Reduto L, Gulotta S, Morrison J: Ineffectiveness of glucose-insulin-potassium infusion on ischemic myocardium [abstr]. Clin Res 22:685A, 1974.

118. Stanley AW Jr, Willis WH Jr, Kreisberg RA, Russell RO Jr, Rackley CE: Pulmonary infiltration (PF) with glucose-insulin-potassium (GIK) infusion during acute myocardial infarction [abstr]. Clin Res 21:425A, 1973.

119. Gerish RA, Compeau L: Treatment of acute myocardial infarction in man with cortisone. Am J Cardiol 1:535–536, 1958.

120. Dall JLC, Peel AAF: A trial of hydrocortisone in acute myocardial infarction. Lancet 2:1097, 1963.

121. Scottish Society of Physicians Trial: Hydrocortisone in severe myocardial infarction. Lancet 2:785, 1964.

122. Barzilai D, Plavnick J, Hazani A, Einath R, Kleinhause N, Kanter Y: Use of hydrocortisone in the treatment of acute myocardial infarction. Chest 61:488, 1972.

123. Morrison J, Reduto L, Pizzarello R, Geller K, Maley T, Gulotta S: Modification of myocardial injury in man by corticosteroid administration. Circulation [Suppl 1] 53:I-200–203, 1976.

124. Selwyn AP, Ogunro EA, Shillingford JP: Natural history and evaluation of ST segment changes and MB CK release in acute myocardial infarction. Br Heart J 39:988, 1977.

125. Roberts R, DeMello V, Sobel BE: Deleterious effects of methyl-prednisolone in patients with myocardial infarction. Circulation [Suppl 1] 53:I-204–206, 1976.

126. Peters RW, Norman A, Parmley WW, Emilson BB, Scheiman MM, Cheitlin M: Effect of therapy with methylprednisolone on the size of myocardial infarcts in man. Chest 73:483–488, 1978.
127. Bulkley BH, Roberts WC: Steroid therapy during acute myocardial infarction: a cause of delayed healing and of ventricular aneurysm. Am J Med 56:244–250, 1974.
128. Baroody NB, Baroody WG: Adrenocorticosteriods in acute myocardial infarction. Am J Med Sci 250:402–405, 1965.
129. Jugdutt BI, Hutchins GM, Bulkley BH, Becker LC: Salvage of ischemic myocardium by ibuprofen during infarction in the conscious dog. Am J Cardiol 46:74, 1980.
130. Darsee JR, Kloner RA, Braunwald E: Dependency of the location of salvageable myocardium on the type of intervention. Circulation [Suppl 3] 62:III-314, 1980.
131. Morgan HE, Swan HJC, Sobel BE, Braunwald E: Assessment of future directions by session chairman. Circulation [Suppl 1] 53:I-213–217, 1976.

INDEX